INVASIVE CARDIOLOGY

A MANUAL FOR CATH LAB PERSONNEL

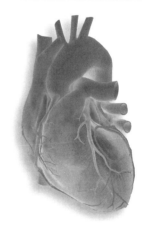

THIRD EDITION

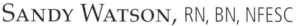

SANDY WATSON, RN, BN, NFESC
Swiss Cardiovascular Centre
University Hospital
Bern, Switzerland

KENNETH A. GORSKI, RN, RCIS, RCSA, FSICP
Cardiovascular Laboratories
Cleveland Clinic Heart and Vascular Institute
Cleveland, Ohio

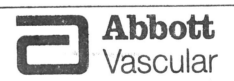

Courtesy of
Sales Training and Development

JONES & BARTLETT
LEARNING

World Headquarters
Jones & Bartlett Learning
40 Tall Pine Drive
Sudbury, MA 01776
978-443-5000
info@jblearning.com
www.jblearning.com

Jones & Bartlett Learning Canada
6339 Ormindale Way
Mississauga, ON L5V 1J2 Canada

Jones & Bartlett Learning International
Barb House, Barb Mews
London W6 7PA
United Kingdom

Jones & Bartlett Learning books and products are available through most bookstores and online booksellers. To contact Jones & Bartlett Learning directly, call 800-832-0034, fax 978-443-8000, or visit our website at www.jblearning.com.

Substantial discounts on bulk quantities of Jones & Bartlett Learning publications are available to corporations, professional associations, and other qualified organizations. For details and specific discount information, contact the special sales department at Jones & Bartlett Learning via the above contact information or send an email to specialsales@jblearning.com.

The authors, editor, and publisher have made every effort to provide accurate information. However, they are not responsible for errors, omissions, or for any outcomes related to the use of the contents of this book and take no responsibility for the use of the products and procedures described. Treatments and side effects described in this book may not be applicable to all people; likewise, some people may require a dose or experience a side effect that is not described herein. Drugs and medical devices are discussed that may have limited availability controlled by the Food and Drug Administration (FDA) for use only in a research study or clinical trial. Research, clinical practice, and government regulations often change the accepted standard in this field. When consideration is being given to use of any drug in the clinical setting, the healthcare provider or reader is responsible for determining FDA status of the drug, reading the package insert, and reviewing prescribing information for the most up-to-date recommendations on dose, precautions, and contraindications, and determining the appropriate usage for the product. This is especially important in the case of drugs that are new or seldom used.

Production Credits
Executive Publisher: Christopher Davis
Senior Acquisitions Editor: Alison Hankey
Editorial Assistant: Sara Cameron
Production Editor: Daniel Stone
Assoc. Marketing Manager: Marion Kerr
V.P., Manufacturing and Inventory Control: Therese Connell
Cover Design: Scott Moden
Cover Image: © MedicalRF.com/age fotostock
Composition: Auburn Associates, Inc.
Printing and Binding: Malloy, Inc.
Cover Printing: Malloy, Inc.

Library of Congress Cataloging-in-Publication Data Application submitted.
Invasive cardiology : a manual for cath lab personnel / Sandy Watson, Kenneth A. Gorski. — 3rd ed.
    p. ; cm.
  Includes bibliographical references and index.
  ISBN 978-0-7637-6468-5
  1. Cardiac catheterization--Handbooks, manuals, etc. I. Watson, Sandy, RN. II. Gorski, Kenneth A.
  [DNLM: 1. Heart Catheterization. 2. Allied Health Personnel. 3. Cardiovascular Diseases—diagnosis. 4. Cardiovascular Diseases—therapy. WG 141.5.C2 I625 2011]
  RD598.35.C35I587 2011
  616.1'20754—dc22
                                                                    2010011064

6048

Printed in the United States of America
14 13 12 11 10   10 9 8 7 6 5 4 3 2 1

CONTENTS

PREFACE

The cardiac catheterization laboratory is one of the most fascinating areas of medicine to work in. In these small procedure rooms, a team of physicians, nurses, and cardiovascular invasive specialists perform diagnostic examinations and therapeutic procedures on patients' hearts with plastic tubes and wires. The level of technology used in modern cardiovascular labs provides a continual challenge to the cath lab professional. Despite this, patient care is the central pillar upon which our work rests. The patient is the common denominator in each of the areas covered in this book.

Many excellent textbooks dedicated to the field of cardiac catheterization are available, but very few have been written to address the training needs of nonphysician members of the team. This text was been written by cath lab nurses and technicians for cath lab nurses and technicians. It has been designed not only to be a helping hand to those just starting out in the specialty but also to serve as a reference for those who have been working in our field for some time

We would like to thank the Swiss Cardiovascular Centre at the University Hospital of Bern, Switzerland, and the Cleveland Clinic in Cleveland, Ohio, for providing an environment in which such an undertaking can be nurtured.

SANDY WATSON AND KENNETH A. GORSKI

FOREWORD

The nurses and technicians working in cardiac catheterization laboratories and the postinterventional care units have played a pivotal role in coronary angioplasty from the very first case on September 16, 1977, in Zürich. The inventor of the method, Andreas Grünzig, relied heavily on their background work, their help with the equipment, and their attention to the needs of the patients.

Originally, it was the preparation of the balloons and the sophisticated pneumatic inflation device that took up most of the time of the assistant nurse or technician. Over the years, inflation devices became simpler and balloon preparation unnecessary. The catheterization laboratory technicians and nurses have become more and more intimately involved in the procedure itself. In many places, they assist the responsible physician with sterile manipulations at the table, either as a sole assistant or as a member of a team of nurses, technicians, and physicians.

In the beginning, angioplasty was an elective procedure, performed in a generous time frame during office hours. Today, it is often an emergency procedure, performed at odd hours, on patients for whom every minute counts, and in an environment where the emphasis is on efficiency.

New techniques and devices constantly come and go. Some of them need little preparation, as does the stent that is now an integral part of the angioplasty procedure in virtually all cases. Some, however, are intricate and only manageable by an experienced and well-trained hand; these include lasers, atherectomy devices, intracoronary filters and clot removers, ultrasound equipment for 2D or 3D imaging, Doppler flow or intracoronary pressure assessments, or invasive tools used to assess plaque vulnerability. Drugs need to be prepared in specified dilutions to be injected either manually into the coronary artery, another vessel, or through infusomats or pressurized fluid lines.

Customization, calibration, and initial trouble-shooting of the X-ray equipment and equipment that monitors the patient's vital signs also fall into the responsibilities of nurses and technicians at many invasive-interventional cardiac laboratories. Finally, percutaneous left ventricular assist devices, such as the Tandem Heart or the Impella pump, can only act as true lifesavers with a team of doctors, nurses, and technicians who are highly qualified, motivated, and available around the clock.

Moreover, most laboratories extend their range of action to peripheral vessels, such as the aorta leg, renal, and carotid arteries. New techniques for procedures in and around the heart emerge that again need expert knowledge and manual dexterity. Such interventions include diagnostic and therapeutic electrophysiology; implantation or exchange of complex pacemaker systems or percutaneous cardioverter-defibrillator-pacers; percutaneous valve repairs or replacements; shunt closure devices for patent foramen ovala, atrial septum defects, ventricular septum defects, or the patent ductus arteriosus; embolizations of fistulae; septal alcohol injection for ablation of obstructive hypertrophic cardiomyopathy; and pericardial balloon fenestrations. The preceding list is not exhaustive and is growing virtually by the year.

Because many physicians practicing interventional cardiology and associated procedures have a relatively large caseload, there is no way that they can keep abreast of all the minute details of the different techniques and devices. That is where the importance of the laboratory assistants comes into play most conspicuously. They typically participate in all the cases performed at the institution. They assimilate the experience of all physicians practicing in the particular institution collectively, and they add their own continued professional education and brainpower. They are the living reference book and equipment manual for the physician.

It has been shown conclusively that low-volume operators produce inferior results with interventional cardiology compared with high-volume operators. It has also been shown conclusively that this deficiency is corrected when low-volume operators work in the realm of an experienced catheterization laboratory (with the help of experienced catheterization personnel).

The book that you are holding in your hands is the product of a tremendous amount of individual and collective brain work, sweat, and dedication. While being created, it had to be constantly adapted to new knowledge, new data, and new ideas. Once printed, these adaptations have to take place in the minds of the reader—at least until the next edition.

Each individual chapter can and should be used independently. Each reflects primarily the experience, the policies, the techniques, and the thoughts of its author. There may be significant divergence from the reader's personal view of the topic as formed by his or her teachers and places of work. This is intentional and overediting of the chapters has been carefully avoided because this would transform them into a confusing enumeration of possible ways to do things. Marrying the described technique, which invariably is a valid and seasoned one, with the technique used by the reader, should improve the overall performance.

Thanks go to all the contributors whose names are listed, but also to all those that remain anonymous. They made invaluable suggestions to the authors either before or after seeing the text or they simply trained the authors, thereby imparting their expertise, style, and knowledge on their disciples.

We are convinced that this book harbors a wealth of valuable information and teaching material. We are hopeful that it will be a captivating reading experience and some fun, too. It is quite likely that many a young doctor in training in this field will grab the book, flip a few pages, and wind up reading it all and learning more than she or he might wish to admit.

BERNHARD MEIER

DEDICATION

To the women who surround me: Laura, Eva, and Giuljana;
you are the color in my days. Thank you for sharing your lives with me.
It is a privilege to be here with you. I also thank my mother, Alison Watson,
for this wonderful life that she has given me.

SANDY WATSON

To my wife, Cathy, and my three wonderful boys, David, Kenny, and Jonathan,
who pray for me daily, and to Mom and Dad, Evelyn and Bob Gorski.
I cannot remember you ever putting your personal wants or needs before those
of the family; your examples taught me the values of honesty and hard work.
Thank you all for being there.

KENNETH A. GORSKI

CONTRIBUTORS

Monica Arpagaus-Lee, RN, MN, MHA
Delegate
International Committee of the Red Cross
Afghanistan

Charles C. Barbiere, RN, CCRN, RCIS, CCT, CRT, EMT, FSICP
Technical Director
Cardiac Catheter Laboratory
Department of Cardiology
VA Northern California Health Care System
Sacramento, California

Ryan Bickel, PharmD
Clinical Pharmacy Specialist
Department of Pharmacy
Denver Veteran's Affairs Medical Center
Denver, Colorado

Henry L. Blair, C-CPT
Clinical Assistant Electrophysiology
Cook Children's Heart Center
Fort Worth, Texas

Lezlie Bridge, BSc, DMS, NASPE Testamur
Senior Regulatory Affairs Specialist
Medtronic Ltd.
United Kingdom

Loren D. Brown, RN, BSN, CCRN
Nursing Educator
Cardiovascular Catheterization Lab
Children's Hospital
Boston, Massachusetts

Elizabeth A. Ching, RN, CCDS, FHRS
Nurse Manager
Electrophysiology and Pacing
Heart and Vascular Institute
The Cleveland Clinic Foundation
Cleveland, Ohio

Joan M. Craney, RN, PhD
Principal Clinical Specialist
Medtronic USA
North New Jersey

Murray Crichton, HDCR(R)
Sector Superintendent Radiographer
NHS Greater Glasgow and Clyde
Glasgow Royal Infirmary
Glasgow, Scotland

Jeff Davis, RRT, RCIS, FSICP
Program Director Coordinator
Cardiovascular Technology
Edison State College
Fort Myers, Florida

Regina Deible, RN, BSN
Clinical Nurse Specialist
Cardiac Cath Lab
NIH Heart Center
Suburban Hospital
Johns Hopkins Medicine
Baltimore, Maryland

Sherri L. Derstine-Hawk, BSPharm, BCPS
Clinical Pharmacy Specialist
Pharmacoeconomics
Department of Pharmacy
Denver Veteran's Affairs Medical Center
Denver, Colorado

Arlene Ewan, RN
Cardiology Research Nurse
Harefield Hospital
Middlesex, England

Matin Ghorbati, MS, RN
Educational Supervisor and Research Officer
Interventional Cardiovascular Department
Day General Hospital
Tehran, Iran

Kenneth A. Gorski, RN, RCIS, RCSA, FSICP
Assistant Manager, Cardiovascular Laboratories
Cleveland Clinic Heart and Vascular Institute
Cleveland, Ohio

Phyllis J. Gustafson, RN, BSN
Clinical Specialist
Medtronic, Inc.
Kansas City, Missouri

John E. Hawk, PharmD, BCPS
Clinical Pharmacy Specialist
Anesthesiology/Critical Care/Nutrition Support
Department of Pharmacy
Denver Veteran's Affairs Medical Center
Denver, Colorado

Patrick Hoier, BS, RCSA, RCIS FSICP
Invasive Cardiovascular Program Director
Southeast Technical Institute
Sioux Falls, South Dakota

Sharon Holloway, RN, MSN, ACNP-CS, CCRN
Cardiology Nurse Practitioner
Mercy Hospital and Medical Center
Chicago, Illinois

Marsha Holton, CCRN, RCIS, FSICP
President and Founder
Cardiovascular Orientation Programs
Indian Head, Maryland

Neil E. Holtz, BS, EMT-P, RCIS
Cardiac Cath Lab Technician
Emory University Hospital
Atlanta, Georgia

Jeff Hunter, RTR, BS
Cardiac Catheter Laboratory Technician
West Pennsylvania Hospital
Pittsburgh, Pennsylvania

Jane M. Kasper, RN, BSN
Research Nurse Coordinator
Cardiovascular Imaging
Division of Radiology
The Cleveland Clinic Foundation
Cleveland, Ohio

Stephanie Lavin, RN, BSN
Arrhythmia Case Manager
Cook Children's Heart Center
Fort Worth, Texas

Thomas H. Maloney, MS, RCIS, RT(N), FSICP
Memorial Regional Medical Center
Richmond, Virginia

Brenda McCulloch, RN, MSN, CNS
Cardiovascular Clinical Nurse Specialist
Sutter Heart and Vascular Institute
Sutter Medical Center
Sacramento, California

Rick Meece, CCT, RCS, RCIS, FSICP
Staff Invasive Cardiovascular Technologist
St. Thomas Health Services
Nashville, Tennessee

Michela Mordasini, RT
Leading Radiographer
Institute of Diagnostic and Interventional
    Neuroradiology
University Hospital
Bern, Switzerland

Carl F. Moxey, PhD
Associate Professor of Biology
Anna Maria College
Paxton, Massachusetts

Laura Nyren, RN, MS, ACNP
Certified EP Specialist-Allied Professional
Cardiology Nurse Practitioner
UMass Memorial Health Care
Worcester, Massachusetts

Corissa Pederson, BS, RCIS
Invasive Cardiology Technologist
Sutter Memorial Hospital
Sacramento, California

Darren Powell, RCIS, FSICP
Program Director
Cardiovascluar Technology
Spokane Community College
Spokane, Washington

Rachael Ramsamujh, RN
Research Coordinator
Interventional Cardiology
The University Health Network
Toronto, Canada

Stephanie Ray, RN
Nurse Coordinator
Cardiac Catheterization Laboratory
Mercy Hospital and Medical Center
Chicago, Illinois

Brenda Ridley, RN, BScN, MA Ed(C), CCN(C)
Clinical Educator
Interventional Cardiology
The University Health Network
Toronto, Canada

Gerhard Schroth, MD
Professor and Chairman
Institute of Diagnostic and Interventional
    Neuroradiology
University Hospital
Bern, Switzerland

Rena L. Silver, RN, MSN, ACNP-C
Nurse Practitioner
Department of Cardiology
North Shore University Health Systems
Evanston, Illinois

Leslie C. Sweet, RN, BSN
Clinical Research Coordinator
Department of Cardiac Surgery
Washington Hospital Center
Washington, DC

Ilcias G. Vargas, RCES, RCIS, HM2
Cath Lab Invasive Specialist
Cardiac Electrophysiology Specialist
Hamilton Medical Center
Dalton, Georgia

Daniel Walsh, RT
Lead Radiology Technologist
Mercy Hospital and Medical Center
Chicago, Illinois

Sandy Watson, RN, BN, NFESC
Swiss Cardiovascular Centre
University Hospital
Bern, Switzerland

J. David Wilson, RCIS
Adult and Pediatric Cardiac Cath Lab/
    Electrophysiology Lab
Albany Medical Center
Albany, New York

Reviewers

Sue Apple, DNSC, RN
Instructor
Georgetown University School of Nursing
Washington, District of Colombia

Angela M. Calvert, MSN, CRNP, CVN
Nurse Practitioner
Vascular Surgery Division
Georgetown University Hospital
Division, Vascular Surgery
Washington, DC

Ted Feldman, MD
Senior Attending
Mercy Hospital and Medical Center
Chicago, Illinois

Michelle Martin, RN, BSN
Nurse Manager
Cardiac Cath Lab and Cardiac Imaging Center
Children's Hospital
Boston, Massachusetts

Bernhard Meier, MD, FACC, FESC
Professor and Chairman
Swiss Cardiovascular Centre
University Hospital
Bern, Switzerland

Michela Mordasini, RT
Leading Radiographer
Institute of Diagnostic and Interventional
   Neuroradiology
University Hospital
Bern, Switzerland

Gerhard Schroth, MD
Professor and Chairman
Institute of Diagnostic and Interventional
    Neuroradiology
University Hospital
Bern, Switzerland

Thomas Tamlyn, MD
Interventional Cardiologist
Director, Cardiac Care Unit
Mercy Hospital and Medical Center
Chicago, Illinois

Andreas Wahl, MD
Swiss Cardiovascular Centre
University Hospital
Bern, Switzerland

Chapter 1

INTRODUCTION

Sandy Watson, RN, BN, NFESC
Kenneth A. Gorski, RN, RCIS, RCSA, FSICP

THE BEGINNINGS

The concept of catheterization has been around for about 5000 years. Using metal pipes, the Egyptians first performed bladder catheterization around 3000 BC. The notion of using hollow reeds, pipes, or tubes to examine the valves of a cadaver heart occurred around 400 BC. In 1711, Hales fashioned a contraption with brass pipes, a glass tube, and the trachea of a goose to perform the first cardiac catheterization on a horse. Claude Bernard is credited with first applying the term cardiac catheterization when he used the technique to record both right and left ventricular pressures in a horse. It was not until the early part of the 20th century that this idea was applied to humans.

In 1929, a 25-year-old resident physician by the name of Werner Forssman, studying surgery in Eberswalde, Germany, theorized that it was possible to safely insert a tube through a vein in the arm and navigate into the heart and lungs.

Against the wishes of his superior and with the aid of a nurse assistant, Dr. Forssman inserted a urinary catheter into his left antecubital vein and advanced it 65 cm into his right atrium. Dr. Forssman then walked up a flight of steps to the X-ray department where the catheter position was documented on a chest film. For his insubordination and "dangerous experiments," Dr. Forssman received an official reprimand and was largely ridiculed by the local medical community. Some accounts say the nurse assistant involved was fired. Forssman eventually did insert a catheter into the right atrium of a patient dying of sepsis for the administration of fluids and medication. Although the technique went largely ignored by the medical community, in the 1930s, a few other physicians began to perform some right heart catheterizations. They even passed catheters into the right ventricle, measuring cardiac output with Adolf Fick's methodology.

In 1941, Dr. Andre Cournand began using catheters to study human circulation and pulmonary physiology at the Bellevue Hospital in New York City. Dr. Cournand and another cardiologist, Dr. Dickinson Richards, began to use catheters to measure cardiac output. After World War II, interest in cardiac catheterization rapidly increased. Right heart catheter techniques evolved, and new, valuable information was obtained about the cardiopulmonary system. During this period, much of the drive to develop catheterization techniques came from pediatricians investigating and diagnosing congenital defects such as atrial and ventricular septal defects.

Dr. Zimmerman was the first to demonstrate the retrograde technique by passing a catheter into the left ventricle to measure left-sided pressures in 1949. This was followed by the development of the percutaneous femoral artery technique by Dr. Seldinger in 1953. Other early (and risky) attempts at catheterizing the left heart included puncturing the left main stem bronchus to reach the left atrium and using a supraclavicular puncture through the chest wall. One method, which is used today only on very rare occasions for patients with older mechanical aortic and mitral valves, is a direct apical or parasternal left ventricular puncture.

Until the end of the 1950s, only nonselective visualization of the proximal portions of the coronary vasculature could be documented. This was done by injecting a bolus of contrast medium into the aortic root. In 1959, Dr. F. Mason Sones, Jr., a pediatric cardiologist at the Cleveland Clinic Foundation, performed the first selective coronary angiogram. Prior to this, it was feared that direct contrast injection into the coronary arteries would result in ventricular fibrillation and death. As the story goes, a cardiology fellow working under the supervision of Dr. Mason Sones was performing an aortic angiogram when the catheter accidentally became positioned in the right coronary artery ostium and contrast was injected. The patient did not fibrillate but had only a brief episode of asystole. Dr. Sones thus became known as the father of coronary arteri-

ography. Dr. Sones performed catheterizations via a 1-inch incision in the antecubital space to isolate the brachial artery, an approach now known as the Sones technique.

Present for the first selective coronary angiogram (but left out of cardiology textbooks) was Vae Lucile Van Derwyst, RN. Miss Van Derwyst began working for Dr. Sones at the Cleveland Clinic in 1952 and initially was his only nurse assistant. Shortly after performing that first coronary angiogram, adults became Dr. Sones's primary patient load, and his workload mushroomed. His practice began by sharing one radiology suite off hours but grew quickly into six dedicated catheterization laboratories, and Miss Van Derwyst trained and supervised the staff of more than 40 nurses. Miss Van Derwyst thus became a pioneer as well, developing a new area of nursing practice. Nurses came from all over the country to train under her, and they, in turn, went back to their hospitals to train and educate other nurses.

Other advancements in diagnostic techniques occurred regularly over the following years. Transseptal catheterization, first described in 1959 by Ross and Cope, was further developed by Drs. Ross and Brockenbrough at the National Institutes of Health and later refined by Dr. Mullins. Their techniques, and the devices that they developed, are still used in everyday practice today.

In 1964, Dr. Charles Dotter and Dr. Melvin Judkins began working with patients who had severe peripheral vascular disease. They found that by inserting a series of stiff dilators, gradually increasing in diameter, through the diseased sections of the vessels, blood flow was improved. Dotter called this technique transluminal angioplasty though it also become known as the Dotter technique. As was the case with Dr. Forssman, Dotter was ridiculed by his peers, and his technique was largely ignored in the United States for the following 15 years.

In 1967, Dr. Judkins, a radiologist, began using Seldinger's technique and catheters with preformed curves to visualize the coronary anatomy. Dr. Judkins took straight catheters and inserted stylets into them to form curves. Through trial and error, he found the most appropriate shapes for reaching the ostium of the coronary arteries. Because the preformed catheters made cannulation of the coronary arteries easier, the Judkins technique eventually surpassed the Sones technique as the preferred method of catheterization.

The era of modern coronary artery bypass (CABG) surgery began in 1967 when Dr. Rene Favaloro conducted the first modern saphenous vein bypass graft at the Cleveland Clinic. It was no accident that modern CABG was developed at the same institution as coronary angiography. It was necessary to have an accurate map of a patient's coronary anatomy before CABG could be performed. Dr. Favaloro would often spend hours each evening reviewing and discussing angiographic studies with Dr. Sones, an interaction that continues today between cardiologists and cardiac surgeons.

Drs. Swan and Ganz introduced a flow-directed, balloon-tipped catheter for monitoring right heart pressures and thermodilution cardiac outputs in 1970. This transformed the catheter into a tool that could be used at the bedside in an intensive care unit. Intra-aortic balloon pumps also became available, but the early, handwrapped catheters were high-profile devices, and could only be inserted after a surgical cutdown had been performed.

The field of interventional cardiology was born in September 1977 when Andreas Gruentzig performed the first percutaneous transluminal coronary angioplasty (PTCA) in Zürich, Switzerland. The patient was a 37-year-old man with a stenosis of his proximal left anterior descending artery. When the patient was restudied 24 years later, the lesion was still patent. The patient is still alive as of 2009 and has not had any subsequent coronary interventions.

In the late 1970s, the only way for a cardiologist to buy a PTCA balloon was to travel personally to Switzerland. There, he or she had to attend a course offered by Andreas Gruentzig. After the course, the cardiologist would receive a small note signed by Dr. Gruenzig, which was then taken to a basement in the Zürich area where the Schneider Company had set up a workshop. The doctor would knock on a window to attract someone's attention and present the note to them. The cardiologist was then permitted to buy one PTCA balloon, but only for cash, and only in Swiss francs.

During the early 1980s, cardiologists were limited by primitive equipment and inadequate materials. Balloons were originally fixed wire and not available in the multitude of diameters and lengths they are today. They would easily break, sometimes rupturing within the patient, resulting in severe vessel dissections. Guide catheters were about 10F and very stiff. It was not uncommon for a catheterization (cath) lab to have a hair dryer or a hot plate with boiling water and a basin of sterile ice water on hand to shape the proper curve.

Cardiologists had to prove to the world (and especially to skeptical surgeons) that balloon dilatation was a safe, viable alternative to standard medical therapy or surgery. Cardiologists would only treat single-vessel, proximal lesions. If a patient had disease in more than one artery, most often they were referred for surgery. On occasion, if the cardiologist was bold, he or she would treat one diseased vessel in a patient, and the patient would be invited to come back at a later date to dilate an additional artery. Angioplasties were only performed with surgical stand-by, with surgeons and their staff waiting within the cardiac catheterization laboratory during every scheduled angioplasty. Patients were often kept hospitalized for several days after an angioplasty procedure for observation and anticoagulation therapy.

Improved devices led to greater initial procedural success, and PTCA gradually became accepted as a valid alternative to surgery. The differentiation between patients suitable for surgery and suitable for dilatation was constantly being reviewed, a process that continues today.

With the success of angioplasty and its rapid international acceptance came a new disease process named restenosis. It occurred in roughly 40% of the lesions treated. Restenosis became known as the Achilles' heel of angioplasty. Cardiologists began to speculate about catheter-based options other than balloon dilatation. Directional atherectomy, lasers, the rotablator, and other techniques were developed in an attempt to find a more effective way to treat coronary artery disease. The balloons themselves improved quickly, becoming available in a wider range of diameters and lengths with lower crossing profiles.

Interventional cardiology took its next step forward with the development of the intracoronary stent. Dotter and Gruentzig had both speculated on the concept of stenting in the 1960s, and Dotter even reported placing a crude, coiled stent following a percutaneous transluminal angioplasty in 1969. When the U.S. Food and Drug Administration (FDA) approved the Gianturco-Roubin Coil Stent (Cook) in 1993, it was little more than a stainless steel coil resembling the spring in a ballpoint pen. The device was only approved for acute and threatened closure by vessel dissection following balloon angioplasty. The Palmaz-Schatz Stent (Johnson & Johnson) arrived shortly thereafter and became the first device to show any significant reduction in restenosis.

It was found, however, that stent placement also produced restenosis, although at rates lower than with PTCA. Localized delivery of radiation (vascular brachytherapy), drugs, cryotherapy, microwaves, lasers, and ultrasound have been developed, some even clinically approved, to treat this phenomenon. In 2002, the first drug-eluting stent received FDA approval. It combined a proven stent design with a pharmaceutical agent that inhibits smooth-muscle proliferation. The Cypher Stent (Johnson & Johnson) was the first technique/device ever to have 0% angiographic restenosis at 6-month follow-up in a clinical trial.

Other stent companies, using other drugs, were not far behind in their development of coated stents. Only time will tell whether the Achilles' heel of interventional cardiology has been overcome.

THE EVOLVING ROLE OF THE INVASIVE CARDIOVASCULAR SPECIALIST

In the early days of the catheterization laboratory, three primary roles developed for the support staff of nurses and technologists. The monitoring person observed and recorded the ECG, measured hemodynamic waveforms, and communicated to the medical staff any changes observed. Since the older X-ray systems did not automatically adjust to the dose rate needed for every shot, the monitoring staff adjusted the kV and mA before each shot. The circulator was present to record procedural events, administer medication, run blood samples on the oximeter, retrieve and open supplies, and assist as needed should an emergency situation arise. The scrub person worked at the table with the physician, helping to exchange catheters and assisting with contrast injections. At a few facilities, nurses were trained to perform brachial cutdowns (isolating the artery and vein for the staff cardiologist performing the catheterization) and suture the skin closed at the conclusion of the case.

As interventional therapies were introduced in the late 1970s and early 1980s, staff at some institutions took on new responsibilities. The scrub assistant's new duties included helping in the complicated process of positioning catheters, advancing wires and balloons across lesions, and inflating and deflating balloons. The monitoring staff were expected to be even more vigilant in observing ischemia brought about by balloon inflations. The monitoring role developed to include selecting a good cardiac roadmap image; documenting all events during the procedure, including inflation times, ischemic changes, and equipment changes; calculating left ventricular ejection fractions; and performing quantitative coronary analysis. The circulating person became more involved with medical management as patients began to receive more sedation, activated clotting times were used for point-of-care anticoagulation management, thrombolytic agents, and glycoprotein IIb/IIIa inhibitors worked their way into the lab. The circulator also could be responsible for setting up, operating, and interpreting results of intravascular ultrasound, doppler flow, and fractional flow devices. A physician entering a lab run by an experienced team can expect the patient to be appropriately sedated; arterial, venous, or both sheaths inserted as appropriate; and the patient's old film ready for viewing. These changes in the role of the support staff have not been universally adopted, however. The difference between the skill levels that cath lab personnel are expected to possess varies greatly between countries, and even from institution to institution within a single city.

As further refinements in techniques are developed, there is a tendency toward specialization. For example, when electrophysiology was first introduced to the cardiac catheterization laboratory, it was performed during the slow periods in the week, between cardiac catheterizations. In most modern facilities, electrophysiology now has its own laboratory and its own team. Many cardiac catheterization laboratories have grown into "heart and vascular institutes," performing not only cardiac procedures but also endovascular procedures (peripheral, carotid, and cranial).

The knowledge base required for this work is broad, and it must be coupled with a high degree of manual dexterity and the ability to work well in emergency situations. For most employees new to the cath lab, it is initially a very intimidating environment. The length of the orientation period varies from facility to facility, but realistically, it takes 12–18 months before a new employee is comfortable with the knowledge and skills required in the cath lab and is familiar with all the material and procedures performed there. The focus of the work, however, is not the technical skills needed to treat the lesion, but the patient on the procedure table. The patient's welfare is the focus of all work in the cath lab.

Chapter 2

CARDIOVASCULAR ANATOMY AND PHYSIOLOGY

Jeff Davis, RRT, RCIS, FSICP

The cardiovascular system maintains the body's homeostasis by delivering oxygen and nutrients to, and removing waste products from, all the cells in the body. This system is comprised of three major components: a circulatory pump (the heart); a distribution network (the vascular beds); and blood, with all of its components.

Interventional cardiology usually focuses on one small section of this network, but knowledge of the entire system is necessary to work in the cardiac catheterization laboratory. The circulatory system is networked with myriad compensatory mechanisms that can complicate a diagnostic procedure or change a patient's cardiovascular status rapidly.

CARDIAC ANATOMY AND PHYSIOLOGY

The heart is a remarkable pump, beating about 70 times per minute, one hundred thousand times a day, 37 million times each year. The adult human's heart is roughly the size and shape of a clenched fist. It is located slightly behind and to the left of the sternum (Figure 2-1). The base of the heart lies behind the second rib, and the apex of the heart is at the midclavicular line of the fifth intercostal space.

The heartbeat can be felt where the apex contacts the internal chest wall during systole. This site is called the point of maximum impulse (PMI) or apical impulse. The PMI is useful in evaluating the size of the heart, and it may shift due to certain conditions. For instance, cardiomegaly displaces PMI downward and laterally, and left ventricular hypertrophy shifts the PMI to the left.

The four-chambered heart consists of two upper collecting chambers, the right and left atria, and two lower pumping chambers, the right and left ventricles. The right side of the heart receives the body's venous deoxygenated blood from the tissues of the systemic circulatory system through the inferior and superior vena cava, and from the cardiac muscle through the

Figure 2-1. Position of the heart

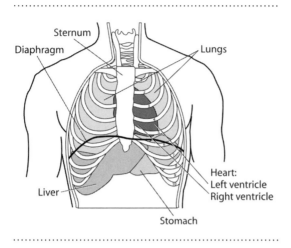

Sternum
Diaphragm
Lungs
Liver
Heart:
Left ventricle
Right ventricle
Stomach

coronary sinus. The blood moves from the right atrium, through the tricuspid valve, into the right ventricle (Figure 2-2). From there, it is pumped through the pulmonic valve into the pulmonary artery and pulmonary circulatory system.

The pulmonary capillary bed is where external respiration occurs. Deoxygenated venous blood comes in contact with the alveoli of the lungs. Oxygen diffuses from the alveoli into the blood in the pulmonary capillaries, and CO_2 and water vapor diffuse from the blood to the alveoli. This causes the blood's oxygen saturation to increase to almost 100%.

This oxygenated blood flows through the pulmonary veins, into the left atria, through the mitral valve and into the left ventricle. The left ventricle is the main pumping chamber of the heart. It pumps oxygenated blood through the aortic valve into the aorta, and then out to the rest of the body.

The aorta branches into many arteries. In turn, the arteries branch into arterioles that ultimately divide into the systemic tissue capillary bed where internal respiration occurs. Here oxygen and nutrients diffuse out of the blood into the tissues, and CO_2 and waste products diffuse from the tis-

sues into the blood. As this exchange occurs, the blood becomes deoxygenated; oxygen saturation drops to between 60%–75%. This blood then travels through venules, veins, and the inferior and superior vena cava back to the right side of the heart to complete the cycle.

CONGENITAL CARDIAC ANOMALIES

The embryonic development of the human heart is a remarkably complex process. A wide array of congenital cardiac anomalies can occur. A detailed description of congenital anomalies is beyond the scope of this chapter; what follows is a basic description of some of the more common cardiac anomalies.

Patent Foramen Ovale (PFO)

While in the womb, a neonate's blood is oxygenated in the placenta, and most of the blood bypasses the undeveloped pulmonary system by flowing directly from the right atrium into the left atrium through an opening called the foramen ovale. The wall between the atria (the atrial septum) is made up of two structures: the fibrous septum primium coming from the direction of the ventricles and the muscular septum secundum coming from the direction of the aorta. After birth, the pressures in the left atrium become higher than those in the right, pushing these flaps together, and they fuse in about 75% of the population.[1]

Atrial Septal Defect (ASD)

The atrial septum can have a hole (or several holes) in it, which permits the flow of blood between the left and right atria.

Ventricular Septal Defect (VSD)

The ventricles are separated by the muscular, thick-walled interventricular septum. If the neo-

Figure 2-2. The circulation system.

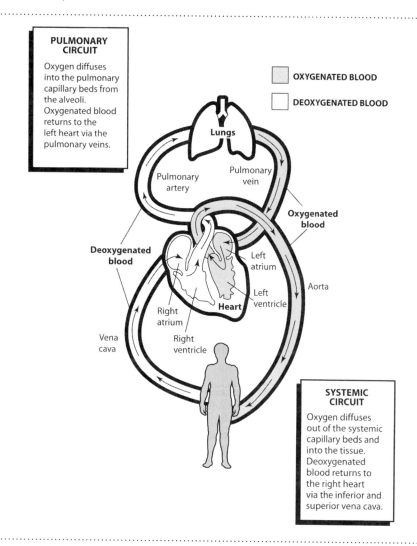

PULMONARY CIRCUIT

Oxygen diffuses into the pulmonary capillary beds from the alveoli. Oxygenated blood returns to the left heart via the pulmonary veins.

OXYGENATED BLOOD

DEOXYGENATED BLOOD

Lungs

Pulmonary artery

Pulmonary vein

Oxygenated blood

Deoxygenated blood

Left atrium

Aorta

Left ventricle

Heart

Right atrium

Vena cava

Right ventricle

SYSTEMIC CIRCUIT

Oxygen diffuses out of the systemic capillary beds and into the tissue. Deoxygenated blood returns to the right heart via the inferior and superior vena cava.

natal tissues that make up the ventricular septum fail to fuse with one another during development, a shunt can manifest, allowing venous and arterial blood to mix.

ASDs, PFOs, and VSDs usually lead to an increase in pulmonary blood flow and pulmonary congestion. The additional volume of blood in the right heart will overload the lungs and can lead to heart failure. An anterior septal or septal MI can also cause a ventricular septal defect, although this is uncommon.

Patent Ductus Arteriosus (PDA)

As part of the fetal circulation is a short vessel connecting the pulmonary artery to the aorta, bypassing the lungs, through the PDA. This normally closes shortly after birth, but when it remains open, arterialized blood from the aorta can flow through the PDA into the lungs, resulting in pulmonary congestion. What is left of the ductus arteriosis becomes a ligament holding the left pulmonary artery and the aortic arch together.

The direction of blood flow through a shunt is a function of blood pressures and vascular resistances, so the direction of the shunt can change. In the event of very high pulmonary vascular resistance and lower systemic vascular resistance, the right heart pressures can exceed left heart pressures. This can cause blood to shunt from the right heart to the left heart, resulting in venous blood entering the left heart and systemic circulation, resulting in cyanosis.

Tetrology of Fallott (TOF)

The four characteristics of TOF are (1) pulmonary (infundibular) stenosis, (2) right ventricular hypertrophy, (3) VSD, and (4) an overriding aorta that receives blood from both right and left ventricles. Cyanosis is secondary to the venous blood from the right ventricle entering the aorta. A variety of palliative and corrective procedures are required to treat a child born with TOF.

Transposition of the Great Vessels (TGV)

When the left ventricle gives rise to the pulmonary artery and the right ventricle (RV) gives rise to the aorta, it is known as transposition of the great vessels. Venous blood returns to the right heart, and the RV ejects this venous blood into the aorta and the systemic circulation. Meanwhile, arterialized blood returning from the lungs enters the left heart and the left ventricle ejects this arterialized blood into the pulmonary artery, back to the lungs. This creates two separate circulatory circuits, and the child cannot survive without some mixing of arterialized and venous blood. Opening two fetal shunts, the foramen

ovale and the ductus arteriosis, will allow some mixing of blood and increase the amount of oxygen in the systemic circuit. This buys time for other palliative and corrective procedures to be undertaken as the child grows.

Persistent Trunctus Arteriosus

The trunctus arteriosus is a part of the embryonic anatomy that becomes (among other things) the wall between the aorta and the pulmonary artery. In this condition, the one large vessel, trunctus arterosis, receives blood from both the RV and LV, and delivers this mixed blood to both the pulmonary and systemic circuits, leading to cyanosis. This is usually associated with a VSD.

Tricuspid Atresia

When the tricuspid valve fails to form properly, the right atrium cannot deliver blood to the right ventricle and the pulmonary circulation. Tricuspid atresia can lead to a hypoplastic right ventricle and diminutive pulmonary artery with a reduction in pulmonary blood flow. An ASD and a VSD are usually present. Venous return to the right atrium is directed to the left heart through the ASD, and out to the systemic circuit, leading to cyanosis.

Total Anomalous Pulmonary Venous Return (TAPVR)

In TAPVR, the pulmonary veins empty into either the superior or inferior vena cava instead of the left atrium. There are several varieties of TAPVR that can result in either cyanosis or pulmonary congestion.

Congenital Aortic Stenosis

Stenosis of the aortic valve will place a pressure overload on the left ventricle, resulting in a decrease in cardiac output and pulmonary congestion.

Coarctation of the Aorta

Aortic coarctation is a congenital narrowing in the descending aorta, creating a gradient between the ascending and descending aorta. This places a high pressure overload on the left ventricle and can lead to pulmonary congestion and damage the aortic valve. The blood pressure in the arms can be higher than blood pressure in the legs in children with coarctation of the aorta.

Advances in medicine and technology have resulted in better diagnosis and treatments for children born with cardiac congenital anomalies. As these children become adults, they may need to be followed for the rest of their lives. This will certainly increase the need for cath lab professionals who choose to work in this rewarding specialty.

CARDIAC VALVES

The four one-way valves in the heart provide unidirectional blood flow through the heart and lungs. Pressure changes cause the valves to open and close in a regular fashion.

The right atrium is not very muscular and acts essentially as a reception area for blood flowing in from the superior and inferior vena cavae. The tricuspid valve, which has three leaflets, is located between the right atrium and right ventricle. This valve allows blood, under low pressure, to flow into the right ventricle, and then prevents the blood from flowing back out when the ventricle contracts. Tough fibrotic cords, called chordae tendinae, attach the free edges of the valve leaflets to the papillary muscles in the right ventricle (Figure 2-3). These cords ensure that the valve flaps do not invert, which would allow blood to flow in the wrong direction.

Between the right ventricle and the pulmonary artery lies the pulmonic valve. It consists of three thin leaflets that coapt, or come together, when closed, sealing off the exit. This valve ensures that the blood ejected out of the right ventricle does

Figure 2-3. Internal view of the heart.

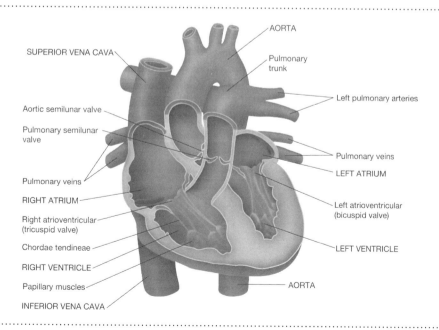

not flow back in during diastole. Each contraction of the ventricle pushes more blood into pulmonary circulation, where it is oxygenated.

This oxygenated blood then flows into the left atrium via the pulmonary veins. Between the left atrium and the left ventricle lies the mitral valve. This valve has two leaflets that are also held by chordae tendinae. The job of the mitral valve is similar to that of the tricuspid: It permits blood to flow into the left ventricle during diastole and prevents it from flowing back in to the left atrium when the left ventricle contracts.

The aortic valve is located between the left ventricle and the aorta. Though usually made up of three leaflets, occasionally it has only two. In this case, it is referred to as a bicuspid aortic valve. The left ventricle is by far the most muscular of the four heart chambers, and its contraction causes the blood to leave under great pressure. The aortic valve ensures that this blood, which is being pumped throughout the entire body, leaves the ventricle efficiently during systole and doesn't flow back when the ventricle relaxes.

The tricuspid and mitral valves are also called atrioventricular (AV) valves. The pulmonic and aortic valves are also known as semilunar valves, and they consist of three very thin half-moon–shaped cusps.

The function of heart valves is straightforward: They open and close. When they are unable to open all the way, they are considered to be stenotic. This stenosis can impose a high-pressure load on the involved heart chamber, resulting in congestion in the chamber, or in vessels upstream from the valve. It can also result in a flow decrease and, therefore, a decrease in cardiac output downstream from the valve. The resulting pressure gradient can be analyzed in the cath lab and used to calculate the size of the valve opening.

In aortic stenosis, the diseased valve decreases the left ventricle's ability to eject blood into the aorta. It can result in decreased blood volume and pressures distal to the aortic valve, and con-gestion proximal to it, in the left ventricle. This can be clearly seen in the systolic pressure gradient between the left ventricle and aorta. The increase in left ventricular blood volume and pressure can ultimately lead to similar increases in the left atrium and pulmonary circulation, resulting in pulmonary congestion.

Mitral stenosis will decrease blood flow and preload in the left ventricle, and ultimately out to the systemic circuit. It can also lead to an increase in blood volume and pressure in the left atrium and pulmonary circulation. It is not unusual for a patient with mitral valve disease to develop atrial fibrillation and pulmonary congestion.

Pulmonic valve disease can decrease forward flow and pressure in the pulmonic circuit, and ultimately to the systemic circuit. Blood volume and pressure will initially increase in the right ventricle and can lead to a similar increase in the right atrium and systemic venous system.

Tricuspid valve disease results in decreased filling of the right ventricle forward flow to the lungs, left heart, and systemic circuit. An increase in blood volume and pressure will initially occur in the right atria and may ultimately be transmitted back to the systemic venous system, leading to venous congestion.

When valves do not close all the way, they leak and are considered to be regurgitant or insufficient. Regurgitant valves can cause an increase in blood volume and pressure in the upstream chamber or vessel. This can lead to congestion in the chamber before the valve, and can decrease forward cardiac output after it. The degree of regurgitation also can be quantified in the cath lab.

LAYERS OF THE HEART WALL

The walls of the heart are comprised of three layers. The serous lining on the heart's outer surface is called the epicardium, or the visceral pericardium; the middle layer is known as the myocardium; and the inner surface of the heart, the endocardium.

The inner surface of the heart is the endocardium, a sheet of squamous epithelium on a thin layer of connective tissue. It is continuous with the endothelium that lines all the arteries, veins, and capillaries of the body, creating a single, closed system.

The middle layer of the heart, the myocardium, is the heart muscle. It is comprised of linearly arranged myofibrils made up of sarcomeres, the actual contracting units of the heart. The sarcomeres are comprised of myosin (thick) myofilaments and actin (thin) myofilaments. These contractile proteins slide over each other, shortening the sarcomere and contracting the heart. As the heart contracts, the myosin heads of the myosin myofilaments bind to the binding sites on the actin myofilaments, forming crossbridges. The myosin pulls the actin toward the center of the sarcomere causing it to shorten, and ultimately, contraction occurs.

The pericardium is a double-walled sac that completely encloses the heart. It serves to anchor and protect the heart and to prevent the heart from overdistending. This double-walled sac consists of parietal and visceral layers separated by the pericardial space, which normally contains 15–50 cc of pericardial fluid. The fluid lubricates the parietal and visceral layers, enabling them to slide over one another with a minimum of friction as the heart beats. The parietal pericardium is attached to the sternum, diaphragm, spine, and the great vessels. The visceral pericardium is attached to the myocardium. Pressure in the pericardium varies with respiration, becoming slightly negative with inspiration and positive with exhalation. The negative intrapericardial pressure during inspiration acts to increase venous return to the heart at the same time as oxygen-rich gas is entering the lungs.

PERICARDIAL EFFUSION

An excess of fluid in the pericardium, known as a pericardial effusion, can prevent the ventricles from distending during diastole, causing cardiac tamponade. Intrapericardial pressure can get so high that it actually causes the ventricles to collapse, a life-threatening emergency. Treatment for cardiac tamponade is called pericardiocentesis, and consists of inserting a needle and/or catheter into the pericardial space to release the pressure and drain off excess fluid.

Constrictive pericarditis is an inflammatory condition that causes the parietal and visceral layers of the pericardium to adhere to each other, obliterating the pericardial space. This inhibits ventricular relaxation and distention during diastole, which can impede ventricular filling and reduce cardiac output.

ELECTRICAL CONDUCTION

The heart has its own electrical conduction system. Electrical impulses originate in the pacemaker of the heart, the sinoatrial (SA) node. The SA node is comprised of specialized tissues and is located in the high posterior right atrium wall near the inflow track of the superior vena cava (Figure 2-4). The SA node normally initiates each cardiac cycle, leading to a wave of depolarization. The impulse travels from the SA node to the AV node, through the anterior, medial, and posterior intranodal pathways, and to the left atria via an intra-atrial pathway known as Bachmann's bundle.

The AV node lies in the bottom part of the right atrial septal wall, near the tricuspid valve. When the impulse arrives at the AV node, it is delayed for about 0.04 seconds to allow time for the ventricles to finish filling.

From the AV node, the impulse flows through the common bundle of His (pronounced "hiss"). The bundle of His allows for electrical communication from the atria to the ventricles through the fibrous skeleton of the heart, an electrically inert wall separating the atria and the ventricles. As the impulse travels through the bundle of His, the impulse is conducted through the right and

Figure 2-4. The electrical system of the heart.

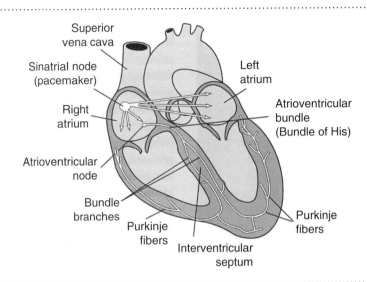

left bundle branches, and ultimately to every contractile cardiac cell in the ventricles via the Purkinje fiber network. Problems can develop in the electrical conduction system and in the electrical properties of the myocardial cells, which can lead to a wide array of dysrhythmias.

CONDUCTION ABNORMALITIES

When abnormalities occur in the heart's electrical conduction system, a wide array of complex dysrhythmias can occur. Problems in the SA node, the AV node, bundle of His, bundle branches, changes in conduction velocity, refractory periods, automaticity, reentry loops, and accessory pathways all can contribute to dysrhythmia development.

The SA node is usually the pacemaker of the heart. Sinus bradycardia occurs when it paces at rates of <60 beats/min, and sinus tachycardia occurs when it paces at rates >100 beats/min. Sick sinus syndrome is characterized by periods of bradycardia and tachycardia. Supraventricular tachycardia results in heart rates >160 beats/min,

and may originate from a reentry loop initiated by changes in conduction velocity and refractory periods.

The purpose of the AV node is to delay the electrical impulse long enough for the atria to contract and top off the ventricles. AV node abnormalities can result in a variety of heart blocks. In first-degree heart block, the AV node delays the impulse longer than 0.2 sec. In second-degree type-one (Wenckebach) heart block, the AV node delays the impulse for progressively longer periods of time until it totally blocks (drops) an impulse; then the cycle repeats. In second-degree type-two heart block, the block is below the AV node in the bundle of His; some impulses are conducted while others are blocked, causing a ventricular rate that is usually 20–40 contractions/min. Third-degree heart block is a condition in which every impulse from the atria is blocked from the ventricular conduction system. The atria may have a normal rate 60–80 contractions per minute, but the ventricles are not stimulated from above, and depolarize at their escape rate of less than 40 contractions/min.[2]

Bundle branch block occurs when one of the bundle branches does not conduct, normally resulting in delayed depolarization of one of the bundle branches. This prevents the right and left ventricles from contracting simultaneously and may reduce cardiac output. Some patients in heart failure with bundle branch block benefit from a biventricular pacemaker that can resynchronize ventricular contraction.

Ventricular tachycardia can be caused by an abnormal reentry loop in the ventricles, causing them to depolarize and beat at rates >160/min. These fast rates prevent the ventricles from filling, and can cause a rapid drop in cardiac output and blood pressure.

Ventricular fibrillation is a life-threatening emergency caused by the ventricles quivering instead of contracting, causing cardiac output and blood pressure to fall rapidly. Immediate defibrillation is required to attempt to resolve ventricular fibrillation. Atrial fibrillation is common in cath lab patients, and may be caused by problems with the mitral valve. The lack of atrial contraction may decrease cardiac output by 30%, and lead to thrombus formation in the atrium. The AV node is bombarded with hundreds of impulses each minute, and in time it is unable to block as many of them. This causes the ventricular rate to increase as well. As the ventricular rate increases to >100 beats/min, cardiac output may drop even further.[3]

HEMODYNAMICS

Blood, like any fluid, flows according to a pressure gradient. Systolic pressures are created when the heart is contracting, and diastolic pressures are created when the heart is resting. The left ventricle is the main pumping chamber of the heart, so it generates the highest pressures. Left ventricular systolic pressure equilibrates with aortic systolic pressure at around 120–130 mmHg.[4]

The pressure gradually drops as blood travels through the systemic circulatory system, and blood returns to the right atria with pressures of approximately 2–6 mmHg. This low-pressure blood flows rather passively from the right atrium into the right ventricle. The right ventricle normally generates systolic pressures of 20–30 mmHg, enough to deliver blood to the lungs and then to the left atria. The pressure gradually drops as blood travels through the pulmonary circuit. Ultimately, blood returns to the left atria with pressure of 2–12 mmHg. The left atrium then empties into the left ventricle and the cycle repeats.

OXYGEN SATURATION

Blood oxygen saturation represents the percent of hemoglobin (the oxygen-carrying component of red blood cells) that is saturated with, or bound to, oxygen. Mixed venous oxygen saturation analysis and monitoring is used to calculate the cardiac output, identify left-to-right shunts, monitor patients, and assess cardiovascular response to treatments.

Blood in the inferior vena cava has a higher oxygen saturation than blood in the superior vena cava, and a much higher saturation than blood from the coronary sinus, so oxygen saturation levels in the right atrium can vary depending on the sampling site. The right ventricle acts as a mixing chamber when it contracts and propels venous blood into the pulmonary artery. Blood in the pulmonary artery is therefore considered to be true mixed venous blood. Venous blood in the right side of the heart and the pulmonary artery normally has an oxygen saturation ranging from the upper-60s to the mid-70s.

As blood travels through the pulmonary capillary bed, oxygen diffuses into the blood, and CO_2 and water vapor diffuse out of the blood. The oxygen saturation of the blood increases to the high 90s, usually 96%–98%. This oxygenated, or arterialized, blood then travels to the left heart, the aorta, and on to the tissues of the systemic circulatory system.

CARDIAC OUTPUT

Cardiac output is the blood that is ejected from the left ventricle into the aorta, measured in L/min. A normal cardiac output is 4–8 L/min. Cardiac output is calculated by multiplying stroke volume by heart rate. Stroke volume is the amount of blood ejected from the left ventricle each heartbeat. It is influenced by preload, afterload, and contractility.

Cardiac output divided by the person's body surface area equals the cardiac index (CI), The CI provides a comparison between individuals' cardiac function, regardless of their body size. A normal CI is 2.5–4.0 L/min/m².[5]

Preload

Preload is the volume of blood still in the ventricle at the end of diastole. This blood stretches the myocardium's sarcomeres and influences contractility. Preload is quantified by measuring the left ventricle end diastolic pressure (LVEDP). Because pulmonary capillary wedge pressure approximately equilibrates with LVEDP, pulmonary capillary wedge pressure is often used to quantify preload.

The Frank-Starling mechanism describes the relationship between preload and contractility, stating that the strength of muscle contraction tends to increase when it is stretched. As preload increases, contractility also increases, causing stroke volume and cardiac output to increase. This is true until a critical point is reached, from which any further preload results in decreased contractility.

Increases in preload may be secondary to many causes, including myocardial infarction (MI), aortic stenosis, and hypervolemia. Elevations in preload that have exceeded the critical point, and resulted in decreased contractility, can lead to increased left atrial and pulmonary artery pressures. This can lead to congestive heart failure, as osmotic pulmonary pressure exceeds oncotic pulmonary pressure, causing fluid to leak from the pulmonary capillary bed into the interstitial and interalveolar spaces of the lung. By decreasing the heart's fluid volume (e.g., with diuretics), preload decreases to a more favorable level. This can result in an increase in contractility, leading to an increase in stroke volume and cardiac output.

Conversely, decreases in left ventricular preload may also cause a reduction in contractility. This may be secondary to hypovolemia, decreased venous return, or right heart MI. A decrease in preload that leads to a reduction in cardiac output may be treated with fluids or venous vasoconstrictors.

Afterload

Afterload is the pressure that the chamber has to generate to eject blood. It represents impedance to ventricular ejection. It is influenced by several factors including the radius of the blood vessels, blood viscosity, and mean arterial pressures (MAP).

Left ventricular afterload is quantified with systemic vascular resistance (SVR), and right ventricular afterload is quantified with pulmonary vascular resistance (PVR). Vascular resistance is calculated by dividing the pressure drop through of a vascular bed by the cardiac output for that vascular bed.

$$\text{SVR (mmHg/L/min)} = [(\text{MAP} - \text{right atrial pressure})/\text{systemic cardiac output}]$$

$$\text{PVR (mmHg/L/min)} = [(\text{mean pulmonary artery pressure} - \text{pulmonary capillary wedge pressure})/\text{pulmonary cardiac output}]$$

This results in vascular resistance being expressed in mmHg/L/min, called Wood or Hybrid units. To convert to SI units, multiply by 80.

$$\text{SVR (dynes/sec/cm}^{-5}) = [(\text{MAP} - \text{right atrial pressure})/ \text{systemic cardiac output}] \times 80$$

PVR (dynes/sec/cm^{-5}) = [(mean pulmonary artery pressure − pulmonary capillary wedge pressure)/ pulmonary cardiac output] × 80

In SI units, vascular resistance is expressed in dynes/sec/cm^{-5}. Normal SVR is 900–1400 dynes/sec/cm^{-5} and normal PVR is 30–100 dynes/sec/cm^{-5}.[2]

As vascular resistance increases, the heart must work harder, and stroke volume may decrease. Vascular resistance can be influenced by vasoconstriction or vasodilatation at the arteriole level.

The precapillary sphincter muscles are located on arterioles just before they divide into capillaries. By constricting and relaxing, they can influence blood flow distribution and afterload. An increase in PVR increases afterload of the right heart, and as the right heart must work harder, it may eventually fail.

Patients with chronic obstructive pulmonary disease (COPD) may be hypoxemic, and develop a compensatory increase in the number of red blood cells (polycythemia). This can thicken the blood, increasing afterload. COPD patients may also have high PVR due to pulmonary vasoconstriction. This can increase the work of the right ventricle and may lead to right side heart failure secondary to lung disease (cor pulmonale).

Contractility

Contractility is the inherent ability of the sarcomeres to shorten. It is influenced by preload, the sympathetic nervous system, circulating catecholamines, metabolic abnormalities (hypoxemia, hypercapnia, and metabolic acidosis can all decrease contractility), and pharmacologic agents. Other important factors include the viability of the heart muscle itself; cardiac ischemia, injury, or infarction can all decrease contractility. Most cardiac patients with decreased contractility have a decreased cardiac output secondary to decreased stroke volume.

CARDIAC INSUFFICIENCY—HEART FAILURE

Damage to the heart decreases its ability to deliver the appropriate cardiac output to meet the metabolic needs of the body. When cardiac output from the left heart is decreased, patients may suffer the effects of decreased systemic perfusion including weakness, exercise intolerance, fatigue, mental confusion, and renal insufficiency.

As the left ventricular ejection fraction decreases, the left ventricular diastolic volumes and pressures increase. The increase in blood volume and pressure is transmitted back to the pulmonary circulatory system. As pressure in the pulmonary capillary bed increases, it reaches a point when fluids seep out of the capillary vessels into the interstitial and alveolar spaces of the lung. This results in pulmonary congestion and subsequent pulmonary edema. Signs and symptoms of pulmonary congestion include dyspnea, orthopnea, hemoptysis, shortness of breath, interstitial and alveolar edema, S3 and S4 heart sounds, moist crackles, increased pulmonary pressures, and hypoxemia.[6] Treatment is directed at correcting the underlying cause of the left heart failure. Patients may also benefit from diuretics, ace inhibitors, beta blockers, oxygen, and digitalis.

Some cardiac or pulmonary disease processes can decrease the right heart's ability to deliver the appropriate cardiac output to the pulmonary and systemic circulatory systems. When this happens, patients exhibit signs and symptoms of decreased pulmonary and systemic perfusion including tachypnea, hypoxemia, weakness, exercise intolerance, confusion, and renal insufficiency.

If the right heart is unable to unload, congestion occurs in the right heart and the systemic venous system. Signs and symptoms of systemic venous congestion include jugular venous distension, peripheral edema, ascites, heptojugular reflex, Kussmaul's sign, and elevation of right heart and central venous pressures. Treatment is directed at correcting the underlying cause, and alleviating the effects, of heart failure. Left heart failure commonly causes right heart failure.

VASCULAR ANATOMY

The body's vascular beds act as a distribution network to deliver blood from the heart to all tissues of the body. They are dynamic; local and systemic mediation enables them to constrict and dilate based on the metabolic needs of the tissues served.

Vessels are comprised of three layers: intimal, medial, and adventitial. The intimal layer (tunica intima) endothelial cells modulate changes in vascular resistance in the systemic and pulmonic vascular beds. The endothelium secretes both nitric oxide (NO), which leads to vasodilatation, and endothelin-1, which leads to vasoconstriction. To maintain normal vascular tone and regulate vascular tone in response to metabolic requirements, a balance must exist between NO and endothelin-1.

Endothelial cells also secrete chemicals to enhance or inhibit platelet aggregation, and smooth-muscle cell proliferation and migration from the medial layer. In the event of vascular injury, vasoconstriction, platelet aggregation, thrombus formation, and smooth-muscle proliferation all act to decrease blood loss and promote healing. The healthy endothelium promotes appropriate vascular tone and platelet and smooth-muscle cell activity to maintain hemostasis.

Because of the low pressures in the venous system, veins have valves in them, preventing the blood from running to our feet when we stand up. These valves are made from thin folds of tunica intima, providing one continuous smooth surface.

The medial layer (tunica media) is comprised of smooth-muscle cells innervated by the nervous system and influenced by hormones and chemicals. These smooth-muscle cells have the ability to constrict or relax, leading to vasoconstriction or dilatation that modulates blood-flow distribution, blood pressure, and vascular resistance. Arteries have a much thicker medial layer than veins.

The adventitial layer (tunica adventitia) is comprised of tough connective tissue that serves as the protective outer layer of the blood vessel.

CORONARY ARTERIES

Like fingerprints, the coronary arteries are unique to every individual. As a general rule, the right coronary artery (RCA) rises from the right coronary cusp of the aortic valve and travels in the right AV groove (Figure 2-5). It usually first gives rise to a conus branch which feeds the right ventricular outflow track, an area of the heart where many arrhythmias are generated. Sometimes, however, the conus branch rises from a separate ostia in the aorta. The RCA also gives rise to the SA nodal artery, perfusing the SA node in 60% of the population and the right atrium. It then gives rise to acute marginal arteries that supply the right ventricle.

The RCA then courses around the heart's right side in the right AV groove, ultimately reaching the posterior heart, where it meets the crux of the heart. The crux is the cross in the posterior heart where the interventricular and interatrial septa meet at the posterior atrioventricular AV groove. In the area of the crux, the RCA gives rise to a posterior descending coronary artery (PDA) that perfuses the posterior one-third of the interventricular septum. It then usually gives rise to an AV nodal artery, perfusing the AV node in 90% of the patients and the interatrial septum. Distal to the AV nodal artery, the RCA gives rise to posterolateral arteries (PLAs), also known as diaphragmatic or left ventricular branches, which perfuse the inferior or inferior posterior left ventricle wall.

The left coronary artery (LCA) rises from the left coronary cusp of the aortic valve, and gives rise to the left main coronary artery, which then bifurcates into the left anterior descending (LAD), the circumflex (CX), and sometimes with an intermediate branch between them. The LAD

Figure 2-5. Schematic diagram of the coronary arteries.

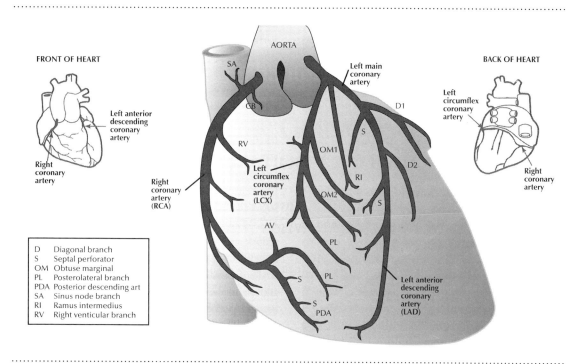

D	Diagonal branch
S	Septal perforator
OM	Obtuse marginal
PL	Posterolateral branch
PDA	Posterior descending art
SA	Sinus node branch
RI	Ramus intermedius
RV	Right venticular branch

courses over the anterior interventricular groove and gives rise to septal perforators, perfusing the anterior two-thirds of the interventricular septum. The LAD also gives rise to the diagonal branches coursing over the anterior surface of the left ventricle. Some of these branches may course down to the heart apex. The distal end of the LAD may also wrap around the apex of the heart.

The CX courses over the left AV groove, and gives rise to obtuse marginals, arteries that perfuse the left ventricle's lateral wall. In addition, the CX gives rise to a left atria branch that perfuses the left atrium. The distal CX gives rise to the vessels that perfuse the left ventricle's posterior wall. Sometimes the LCA trifurcates, with a ramus branch originating between the LAD and the CX.

The dominant coronary artery is the one that supplies both the posterior descending artery and the posterolateral branches supplying the inferior wall of the left ventricle. The RCA is dominant in about 85% of the population. The LCA is dominant in about 8% of the population. About 7% of the population has a codominant system in which the RCA gives rise to the PDA and the distal circumflex gives rise to the PLAs.

CORONARY BLOOD FLOW

Blood traveling through the heart passes through without delivering oxygen and nutrients directly to the surrounding heart muscle. The heart receives its oxygen and nutrients from its own circulatory system made up of the coronary arteries and cardiac veins.

The coronary arteries rise off the root of the aorta, making the heart the first organ in the body to be perfused with oxygenated blood.

The arteries branch into capillaries, where gas exchange occurs. The capillaries run through the myocardium, and when the myocardium contracts, the capillaries are squeezed, and no blood can flow through them. The coronary arteries therefore supply oxygen to the heart muscle mainly during diastole, when the heart is in its resting phase.

The capillaries merge into cardiac veins, then into the coronary sinus, which empties into the right atrium. Because of the high oxygen-extraction rate of the myocardium, the blood in the coronary sinus has the lowest oxygen saturation of any blood in the body, usually about 40%.

The pressure under which the blood enters the coronary arteries (the coronary perfusion pressure) is influenced by the aortic diastolic pressure, left ventricular diastolic pressure, right atrial pressure, and coronary artery disease. Decreases in coronary perfusion pressure can reduce blood flow through the coronary arteries, leading to a decrease in the myocardial oxygen supply and resulting in myocardial ischemia.

The myocardial oxygen supply should equal myocardial oxygen demand. Mismatches in this relationship can lead to ischemia, injury, or infarction. The myocardial oxygen supply is influenced by the radius of the coronaries, coronary perfusion pressure, and oxygen and hemoglobin levels. Myocardial oxygen demand is influenced by heart rate, preload, afterload, and contractility.

ARTERIOSCLEROSIS

Atherosclerosis results in blockages (lesions or stenoses) in the coronary arteries. The stenosis can decrease blood flow and oxygen delivery to heart muscle. This may lead to myocardial ischemia, injury, or infarction. The progression of arteriosclerosis is complex and not well understood. It is thought to begin with damage to the endothelium, leading to endothelial dysfunction that causes the development of fatty streaks and, ultimately, plaque formation (Figure 2-6). Vessel inflammation and inflammatory changes also play a role in the process.

Endothelial injury increases the permeability of the endothelium, allowing the blood's low-density lipoproteins to invade the arterial wall and accumulate in the subendothelial spaces. Those lipoproteins become oxidized, and chemoattractants are released, causing monocytes (a type of white blood cell) to migrate to the injury site. The monocytes differentiate into macrophages and phagocytize (ingest) the low-density lipoproteins. These lipid-laden macrophages, known as foam cells, contribute to the initial bulging of the fatty streak from the subendothelium into the lumen of the vessel.

The stenosis can be exacerbated by endothelial dysfunction, leading to vasoconstriction, platelet aggregation, and smooth-muscle cell proliferation in the stenotic segment, compromising blood flow even further. At this stage in the process, the atherosclerotic lesion is complex mixture of low-density lipoproteins, macrophages, foam cells, smooth-muscle cells, collagen, calcium, and platelets. Inflammatory changes complicate the situation and may result in plaque rupture and thrombus formation.

Coronary artery disease can ultimately lead to ischemia, injury, or MI (Figure 2-7). Some of the risk factors include family history, advancing age, male gender (women quickly catch up after menopause), hypertension, hyperlipidemia, obesity, stress, physical inactivity, smoking, and diabetes mellitus.

Arteriosclerosis can occur in vessels other than coronary arteries. Peripheral vascular disease causes decreased blood flow and oxygen delivery to tissues supplied by the stenotic vessels. For example, when the arteries supplying the legs are affected, patients may feel leg pain, known as intermittent claudication, when walking.

ANGINA

Angina is the chest pain patients feel secondary to atherosclerotic coronary artery disease and

Figure 2-6. Development of coronary atherosclerosis: the Stary classification. Atheriosclerosis is due to endothelial injury leading to a localized inflammatory response. Initially plaques evolve slowly, but may acutely rupture or gradually stenose over time. SMC = smooth muscle cells.

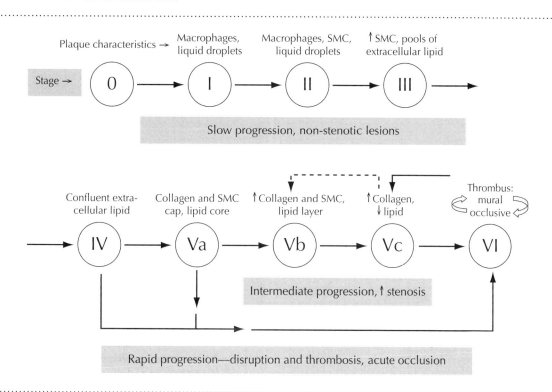

cardiac ischemia. It results from the mismatch between myocardial oxygen supply and demand. The demand for oxygen exceeds the supply due to decreased oxygen delivery distal to a coronary artery restriction or blockage.

Stable angina is characterized by chest pain that is predictable in nature and onset. It is secondary to a fixed lesion that causes a temporary oxygen demand-supply mismatch. The symptoms are directly related to cardiac activity, such as when the heart must work harder during physical exercise. Stable anginal pain does not occur without increased activity (it does not occur at rest), and pain should recede with rest or administration of nitroglycerin.

Unstable angina is basically aggravated stable angina. The onset of chest pain is not predictable; it may occur suddenly, while at rest, or with a low level of activity. The chest pain may be more intense and last longer. It is not as easily relieved and additional nitroglycerin administration or other coronary interventions may be required. Unstable angina may be caused by a thrombus formation that totally occludes the vessel for a period of time. The body's own thrombolytic system may lyse the clot, restoring blood flow to the compromised heart wall.

Prinzmetal's angina is caused by coronary artery spasm. The spasm usually occurs at rest and compromises coronary blood flow distal of the spasm. Nitroglycerin, calcium channel blockers, or both help to relax the smooth muscles in the vessel wall to break the spasm. Prinzmetal's angina can be provoked in susceptible patients in the cath lab

Figure 2-7. Progression of coronary atherosclerosis. Atherosclerosis is a dynamic, repetitive process of injury, inflammation, and repair. The resulting atherosclerosis plaque through phases leading to progressive stenosis or acute plaque rupture and thrombosis.

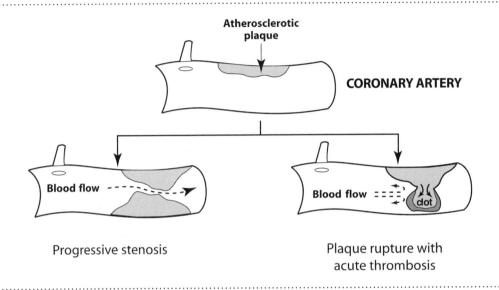

using intracoronary ergonovine or methergine.[7] Some patients have atherosclerotic coronary artery disease and Prinzmetal's angina.

MYOCARDIAL INFARCTION

The progression of coronary artery disease, angina, or unstable angina may culminate in a myocardial infarction (MI). MIs are characterized by plaque rupture leading to thrombus formation and total coronary artery occlusion. Some plaques (stenoses) are more likely to rupture than others. Known as vulnerable plaques, these are characterized by a thin cap over a relatively liquid lipid core. Stable plaques have a thick cap over a more solid core. Plaque rupture may be caused by inflammatory changes and/or shear stresses.

When plaque ruptures, cells within the lesion come in contact with circulating platelets, causing them to become activated. The platelet activation/clotting cascade is initiated, resulting in thrombus formation. In a coronary artery, this can stop blood from reaching the myocardium. If blood flow is not restored, the myocardial cells can die.

The chest pain from an MI is more intense and lasts longer than anginal pain. MI chest pain is not relieved with rest or nitroglycerin. Cardiac markers, proteins, and enzymes such as troponins, CKMB, and LDH1 and 2 are released from the injured and dying myocardium. Laboratory tests for these substances can be used as markers for acute MI. Changes in the patient's ECG, including ST-segment elevation and the development of Q-waves in the leads looking at the infarcting wall, may also occur. Correlation of ECGs, laboratory tests, and patient symptoms are important in the diagnosis and treatment strategies of MI.

The prognosis for patients suffering an MI depends on the extent of left ventricular damage: the greater the damage, the poorer the patient's prognosis. If patients are able to receive medical attention rapidly, the damage caused by an MI can be limited. Opening the vessel up (revascularization) can be performed with thrombolytic administration or with percutaneous coronary intervention (PCI).

A left heart MI can result in decreased forward blood flow to the systemic circulation. The inability of the left heart to move blood forward also will result in an increase in volume and a high diastolic pressure. This can impede the left atria's ability to empty into the ventricle, increasing blood volume and pressure in the left atrium and lungs, resulting in pulmonary congestion.

A right ventricular MI can result in decreased right ventricular ejection to the lungs, decreasing pulmonary blood flow and left heart filling, and the systemic venous system will become congested.

Instead of infarcting, sometimes myocardial cells that have been subject to severe ischemia may become stunned or hibernate if blood flow is reestablished in time. Myocardial stunning occurs when, after a brief period of severe ischemia and an initial period of cardiac dysfunction, normal contractility gradually returns over a period of hours to days. The myocardium is said to hibernate when patients with severe chronic ischemia and chronically depressed ventricular function experience a return to normal function over a period of days to weeks after the reestablishment of blood flow.

RESTENOSIS

Restenosis is a condition in which the blockage returns to a vessel segment that has been dilated by PCI. The mechanisms of restenosis include elastic recoil, intimal thickening, and vessel remodeling. Elastic recoil is a function of changes in the atherosclerotic plaque and the elastic properties of the arterial wall. Intimal thickening is the vessel's healing response to injury caused by the coronary intervention. Vessel remodeling is vessel constriction or shrinkage that decreases lumen diameter in the area of the intervention.

Neointimal hyperplasia (NIH) is another cause of restenosis. It is the most common cause of restenosis following coronary stent implantation. NIH describes the migration of smooth-muscle cells into the artery's walls in response to vessel injury. Once there, the smooth-muscle cells proliferate and produce a connective tissue matrix, which becomes bulky, restricting flow within the artery.

PERIPHERAL ARTERIAL SYSTEM

The left ventricle ejects arterialized blood into the aorta for distribution to the systemic circulatory system. The aorta is the largest artery in the body, with a diameter of 2–3cm (1 inch). It can be divided into four parts: the ascending aorta, the arch of the aorta, the descending thoracic aorta, and the abdominal aorta (Figure 2-8).

As the aorta ascends from the left ventricle, it gives rise to the coronary arteries, so the heart is the first organ to be perfused with oxygenated blood. The ascending aorta continues upward a short distance until it turns left, creating the aortic arch. The aortic arch gives rise to three major arteries supplying the head and upper extremities: the brachiocephalic (innominate), left common carotid, and left subclavian. The brachiocephalic divides into the right subclavian and the right common carotid arteries.

The right subclavian continues in the right upper thorax and into the right arm where it becomes the right axillary artery. It continues down the arm as the right brachial artery, and in the area of the elbow, it bifurcates into the right radial and right ulnar arteries. These two arteries continue down the forearm to the wrist where they anastomose back together via the superficial and deep palmar arches. This creates a dual-perfusion system to the hand. Whenever the radial artery is to be punctured, an "Allen's test" should be done to ensure the patient has a patent palmar arch.

The third major artery off the arch of the aorta is the left subclavian. The left subclavian becomes

Figure 2-8. Aorta and the main arteries branching off it.

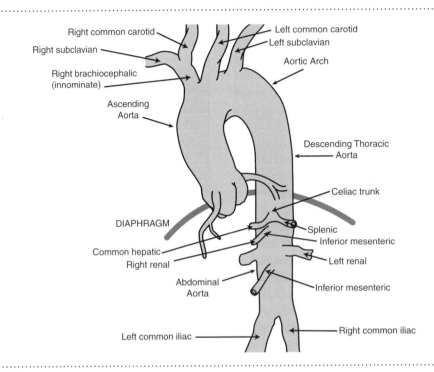

the left axillary, left brachial, and continues to the left hand and the branches are named the same as the branches of the right subclavian. Perfusion to the left arm is similar to that of the right.

The right and left subclavian arteries also give rise to two other significant arteries: the vertebral and internal mammary arteries. The right and left internal mammary arteries arise off their respective subclavian arteries to contribute blood supply to the anterior chest. The internal mammary arteries have proven to be excellent conduits and are commonly used as coronary artery bypass grafts.

The right and left vertebral arteries arise off their respective subclavian arteries to contribute blood supply to the brain. The two vertebral arteries unite at the inferior surface of the brain to become the basilar artery.

Blood flow to the head and brain occurs through the right and left common carotid arteries and their branches. The right common carotid arises as a major branch from the brachiocephalic

artery, and the left common carotid arises as the second branch from the arch of the aorta. Both common carotids divide in the neck into the internal and external carotid arteries. The right and left external carotids provide blood supply to the thyroid gland, tongue, throat, face, ears, scalp, and dura mater. The right and left internal carotids supply the brain, eyes, forehead, and nose. Anastomoses of the right and left internal carotids and the basilar artery form a vascular circle at the base of the brain known as the circle of Willis. This creates alternate routes for blood flow to the brain in the event of cerebral vascular disease. Additional arteries supplying the brain arise from this circle.

After supplying blood to the upper extremities and the head from the arch, the aorta turns and descends through the thorax as the thoracic aorta, which supplies the organs and skeletal muscle in the chest. Some of the significant vessels include the pericardial arteries supplying the pericardium, the bronchial arteries feeding the airways of the lungs, and the esophageal arteries supplying the esophagus.

As the thoracic aorta passes through the diaphragm, it becomes the abdominal aorta. The abdominal aorta provides blood flow to the organs and walls of the abdominal cavity. Some of the principal arteries of the abdominal aorta include the celiac trunk supplying the liver, stomach, spleen, and pancreas, the superior mesenteric artery feeding the small intestine and part of the large intestine, the right and left renal arteries feeding the right and left kidneys, and the inferior mesenteric artery supplying the major part of the large intestine and rectum.

AORTIC ANEURYSM AND DISSECTION

An aneurysm is a localized dilatation of the blood vessel wall, usually caused by atherosclerosis and hypertension. True aortic aneurysms involve a weakening of all three layers of the aorta to create a localized bulge of the vessel. These aneurysms are classified as being fusiform or saccular (Figure 2-9). A fusiform aneurysm is one that involves the entire circumference of an aortic segment, resulting in a cylindroid dilatation in that segment. A saccular aneurysm involves only a portion of the circumference, resulting in a dilatation, or

outpouching, in part of the aortic circumference. In either case, all three layers of the aortic wall remain intact.

Dissections occur when the three layers of the aortic wall are no longer intact. A tear or longitudinal disruption occurs between the medial and intimal layers of the vessel, creating a false channel into the vessel wall through which blood may travel. The DeBakey classification of aortic dissections describes dissection locations.

Type I dissections are the most common and begin just above the aortic valve. They may involve the leaflets of the valve and extend up the ascending aorta, around the arch, and down the descending aorta as far as into the abdominal aorta.

Type II dissections begin in the same location as type I, but they stop in the ascending aorta and do not extend into the aortic arch. These are seen in pregnant patients and patients with Marfan's syndrome.

Type III dissections begin past the aortic arch, distal to the left subclavian artery. They can extend a variable distance down the thoracic aorta and may extend into the abdominal aorta.

Both aneurysms and dissections can rupture, leading to fatal hemorrhage. Patients need to be

Figure 2-9. Aortic aneurysms.

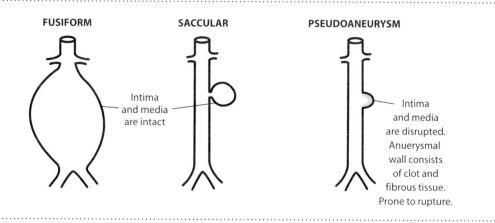

followed closely for any signs of aortic enlargement or extension. Maintenance of normal blood pressure is essential. Surgery may be necessary to repair the aorta, and new devices are emerging for minimally invasive endovascular repairs.

Sub-Aortic Arteries

The abdominal aorta terminates in the lower abdominal cavity as it divides to become the right and left common iliac arteries. The right and left common iliacs branch into the right and left internal and right and left external iliac arteries. The internal iliacs provide blood to the thigh, urinary bladder, rectum, prostate, uterus, and vagina. The right and left external iliac arteries and its branches carry blood to the lower extremities.

The right and left external iliac arteries continue through the thigh area, where they become the right and left common femoral arteries. The common femoral arteries branch into the deep and superficial femoral arteries. As the superficial femoral arteries reach the knee, they become the right and left popliteal arteries. The popliteal arteries become the tibioperoneal trucks below the knees, and divide into the anterior and posterior tibial arteries. The right and left posterior tibial arteries feed the lower legs and feet. The right and left anterior tibial arteries continue through the calf to the ankle where they become the right and left dorsalis pedis arteries and also provide blood flow to the feet.

VENOUS SYSTEM

After supplying oxygen and nutrient-rich blood to the systemic tissues via the arterial circulatory system, gas exchange (internal respiration) occurs in the capillary system. The venous system returns blood to the right heart through a system of veins that basically parallels the arterial circulation. The veins are usually, but not always, named for their companion arteries. All of the systemic veins ultimately flow into either the superior or inferior venae cavae that, in turn, empty into the right atrium. The

right ventricle ejects venous blood into the lungs through the pulmonary trunk, then the right and left pulmonary arteries.

Gas exchange (external respiration) occurs in the lungs. Oxygenated blood now travels through the pulmonary veins back to the left atrium and left ventricle. The left ventricle ejects oxygenated blood into the aorta and systemic circulatory system and the cycle continues.

SUMMARY

The components of the cardiovascular system work in concert to circulate blood throughout the body, delivering oxygen and other nutrients essential to life and removing CO_2 and other waste products. Unfortunately, many disease processes compromise the integrity of the cardiovascular system. The cardiac cath lab is an ideal environment to diagnose and quantify the severity of these diseases and to perform interventional procedures in an effort to restore a healthy balance to a patient's cardiovascular system.

REFERENCES

1. Hagen PT, Scholz DG, Edwards WD. Incidence and size of patent foramen ovale during the first 10 decades of life: an autopsy study of 965 normal hearts. *Mayo Clin Proc* 1984;59:17–20.
2. Conover M. *Understanding Electrocardiography*, 8th ed. St. Louis, MO: Mosby; 2002.
3. Grauer K. *A Practical Guide to ECG Interpretation*, 2nd ed. St. Louis, MO: Mosby; 1998.
4. Daily E, Schroeder J. *Techniques in Bedside Hemodynamic Monitoring*, 5th ed. St. Louis, MO: Mosby; 1994.
5. Lilly LS. *Pathophysiology of Heart Disease*, 3rd ed. Philadelphia: Lea & Febiger; 2002.
6. Canobbio MM. *Cardiovascular Disorders*. St. Louis, MO: Mosby; 1990.
7. Baim DS, Grossman W. *Cardiac Catheterization, Angiography and Intervention*, 6th ed. Philadelphia: Lippincott Williams & Wilkins; 2000.

SUGGESTED READING

Braunwald E, Zipes DP, Libby P. *Heart Disease: A Textbook of Cardiovascular Medicine*, 6th ed. Philadelphia: W. B. Saunders; 2001.

Des Jardins T. *Cardiopulmonary Anatomy and Physiology*, 4th ed. Clifton Park, NY: Delmar; 2002.

Guyton AC, Hall JE. *Textbook of Medical Physiology*, 10th ed. Philadelphia: W.B. Saunders; 2001.

Hurst JW, Alpert JS. *Diagnostic Atlas of the Heart*. New York: Raven Press; 1994.

Kern MJ. *The Cardiac Catheterization Handbook*, 4th ed. St. Louis, MO: Mosby; 2003.

Safian RD, Freed MS. *The Manual of Interventional Cardiology*, 3rd ed. Royal Oak, MI: Physicians' Press; 2001.

Tortora G, Grabowski SR. *Principles of Anatomy and Physiology*, 10th ed. Indianapolis, IN: John Wiley & Sons; 2003.

Chapter 3

Electrocardiography and Rhythm Interpretation

Rick Meece, CCT, RCS, RCIS, FSICP
Neil E. Holtz, BS, EMT-P, RCIS

In practice, electrocardiography is a very important diagnostic component that involves an electronic mapping how well the heart generates and conducts electrical impulses and a monitoring of changes in its ability to do so. Learning to identify ECG changes and understanding their implications for the patient's condition are critical skills necessary for all personnel who work in environments such as acute cardiac care, post surgical care and cardiac catheterization laboratories.

The 12-lead ECG along with specific blood enzyme analysis can accurately detect myocardial injury, ischemia and infarction, as well as indicate the area in the myocardium where these conditions exist. The 12-lead ECG may also indicate conditions related to cardiac chamber enlargement, abnormal blood levels of electrolytes, and conduction defects secondary to other pathophysiological conditions.

Arrhythmia recognition by ECG is a dynamic process involving continual assessment over time for ECG changes related to rhythm, rate, and conduction.

ELECTROCARDIOLOGIC ANATOMY

The heart has specialized muscular cells which create and conduct electrical impulses that produce the rhythmic pumping action of the heart. These cells are called sarcomeres, and they contain a multitude of fibers called actin and myosin which, when stimulated by chemical reaction, will contract and relax, producing what is known as the cardiac cycle. Sarcomeres are the contractile cells of the human heart.

A small group of cardiac cells, the P cells, are located in the sinoatrial (SA) and atrioventricular (AV) nodal areas. They are responsible for impulse formation and conduction of electrical activity. Similar types of conductive cells located around the nodal areas are called transitional; they aid with the production of electrical impulses when demanded by certain conditions. Both types of cardiac cells work in unison to function automatically, without any external stimulus.

In the normal heart, cardiac electrical impulses originate from the SA node, which cause the atria to contract and expel their blood into the ventricles (Figure 3-1). The impulses then travel along the internodal pathways, and converge at the AV node. The primary function of the AV node is to delay the impulse long enough (0.04 seconds) to allow the atria to complete contraction from the SA nodal impulse and push blood into the ventricles before they begin contracting themselves. With its specialized cells, the AV node also protects the ventricular conduction pathways from being overstimulated by extra impulses from the atria. The extra impulses are found in some disease conditions, and can possibly produce dangerous and even fatal arrhythmias such as ventricular tachycardia (VT) or ventricular fibrillation (VF).

From the AV node, the impulses move through the bundle of His along the interventricular groove and divide into the right and left bundle branches. The left bundle branch further bifurcates into the left anterior and posterior hemifascicles and terminates in the complex system of the Purkinje network, which covers the whole of the myocardium.

Cardiac impulses stimulate ventricular systole moving from the apex towards the base. This design maximizes effective stroke volume and prevents pooling of blood in the apex, as may occur following an anteroapical myocardial infarction (MI).

After depolarization, the cardiac cells must then recharge, or repolarize, to prepare and clear the electrical pathway for the next impulse. These cycles are initiated and carried out through continual chemical changes, as positively and negatively charged ions (primarily Na^+, K^+, and Ca^+)

Figure 3-1. Electrical system of the heart.

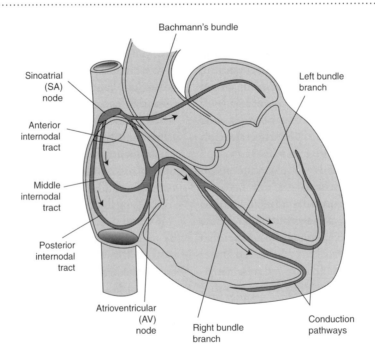

are gated back and forth by osmosis within the cardiac cellular structure.

BASIC ECG ANALYSIS

As the ECG tracing moves in real time, it displays cardiac electrical impulses moving through the cardiac pathways from atrial contraction through depolarization (ventricular systole).

An ECG recording without an electrical impulse appears as a flat (isoelectric) line. Deflections that record above the isoelectric line are considered positive deflections. Deflections recorded below the isoelectric line are negative deflections.

It is critical to understand that upward or positive ECG deflections demonstrate where the majority of electrical depolarization (positive ionic movement) is occurring in the general direction of that particular ECG lead, thus quantifying the location where the largest mass of myocardium is effectively conducting the impulse(s). Understanding this principal will rapidly increase your ability to quickly and accurately diagnose ECG changes.

The ECG is normally recorded on graph paper that is automatically fed from the recorder on demand for baseline measurement and analysis.

The recording strip (Figure 3-2) consists of a grid background with larger boxes outlined and filled with smaller boxes. The paper is usually discharged from the machine at a rate of 25mm/sec. Along the horizontal time line, time is measured in seconds. Each larger square represents 2/10 of a second, or 0.2 seconds. Each smaller square represents 0.04 seconds. Along the vertical axis of the recording, the deflection above or below the isoelectric line is measured as mV, or the intensity of the impulse. The larger square represents 0.5 mV, and the smaller square 0.1 mV. The standardization mark on a calibrated ECG is 1 mV or 10 mm.

The ECG is obtained by placing both limb and pre-cordial leads or electrodes on and around the thoracic area of the patient at the fourth intercostal space right sternal border (V1), the fourth intercostal space left sternal border (V2), the mid-clavicular line fifth intercostal space (V3), the axillary line sixth intercostal space (V4), and the mid-axillary line sixth intercostals space (V6). V5 is placed halfway between V4 and V6.

Through these electrodes, cardiac impulses can be observed and recorded from a number of different angles (vectors of conduction). There are two basic types of leads, bipolar and unipolar. With the bipolar leads (I/II/III), the impulse is

Figure 3-2. ECG strip on usual graph paper with measurements marked vertically and horizontally.

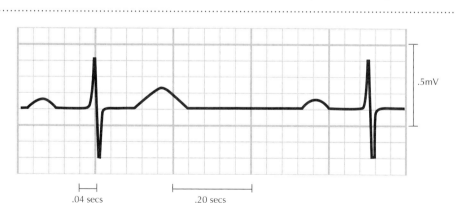

tracked as it travels from a negative (−) pole to a positive (+) pole from different perspectives across the myocardium. Augmented, or unipolar, leads (aVR/aVL/aVF) combine the leads to form the third pole, with a third lead representing the positive pole (e.g., right arm and left arm against the legs for aVF). The precordial leads (V1 to V6) are unipolar, but generally not used in the catheterization laboratory for monitoring except for patients undergoing an electrophysiology procedure. However, they are essential for a complete picture of cardiac activity when obtaining a 12-lead ECG.

The electrodes, or lead wires, that connect the monitoring system to the patient are usually marked and/or color coded to assist with proper placement. It is extremely important to double check that the lead wires are in the correct positions to avoid inaccurate interpretation of the ECG (Figure 3-3).

DETERMINING HEART RATE FROM THE ECG

The heart rate is the number of times the heart depolarizes in the space of one minute. Most equipment used today is digitally enhanced, and automatically displays the rate on the monitor. If this is not available, a simple method can be used to calculate the rate.

The cardiac rate in beats per minute (bpm) is calculated by comparing the distance over time, usually measured from one R wave to the next R wave, or from depolarization to depolarization, assuming that the ventricular response is regular. Find an R wave (the upward point) that occurs on or very close to a

Figure 3-3. Chest diagram of lead replacement.

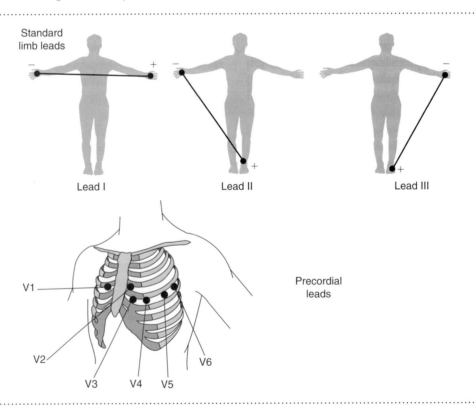

Figure 3-4. Countdown method.

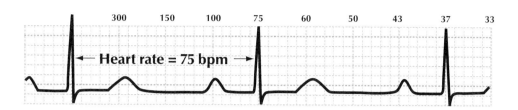

darker black line on the larger squares. From there, count the number of darker lines to the next R wave. The first dark line would be 300 bpm, the next 150 bpm, the next 100 bpm, the next 75 bpm, the next 60 bpm, and the next 50 bpm. This is called the countdown method (Figure 3-4). Committing the sequence to memory will make calculating the basic rate a quick and easy procedure.

The normal heart will display a normal sinus rhythm (NSR) at a rate between 60 and 100 bpm. Rates slower than 60 bpm are considered to be bradycardic. Bradycardia may not be detrimental, however, to individuals who are athletic or who are taking medication such as beta blockers. Rates that are greater than 100 bpm are faster than normal, or tachycardic. Again, certain tachycardia rhythms may not be a serious threat, and

can occur with anxiety or exercise, and in febrile or dehydrated patients. Tachycardia is not benign though; the earliest signs of patient distress often will be sinus tachycardia. Sinus tachycardia may be also associated with hypoxemia, hypoglycemia, and acute pulmonary embolus.

UNDERSTANDING ECG WAVEFORM MEASUREMENTS

The ECG tracing is a series of deflections that construct themselves into identifiable patterns along a timeline based on the received electrical impulse. They may be demonstrated in rhythmic or arrhythmic intervals. Each component (Figure 3-5) represents a segment of the cardiac electromechanical cycle and has unique terminology and assessment associated with it.

Figure 3-5. ECG waveforms and intervals.

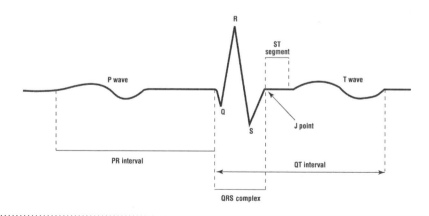

P WAVE

Contraction of the atria is displayed as a short positive deflection, and is called the P wave. The first and second halves of the P wave (if seen) roughly correspond to right and left atrial activation, respectively. Normal P-wave values are as follows.

Normal P wave: 0.08–0.11 seconds duration.

Amplitude (mm): P-wave amplitude is measured from the baseline to the top (or bottom) of the P wave. Positive and negative deflections are determined separately. Limb leads are <2.5 mm, and V1 has a positive deflection <1.5 mm and a negative deflection <1 mm.

Morphology: Upright in I, II, aVF; upright or biphasic in III, aVL, V1, V2; small notching may be present (Figure 3-6).

PR INTERVAL

The PR interval (Figure 3-7) is the amount of time between an atrial contraction (P) and ventricular depolarization (systole). It is measured from the beginning of the P wave to the Q wave. Measure the longest PR interval seen.

Normal PR Interval: 0.12–0.20 seconds duration. PR intervals > 0.20 seconds are considered abnormal, and indicate some level of blockade at the atrioventricular node. These elongated PR intervals are called first degree heart block. They occur because an abnormal condition is slowing down, or blocking the SA node impulse from reaching a ventricular response in due time. This can also be an iatrogenic affect of the drugs given during a procedure, or as part of the patient's normal medication regime. Calcium channel blockers, beta blockers, and opiates may induce slower conduction to the AV node.

The PR segment represents atrial repolarization. On the ECG it is the amount of elevation or depression (Figure 3-8) compared to the TP segment (end of T wave to beginning of P wave).

Morphology: The normal PR segment is usually isoelectric. It may be displaced in a direction opposite to the P wave.

Figure 3-6. P-wave morphology.

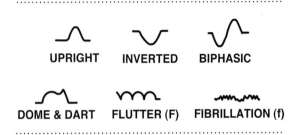

Figure 3-7. The PR Interval.

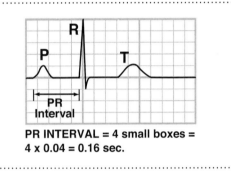

PR INTERVAL = 4 small boxes = 4 x 0.04 = 0.16 sec.

Figure 3-8. The PR segment.

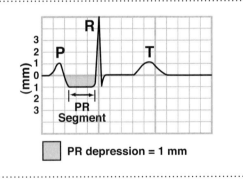

PR depression = 1 mm

Amplitude (mm): The elevation is usually <0.5 mm; depression usually <0.8 mm.

PR segments can be elevated or depressed in some pathological conditions. PR depressions are associated with pericarditis. PR elevations are rare but are associated with atrial infarction.

Q WAVE

The QRS complex (Figure 3-9) represents ventricular depolarization. A Q wave is present when the first deflection of the QRS is negative. If the QRS consists exclusively of a negative deflection, that defection is considered a Q wave but the complex is referred to as a QS complex.

Duration: Measured from beginning to end of Q wave (when it returns to baseline).

Normal Q waves: Small Q waves (duration <0.03 seconds) are common in most leads except aVR, V1, and V2.

Abnormal Q waves: Duration "0.04 seconds in leads III, aVL, aVF, and duration "0.03 seconds for all other leads. An abnormal Q wave is also defined as an initial downward deflection if it is >1/3 of the R-wave height. Abnormal Q waves indicate a blockade of normal electrical conductivity through or around damaged myocardium. Observed in specific ECG lead groups, they indicate areas of damaged heart muscle.

R WAVE

The Q is always a negative deflection before the R wave (Figure 3-10), and the R wave is always the positive peak of the QRS complex, with the S wave being the concurrent negative deflection following the R wave. Depending on where the greatest area of depolarization occurs, the R or the S may be exhibit the greater deflection in the complex.

Figure 3-10. R-wave progression.

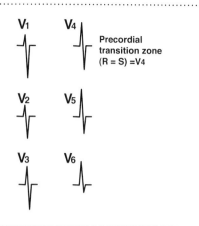

QRS COMPLEX

The QRS complex displays the period of ventricular electrical depolarization. It is important to remember that mechanical events (systole) follow electrical impulses to that area of myocardium. Duration of electrical cardiac events should not be confused with the duration of mechanical events, such as left ventricular ejection time.

Duration: The total QRS time interval (Figure 3-11) is normally 0.06–0.11 seconds. Intervals longer than this indicate an interventricular conduction delay (IVCD). This delay can caused by several etiologies, some of which are lethal. The most worrisome IVCD is associated with

Figure 3-9. The Q wave.

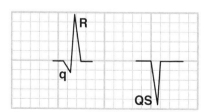

Q-wave duration = 1 small box
= 0.04 seconds

Figure 3-11. QRS duration.

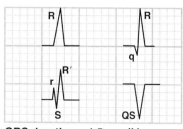

QRS duration = 1.5 small boxes =
0.06 seconds

hyperkalemia; electrolyte abnormalities can give rise to lethal arrhythmias very quickly. A second cause of IVCDs is bundle branch blocks, either left or right. IVCDs can also be due to paced rhythms, ventricular rhythms, as an iatrogenic affect associated with cardiac medicines (Procainamide) or prior cardiac surgeries. For the purposes of establishing a differential diagnosis, it is often useful to distinguish moderate prolongation of the QRS (0.10–0.12 seconds) from marked prolongation of the QRS (>0.12 seconds)

QT INTERVAL

The QT interval (Figure 3-12) measures the amount of time between the beginning of ventricular depolarization (Q wave) to the endpoint of ventricular repolarization, demonstrated by the T wave. Elongated QT segments can give rise to lethal arrhythmias such as VF and torsade de pointes (Figure 3-13).

Duration: The normal QT segment is usually from 0.25–0.40 seconds when measured from the beginning of depolarization to the beginning of repolarization. The QT interval can be varied, and it is dependant upon the patient's heart rate, gender, and age. Adjusting for these factors give the QT corrected.

ST SEGMENT

The ST segment comprises the interval of time between the end of ventricular depolarization and the beginning of repolarization at the T wave. It begins at the junction point (J point) of the S wave and the beginning of the ST segment (Figure 3-14).

Duration: Normal ST segments are from 0.10–0.16 seconds, depending on the heart rate.

Morphology: A normal ST segment is usually isoelectric, but it may vary from 0.5 mm below to 1 mm above baseline in limb leads. In the precordial leads, up to 3 mm concave upward elevation may be seen (early repolarization). The amount

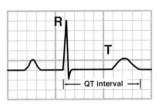

Figure 3-12. QT interval.

QT interval = 8 small boxes =
8 x 0.04 sec. = 0.32 sec.

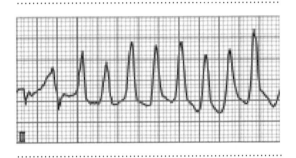

Figure 3-13. Polymorphic ventricular tachycardia (Torsade de Pontes).

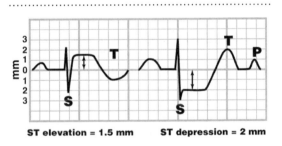

Figure 3-14. ST segment.

ST elevation = 1.5 mm   ST depression = 2 mm

of elevation or depression, in mm, relative to the TP segment (end of T wave to beginning of P wave) is measured, and its shape is evaluated (Figure 3-15).

While mild ST segment depression or elevation may be seen in normal ECGs, it may also

Figure 3-15. ST segment morphology.

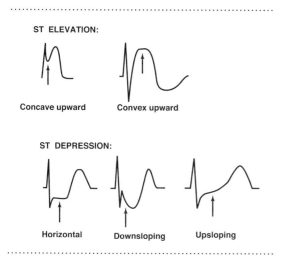

Figure 3-16. T-wave morphology.

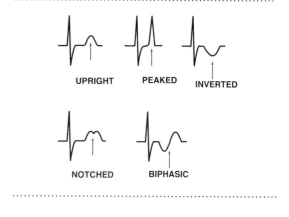

Figure 3-17. T-wave amplitude.

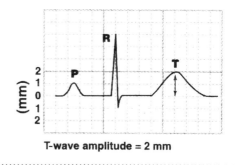

T-wave amplitude = 2 mm

indicate subendocardial ischemia, injury, or pericarditis. A thorough history and physical is essential for clinical correlation and differential diagnosis of nonspecific ST segment changes.

T WAVE

The T wave is generated by the final phase of ventricular myocyte chemical exchange, or repolarization. Here, the now positively-charged cell has dissipated its energy and is reinfused and repolarized, ready for the next cycle. T waves generally have an asymmetrical deflection, with the upward slope less acute than the downward slope. The T wave may appear more sharply pointed in patients with hyperkalemia.

Morphology: The normal T wave is upright in I, II, V3-V6, inverted in aVR, and may be upright, flat, or biphasic in III, aVL, and aVF (Figure 3-16). T-wave inversion may be present in V1-V3 in healthy pre-adult juveniles.

Amplitude (mm): T-wave amplitude is measured from the baseline to the peak or valley of the T wave (Figure 3-17). It is usually <6 mm in limb leads and <10 mm in precordial leads.

NORMAL AND ABNORMAL CARDIAC RHYTHMS

The normal ECG will demonstrate normal deflections and electrical event durations with a rate of 60–100 bpm originating from the SA node. The diseased or abnormal heart is capable of presenting many different rhythm and functional disturbances that can be assessed by looking at the EGG.

One common rhythm disturbance is premature beats or impulses. These impulses may originate from the atria (premature atrial contraction or PAC) (Figure 3-18) or the AV node junction (premature junctional contraction). Premature impulses also may originate from ventricular foci below the AV node. These rhythms include premature ventricular contractions (PVC), VT, and VF. Careful analysis of premature beats to assess their origin is important to determine whether they present a danger to the health of the patient. PVCs that show unique QRS complexes originate from different areas of the ventricle or are multifocal in nature.

A PAC has a P wave and normal QRS, but the P wave appears different from the P waves present in the NSR. PACs are rarely of concern, but they do indicate a certain amount of increased excitability in the atria due to various intrinsic or pharmacological effects, such as caffeine intake.

Sometimes young and active persons experience sudden but relatively short runs of very fast atrial rhythms called paroxysmal atrial tachycardia (PAT). PAT is generally considered benign, but it may cause chest pain or breathlessness.

Another relatively common type of atrial dysrhythmia is atrial fibrillation (AF) (Figure 3-19). AF may result from atrial enlargement secondary to a regurgitant AV valve (tearing normal conduction pathways), or chronic hypervolemia. Stress, adrenergic stimulants, alcoholism, or a malfunctioning SA node may also cause AF.

AF is caused by a multitude of impulses being sent from various locations in the atria. Because the AV node only accepts one impulse at a time to safeguard ventricular response, the impulses are conducted to the ventricles with an erratic, irregular cardiac rate on the ECG. AF is easily identified by its regularly irregular heart rate, normal QRS, and an absence of discernable P waves. A major risk of AF is the pooling of blood within the atria due to the lack of effective atrial contraction. Without appropriate antithrombin agents, a large clot can form and be ejected into the ventricles, creating a risk of pulmonary emboli, acute outflow tract occlusion, and stroke. Patients with AF generally feel increased fatigue and dyspnea on exertion.

PVCs, may be essentially benign or clinically significant in nature. Like PACs, PVCs arise from

Figure 3-18. Premature junctional contractions.

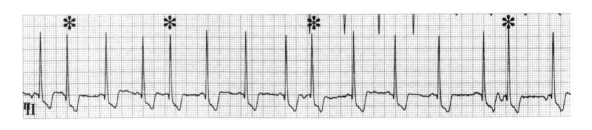

Figure 3-19. Atrial fibrillation.

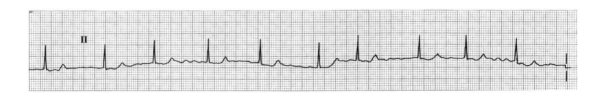

over-excited foci of the ventricular myocardium outside normal conduction pathways. Often this is caused by the lack of adequate blood flow to the myocardium secondary to coronary artery disease. PVCs exhibit wide and bizarre deflections on the ECG (Figure 3-20). No P wave is present, and the QRS will be large and of excessive time duration. Patients experiencing frequent episodes of PVC or "skipping" of the heart should be evaluated by a physician to determine any clinical significance.

PVCs that occur frequently with unique morphology are called multifocal, because the beats arise from many different areas within the ventricular myocardium (Figure 3-21). Multi-focal PVCs often indicate a deterious condition within

Figure 3-20. PVC.

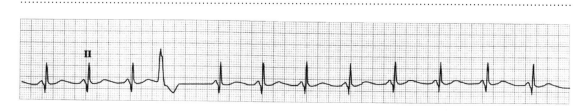

Figure 3-21. Multifocal PVCs.

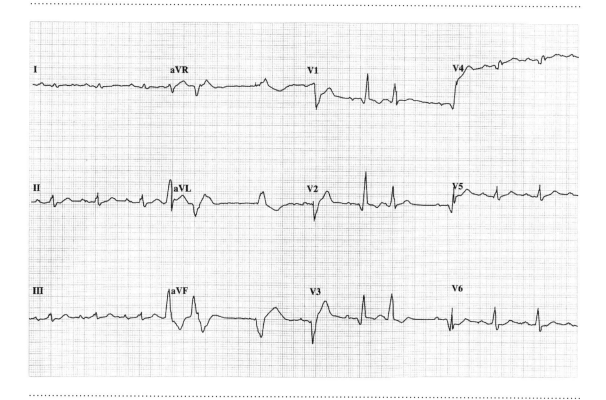

the ventricular myocardium, particularly if they occur as couplets or triplets or fall on the T wave of the preceding depolarization.

PVCs occurring in a run of three or more at a rate greater than 100 bpm is VT (Figure 3-22). Because of the lack of filling time for the ventricles at this high rate, blood flow to vital organs is compromised. VT can be dangerous and even cause death if untreated because of lack of effective stroke volume and cardiac output.

In a setting of acute myocardial infarction (AMI) or coronary syndrome, VT may further deteriorate into the lethal rhythm VF (Figure 3-23). VF produces no coordinated blood flow forward to vital organs, and death will invariably occur if not quickly terminated by electrical cardiac defibrillation. In rare cases, VF can be in-

duced in the catheterization lab when selectively introducing contrast dye into the right coronary sinus or conus branch by temporarily denying normal perfusion to vital conduction nodes.

HEART BLOCKS

Heart blocks occur with interruption of the normal conduction pathways from the SA node all the way down the main branches (fasciles) to the Purkinje network. These blocks may result from changes in chemical exchange, action potential or physical injury to the conduction lines themselves. Some medications may cause or prevent heart block and should be adjusted accordingly. Heart blocks may cause any level of mechanical failure, from diastolic dysfunction to asystole, de-

Figure 3-22. Ventricular tachycardia.

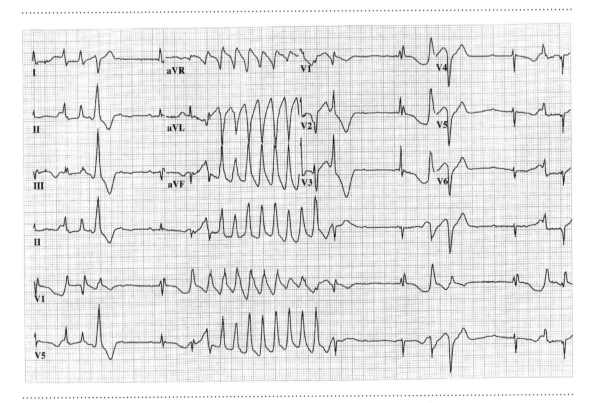

Figure 3-23. Ventricular fibrillation.

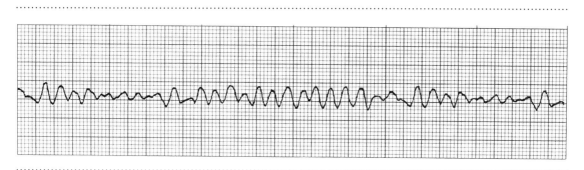

pending on origin and severity. Most common blocks occur at the AV node (Table 3-1).

Another type of heart block is bundle branch block, or fascicular block. These are sometimes idiopathic, but many times fascicular blocks are associated with left ventricular hypertrophy and MI. Bundle branch block occurs where the main conduction branches bifurcate. One or both branches are damaged and will not conduct properly. Instead, the impulse will continue down the healthy branch with the remaining myocardium being activated passively by other pathways. This slows overall contraction time for the myocardium. The delay causes inhibition of pumping action and lowers effective cardiac output. Due to this longer conduction duration, bundle branch block can be diagnosed by

a widened QRS, usually 0.12–0.30 seconds. The wider the complex becomes, the more likely unstable ventricular rhythms may occur as an escape mechanism. Also important is the fact that MI and ischemia may not be detected in the presence of left bundle branch block (LBBB). LBBB may be a contraindication in some diagnostic laboratories for certain testing for coronary ischemia.

A last type of block involves a sick sinus node arrhythmia. This can be found in elderly people who may complain of increased breathlessness and fatigue. The SA node simply loses its ability to create normal impulses and may conduct irregularly combined with other atrial impulses. This and certain ventricular arrhythmias are generally treated with a permanent pacemaker or electrophysiology study.

Table 3-1. Common Heart Blocks

Type	Description
First degree AV	PR interval is increased to >0.20 seconds. The rate is regular.
Second degree AV Mobitz I	Wenkebach. PR becomes longer and longer until one is dropped, leaving an unconducted beat. Less dangerous than Mobitz II.
Second degree AV Mobitz II	PR elongated and regular until one unconducted beat is seen. It represents a true blockade, and the risk of complete heart block and lethal rhythms increases.
Third degree AV	Complete heart block. No supraventricular impulses conduct past the AV node, leading to independent atrial and ventricular rhythms. Also known as AV disassociation. Look for regular P waves mixed with slower rate of QRS.

MYOCARDIAL INFARCTION

The ECG provides gross assessment of both acute and old MI or injury to the heart muscle. MI describes ongoing or completed death to vital myocardium. By observing ST waves, Q waves, or both and changes from baseline in certain groupings of leads, a 12-lead ECG can indicate both the area and extent of injury that has occurred (Figure 3-24). It is important to note that MI can occur without dramatic presentation by ECG, as happens in subendocardial infarctions and some lateral infarctions. All suspected MI by clinical presentation should be investigated by a lab measurement of cardiac enzymes, such as troponin levels.

ABNORMAL ST SEGMENT AND T WAVE DEVIATIONS

As previously described, the ST segment represents the period between depolarization and repolarization. A decrease in effective coronary blood flow to the myocardium, or ischemia, can have a significant effect on the appearance of the ST segment on the ECG. It is vital to assess changes in the ST segment in patients at risk for ischemic events, such as in the cardiac catheterization laboratory.

When myocardial blood flow is impaired, regardless of the cause, the ability for the heart to repolarize is affected. When viewing the ST on a normal ECG, the ST runs along the isoelectric line, or is baseline in comparison with the other deflections. The T wave also has a curve upward with a positive deflection and returns to baseline fully repolarized.

In the heart with myocardial ischemia, the T wave can become flattened or inverted with a negative deflection. This is called T-wave inversion. Another sign is the downward shift of the ST segments, called ST depression (Figure 3-25). The more depressed the ST deflection, the more ischemia there is; the more leads involved, the larger the area concerned.

Myocardial ischemia that involves the entire depth of the ventricle wall is represented by an upward shift of the ST segment, called ST elevation (Figure 3-26). This is called transmural ischemia, or MI if it lasts longer than a few minutes. The ST rises because the blood flow has been virtually cut off, and the portion of the myocardium affected cannot repolarize effectively enough to return to baseline. This ST elevation indicates that permanent damage or injury is occurring to the heart, and immediate treatment is necessary. It is at this stage that many patients present themselves to the emergency department with ongoing chest pain (angina), shortness of breath (dyspnea), profuse sweating (diaphoresis), and sometimes nausea and vomiting. These same symptoms may suddenly appear in any patient

Figure 3-24. Myocardial infarction.

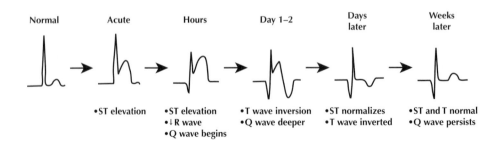

Normal	Acute	Hours	Day 1–2	Days later	Weeks later
	• ST elevation	• ST elevation • ↓ R wave • Q wave begins	• T wave inversion • Q wave deeper	• ST normalizes • T wave inverted	• ST and T normal • Q wave persists

Figure 3-25. ST depression.

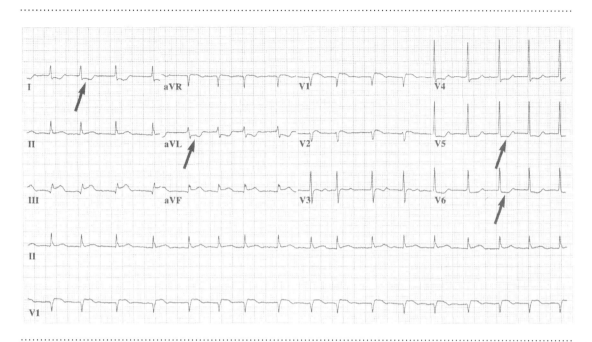

being prepared for a cardiac catheterization, and should be assessed and reported to the attending physician immediately.

As with ST depression, the higher the ST segment is above baseline, the more significant or acute the injury to the myocardium, and the more leads involved, the greater the area concerned. The usual frontline treatment or intervention for MI is the use of thrombolytics (see Chapter 26) or percutaneous transluminal coronary angioplasty (PTCA) in the catheterization laboratory. If performed quickly enough, usually one or both of these approaches is successful and will reopen closed blood vessels to reperfuse the affected heart area.

Ischemia and infarction also cause changes in the T wave, with the T waves becoming flattened or inverted as a negative deflection. T-wave inversion indicates a serious inhibition in the chemical exchange of repolarization, "flipping" the T wave on the ECG. Again, as ischemia deteriorates to

myocardial death, the rising ST will "pull" the T wave up above baseline. In acute infarctions, this melding of the R, S, and T waves above baseline is sometimes referred to as "tombstones," an ominous but accurate description of acute myocardial injury requiring immediate intervention by thrombolytics, emergent catheterization involving PTCA, or other available modalities described elsewhere in this text.

A subendocardial infarction may be virtually undetectable by ECG, and usually will be termed as a non-Q wave infarction. This type is usually detected by an increase in the cardiac enzymes troponin and creatine kinase MB. T wave changes appear in reciprocal leads to the area affected.

Dangerous rhythms can present themselves with no warning during any stage of infarction or intervention, and require immediate treatment from the cardiac catheterization team. New classes of drugs, such as amiodarone, have enabled physicians to keep tighter rein on lethal

Figure 3-26. ST elevation. ST elevation is seen in leads II, III aVF, and V1; ST depression is seen in leads V2–V6. This patient presented with an acute inferoposterior MI.

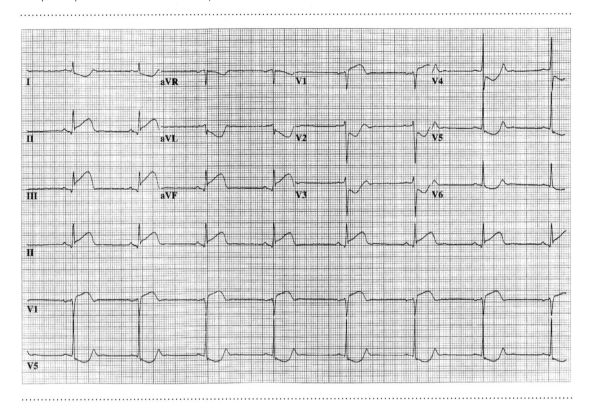

arrhythmias while working to re-establish coronary flow. Different rhythms may appear with dependent on areas ischemia and what parts of the conduction system are denied normal perfusion. Heart blocks and idioventricular rhythms are also seen.

Q WAVE INFARCT

When permanent myocardial death occurs, it can be detected in most cases by a dominant and wide Q wave on the ECG (Figure 3-27). When an impulse passes through or around infarcted myocardium, it causes the impulse to seek alternate pathways to complete its circuit around the dead tissue in order to depolarize. This "delay," in turn, creates a significant Q wave that is >1/3

of the height of the concurrent R wave, or at least 0.04 seconds in duration.

LOCALIZING AN INFARCT

Lack of oxygen or prior infarctions of the left ventricle can be accurately localized by the ECG. The left ventricle is divided into five primary areas of interest for function and blood flow. By scanning across the complete 12-lead ECG, the overall map can be assessed to make a diagnosis, taking into consideration all the components of the cardiac cycle comparison with the areas of the heart represented by the various leads (Table 3-2). ST elevations in leads II, III, aVF indicate the presence of inferior wall MI; V1 and V2 indicate a septal MI; V3 and V4 an anterior MI; and V5 and V6 a

Figure 3-27. Significant Q waves indicated on strip.

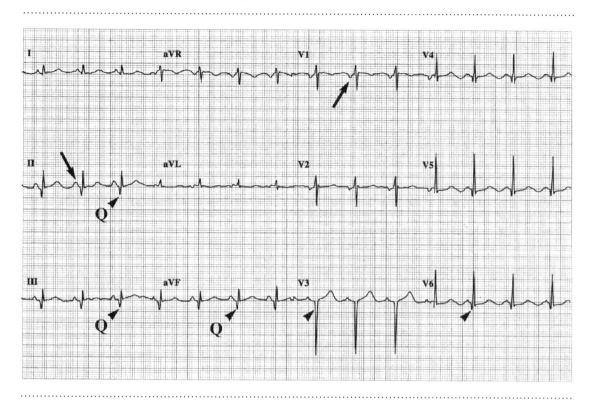

Table 3-2. Five Areas of Left Ventrical

Area	Associated Leads for Observation
Anterior	I, aVL, V2–V5
Septal	V1, V2
Lateral	aVL, I, V5, V6
Inferior	II, III, aVF
Inferolateral	II, III, aVF, V6

lateral MI. ST depression in leads V1 and V2 may indicate the possibility of a posterior wall MI. By scanning across the complete 12-lead ECG, the overall map can be assessed to make a diagnosis, keeping in mind that a normal ECG will usually display waves as described in Table 3-3.

PHARMACOLOGIC EFFECTS ON THE ECG

Many cardiospecific and noncardiac drugs can affect or disturb normal cardiac conduction cycles. Specifically, ventricular anti-arrhythmic agents may prolong the QRS duration >0.12 seconds (Vaughn Williams class 1A). These classes of drugs affect the action potential by blocking Na+ channels and slowing ventricular depolarization. Vaughn Williams class 3 agents can prolong the QT interval and block K+ channels, slowing repolarization. In certain situations these agents may cause torsade de pointes (polymorphic VT) and even VF.

Particularly useful and common are the cardiospecific beta-1 blocking agents, which inhibit the cardiac sympathetic response (Vaughn Williams class 2). Vaughn Williams class 4 agents prolong

Table 3-3. Normal R and S Wave as Represented in Each Lead

Lead	Normal R, S Representations
I	Dominant R wave
II	Dominant R wave
III	Moderate R wave or balanced R and S waves
aVR	Abnormal S wave
aVF	Moderate R wave or balanced R and S waves in old age
aVL	Dominant R wave
V1–V6	Small R waves progressing to dominant R waves

the PR interval by inhibiting Ca+ channel flow. Some anti-arrhythmic drugs may become arrhythmogenic in therapeutic doses, specifically digitalis (Digoxin, Lanoxin). Care must be taken with patients taking digitalis because it has a very narrow therapeutic window of affect.

Many times drugs will have an indirect affect on the heart. Diuretics can cause electrolyte abnormalities, especially hypokalemia. Opiates can induce excessive stimulus of the vagus nerve, causing bradycardia.

EMERGENCY TREATMENT FOR ARRHYTHMIAS

Many arrhythmias can be readily treated if recognized early. The treatment chosen will be based upon the hemodynamic and clinical status of the subject, as well as the particular rhythm presented.

VF will always result in detrimental decrease of blood pressure. VF appears as an erratic reading with no pattern (see Figure 3-23). VF must be converted with defibrillation quickly or death will result with or without CPR. Pulseless VT also needs to be immediately defibrillated.

Ventricular asystole is noted by the presence of P waves, but no corresponding QRS complexes. Immediate treatment, particularly for complete heart block (third degree) may require transthoracic (external) or transvenous pacing. The patient's ventricles needs to stimulation immediately.

A second form of asystole occurs when the patient has no conduction and displays no wave forms on the ECG monitor. This condition must be confirmed by switching the lead selector to another lead to confirm that the patient is not in fine VF and should be immediately be defibrillated. CPR and emergency medicines may be administered as according to physician direction.

Pulseless electrical activity presents with a normal or acceptable ECG but without detectable active blood flow by palpation or Doppler. The loss of pulses can have several causes. The primary cause is the loss of fluid or blood in the body. This can occur with trauma, retroperitoneal bleeding, extreme vomiting, or diarrhea. A second reason for a loss of blood pressure is pump failure. This can occur as a result of AMI, ventricular rupture, or flaccidity of the left ventricle associated with hyperkalemia. Increased intrathoracic pressure can also cause a loss of blood pressure. Tension pneumothorax can readily decrease venous return and thereby reduce cardiac output significantly. Another reason for loss of blood pressure is the presence of pericardial tamponade. This condition can be recognized by the presence of Beck's Triad: narrowed pulse pressure, distended neck veins and muffled heart tones. An ECG finding associated with pericardial tamponade is called electrical alternans (Figure 3-28). Electrical alternans is noted when the size of the QRS complex varies from beat to beat. It is generally seen in the percordial leads V3 and V4.

A decrease in blood pressure may occur with tachyarrhythmias. Symptomatic bradycardia can occur due to increased vagus nerve stimulus, which can be treated with atropine. The dose of atropine will vary between physicians, but generally and initial bolus of 0.5 mg or 1 mg is given and then repeated until an adequate rhythm is re-

Figure 3-28. Electrical alternans.

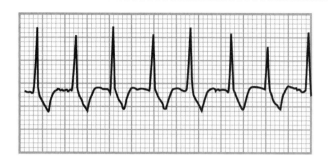 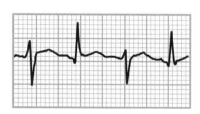

stored. If an adequate rhythm cannot be restored with the use of atropine, it might be necessary to pace the patient, either transthoracicly or transvenously. The use of atropine in the presence of high grade heat blocks (second degree type 2 and third degree) is contraindicated, and the clinician must proceed immediately with pacing.

Tachyarrhythmias are a complex and a problematic cause of decreased blood pressure. Emergently, a tachycardia that is symptomatic may be treated with a synchronized cardioversion. This is a technique whereby the defibrillator is used in conjunction with a monitoring ECG machine to avoid defibrillating on the R wave (which could lead to VF). Medical treatment for tachyarrhythmias is varied and should be left to the discretion of the attending physician.

ELECTROLYTE ABNORMALITIES

Many electrolyte abnormalities are benign, although some can cause sudden death. Hyperkalemia and hypomagnamesia specifically are associated with lethal arrhythmias. A reduction in the magnesium level will cause a prolongation of the QT interval and may lead to polymorphic VT (torsade de pointes). Provision of magnesium by the technician or nurse will reduce the chance of lethal arrhythmias.

Hyperkalemia usually has its root cause in acidosis. This acidosis can be either metabolic or respiratory in nature, and the condition must be treated at its underlying cause. The immediate treatment for hyperkalemia may include the use of $Ca+$, $NaHCO3$, insulin, and IV dextrose 50%. The widening of the QRS complex can be an ominous sign and should be treated immediately.

QUICK GUIDE TO ECG INTERPRETATION

Each ECG should be read in a thorough and systematic fashion. It is important to be organized, compulsive, and strict in your application of the ECG criteria. Analyze the following 13 features on every ECG:

Once these features have been identified, ask the following questions:

1. Is an arrhythmia or conduction disturbance present?
2. Is chamber enlargement or hypertrophy present?
3. Is ischemia, injury, or infarction present?
4. Is a clinical disorder present?

Be sure to consider each ECG in the context of the clinical history. For example, diffuse ST segment elevation in a young asymptomatic patient without a previous cardiac history is likely to represent early repolarization abnormality, whereas the same finding in a patient with chest pain and a friction rub is likely to represent acute pericarditis.

1. HEART RATE

The following method can be used to determine heart rate. (Assumes a standard paper speed of 25 mm/sec.)

Regular Rhythm

- Count the number of large boxes between P waves (atrial rate), R waves (ventricular rate), or pacer spikes (pacemaker rate)
- Beats per minute = 300 ÷ # large boxes

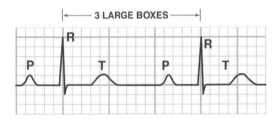

Heart Rate = 300 √ no. large boxes between "R" Waves = 300 √ 3 = 100 bpm

Note: It is easier to memorize the heart rates associated with each of the large boxes, rather than count the number of large boxes (1, 2, 3, etc.) and divide into 300:

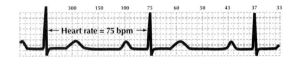

Note: If the number of large boxes is not a whole number, either estimate the rate (this is routine practice) or divide 1500 by the number of small boxes between P waves (atrial rate), R waves (ventricular rate), or pacer spikes (pacemaker rate):

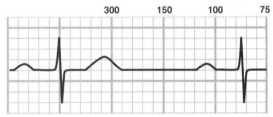

ESTIMATED Heart Rate = halfway between 100 and 75 = ~87 bpm (or 1500 √ 17.5 small boxes)

Note: For tachycardias, it is helpful to memorize the rates between 150 and 300 BPM:

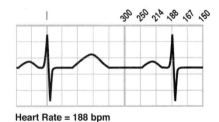

Heart Rate = 188 bpm

Slow or Irregular Rhythm

- Identify the 3-second markers at top or bottom of ECG tracing
- Count the number of QRS complexes (or P waves or pacer spikes) that appear in 6

seconds (i.e., two consecutive 3-second markers)
* Multiply by 10 to obtain rate in BPM

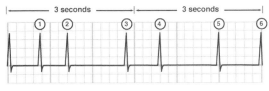

ESTIMATED Heart Rate = number of QRS complexes in 6 seconds x 10 = 6 x 10 = 60 bpm

2. P WAVE

What It Represents

Electrical forces generated from atrial activation. The first and second halves of the P wave roughly correspond to right and left atrial activation, respectively.

What to Measure

* Duration (seconds): Measured from beginning to end of P wave.
* Amplitude (mm): Measured from baseline to top (or bottom) of P wave. Positive and negative deflections are determined separately. One small box = 1 mm on ECGs where 10 mm = 1 mV (standard)

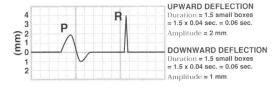

* Morphology:

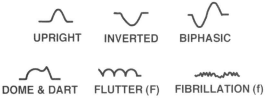

UPRIGHT   INVERTED   BIPHASIC

DOME & DART   FLUTTER (F)   FIBRILLATION (f)

Normal P Wave Characteristics

Duration/Axis: 0.08–0.11 seconds/0–75°
Morphology: Upright in I, II, aVF; upright or biphasic in III, aVL, V1, V2; small notching may be present
Amplitude: Limb leads: <2.5 mm; V1: positive deflection (<1.5 mm and negative deflection <1 mm)

3. ORIGIN OF THE RHYTHM

Determining the origin of and identifying the rhythm is one of the most difficult and complex aspects of ECG interpretation (and one of the most common mistakes made by computer ECG interpretation programs). To determine the rhythm, several key features must be discerned and integrated: heart rate, RR regularity, P wave morphology, PR interval, QRS width, and the P:QRS relationship. No single algorithm is able to simply describe all the various permutations; however the following rhythm-recognition tables, based initially on the P:QRS relationship and heart rate, provide a useful frame of reference:

P:QRS Relationships
P:QRS <1: JPCs or VPCs; junctional or ventricular rhythms (escape, accelerated, tachycardia) **P:QRS = 1** • **P precedes QRS:** Sinus rhythm; ectopic atrial rhythm; multifocal atrial tachycardia; wandering atrial pacemaker; SVT (sinus node reentry tachycardia, automatic atrial tachycardia); sinoatrial exit block, 2°; conducted APCs with any of the above • **P follows QRS:** SVT (AV nodal reentry tachycardia, orthodromic SVT); junctional/ventricular rhythm with 1:1 retrograde atrial activation **No P Waves:** Atrial fibrillation; atrial flutter; sinus arrest with junctional or ventricular escape rhythm; SVT (AV nodal reentry tachycardia, AV reentry tachycardia), junctional tachycardia or VT with P wave buried in QRS; VF

RATE <100 BPM: Differential Diagnosis

Narrow QRS (<0.12 sec)—Regular R-R

- **Sinus P‡; rate 60–100:** Sinus rhythm
- **Sinus P; rate <60:** Sinus bradycardia
- **Nonsinus P; PR 0.12:** Ectopic atrial rhythm
- **Nonsinus P, PR ≥0.12:** Junctional or low atrial rhythm
- **Sawtooth flutter waves:** Atrial flutter usually with 4:1 AV block
- **No P; rate <60:** Junctional rhythm
- **No P; rate 60–100:** Accelerated junctional rhythm

Narrow QRS—Irregular R-R

- **Sinus P, P-P varying >0.16 sec:** Sinus arrhythmia
- **Sinus and nonsinus P:** Wandering atrial pacemaker
- **Any regular rhythm** with 2°/3° AV block or premature beats
- **Fine or coarse baseline oscillations:** AFIB with slow ventricular response
- **Sawtooth flutter waves:** Atrial flutter usually with variable AV block
- **P:QRS ratio >1:** 2° or 3° AV block or blocked APCs
- **P:QRS ratio <1:** Junctional or ventricular premature beats or escape rhythm

Wide QRS (≥0.12 sec)

- **Sinus or nonsinus P:** Any supraventricular rhythm with a preexisting IVCD (e.g., bundle branch block) or aberrancy
- **No P†; rate <60:** Idioventricular rhythm
- **No P†; rate 60–100:** Accelerated idioventricular rhythm

* Sinus P wave: Upright in I, II, aVF; inverted in AVR
† AV dissociation may be present.

RATE >100 BPM: Differential Diagnosis

Narrow QRS (<0.12 sec)—Regular R-R

- **Sinus P*:** Sinus tachycardia
- **Flutter waves:** Atrial flutter
- **No P:** AV nodal reentrant tachycardia (AVNRT), junctional tachycardia
- **Short R-P (R-P <50% of R-R interval):** AVNRT, orthodromic SVT (AVRT), atrial tachycardia with 1° AV block, junctional tachycardia with 1:1 retrograde atrial activation
- **Long R-P (R-P >50% of R-R interval):** Atrial tachycardia, sinus node reentrant tachycardia, atypical AVNRT, orthodromic SVT with prolonged V-A conduction

Narrow QRS—Irregular R-R

- **Nonsinus P; >3 morphologies:** Multifocal atrial tachycardia
- **Fine or coarse baseline oscillations:** Atrial fibrillation
- **Flutter waves:** Atrial flutter
- Any regular rhythm with 2°/3° AV block or premature beats

Wide QRS (≥0.12 sec)

- **Sinus or nonsinus P:** Any regular or irregular supraventricular rhythm with a preexisting IVCD or aberrancy
- **No P; rate 100–110:** Accelerated idioventricular rhythm
- **No P, rate 110–250:** VT, SVT with aberrancy
- **Irregular, polymorphic, alternating polarity:** Torsade de Pointes
- **Chaotic irregular oscillations; no discrete QRS:** Ventricular fibrillation

*Sinus P wave: Upright in I, II, aVF; inverted in AVR

4. PR INTERVAL AND SEGMENT

What It Represents

- PR interval: Conduction time from the onset of atrial depolarization to the onset of ventricular repolarization. It does not reflect conduction from the sinus node to the atrium.
- PR segment: Represents atrial repolarization.

How to Measure

- PR interval (seconds): From beginning of P wave to first deflection of QRS. Measure longest PR seen.

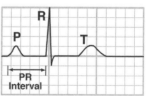

PR INTERVAL = 4 small boxes =
4 x 0.04 = 0.16 sec.

- PR segment (mm): Amount of elevation or depression compared to the TP segment (end of T wave to beginning of P wave).

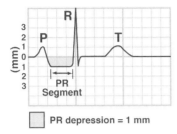

PR depression = 1 mm

Definitions

PR Interval

- Normal PR interval: 0.12–0.20 seconds
- Prolonged PR interval: >0.20 seconds
- Short PR interval: <0.12 seconds

PR Segment

- Normal PR segment: Usually isoelectric. May be displaced in a direction opposite to the P wave. Elevation usually <0.5 mm; depression usually <0.8 mm.
- PR segment elevation: Usually ≥0.5 mm
- PR segment depression: Usually ≥0.8 mm

5. QRS DURATION

What It Represents
Duration of ventricular activation

How to Measure
In seconds, from the beginning to the end of the QRS (or QS) complex

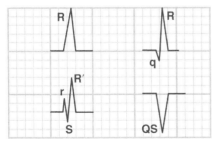

QRS duration = 1.5 small boxes = 0.06 sec.

Definitions

- Normal QRS duration: <0.10 seconds
- Increased QRS duration: ≥0.10 seconds.

Note: For the purposes of establishing a differential diagnosis, it is often useful to distinguish moderate prolongation of the QRS (0.10 to ≤0.12 seconds) from marked prolongation of the QRS (>0.12 seconds)

6. QT INTERVAL

What It Represents

Total duration of ventricular systole (depolarization [QRS] and repolarization [T wave])

How To Measure

- QT interval: In seconds, from the beginning of the QRS (or QS) complex to the end of the T wave. It is best use a lead with a large T wave and a distinct termination.

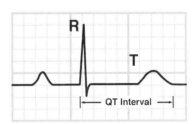

QT interval = 8 small boxes = 8 x 0.04 sec. = 0.32 sec.

- Corrected QT interval (QTc): Since the normal QT interval varies inversely with heart rate, the QTc, which corrects for heart rate, is usually determined
  - QTc = QT interval divided by the square root of the preceding RR interval. **Example:** For heart rate of 50 bpm, RR interval = 1.2 seconds, and QTc = $QT \div \sqrt{1.2} = QT \div 1.1$

○ Alternative method: Use 0.40 seconds as the normal QT interval for a heart rate of 70. For every 10 BPM change in heart rate above (or below) 70, subtract (or add) 0.02 seconds. The measured value should be within ± 0.035 seconds of the calculated normal. **Example:** For a HR of 100 BPM, the calculated normal QT interval = 0.40 seconds − (3 × 0.02 seconds) = 0.34 ± .035 seconds. For a HR of 50 BPM, the calculated normal QT interval = 0.40 seconds + (3 × 0.02 seconds) = 0.44 ± .035 seconds.

Definitions

- Normal QTc: 0.35–0.43 seconds for heart rates of 60–100 bpm. (The normal QT should be <50% of the RR interval)
- Prolonged QTc: ≥0.44 seconds
- Short QTc: <0.35 sec for heart rates of 60–100 bpm

7. QRS AXIS

What It Represents

The major vector of ventricular activation

How to Determine

- Determine if net QRS voltage (upward minus downward QRS deflection) is positive (>0) or negative (<0) in leads I, II, aVF:

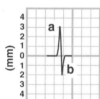

NET QRS VOLTAGE =
upward − downward deflection (mm)
= a − b = 3 − 2 = 1 (positive)

- Determine axis category according to the chart below:

Axis	Lead I	aVF	Lead II
−Normal axis (0° to 90°)	+	+	
−Normal variant −(0° to −30°)	+	−	+
−Left axis deviation −(−30° to −90°)	+	−	−
−Right axis deviation −(>90°)	−	+	
−Right superior axis −(−90° to +180°)	−	−	

\+ = positive (>0) net QRS voltage
− = negative (<0) net QRS voltage

8. QRS VOLTAGE

How to Measure

In millimeters, from baseline to peak of R wave (R wave voltage) or S wave (S wave voltage) (See preceding QRS axis)

Definitions

- Normal voltage: Amplitude of the QRS has a wide range of normal limits, depending on the lead, age of the individual, and other factors
- Low voltage (from peak of R wave to peak of S wave): Limb leads: <5 mm in all leads; precordial leads: <10 mm in all leads
- Increased voltage: See LVH, RVH

9. R-WAVE PROGRESSION

How to Identify

Determine the *precordial transition zone,* i.e., the lead with equal R and S wave voltage (R/S = 1)

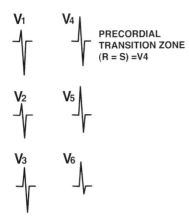

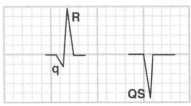

**Q wave duration = 1 small box
= 0.04 seconds**

Definitions

- Normal R wave progression: Transition zone = V2–V4; increasing R-wave amplitude across the precordial leads (exception: R wave in V5 often exceeds R wave in V6)
- Poor R wave progression: Transition zone = V5 or V6
- Reverse R wave progression: Decreasing R wave amplitude across the precordial leads

10. Q WAVES

How to Identify

A Q wave is present when the first deflection of the QRS is negative. If the QRS consists exclusively of a negative deflection, that defection is considered a Q wave, but the complex is referred to as a QS complex

What to Measure

Duration, in seconds, from beginning to end (i.e., when it returns to baseline) of Q wave. **Note:** When the QRS complex consists solely of a Q wave, a QS designation is used.

Definitions

- Normal Q waves: Small Q waves (duration <0.03 seconds) are common in most leads except aVR, V1 and V2.
- Abnormal Q waves: Duration ≥0.04 seconds in leads III, aVL, aVF, and V1; duration ≥0.03 seconds for all other leads

11. ST SEGMENT

What It Represents

The ST segment represents the interval between the end of ventricular depolarization (QRS) and the beginning of repolarization (T wave). It is identified as the segment between the end of the QRS and the beginning of the T wave.

What to Identify

- Amount of elevation or depression, in millimeters, relative to the TP segment (end of T wave to beginning of P wave)

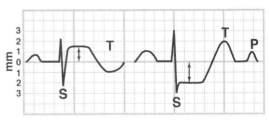

ST elevation = 1.5 mm   ST depression = 2 mm

- ST segment morphology

ST ELEVATION:

Concave Upward

Convex Upward

ST DEPRESSION:

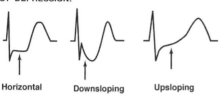

Horizontal   Downsloping   Upsloping

Definitions

- Normal ST segment: Usually isoelectric; may vary from 0.5 mm below to 1 mm above baseline in limb leads; in the precordial leads, up to 3 mm concave upward elevation may be seen (early repolarization). **Note:** While some ST segment depression and elevation can be seen in normals, it may also indicate myocardial infarction, injury, or some other pathological process. It is especially important to consider the clinical presentation and compare to previous ECGs (if available) when ST segment depression or elevation is identified.
- Nonspecific ST segment: Slight (<1 mm) ST segment depression or elevation.

12. T WAVE

What It Represents

The electrical forces generated from ventricular repolarization

What to Identify

- Amplitude: In millimeters, from baseline to peak or valley of T wave:

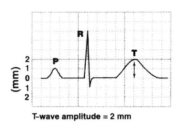

T-wave amplitude = 2 mm

- Morphology:

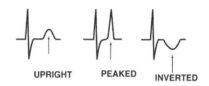

UPRIGHT   PEAKED   INVERTED

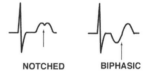

NOTCHED   BIPHASIC

Definitions

- Normal T waves:
  Morphology: Upright in I, II, V3–V6; inverted in aVR, V1; may be upright, flat or biphasic in III, aVL, aVF, V1, V2; T wave inversion may be present in V1–V3 in healthy young adults (juvenile T waves)
  Amplitude: Usually <6 mm in limb leads and ≤10 mm in precordial leads
- Tall T waves: Amplitude >6 mm in limb leads or >10 mm in precordial leads

- Nonspecific T waves: Flat or slightly inverted

13. U WAVE

What it Represents

Controversial: Afterpotentials of ventricular muscle vs. repolarization of Purkinje fibers.

How to Identify

When present, the U wave manifests as a small (usually positive) deflection following the T wave. At faster heart rates, it may be superimposed on the preceeding T wave.

What to Determine

- Morphology: upright, inverted, or absent
- Height, in millimeters, from baseline to peak or valley

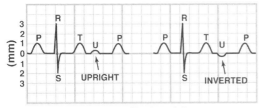

U wave amplitude = 0.3 mm

Definitions

- Normal U wave: Not always present; morphology: Upright in all leads except aVR; Amplitude: 5%–25% the height of the T wave (usually <1.5 mm); usually most prominent in V2, V3
- Prominent U wave: Amplitude >1.5 mm

14. PACEMAKERS

Overview

Pacemakers are described by a 4 letter code:

- First letter: Refers to the chamber(s) PACED (**A**trial, **V**entricular, or **D**ual)
- Second letter: Refers to the chamber SENSED (**A**, **V**, or **D**)
- Third letter: Refers to the pacemaker MODE (**I**nhibited, **T**riggered, **D**ual).
- Fourth letter: Refers to the presence (**R**) or absence (no letter) of RATE RESPONSIVENESS. Rate-responsive (or rate-adaptive) pacemakers can vary their rate in response to sensed motion or physiologic alterations (e.g., QT interval, temperature) produced by exercise by increasing their rate of pacing.

For example, a **VVIR** pacemaker PACES the **V**entricle, SENSES the **V**entricle, ventricular pacing **I**NHIBITS a sensed QRS complex, and is **R**ate responsive. A DDD pacemaker PACES and SENSES the atria and ventricle; the DUAL MODE indicates that sensed atrial activity will inhibit atrial output and trigger a ventricular output after a designated AV interval, and that sensed ventricular activity will inhibit ventricular output and trigger atrial output.

- Typical single chamber pacemakers include VVI and AAI
- Typical dual chamber pacemakers include DVI and DDD

APPROACH TO PACEMAKER EVALUATION

1. **Assess underlying rhythm** (100% paced vs. nonpaced intrinsic rhythm with pacemaker in demand mode)

- 100% ventricular paced

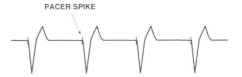

PACER SPIKE

- Ventricular pacing in *demand mode* (inconstant ventricular pacing from output inhibition by intrinsic sinus rhythm)

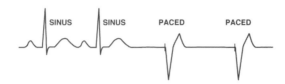

2. **Determine the chamber(s) PACED**
   Determine relationship of pacing spike to P wave and QRS complex: A spike preceding the P wave typically represents atrial pacing; a spike preceding the QRS complex typically represents ventricular pacing.

   - Atrial (A) paced beat

   - Ventricular (V) paced beat

   - Atrial (A) and ventricular (V) paced beat

3. **Determine timing intervals** from two consecutively paced beats:

   - For atrial pacing, determine the A-A interval

- For ventricular pacing, determine the V–V interval

- For dual chamber pacing, determine the A–V and V–A intervals

4. **Determine the chamber(s) SENSED**
   - **Atrial pacemaker:** Proper atrial sensing is present when intrinsic atrial activation (native P wave) is always followed by 1) a native P wave that occurs at an interval less than the A-A interval; or 2) an atrial-paced beat that occurs after an interval equal to the AA interval

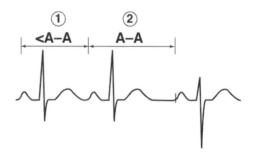

   - **Ventricular pacemaker:** Proper ventricular sensing is present when intrinsic ventricular activation (native QRS complex) is always followed by: 1) a native QRS complex that occurs at an interval less than the V–V interval; or 2) a ventricular-paced beat that occurs after an interval equal to the V–V interval

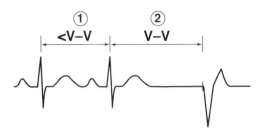

- **Dual chamber pacemaker:**
  - *Atrial sensing* is evident when intrinsic atrial activation (native P wave) is always followed by: 1) a native QRS complex that occurs at an interval less than the A–V interval; or 2) a ventricular-paced beat that occurs at an interval equal to the A–V interval

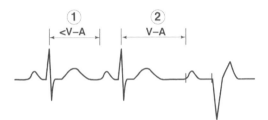

  - *Ventricular sensing* is evident when intrinsic ventricular activation (native QRS complex) is always followed by: 1) a native P wave that occurs at an interval less than the V–A interval; or 2) an atrial-paced beat that occurs at an interval equal to the V–A interval

|← V–V →|← V–V →|← V–V →|

5. **Determine the sequence of complexes** representing normal pacing function. (Keep in mind that single-chamber pacing on the surface ECG does not exclude the possibility that a dual-chamber pacemaker is present ventricular-paced beats may be due to a single-

chamber ventricular pacemaker or a dual-chamber pacemaker in which ventricular spikes are timed to follow P waves [DDD pacemaker])

Pacing Mode	Atrial pacing spike	Ventricular pacing spike
−Atrial pacing	+	−
−Ventricular pacing	−	+
−Dual-chamber (DDD) pacing	+	+
	+	−
	−	+
	−	−

+ Pacing spike present on surface ECG
− Pacing spike absent on surface ECG

6. **Look for pacemaker malfunction**
   A. **Failure to Capture**: Are any pacing spikes not followed by a depolarization?

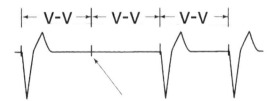

   B. **Sensing Abnormalities**
   - **Undersensing:** Based on timing intervals, are there pacing spikes that should have been inhibited by a native P wave or QRS complex but were not? This results in a paced beat that appears EARLIER than expected.
     - *Example:* For ventricular pacing, undersensing is evident when a native QRS complex is followed by a ventricular-paced beat at an interval <V–V interval.

|← V–V →|

PACEMAKER
FIRES EARLY

- **Oversensing:** Based on timing intervals, are there pacing spikes that should have been initiated after a native P wave or QRS complex but were not? This results in a paced beat that appears LATER than expected.
  - *Examples:*
    For ventricular pacing, oversensing occurs when a native QRS is followed by a ventricular-paced beat at an interval much greater than the V–V interval. Causes include:
    - Oversensing of the T wave, in which the T wave is sensed as (mistaken for) a QRS complex:

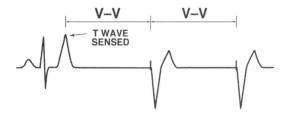

  - Or muscle contractions (myopotential inhibition; in which a myopotential is sensed as (mistaken for) a QRS complex:

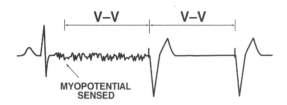

C. **Others:** Less common types of pacemaker malfunction include pacemaker not firing, pacemaker slowing, and pacemaker-mediated tachycardia.

SUMMARY

Every ECG represents a unique electrical map of a patient's heart. Using a disciplined and methodical approach, you can learn to interpret the most important elements quickly.

Look at each ECG and ask:

Is the rhythm regular or irregular? What is the relationship between the P and QRS waves?

How fast is the rate? Is this rate normal or abnormal given the clinical situation?

Is the PR interval of normal duration and does it vary in length? Is there a pattern?

What is the QRS time duration? Do all the QRS complexes look alike?

What is the patient's frontal electrical axis?

Is there hypertrophy indicated in the ECG?

What about the T waves and ST segments? Are they baseline?

Are the ST-T changes in particular lead groups? What segment of the myocardium is it?

Asking these basic questions with each and every ECG you encounter will ensure an adequate interpretation. Your expertise will increase with time and practice.

Having a good ECG interpretation booklet on hand in the catheterization laboratory is also a good idea, no matter how experienced you are. Collect interesting rhythm strips when you come across them, and always be prepared to share your knowledge and questions with your colleagues.

RECOMMENDED READING

Garcia TB, Holtz NE. *12 Lead ECG: The Art of Interpretation.* Sudbury, MA: Jones and Bartlett; 2000.

Gertsch M. *The ECG: A Two-Step Approach to Diagnosis.* Berlin: Springer; 2004.

Hampton JR. *The ECG Made Easy.* 5th ed. New York: Churchill Livingstone; 2003.

Marriot HJL. *Pearls and Pitfalls in Electrocardiology.* 2nd ed. Baltimore: Williams & Wilkins; 1998.

O'Keefe JH, Hammill SC, Freed MS, Pogwizd SM. *The Complete Guide to ECGs.* 3rd ed. Sudbury, MA: Jones and Bartlett; 2008.

Taylor GJ. *150 Practice ECGs: Interpretation and Board Review.* Malden, MA: Blackwell Science; 1997.

Chapter 4

RADIOGRAPHY

Murray Crichton, HDCR(R)

HISTORY

While working in his laboratory on the 8th of November 1895, Wilhelm Conrad Roentgen noted a strange phenomenon. He had been investigating the conduction of electricity through low pressure gas and discovered that invisible rays were being emitted from the positive electrode.

He also found that these rays blackened a photographic plate. Because the nature of these rays was unknown, he called them X-rays. Later that year, he took the first "diagnostic" X-ray of his wife's hand.

Rapid progress was aided by the fact that it was very fashionable among Victorian gentlemen to carry out electrical experiments. The use of evacuated gas tubes and the apparatus required had been common for several years and demand was easily satisfied. Thus Roentgen's experiments could be quickly reproduced and confirmed. In 1901, Roentgen was awarded the first Nobel Prize for physics. Like all German scientists at that time, Roentgen believed that discoveries belong to the world. Thus, his X-ray production was never patented.

Cardiac Catheterization

The history of cardiac catheterization dates back to around 1929, when a German, Dr. Forssman, inserted a urinary catheter into his arm and advanced it.[1] A chest X-ray was then taken, which demonstrated that the catheter was indeed positioned within the doctor's heart. In the 1930s, right heart catheterization quickly became an important diagnostic tool, although it was limited to hemodynamic studies and blood sampling. Two milestones in the 20th century were important in the advancement of X-ray technology. First, World War II brought with it the development of the cathode-ray tube (television) and image-intensifier (light amplification) tubes. Prior to this, images were viewed on a fluorescent screen that exposed the viewer to a high-radiation dose. Images were very poor quality, and examinations had to be performed in a darkened room, requiring operators to wear dark red glasses for 30 minutes beforehand to adequately adapt themselves to the darkness. The second milestone was the development of sophisticated computers that enabled large volumes of information to be processed very quickly. This also facilitated the development of digital image production and handling.

During the 1950s, X-ray equipment was improved with the development of the first image intensifiers and cineangiography. Over the next few years, radiographic equipment was improved further to allow imaging at frame rates of up to 100 per second and thus dynamic structures could be imaged. It was not until the 1960s, after Dr. Mason Sones had developed the brachial technique, that left heart cardiac catheterization became practical as a diagnostic tool. In 1967, Judkins developed catheters for use in the femoral technique, the most widely used technique today. Developments in computers for medical imaging, especially CT scanning, have allowed manufactures to continually increase image quality and resolution.

In 1977, digital subtraction angiography (DSA) was developed. This revolutionized vascular imaging and the quality of the image produced, although cardiac applications were limited. Thirty years later, equipment has become more advanced, especially with developments in image receptors and in the Patient Archive and Communications System (PACS).

PHYSICS AND OPERATION

X-rays are generated when electrons traveling at a very high velocity are abruptly stopped. The X-ray emission is controlled electrically, and thus the system is inactive when the power is switched off. An X-ray tube is a device in which electrons can be produced, accelerated, and stopped (Figure 4-1).

Production

Inside the X-ray tube is a coil of tungsten wire (the filament) that is part of the cathode assembly. Basically, it operates like a light bulb. As the filament is heated by increasing the current, electrons are liberated. The key factor to remember is the relationship between current (mA) and the amount (quantity) of X-rays produced, because this determines exposure factors.

Acceleration

Electrons are accelerated by introducing a high potential difference between the cathode and anode. The potential difference is measurable in kilovoltage (kV). It is the level of kV that dictates the quality of X-rays produced and defines the density of tissue that can be penetrated. Therefore, the kV level needs to be increased in order to penetrate a large volume of tissue.

Stopping

X-rays are formed from the energy released when the electrons are suddenly stopped as they collide with the anode. This energy is released as 99%

Figure 4-1. Components of an X-ray tube.

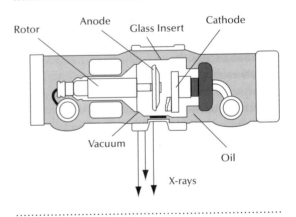

heat and only 1% X-rays. Although this process is not efficient, it is an effective way of generating a controlled quantity of radiation. The material used to form the anode will govern the characteristics of the radiation produced. Generally tungsten is used, but molybdenum can be used in tubes specifically designed for soft issue imaging.

TUBE DESIGN

An X-ray tube is basically a metal cylindrical case that protects the contents from damage and supports the necessary voltage and cooling supplies. The entire assembly is accommodated in an evacuated glass bulb. The X-ray tube must withstand extremes of heat and voltage, so the construction is very important.

Internal Components

Oil

The tube insert is surrounded by a thin, purified, insulating oil. This has two purposes: to act as an insulator between the cathode and anode supplies and to provide a medium for effective heat dissipation.

Tube Cooling

X-ray tubes generate a substantial amount of heat, and if the heat dissipation process is not efficient, damage, including crazing and pitting of the anode surface, will result. This will adversely affect the quality of the radiation produced and increase the size of the focal spot, resulting in poor image quality. Cooling is achieved by pumping the oil through a heat exchanger to improve dissipation. Most modern tubes cool the anode directly by pumping oil through the anode block. This is necessary for tubes with high work loads, like those used in CT scanning and in cardiology.

Rotor

Early tubes generated X-rays from a fixed anode, and only a small target area was used; these overheated very quickly. Overheating or overloading lead to electrical and mechanical breakdown that ruin the tube. Thus, X-ray production is limited by tube loading, which is a function of heat dissipation. Localized heating to a small area of anode will cause the anode to melt and become distorted. This is reduced by increasing the area of anode involved in X-ray production by rotating the anode. To achieve this, the anode disc is rotated at a very high speed. Therefore, instead of using a single focal spot, a tract on the circumference of the disc is used. It is this action that causes the noise prior to exposure in most units (one manufacturer employs a liquid bearing that rotates continually and silently).

Tube Focus

The tube focus is the area on the anode that is struck by electrons. The larger the area used, the more effective the heat dissipation. Unfortunately, image sharpness decreases correspondingly. A solution to this problem is altering the anode angle. This increases the effective focal spot size while decreasing the actual focal spot size. This is known as the line focus principle. However, this arrangement is achieved to the detriment of total field coverage. This is not a problem for cardiac work, but it limits the uses of the equipment.

Other Features

- The tube needs to be lined with lead to prevent X-ray leakage.
- The primary X-ray beam is filtered to remove low-energy radiation. This radiation would be noxious for the patient's skin (though would not penetrate the patient's body), and it would reduce the quality of the resulting picture.

- The size of the tube is relative to the load to be applied (i.e., dental work needs only a small tube, and in cardiology a larger tube is required).

Collimation

The actual imaging field size can be reduced to the specific area of interest by introducing lead leaves, or collimators, to limit the beam. The dose received is proportional to the area of tissue irradiated; thus, accurate collimation by the radiographer will reduce the total dose to both staff and patient as well as improve the image quality.

Diaphragms

Cardiac units have an arrangement of diaphragms (often crescent shaped) situated in the collimator box. The filter is used to mask the image and effectively equalize densities within the radiation field. This is essential when lung fields are included in the image. Lung fields may be overpenetrated by the X-ray beam, and image flaring may occur that is detrimental to the image. Correct positioning of the diaphragms will prevent this.

X-ray Control

The amount of X-rays being produced has to be known, reproducible, and consistent. The kV and mA factors need to be controlled, and the operator must be able to pulse the X-ray beam at high speeds. Modern units are controlled by a computer, and this allows efficient operation and fault finding.

The heart is a three-dimensional dynamic structure with the coronary arteries spreading over its surface. The arteries are small in caliber, 3–4 mm proximally, and the blood flow through them is rapid. These factors cause several technical problems for imaging: movement, magnification, and complexity.

Movement

The duration of X-ray exposure has to be very short to enable a clear, motion-free image to be formed. These are typically flashes of 5–8 msec duration. In Europe, images are acquired at 50, 25, or 12.5 frames per second, depending on the temporal resolution required. Equipment in the United States films at 60, 30, or 15 frames per second, with 30 being the most common.

Quality still images can then be reviewed at the operator's preference frame by frame or dynamically at variable speeds.

Magnification

By using an image intensifier, the image can be electrically magnified to allow accurate visualization of the arteries. Further magnification is possible digitally, but the results depend on the quality of the initial acquisition.

Complexity

Because of the complexity of the coronary arteries and the need to demonstrate pathology, it is necessary to image them from several different angles. This is achieved by mounting the X-ray tube and image intensifier on a movable gantry.

Image Production

The primary beam emerging from the X-ray tube has no image pattern and is said to be of homogenous intensity. When X-rays strike a material, they either pass through unchanged or are partially or wholly absorbed. This process is termed attenuation. The resultant X-ray beam is composed of differing, or heterozygous beam intensities, which are dependent on the degree of attenuation. It is this difference in the beam intensities that forms an X-ray image. It is useful to consider the formation of the X-ray image as a series of events.

Patient

X-rays are attenuated by the patient. This attenuation is relative to the density and size of the structures in the path of the X-rays.

Image Intensifier

The image intensifier converts the X-ray pattern into a luminescent image that is recorded by a camera. The size of the image intensifier required is dictated by the procedure. For cardiology, a 23-cm maximum field size is adequate, but a 40-cm field is required for general vascular work.

Camera

In cineradiography, an image is recorded onto film, the frames of which represent the pattern of X-ray attenuation. In digital radiography, these patterns are displayed as a series of pixels (tiny spots on a monitor screen that are individually either black or white). All together, the pixels make up the image that represents the object being filmed. The pixels are presented as a matrix on the screen, usually 512 × 512. This means that there are over half a million units of information on the screen at any one time. The image is then in a form that a computer can recognize, store, and manipulate.

Flat Digital Plate Detector

The next generation of image receptors is already widely available. These are composed of a scintillation layer of thallium-doped cesium iodide that coverts the X-ray image to green light. The light is then channeled to an amorphous silicon photodiode array. A digital image in the form of a 10,242 matrix and 14 bits is generated by this array. Acquisition speeds of up to 30 f/sec are achievable with a resolution of around 184 microns and detective quantum efficiency (DQE)

of 75%. The major advantage is the production of a digital image comparable to DICOM XA MF standards that can be viewed and processed using the same quality of data at any time. As with all scintillation, there is slight afterglow, and this is compensated by "refreshing" the plate between exposures.

Flat plate detectors are smaller than an image intensifier, allow easier movement of the gantry, and can achieve steeper angulations. They also take up a lot less room in the lab and are less obtrusive in an emergency situation.

Gantry

The gantry allows the X-ray tube and image intensifier to be mounted opposite each other. Thus they are always in alignment although the distance between them can be altered (Figure 4-2). The gantry can be ceiling or floor mounted and is designed to allow free movement of the table within the X-ray field while maintaining access to the patient. Gantry movement is controlled by motors that allow fast, accurate, and reproducible positioning of the X-ray apparatus over the patient. This is a definite improvement over the early systems in which the X-ray equipment was static, and the patient was strapped to the table and tilted as necessary. Obviously, this made many projections impossible to achieve. The size and movement of the system can be a source of anxiety to some patients. When necessary, time should be taken to explain the equipment and the need for its complexity.

Exposure Factors

Exposure factors are made up of three components: kV, mA, and time. Usually, mA and time are combined to form mAs. Exposure factors are selected dependent upon the characteristics required for the resultant image. This may necessitate high radiation intensity for a quality digital image or less radiation for a relatively low-quality

Figure 4-2. Monoplane gantry.

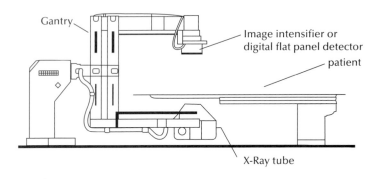

fluoroscopy image. The radiation dose should be kept as low as reasonably practical (ALARP) while still consistent with good image quality.

Kilovoltage

X-ray energy is measured in terms of kV. It is the potential difference applied across the X-ray tube, and it affects the quality (penetration) of the X-ray beam. The kV can be altered to accommodate the density of tissue the beam has to penetrate. Tissue density is dependent on the projection and patient size. Thus for larger patients and oblique projections, the kV is increased to allow adequate visualization, even though an increase in the kV applied also increases scatter radiation.

Milliampere Seconds

The mAs is a product of tube mA and the time that this is applied. To image a fast-moving structure, it is necessary to use as short an exposure time as possible. This effectively freezes the motion and allows a clear image to be generated. The mA controls the quantity of radiation that is generated, thus controlling the image intensity. To produce a short enough exposure time to image the coronary arteries, the mA needs to be increased. This controls the amount of radiation required to form the image.

Other Factors

Tube Focus

The tube focus is the area of anode that is used to produce X-rays. The smaller the focus selected, the better the image sharpness. However, there is a compromise with tube rating: the smaller the selected focus, the poorer the tube rating. If the rating is exceeded, overheating will occur, and the procedure will be held up while the tube cools.

Frame Rate

To further reduce the radiation dose, the X-ray beam is pulsed. Short bursts of radiation (typically 5–8msec duration in cardiology) are emitted instead of a continuous beam. These pulses are coordinated with the frames being filmed. Standard cine systems are set at 25 frames per sec. Digital acquisition can be set at anywhere from 1–50 frames per sec, reducing the radiation dose even further.

Field Size

The area and magnification of the image is controlled by the image intensifier field size selection. In general, the largest field consistent with the information required is selected (Table 4-1).

Table 4-1. Example Field Sizes

Imaging	Field Size
Vascular Fluoroscopy	40 cm (16 in)
Cardiac Fluoroscopy	23 cm (9 in)
Flat Detector	30 × 40 cm (12 × 16 in)
Coronary Arteriography	18 cm (7 in)
Increased Detail	13 cm (5 in)

The stated field size is the diameter of the circle forming the image. Selection of a smaller field size requires a relative increase in radiation to provide sufficient image density but a decrease in the absolute dose.

Automatic Exposure Settings

Modern equipment automatically controls the exposure factors to achieve a preset level. This is done by the electronic analysis of the beam, and the image and adjusting factors are set accordingly. Sensing of the image occurs in real time, so as the table is panned to follow contrast flow, the radiation characteristics will alter to accommodate this. The automatic exposure settings are calculated on the central part of the image. It is therefore important that target structures are in the center of the picture.

There is a large increase in image contrast when imaging the left ventricle, and the automatic exposure control will attempt to penetrate this by increasing the settings. Thus it is possible to "lock" the kV at a specific level to avoid over-penetration of the contrast bolus.

Image Storage

An X-ray image can be stored as a series of black, gray, and white dots (analog) or as a computerized matrix with a number assigned relative to the density (digital). Analog images can only be viewed, and are typically stored on cine film, videotape, or videodisc. Digital images can be reviewed and manipulated and are stored on digital tape, compact disc, or the hard drive of a computer.

Patient Identification

Correct image identification has always been an important issue in all forms of patient documentation, and it is essential to be able to correctly collate a patient to the images taken. This process has been done, and continues to be done, by imaging the patient's details onto a header on a cine film, or recording it digitally on each image. Hard-copy images are then stored with the patient's details and retrieved when necessary.

The medical field is now in the age of soft-copy image storage and image retrieval. This has many advantages, especially regarding remote multisite access to images—no more lost films! PACS is now widely available, allowing images to be reviewed on a workstation almost immediately after they have been captured. The review of cine images was previously limited to the rate at which they were projected. Digital systems allow images to easily be manipulated to the operator's own preferences, and several applications are available for review. Images can be viewed at varying speeds, contrast, magnification, and brightness. They can also be accurately calibrated and the results saved for review. Previous procedural reports can also be accessed by the same system.

Correct patient identification is essential to allow the correct file to be pulled from the archive. Care is essential to ensure that the correct numbering system is used. Manual data entry can be flawed by spelling and numerical errors, and the use of worklists is recommended. Digital images contain storage information within the image DICOM header, most of which is generated from a worklist server. The use of correct identification information is essential for the operation of PACS and the retrieval of images. Similar to putting the wrong film in the wrong tin, if the wrong worklist information is used, then it can be very difficult to retrieve the images. However, unlike tins, when two could have been mixed up and retrieval was by simply finding the other one, PACS archives can be hospital-wide, city-wide, or even nation-wide where staff could be looking at many millions of patient entries.

PROJECTIONS

To gain the maximum amount of information and decrease the procedure time, there is a need for standardization of projections. The sequence used may differ from center to center and between individual operators or procedures, but projections should be reproducible and allow uniformity. This will assist in the correct identification of anatomic structures. Nonroutine projections are adopted for specific circumstances such as angioplasty. Additional projections will vary with the operator, pathology, and congenital abnormalities. Modern equipment allows for projections to be preprogrammed, thus further decreasing examination time and increasing the level of standardization.

Naming Projections

Names of projections are taken from the anatomic position. In radiology, projections are named according to the direction of the central ray and the patient's position relative to the imaging device.

For an anterioposterior (AP) projection, the central ray travels through the patient from front to back. The reverse is true for a posterioanterior (PA) projection.

With angulation from the median sagittal plane, the patient's position is described relative to the recording device. Therefore, a right anterior oblique (RAO) is one in which the right anterior aspect of the patient is in contact with the image intensifier.

Angulation across the transverse plane is termed as cranial or caudal angulation. A cranial angulation is one in which the image intensifier is closer to the patient's head.

Naming projections is further complicated when anatomical landmarks or descriptions are used. For example, a "spider" is a left anterior oblique (LAO) angle with caudal tilt used to separate the left coronary bifurcation. The resultant image often resembles a spider.

RADIOGRAPHIC ANATOMY

What should be expected from an angiogram? Anatomically, the coronary arteries branch out from their ostia; therefore, the resultant image appears similar to the roots of a tree, shown in black. Normal anatomy is imaged as vessels with smooth uninterrupted lumen that taper gradually distally. Branches of similar size will demonstrate similar flow rates and patterns. Numerous charts and posters are available that depict the coronary circulation. Although there is agreement on naming the main arteries, this is not so with the smaller vessels, and differences can cause a problem. Each lab usually has a formula that its staff should follow.

Hints for Image Orientation

- In the RAO projection, the spine will always appear on the left side of the image.
- The opposite is true for the LAO.
- In all views, the circumflex artery will be closest to the spine.
- The shape of the right coronary changes from a "C" in the LAO projection to an "L" in the RAO.

RADIOGRAPHIC PATHOLOGY

The most common pathology of the coronary artery (CA) is plaque, a deposit on the vessel's wall that is rich in lipids, cells and, at times, calcium. When imaging the CA by contrast angiography, the negative image of this plaque is seen as a filling defect (Figure 4-3A). If the plaque is small, it is considered to be a wall irregularity. If it is larger, particularly if it is obstructing the lumen of the vessel, then it is referred to as a stenosis of varying degree, length, and shape. If the plaque is fully occluding the vessel, then it is an occlusion (Figure 4-3B).

Other pathologies are spasms, thrombi, and dissections. All of these can occur isolated or in combination, and sometimes it is not possible (even for experts) to tell them apart.

Figure 4-3. (A) Plaque deposit. (B) Total occlusion.

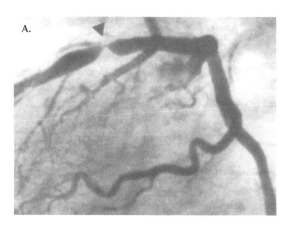

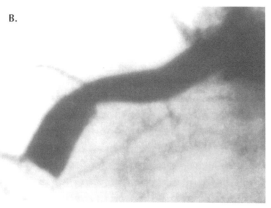

Radiography can only display the shape of the arteries' inner lumens; it cannot give details on the morphology of the vessel wall. However, it is possible to accurately differentiate a calcified lesion from one containing thrombus. This is done by visualizing the blood flow within the vessel and recognizing the structures that are not opaque; the structures themselves are not displayed. Intravascular ultrasound (IVUS) assessment of a coronary vessel (see Chapter 13) can show what is present in the vessel walls, but radiographic pictures, if assessed accurately, are usually considered to provide enough information to guide an intervention.

CORONARY MORPHOLOGY

The assessment of the level of stenosis can be made either by the operator or by a computer.

Subjective Assessment

The degree of lumen obstruction is given in percent diameter reduction according to the formula:

% Stenosis = (Minimum diameter within the stenosis/Diameter of the vessel after the stenosis) × 100.

With some experience, this degree can be assessed accurately within an acceptable degree of observer variability. Bear in mind, however, that a 50% stenosis (i.e., a 50% diameter reduction) will reduce the vessel cross-section by 75% and a 90% stenosis by 99%. The length of the stenosis, the presence or absence of collaterals, the size of the vessel, and prior myocardial infarctions will strongly alter the hemodynamic consequences of a stenosis. Also, a stenosis can become more severe by spasm or thrombotic appositions. Even a minor plaque can occlude a vessel if it ruptures and clogs the vessel by apposition thrombus formation.

A description of a stenosis not only includes its severity in percent, but also its location (in a curve, at a bifurcation, proximal, distal, in a small or large vessel), its shape (smooth, rough, concentric, eccentric, irregular, short, long, calcified, aneurysmatic), its length and the possibility of thrombus or dissection. If a stenosis is (sub)total, there might also be collateral circulation to the distal segments of the vessel. Collateral circulation is provided by branches that arise from a vessel proximal to the stenosis that lead blood to the distal segments of a stenosed artery. This is seen as filling of the peripheral vessel, either in a retrograde direction or through side branches.

Quantitative Assessment

Angiograms provide the clinician with pictures of the coronary arteries, the ventricles, and other structures. Generally these are analyzed visually (subjectively) by the cardiologist. Subjective analyses are usually fast and easy, but they are subject to observer variability and they are of not much value for research. For follow-up studies (such as those used to determine the degree of coronary stenosis and left ventricular function before and after treatment), objective measurements are a must. That is why as many parameters as possible are measured objectively.

The development of high-quality imaging chains and digital-image handling allow computerized analysis of images. The use of quantitative coronary assessment is becoming widespread because there is a need for accurate, objective assessment of data both before and after interventional procedures. To achieve this, several software programs have been developed that allow in-lab analysis for the required quantitative data.

Calibration

As with all analysis, it is necessary to calibrate the image prior to calculation. This can be done by using an object of known size, such as a calibration ball or grid, or by using the guiding catheter on the image. In most modern systems, it is possible to use the radiographic image of the catheter to calibrate for vascular images. The calibration ball is more accurate when large structures, such as the aorta, need to be measured.

Care must be taken to ensure that the object used for calibration is in the same plane, and filmed at the same magnitude, as the object to be measured. Calibration is achieved by defining the object on the computer screen and entering its known size. The computer will then calculate a calibration factor related to the number of pixels that the object fills. This factor is then applied to the structure to be measured, resulting in an actual size calculation.

Stenotic Index

The next stage is to select the vessel to be measured. The method for this differs between programs, but it is usually done by indicating two points, one proximal and one distal to the stenosis. The image is then digitally filtered, and the edges of the artery are detected. These may deviate from the actual course of the artery due to side branches or overlapping arteries in the image, so a correction is possible at this stage.

The contours of the artery are shown, and the point and degree of maximum stenosis are indicated (Figure 4-4). The software then will generate the reference diameter (size of the artery), obstructive diameter (size of stenosis), percentage diameter stenosis, and percentage area stenosis.

Coronary Flow Assessment

At rest, coronary flow is relatively stable and unaltered, even by stenoses up to 90%, and only a subtotal or total occlusion will impede it. A valuable and easy-to-use tool to semiquantitatively grade coronary flow is the thrombosis in myocardial infarction (TIMI)-score,[2] but it works only on (sub)total stenoses (Table 4-2).

Figure 4-4. QCA stenosis calculation.

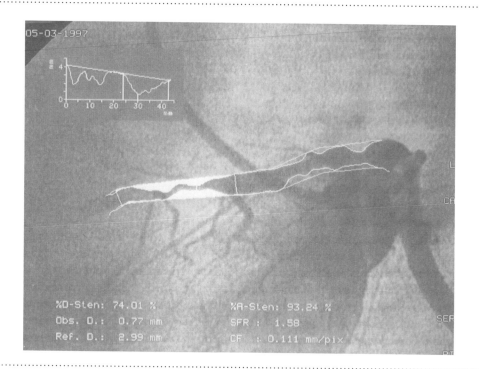

Left Ventricular Analysis

The left ventricle can be visualized by filling it with a large amount of contrast media using an electrically driven power injector. Its size, its global function, and its regional contractions can then be assessed visually or by computerized calculation derived from its angiographic contours.

Table 4-2. TIMI Scores Relative to Coronary Flow.

TIMI Score	Coronary Flow
0	No flow at all through the occlusion
1	Partial flow with incomplete distal filling
2	Delayed filling and washout
3	Normal flow and washout

GLOBAL FUNCTION

As with stenosis assessment, left ventricular function can be assessed either by the operator, or by computer.

Subjective

The ventricle is evaluated as enlarged, normal, or small with normal or abnormal global function. Because it is very easy to measure these parameters objectively, computer measurements of these parameters are common in everyday use.

Objective

Table 4-3 describes measurements commonly performed after every ventriculogram. The most important and most frequently used value is the ejection fraction (EF). It is a simple,

Table 4-3. Objective Ventricle Function Measurements

Measure	Description
End diastolic volume (EDV)*	Volume in mL at the end of diastole
End systolic volume (ESV)*	Volume in mL at the end of systole
Stroke volume (SV)*	Volume in mL ejected during contraction (SV = EDV−ESV)
Ejection fraction (EF)	The percentage of the EDV that is ejected during systole (EF = SV/EDV × 100%)

*Because larger patients have larger hearts, EDV, ESV, and SV are indexed by their body surface area, becoming EDVi, ESVi, SVi. Their units are mL/m².

reproducible, and easily available measurement that has clinical and prognostic value. Unlike the volume measurements, it is independent of the size of the patient. The ventricle is first traced in both systole and diastole, and the position of the aortic valve is indicated. The computer can then generate data based on the relative movement of the ventricular wall and show this graphically.

Accurate image selection is achieved using an ECG trace to identify the exact points of the cardiac cycle. The resulting graphic images (Figure 4-5) are used to calculate the relative volume of blood in the ventricle during diastole compared

Figure 4-5. Example of an automatic ejection fraction calculation with graphic representation.

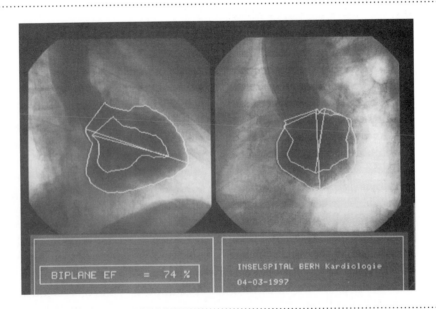

with that during systole. The EF is given as a percentage value.

The following is a rough overview of the implications of an abnormal EF:

<20%	Severe heart failure; very poor prognosis
20–40%	Severe reduction; heart failure, poor prognosis
40–50%	Moderate reduction; patient may have symptoms of heart failure
50–60%	Slight reduction; patient may be asymptomatic
60–80%	Normal
>80%	Hypercontractile; usually found with severe hypertrophy

REGIONAL FUNCTION

Subjective

At least as important as the overall function of the left ventricle is the regional function. The contours of the two ventriculographies (RAO and LAO) are divided into seven regions (depending on the laboratory) that correspond, more or less, to the territories of the different coronary arteries. Each region is then subjectively judged as being hyperkinetic, normal, hypokinetic, akinetic, or dyskinetic.

Objective

There are many geometric models to explain the complex motion of the left ventricle. The Slanger or Sheehan methods are used most commonly. With the aid of the computer, the end diastolic and end systolic frames are drawn. The computer then generates data based on the relative movement of the ventricular wall and shows this graphically. More complex models use several contours during a cardiac cycle and analyze not only the amplitude of a contraction but also its speed and acceleration.

DIGITAL IMAGE ENHANCEMENT

In the early 1980s, when digital image processing came to radiology and cardiology, researchers hoped to be able to enhance the new technology to enable them to perform coronary angiograms by IV contrast injection. During that period, it was recognized that while any kind of processing might increase image crispness or enhance some details, it would also introduce significant artifacts. Two techniques have made their way into everyday use, however: local contrast enhancement (or edge amplification) and subtraction angiography.

Local Contrast Enhancement

In classic angiography, if the filters are not used correctly, parts of the image may be too bright or too dark. The contrast between the background (heart, muscle, bones) and the contrast-filled vessel may be insufficient in these regions to produce a clear image, making assessment difficult. Local contrast enhancement darkens large areas of brightness, brightens large areas of darkness, and enhances differences of brightness in small areas. This results in a more or less uniformly gray image with sharp dark vessels. The artifacts introduced by this kind of treatment are thin, bright lines along any dark structure, which might mimic stenoses when vessels cross or bifurcate. The process of local contrast enhancement is usually built into modern angiography equipment and happens without any user interference.

Digital Subtraction Angiography

An image taken before (mask) contrast medium injection is subtracted from an image taken during contrast filling. On the resulting subtracted image, all background structures are gone; only the contrast-filled vessels stand out crisply against a uniform white or gray background. The technique was performed even before the advent of digital image processing using different analogous and filming techniques. Unfortunately, the process reduces the signal-to-noise ratio, which often makes vessel walls appear rugged, and it is often impossible to tell whether small wall irregularities are plaque or artifact.

Subtraction can be used only if the background does not move between acquisition of the mask and the image. Thus it works for peripheral angiography, aortography, and sometimes for proximal aortocoronary grafts. Subtraction angiograms of the coronary arteries are theoretically possible but only through the use of multiple masks. A mask that was acquired during the same interval of the cardiac cycle is subtracted from each image. The advantages of this technique do not outweigh its complexity and its artifacts, so it is not commonly used.

The method used to perform a DSA depends on the machinery and software available in the cardiac catheterization laboratory. Usually patients are told to hold their breath, then filming is started, and the contrast material is injected as in any angiography, although with a slightly longer pause before injection. When the sequence is terminated, the operator activates the DSA program. The computer directs the operator to choose a mask, which will be the last frame before the contrast material was injected. The whole process of subtraction of this mask from the subsequent images is then performed automatically by the system. The operator can move forward and backward in the subtracted video sequences and can also store or print them.

IV DSA has become standard for angiography of some noncardiac vessels, such as renal arteries or carotids, but so far it has not been possible to image the coronary arteries in this manner with adequate resolution.

RADIATION PROTECTION

Diagnostic radiography uses radiation to benefit the patient. The health risk from the radiation may be insignificant compared to the risks from not obtaining an accurate diagnosis; however, it is essential that an acceptable level of information is achieved by all radiologic procedures to justify the inherent risk. Noninvasive methods of imaging should be employed whenever possible (e.g., ultrasound or MRI).

Sources of Radiation

Patients will encounter both natural and man-made radiation over the course of their lifetime. The natural background radiation accounts for 85% of the average person's lifetime dose.[3] Of the 15% for which mankind is responsible, medical X-rays account for 90%, and nuclear medicine for 4%. The source of the remaining 6% of man-made radiation comes from nuclear fallout, television sets, portable telephones, and other devices.

Electromagnetic Radiation

Electromagnetic radiation is the term given to a group of energies that have similar properties. The spectrum of this type of radiation includes visible light and extends from low-energy radiowaves to high-energy X-rays (Figure 4-6).

Figure 4-6. Electromagnetic radiation spectrum.

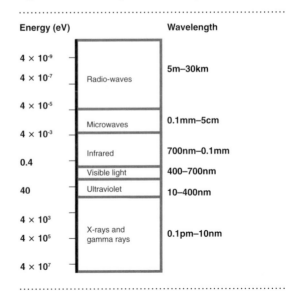

Inverse Square Law

The X-ray beam is divergent from its source, and the intensity of the beam will reduce as a function of the distance from the source due to the increase in beam area. Mathematically, this is described by saying the intensity of the X-ray beam is inversely proportional to the square of the distance between the object and the source of radiation. In practice, this means that if an object is moved from an original location to one twice as far from the source of radiation, it receives only a quarter of the radiation that it did in the original position. Moving it three times as far away results in one-ninth of the radiation, and so forth (Figure 4-7).

Dose Measurement

There are two units of dose measurement: absorbed dose and dose equivalent.

Absorbed Dose

The absorbed dose is the energy absorbed per each unit of mass. This figure is measured in units called grays (Gy), where 1 Gy = 1 J/Kg (SI unit)

In some countries, the most common unit of measurement is the rad, which stands for *radiation absorbed dose*. Conversion is easy: 1 Gy = 100 rad

Dose Equivalent

The absorbed dose does not take into consideration the properties of different types of radiation, and therefore a dose equivalent is used. This figure is derived from the absorbed dose multiplied by a quality factor. For X-rays and gamma rays, the quality factor is 1 (i.e., the absorbed dose and the dose equivalent are the same value for diagnostic radiography). However, when considering alpha particles, the quality factor is 20. The unit used for dose equivalent values is the Sievert (Sv), or, more commonly, the mSv.

Figure 4-7. The inverse square law.

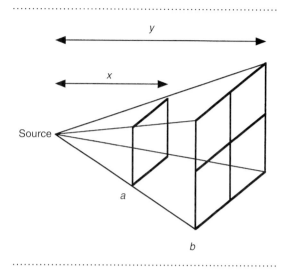

$$1 \text{ Sv} = 1 \text{ Gy} \times \text{Quality factor}$$

When a radiation film badge is developed, a calculated dose is produced. This figure is routinely reported in mSv.

Another unit commonly used to describe dose equivalence is the rem, or *radiation equivalent in man*. Conversion can be made with the formula: 1 Sv = 100 rem.

European legislation from the International Commission for Radiological Protection (ICRP), Ionizing Regulations (IR99), and Ionizing Radiation (medical exposure) Regulations 2000 sets limits for the amount of radiation staff can receive in a year.[4] An employer is expected to ensure that all employees who work in radiation areas are monitored and that records are kept of the doses received.

Staff Dose

Radiation travels in a straight line. However, following interaction with an object, its course and quality are altered (Figure 4-8). This lower quality, attenuated radiation is termed scatter or secondary

Figure 4-8. Effect of an object on primary X-ray beam.

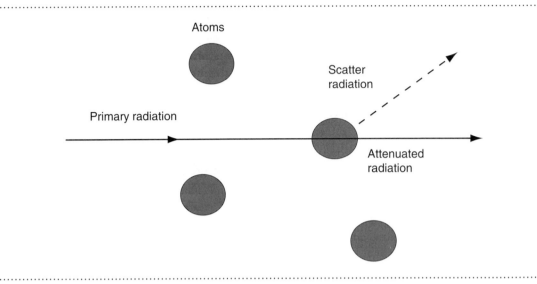

radiation. Primary radiation is the term given to the unattenuated beam (i.e, the beam from the X-ray tube before it interacts with any material). Varying densities of image are achieved through beam attenuation. Total attenuation of the beam occurs when no radiation passes, and scatter is produced as a result of incomplete attenuation. The amount of scatter produced is a product of the quantity and quality of the primary X-ray beam, the density of the tissue, and the time of exposure. Scatter radiation is emitted from the patient in all directions. Due mainly to the high kV used, most scatter will travel in the direction of the primary beam, toward the intensifier (Figure 4-9).

Figure 4-9. Emergence of scatter radiation.

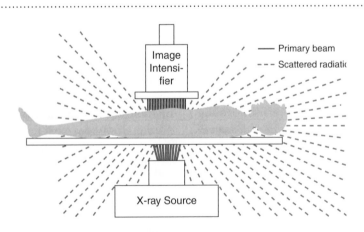

Staff Protection from Scatter Radiation

Conventionally, a nurse will stand to the left of the patient and the operator to the right. There is no need, however, for the nurse to maintain this position for the duration of the procedure. To minimize scatter, staff should choose times when fluoroscopy is not taking place to ask after the well-being of the patient or to administer medication. Scatter can also be minimized by correct usage of the equipment. In an AP projection, less scatter is produced and much of what is produced is blocked by the image intensifier, which is why it is important to have the image intensifier close to the patient. In the RAO position, the operator is shielded from the patient by the image intensifier, but the nurse is exposed to a high level of scatter. With a cranial angulation, the operator is exposed to a high degree of scatter. In an LAO position, the operator receives the highest exposure.

Fluoroscopy requires less radiation to form an image and will produce less scatter, and the mode of fluoroscopy and beam filtration can reduce levels even further. Digital acquisition, however, demands a higher radiation dose and consequently produces a higher degree of scatter formation. During the actual procedure, it is normally necessary for the operator to remain close to the patient while securing the catheter and injecting contrast, so it is not possible for him or her to stand back.

However, during imaging, the nurse should be aware of the radiation dose and move back from the patient. Other staff in the cath lab should also be aware of potential risks of radiation and carry out their duties from as safe a distance as appropriate for patient care. As a rule, only essential staff should be present in the lab during a procedure.

EFFECTS OF RADIATION

In the cath lab, radiation is used to visualize the inner lumen of vessels and other structures. This radiation can have adverse effects on the patient and cath lab staff, however. These adverse effects are minimal, however, and are outweighed by the benefits gained by the procedure.

Biologic Effects

X-rays ionize matter. This means that they remove an electron from the atomic structure of the material, which results in the breaking of atomic bonds. If all ions recombine exactly as they were, there is said to be no radiation damage. Broken bonds, however, can produce free radicals that are chemically reactive and capable of forming new bonds. It is this molecular disruption that can cause chemical changes that may produce biologic cell damage. The chances of these effects occurring can be estimated by examining the deterministic and stochastic effects.

Deterministic Effects

A deterministic effect will result in biologic damage occurring during the individual's lifetime. These effects are limited by a threshold below which the effects will not occur. It is this threshold that limits the radiation doses that both patients and staff can receive during radiologic investigations. A dose of approximately 10 Sv is required to produce deterministic effects including erythema, cataract formation, and gastrointestinal damage.

Stochastic Effects

The occurrence of stochastic effects are governed by the laws of probability rather than absolute values. With an increase in the radiation dose, the probability of a pathologic effect occurring increases. There is no safe dose, however. A reduction in radiation dose will reduce the chance of cellular damage, but the chance will always be greater than zero that something will occur. It should also be noted that the severity of disease is not related to the dose. The effects could be the inducement of cancer, genetic effects, or both.

Cancer

Cancer formation may not be apparent for up to 5–10 years. This is known as the latent period. Risk factors are used to estimate the likelihood of occurrence of a particular radiation-induced effect per unit dose equivalent received by each member of the population. Thus, risk factor = (cases/population) × dose.

Genetic Effects

Biologic damage will affect the body's chromosomes, resulting in an alteration in their code. This can lead to genetic defects that can be passed on to offspring. Thus, there is a special need to reduce the gonadal dose.

Risks

There is a low probability of cancer inducement with the levels of radiation used in diagnostic imaging. However, patients' fear and anxiety are understandable and should be relieved by freely given information. No studies have proven that even low levels of radiation do not cause cellular damage resulting in a cancer development.

It should be noted that the cell-mutation process is complex, and the possibility of a cancer developing as a direct result of radiation exposure is very low. Keep in mind, however, that there is no safe dose where X-rays are concerned. Any amount of radiation is potentially harmful. No statistically significant hereditary defects have been seen in human data.

Mortality

The risk of mortality resulting from a single chest X-ray is 1:1,000,000. A patient receives the equivalent of 100–250 normal chest X-rays during the course of a percutaneous transluminal coronary angioplasty (PTCA).[5] Data published for barium enemas and CT scans can be used as a benchmark by which to assess cardiac catheter-

ization, for which the risks quoted are 1:30,000. It should be noted that the probability of cancer occurring in the population as a whole is 1:4.5, and the risk from background radiation is 1:100. Dosimetry can identify areas and practices that result in a high exposure, and action can subsequently be taken.

Measurement of Dose

Radiation protection can only be effective when the staff and working area have been properly assessed. The first indication of any problem may be an increase in badge readings. Thus if the staff don't wear their badges, this process is hampered. Several devices are used to measure dose. The most common are film badges and thermoluminescent detectors (TLDs).

Film Badges

The film badge consists of two halves that contain various filters. The amount and type of radiation to which the badge is exposed is recorded on a photographic film. The film is sent to be analyzed.

Thermoluminescent Detectors

TLDs are a variation of the film badge. They contain crystals that effectively store the energy created as a result of a radiation exposure. This energy is released as light when the crystal is heated, allowing a dose to be calculated. Because of their size and radiolucency, TLDs can effectively be used for dose surveys.

Guidelines for the Use of Film Badges and TLDs

- Always wear the badge while at work.
- When wearing protective aprons, the badge should remain under the apron at all times.
- Change the badge promptly when a new badge is issued.

- When changing the badge, please check the holder to ensure that all the filters are intact.
- If an unusual dose is suspected, report the incident immediately.

Protective Clothing

Apart from limiting personal exposure to radiation, the most effective way to reduce the amount of radiation that the body receives is by always wearing the protective clothing provided by the institution.

Aprons

Protective aprons consist of lead rubber that basically acts as a shield to protect the wearer from secondary (scatter) radiation. There is a numerical value to each apron that indicates the lead equivalent (LE) value of that apron (i.e., 0.25 mm or 0.35 mm LE). It is recommended in the cardiac catheterization laboratory that the scrub nurse and doctor wear an apron with an LE of at least 0.35 mm.

Maximum protection is achieved when the apron is correctly worn and secured. Care should be taken when using and storing aprons, because any damage to the apron will reduce its effectiveness. Aprons should be stored on hangers when not in use, and any defect should be reported immediately. Lead aprons are only designed to shield the wearer from secondary radiation and offer little protection from primary (unattenuated) radiation. However, the use of increased lead levels will reduce the total dose.

Thyroid Collars

These provide protection for the thyroid gland and should be worn by everyone working in close proximity to the patient.

Shields and Glasses

Glass containing a high LE from mineral content provides the operator with a clear field of vision while maintaining adequate protection from secondary radiation. When protective devices such as shields and glasses are available, it is advisable to make use of them as much as possible.

Basic Protection

The most effective protection from radiation is to avoid it. Exposure is cumulative and increases throughout the lifespan. The surest method of protection is to remain outside the lab whenever possible. It is good practice to have only essential personnel in the lab during a procedure. It is also advisable to alternate staff who need to operate in close proximity to the patient, thus spreading the total dose among several individuals. Any barrier between the staff and the source of radiation will offer protection. This includes standing behind any machines or other people who may be in the cardiac catheterization laboratory.

It is important that the intended use and future development of a room are taken into consideration during the design process. Radiation protection should be a prime concern.

Pregnancy

The neonate is especially sensitive to the adverse effects of radiation exposure, and additional care must be taken wherever pregnancy is suspected.

Patients

All female patients of childbearing age should be questioned about the possibility of pregnancy. A negative answer should be documented, and the procedure should be allowed to continue. In the event of a positive response (or any uncertainty), the patient should be referred to the cardiologist in charge. Depending upon the clinical urgency, the cardiologist has the final decision regarding whether the procedure should continue or not. Ideally this issue should be addressed when patients are seen at the clinic or during preadmission to avoid problems in the cardiac catheterization laboratory later.

Staff

The current recommendation of the ICRP[4] is that fetal dose should not exceed 1 mSv. Few, if any, nurses fall into this category.[6] Pregnancy, or suspected pregnancy, should be reported to the radiation protection supervisor who will arrange a risk assessment to be carried out. This will entail assessment of the individual's previous radiation exposure and the likelihood of a limit being reached should they continue to work in the area. In general, staff in the catheterization laboratory receive some of the highest doses due to their heavy workloads, and they need to wear lead aprons for extended periods. Managers should be encouraged to provide alternate duties for pregnant staff members.

REFERENCES

1. Forssman W. Die Sondierung des rechten Herzens. *Berliner Klinische Wochenschrift* 1929; 8:2085–2087.
2. TIMI Study Group. The Thrombolysis in Myocardial Infarction (TIMI) trial, phase 1: findings. *N Engl J Med* 1985;321:932–936.
3. Dosimetry Working Party of the Institute of Physical Sciences in Medicine, National Radiological Protection Board (of Great Britain). National Protocol for Patient Dose Measurements in Diagnostic Radiology. 1992.
4. International Commission on Radiological Protection. Publication 60. London: ICRP; 1990.
5. Wilks R. *Principles of Radiological Physics*. London: Churchill Livingstone; 1981.
6. British Institute of Radiology. *Work in Diagnostic Imaging*. London: BIR; 1992.

SUGGESTED READING

Baim DS. Angiography: proper utilization of cineangiographic equipment and contrastagents. In: Baim DS, Grossman W, eds. *Cardiac Catheterization, Angiography, and Intervention*, 5th ed. Baltimore, MD: Williams & Wilkins; 2000.

Foster E. *Equipment for Diagnostic Radiography*. Boston: MTP; 1985.

Graham H, Whitehouse B. *Techniques in Diagnostic Imaging*, 2nd ed. London: Blackwell Scientific; 1990.

Moore RJ. *Imaging Principles of Cardiac Angiography*. Bethesda, MD: Aspen; 1990.

Pepine CJ, Allen HD, Bashore TM, et al. ACC/AHA guidelines for cardiac catheterization laboratories. *Circulation* 1991;84:2213–2247.

Wall B. Full protection. *Synergy* 1996;4:41–43.

Chapter 5

CONTRAST MEDIA

Charles C. Barbiere RN, CCRN, RCIS, CCT, CRT, EMT, FSICP

X-RAY ANGIOGRAPHY

Due to the different X-ray absorption rates between bodily structures, X-ray images show these structures as different shades of gray, referred to as grayscale. The more atoms a structure contains, and the heavier the atoms, the more X-rays the structure will absorb, and the whiter the structure will appear on X-ray. Bones, containing calcium in high density, are white in X-ray images, whereas lungs, containing air (a mixture of elements with low atomic numbers), appear dark.

Blood vessels, and the blood flowing within them, have similar X-ray absorption rates to the surrounding body tissues, so they cannot be seen in X-ray images. An exception to this are heavily calcified atherosclerotic vessels, which can often be visualized with sensitive X-ray equipment. To visualize blood vessels with X-ray, it is necessary to pass a liquid with a high X-ray absorption rate through them. This liquid, known as contrast medium or dye, displaces the blood in the vessels long enough for images to be made. These images show the path of blood flowing through the vessel, which provides the inner contours of the vessel walls.

CONTRAST MEDIA

All contrast media used in the cardiovascular catheterization laboratory (CCL) contain iodine, which is an effective absorber of X-rays. Iodine has a high atomic weight, and appears whiter than the surrounding tissues in an X-ray image. The iodine molecules are bound to a very stable Benzoic ring, which allows relatively large amounts of iodine to be injected into a person safely, at levels that would otherwise be toxic. The contrast medium's large molecular size ensures that very little is passed out through the walls of the vascular system and allows it to be very effectively filtered out of the blood by the kidneys and excreted by the renal system.

The ideal angiographic contrast medium permits visualization of blood vessels and is inert; it should pass through the body without producing any undesired side effect.

Definitions

All contrast media function in a similar way, but each one's unique molecular structure gives them slightly different physical characteristics. The contrast medium molecule's side chains generally determine the important physochemical parameters of hydrophilicity, osmolarity, and viscosity (Table 5-1).

Hydrophilicity

The hydrophilicity of a contrast medium is a crucial factor in determining how well patients will tolerate it, because the more hydrophilic the product is, the fewer side effects it will tend to produce. In all modern contrast agents, the side chains carry hydroxyl groups ($-OH$). The number and spatial distribution of these groups determines the hydrophilicity of the contrast medium molecule. These can increase the molecule's water solubility because they interact freely with the surrounding water molecules. The side chains can also be designed in such that the hydrophobic nucleus of the contrast medium is shielded against interactions with the surrounding biologic membranes, which are also hydrophobic.

The octanol-water repartition coefficient is a commonly used method of quantifying hydrophilicity. It is a two-phase system in which octanol (hydrophobic) is layered onto water (hydrophilic), and the amount of contrast medium present in each phase is measured. If a contrast medium has an octanol-water repartition coefficient of 1:3, it means that 25% of the contrast medium remains in the hydrophobic phase (octanol) while the remaining 75% of the product will be dissolved in the water phase (hydrophilic). Ideally, a contrast medium should have a very high hy-

drophilicity in order to stay in the blood in solution and reduce interaction with hydrophobic membranes and proteins.

Osmolarity

Osmotic processes in the body occur through semipermeable membranes. These membranes serve as filters, retaining dissolved particles even though water passes through them freely. An example of such membranes is the vessel wall, which is permeable to water but not to contrast media.

Osmosis describes the movement of water through semipermeable membranes, from an area that has lots of water to an area that has relatively little. Osmolarity is the quantitative expression of the capacity to attract water.

The osmolarity of blood, for example, corresponds to 300 mOsm/kg water. Contrast media can be divided into high osmolarity contrast media (HOCM), which have an osmolarity of 1500–2100 mOsm/kg water (first generation), and low osmolarity contrast media (LOCM), which have an osmolarity of 300–900 mOsm/kg water (second generation). HOCM are all ionic, while LOCM can be either ionic or nonionic.

The excretion rate of contrast media differs somewhat between classes, but approximately 70% of the dose is recovered in urine 6 hours after intravenous injection, and a nonionic medium with low osmolarity is excreted from the body within 24 hours of injection.

Viscosity

The viscosity (fluidity) of a contrast medium affects the ease with which the contrast agent can be injected through catheters, and its capacity to flow through blood vessels. Prewarmed contrast medium is less viscous than that which is stored at room temperature.

Viscosity is measured in millipascal.second (mPa. sec) or centipoise (cP) (1 cP = 1 mPa.sec).

Table 5-1. Contrast Agents used in the CCL

Class	Generic Name	Trade Name	Iodine (mg/ml)	Osmolarity (mOsm/kgH$_2$O)	Sodium Viscosity (37°F)	Content (mEq/L)	Additives
Ionic High Osmolar	Diatrizoate	Renografin-76	370	1940	8.4	190	Na Citrate disodium EDTA
		Hypaque-76	370	2076	8.32	160	Calcium disodium EDTA
		MD 76 R	370	2140	9.1	190	Na Citrate disodium EDTA
		Angiovist 370	370	2076	8.4	157	Calcium disodium EDTA
Low Osmolar	Ioxaglate	Hexabrix	320	600	7.5	157	Calcium disodium EDTA
Nonionic Low Osmolar	Isovue	Omnipaque	350	844	10.4	Trace	Tromethamine Calcium disodium EDTA
	Iopamidol	Isovue 370	370	796	9.4	Trace	Tromethamine Calcium disodium EDTA
	Ioversol	Opitray 320	320	702	5.8	Trace	Tromethamine Calcium, disodium EDTA
	Ioxilan	Oxilian 350	350	695	8.1	Trace	Citric acid edentate calcium disodium
Isosmolar	Iodixanol	Visipaque	320	290	11.8	Trace	Tromethamine, edentate calcium disodium, calcium chloride dehydrate, sodium chloride

It is proportional to iodine content and inversely proportional to the temperature. For nonionic monomers, viscosity at room temperature varies from 16.3 mPa.s for ioxilan 350 to 20.4 mPa.sec for iohexol 350 to 22.0 mPa.sec for iopromide 370. The viscosity of iso-osmolar, nonionic dimers such as iodixanol is greater than that of all other contrast media (26.6 mPa.sec at 320 mgL/mL and 20°C).[1]

Different Contrast Media

The various contrast media differ in the number of iodine molecules, ionic and osmolar composition, sodium content, and other additives that function as preservatives and stabilizers. There are major differences between the various contrast media, and these can have profound sequelae for the patient. These compositional differences also are responsible for the wide range in the cost of the different contrast media.

Iodine Concentration

Iodine content is measured in mg/ml, and the iodine concentration for coronary angiographic procedures range from 300 to 370 mg/ml. The iodine content influences the physicochemical properties of a contrast medium; the greater the iodine content, the more viscous and osmotically active it is. Contrast media with lower iodine concentrations can provide inadequate imaging in older X-rays units.

The iodine content can also determine the cost of a contrast medium, because iodine is very expensive; most of it is extracted from brackish water in Japan. There are relatively few sources for the raw material, so supply and demand dictates the price. HOCM are much less expensive than LOCM because chemical synthesis of the low osmolar compounds is more complicated, requiring extended and therefore expensive processing.

High Osmolarity Contrast Media

Also known as first-generation contrast media, ionic HOCM consist of a negatively charged benzene ring with three iodine atoms and methylglucamine (meglumine), sodium, or both as counterions. They typically have an osmolarity of 1400–2100 mOsm/kg water, given an iodine content of at least 300 mg/mL. HOCM provoke some discomfort in patients because their high osmolarity tends to make the vessel swell (water is attracted from the surrounding tissues), thereby inducing a feeling of heat and can induce pain. HOCM acutely expand intravascular volume and depress myocardial contractile force, leading to a small increase in left ventricular end-diastolic pressure.

Low Osmolarity Contrast Media

The second-generation contrast media have a lower osmolarity than the first generation and are divided into ionic and nonionic. It has been found that nonionic, low-osmolar, and iso-osmolar contrast media are safer to use in high-risk patients than high osmolar contrast media and still provide acceptable image quality.[2,3,4]

Nonionic LOCM

One way of reducing the number of osmotically active particles in a contrast medium is to substitute the ionic carboxyl group ($-COOH$) with a group that does not dissociate in solution, creating a nonionic LOCM. All these compounds consist of three iodine atoms attached to an uncharged benzene ring (Figure 5-1), so a single osmotically active particle is present for three iodine atoms. The resulting osmolarity (290–900 mOsm/kg water) offers greater comfort for the patient.

Ionic LOCM

Only one contrast medium belongs to this class, ioxaglate, which is an ionic dimer. The reduc-

Figure 5-1. Three iodine atoms attached to a benzene ring.

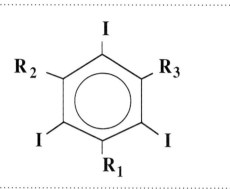

tion of osmolarity is achieved by connecting two benzene rings, creating one negatively-charged particle with six iodine atoms. The osmolarity of ioxaglate at a concentration of 320 mg/mL iodine is about 600 mOsm/kg water.

CONTRAST MEDIA USE

Prior to the start of the catheterization procedure, patients should be instructed on what to expect. They should also be queried again about any allergies they may have with a focus on previous reactions to contrast media and to iodine allergies, including allergies to seafood.

The contrast medium should be warmed to body temperature, and the solution should be examined for any discoloration or sediment. If discoloration or sediment are observed, the contrast should not be used. By warming the contrast to body temperature, patient hypothermia is reduced, and the viscosity of the contrast media is improved, which allows for easier injections.

With the injection of contrast media, patients may develop a flushed sensation; they may also develop nausea and vomiting. Due to the volume of contrast used when imaging the ventricles, aorta, or any other large structures, most patients will complain of feeling flushed or of having a burning sensation and often feel that they may have urinated.

The total volume of contrast medium should be recorded as part of the patient record, and a running total volume should be available at any time during the case. It is good practice that whenever staff hangs a new bottle of contrast medium, that the volume of contrast given up to that point be communicated to the primary operator.[5,6]

Contrast media is currently available in glass or plastic containers. Many labs choose plastic to minimize any possible breakage. It is also common to employ contrast savers in an effort to reduce cost per case and medical waste.

Complications

The administration of contrast media can produce a wide range of symptoms and complications. Due to the side effects and complications that may occur with the injection of contrast, the patient ECG should be continuously monitored. Atropine, antiarrhythmic, and vasopressor drugs should be available for prompt administration if necessary. The equipment for temporary pacing should be readily available (Table 5-2).

With the first contrast injection, it is important to reassess the patient for any signs of contrast reactions; any complaints of shortness of breath or urticaria deserve special attention.

Table 5-2. Contrast Medium Reactions

Mild	Moderate	Severe
flushing	headache	arrhythmias
pruritus	vomiting	hypotension
rhinorrhea	diffuse urticaria	bronchospasm
urticaria	facial edema	laryngeal edema
retching	mild bronchospasm	pulmonary edema seizures
diaphoresis	palpitations abdominal cramps persistent vomiting	death

When the contrast medium is injected into a coronary artery, transient bradycardia and/or hypotension may occur. This occurs more frequently, and more severely, with ionic contrast versus nonionic contrast media, and in patients who have flow-limiting lesions. In some patients, this may become profound. Patients should be instructed at the start of the case in cough CPR. Coughing does not increase coronary blood flow, but it does maintain arterial blood pressure, cerebral blood flow, and influences vagal tone.

Allergies

Patients with preexisting allergies to iodine need to be premedicated with an antihistamine, corticosteroids, H1 and H2 blockers, hydration, and so forth.

Anaphylactic and Anaphylactoid Reactions

To be considered a true anaphylactic reaction, there must be a true antibody-mediated (immunoglobin E) reaction. The majority of reactions are anaphylactoid or pseudoallergic reactions. The exact mechanisms of these reactions are not known, but probably include a combination of factors including direct cellular effects, direct enzyme induction, fibrinolytic, kinin, and others.

Symptoms usually develop within minutes of administration and range from mild to severe. Repeat reactions occur in 15%–40% of patients who have had a prior contrast medium reaction. Treatment guidelines are widely available;[7] it is standard practice to have drugs listed, and the guideline readily available in the laboratory.

HIGH-RISK PATIENTS

Patients with certain disease processes have been determined to be at high risk for adverse outcomes during diagnostic studies and invasive procedures in the cardiac catheterization laboratory. These patients are candidates for low or iso osmolar, nonionic contrast.[8–10] These high-risk factors are:

- Unstable coronary syndromes
- Congestive heart failure
- Diabetes (serum creatinine >1.5 mg/dL)
- Renal insufficiency (serum creatinine >2 mg/dL)
- Hypotension
- Hypovolemia
- Severe bradycardia
- Severe valvular heart disease
- History of previous contrast reaction
- History of any previous reaction to iodine
- Comorbid conditions

CHRONIC HEART FAILURE (CHF)

With the administration of hyperosmolar contrast medium, there is an initial increase in circulating volume due to the contrast volume, and then a decrease in circulating volume as the osmolarity of the contrast forces fluid into the cells. This may make patients with CHF worse and later may cause a diuresis, which may lower the patient's blood pressure. Due to this increased diuresis, all patients who receive contrast media should have their input and output monitored. Any decrease in urine output should be noted and the physician contacted. It is common practice to administer 500 cc to 1000 cc of normal saline intravenously over 4 to 6 hours postcatheterization in patients without contraindications to fluid loading.

When injecting the internal mammary artery or any other peripheral artery, nonionic contrast should be utilized; if not, the patient may experience severe pain.

DIABETES MELLITUS

With patients who are insulin dependent, the dose of insulin is generally cut in half on the morning of the procedure. Patients with diabetes who take metformin (Glucophage) may develop a profound lactic acidosis should contrast-induced nephropathy (CIN) develop. Because the occurrence is rare, metformin is relatively contraindicated in diabetic patients with significant renal insufficiency. The current recommendation is that metformin be discontinued the morning of the procedure and not restarted until the patient's creatinine level is shown to be stable.[11]

RENAL FAILURE

Because the majority of contrast medium is excreted by the kidneys, patients with compromised renal function must be treated with care. Patients on dialysis should be dialyzed soon after any angiographic study where contrast media is used. Biplane systems are beneficial with these patients. With thoughtful positioning of both the AP and LAT imaging chains, two views are obtained with a single injection of contrast medium (panning is often required). The left ventriculogram is not performed, because this can be very well visualized with echocardiography.

CONTRAST-INDUCED NEPHROPATHY

CIN is an acute decline in renal function after the administration of an iodinated contrast medium. It is an adverse event that may occur in up to 15% of all patients undergoing invasive cardiovascular procedures, and may occur in up to 50% of patients with preexisting renal insufficiency and/or diabetes undergoing invasive cardiovascular procedures.[12] The pathogenesis probably involves a combination of ischemic and direct tubulotoxic effects, but the impairment of renal function is normally mild and transient.

CIN is defined as an elevation of serum creatinine (Scr) of 20%–50% from baseline, 48–72 hours after the administration of contrast medium. The serum creatinine will begin to rise within the first 24 hours, peak within 96 hours and return to baseline within 7–10 days.[13,14] This type of renal failure is suspected after the administration of contrast media when no other cause can be determined from the patient's medical history.

Patients with preexisting renal insufficiency, diabetes mellitus, or cardiovascular disease receiving intra-arterial contrast material are at increased risk for CIN. The incidence of CIN correlates with the amount of contrast medium used during a case, so the amount of contrast medium should be minimized in at-risk patients.

Periprocedural hydration has been shown to be the most effective treatment for reducing the incidence of CIN in high-risk patients.[6] A postprocedure fluids regime involving diuretics and intravenous fluids should also be considered. Some centers hydrate at-risk patients with sodium bicarbonate, as a bolus of 3 ml/kg per hour for 1 hour before contrast medium administration, followed by an infusion of 1 ml/kg per hour for 6 hours after the procedure.

In cases of suspected contrast media nephrotoxicity, monitoring the patient's renal function and daily intake and output are vital. However, because contrast media nephrotoxicity is self-limiting, dialysis is rarely needed; renal function normally recovers after a few weeks.

Because CIN develops over several days, patients may have no symptoms when discharged. Patients should be instructed to contact their physician should they experience weight gain of 1 kg per day or excessive oedema. Oral hydration should be encouraged unless the patient has another condition (such as CHF) which contraindicates increased fluid intake.

CARDIAC COMPUTERIZED TOMOGRAPHY

Multislice CT scanners have multiple rows of detectors, enabling a large number of thin image slices (ranging from 2 to 64) to be obtained simultaneously. CT Angiography (CTA) is safer than coronary angiography because it is less invasive and does not have the risks associated with arterial catheterization.

Like coronary angiography, CTA requires the administration of iodinated contrast agents, although the amount of material required is 25% less. When scanning starts, 80–100 ml of contrast medium is injected through an IV line at a rate of 3–5 ml/s. This maintains homogeneous vascular contrast throughout the scan. The same precautions for contrast medium that are taken for coronary angiography apply to patients having CTA. Patients with histories of significant allergic reaction are best avoided or if the creatinine is <2.0 mg/dl.[15,16]

CARDIAC MAGNETIC RESONANCE ANGIOGRAPHY

Unlike conventional angiography, which requires injection of iodine-based contrast media through a catheter in a large artery, cardiac magnetic resonance angiography requires the injection of a noniodine contrast medium, gadolinium (gadopentetate chelates), into a vein. Gadolinium (chemical symbol Gd) is a naturally occurring substance that is slightly magnetic. It is a heavy metal that is encapsulated within a ligand, which makes gadolinium less toxic, and ensures that the contrast medium remains in the bloodstream.

Gadolinium acts as a contrast agent by affecting the time it takes for the hydrogen atoms to return to their original state. This increases the difference in the signal intensity from different types of tissue, increasing the degree of contrast in the image.

The volume of gadolinium required is much less than that used for typical coronary angiograms, and it is rapidly excreted by the kidneys.

Adverse reactions are headache, nausea, pain, and sensation of cold at the site of injection, taste perversion, dizziness, vasodilatation, and reduced threshold for seizures. Severe adverse reactions occur at significantly lower rates than with nonionic iodinated contrast media.[17,18]

REFERENCES

1. Eivindvik K, Sjogren CE. Physicochemical properties of iodixanol. *Acta Radiol* 1995;36(Suppl. 399):32–38.
2. Morcos SK, Thomsen HS. Adverse reactions to iodinated contrast media. *Fur Radiol* 2001;1(1):1267–1275.
3. Goss JE, Chambers CE, Heupler FA Jr, Members of the Laboratory Performance Standards Committee of the Society for Cardiac Angiography and Interventions. Systemic anaphylactoid reactions to iodinated contrast media during cardiac catheterization procedures: guidelines for prevention, diagnosis, and treatment. *Cathet Cardiovasc Diag* 1995;34:99–104.
4. Lasser EC, Lyon SG, Berry CC. Reports on contrast media reactions: analysis of data from reports to the U.S. Food and Drug Administration. *Radiology* 1997;203:605–610.
5. Steinberg EP, Moore RD, Powe NR, et al. Safety and cost effectiveness of high-osmolality as compared with low-osmolality contrast material in patients undergoing cardiac angiography. *N Engl J Med* 1992;326:425–430.
6. Matthai WH Jr, Groh WC, Waxman HL, Kurnik PB. Adverse effects of calcium binding contrast agents in diagnostic cardiac angiography. A comparison between formulations with and without calcium binding additives. *Invest Radiol* 1995;30:663–668.
7. S. Scanlon PJ, Faxon DP, Audet AM., et al. ACC/AHA guidelines for coronary angiography. *J Am Coll Cardiol* 1999;33:1756–1824.
8. Davidson CJ, Laskey WK, Hetmiller JB, et al. Randomized trial of contrast media utilization in

high-risk PTCA: the COURT trial. *Circulation* 2000;101:2172–2177.

9. American College of Cardiology/American Heart Association Ad Hoc Task Force on Cardiac Catheterization. ACC/AHA guidelines for cardiac catheterization and cardiac catheterization laboratories. *J Am Coll Cardiol* 1991;18: 1149–1182.

10. Hill JA, Grabowski EF. Relationship of anticoagulation and radiographic contrast agents to thrombosis during coronary angiography and angioplasty: are there real concerns? *Gather Cardiovase Diagn* 1992;25:200–208.

11. Heupler FA Jr. Guidelines for performing angiography in patients taking metformin. Members of the Laboratory Performance Standards Committee of the Society for Cardiac Angiography and Interventions. *Cathet Cardiovasc Diagn* 1998;43:121–123.

12. Tepel M, van der Giet M, Schwarzfeld C, et al. Prevention of radiographic-contrast-agent-induced reductions in renal function by acetylcysteine. *N Engl J Med* 2000;343(3):180–184.

13. Maeder M, Klein M, Fehr T, Rickli H. Contrast nephropathy: review focusing on prevention. *J Am Coll Cardiol* 2004;44:1763–1771.

14. Tadros GM, Malik JA, Manske CL. Iso-osmolar radio contrast iodixanol in patients with chronic kidney disease. *J Invas Cardiol* 2005;17:211–215.

15. Goldstein JA, Gallagher MJ, O'Neill WW, et al. A randomized controlled trial of multi-slice coronary computed tomography for evaluation of acute chest pain. *J Am Coll Cardiol* 2007;49:863–871.

16. de Feyter PJ, van Pelt N. Spiral computed tomography coronary angiography: a new diagnostic tool developing its role in clinical cardiology. *J Am Coll Cardiol* 2007;49:872–875.

17. Murphy KJ, Brunberg JA, Cohan RH. Adverse reactions to gadolinium contrast media: a review of 36 cases. *Am J Roentgenol* 1996;167:847–849.

18. Dillman J, Ellis J, Cohan R, Strouse P. Frequency and severity of acute allergic-like reactions to gadolinium-containing IV contrast media in children and adults. *Am J Roentgenol* 2007;189:1533–1538.

Chapter 6

CARDIAC COMPUTED TOMOGRAPHY

J. David Wilson, RCIS

INTRODUCTION

Computed tomography (CT) uses X-rays to generate detailed images of an object. Many X-ray images are made, from many different angles, around a single axis of rotation, and processed to produce two- or three-dimensional images that can be viewed from any angle. Cardiac computed tomography is a fast, safe test that gives extremely clear pictures of the heart, its structures, and their functionality.

Tomography is made up of two Greek words: *tomos*, meaning "slice" or "section," and *graphia*, which means "describing." CT is also known as computed axial tomography (CAT) or CT scan.

Cardiac CT is performed, usually with intravenous contrast medium, to visualize cardiac anatomy, including the coronary arteries, great arteries, and veins. The continuous rhythmic movement of the heart and respiratory motion create great challenges for cardiac CT imaging.

To reduce motion artifact, it is necessary to ask the patient to hold their breath and image the coronary arteries during the late diastole phase (lasting between 100 and 300 milliseconds) of the cardiac cycle.

With CT scanning, X-ray beams and X-ray detectors move in a circular pattern around the patient, and the patient is moved through the scanner, so that the radiation passes through the patient in a spiral. A special computer program processes this series of image slices to create two- or three-dimensional pictures.

A CT image does not actually show the heart and the arteries; it shows the effects on the X-rays as they pass through the soft tissue and more dense tissue-like calcium. The CT scanner takes this information and turns it into an image with light and dark areas. The dark areas represent the soft tissue, which lets the X-rays pass through, and the light areas are caused by more solid substances, such as calcium.

HISTORY

The first CT scanner was invented in 1972 by an English engineer named Godfrey Hounsfield and a physicist from South Africa named Dr. Allan Cormack. The men received the Nobel Prize for medicine in 1979 for their invention. The first CT scanner took hours to accumulate the necessary data, and days to put the slices together to give the images. Head-only imaging was available in 1974, and whole-body systems were available in 1976, but it wasn't until about 1980 that CT scanners were widely available.

TYPES OF CT SCANNERS

There are two types of CT scanning: electron beam computed tomography (EBCT) and multislice computed tomography (MSCT).

MSCT scanners use an X-ray tube that rotates around the patient. The quality of MSCT images, and their ability to visualize minute anatomic features, is superior to EBCT. It is also possible to vary the tube current, if necessary, to enhance image quality. This is valuable in imaging obese patients, as well as in detecting small amounts of coronary artery calcification (Fig-

ures 6-1 and 6-2). This function does, however, increase the radiation exposure to the patient. State-of-the-art, dual-source MSCT scanners are capable of acquiring up to 64 slices per rotation with a minimum slice thickness of 0.75 mm and a maximum temporal resolution of 100 msec, independent of heart rate. This enables scanning of the entire heart within one short breath-hold and improves the detection of significant luminal stenoses. MSCT has better spatial resolution, which is the quality of the image and its ability to define smaller structures. Additionally, MSCT is less expensive, more readily available, and can be used more effectively to scan other parts of the body than EBCT.

Instead of rotating an X-ray tube around the patient, the EBCT has a huge vacuum tube, and an electron beam is steered toward an array of X-ray anodes arranged circularly around the patient. As each anode is hit by the electron beam, and emits X-rays that are collimated and detected. The lack of moving parts allows very quick scanning, with single slice acquisition in 50 to 100 ms, making the technique ideal for capturing images of the heart. With EBCT, there is a direct inverse relationship between the num-

Figure 6-1. Non-contrast enhanced axial image displays moderate calcification in the LAD.

Figure 6-2. Calcium deposits.

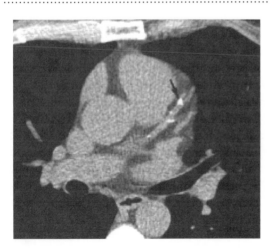

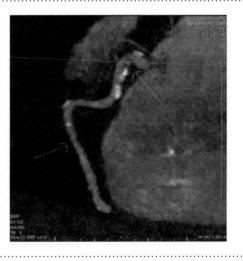

ber of milliseconds that it is set to and the image quality, which is called the temporal resolution.

INDICATIONS FOR CARDIAC CT

Cardiac CT can be used for:

- Patients with a low pretest probability of disease, but with a nonconclusive ECG or stress imaging test.
- Detecting cardiac abnormalities and mapping cardiac masses and thrombus.
- Evaluating the heart and coronary arteries before cardiac surgery.
- Evaluating cardiac wall motion and the function of the cardiac valves. However, an MRI does a better job of imaging the valve orifice and does so without the high-radiation dose of CT. The gold standard diagnostic tool for this, however, is still color Doppler echocardiography.

CALCIUM SCORE

Cardiac EBCT can be used to determine the extent of calcium in the coronary arteries. Calcium scoring is a way of determining a patient's risk of coronary artery disease. There has been shown to be a direct positive correlation between the amount of calcium and the likelihood of coronary artery disease. A higher calcium score in a younger patient is more concerning than if the patient were older, because older people are more likely to have calcium deposits.

Calcium Score Interpretation

0 No plaque is present. The risk of having a heart attack is very low, about 5%. Keep in mind, however, that a score of zero means that *no calcium or hard plaques are present.* This does not rule out soft plaques vulnerable to rupture. If there is soft plaque in the arteries and the score is read as zero,

this is a false positive test. There is a less than 5% likelihood of a coronary stenosis >50%.[1]

1–10 Very little plaque is present. The likelihood of having a heart attack is around 10%. It is advised that these people modify their risk factors.

11–100 There is mild plaque present and the chance of having a heart attack is moderate. The more risk factors a patient has, the more likely they are to have a heart attack. Again, modifying risk factors and any other treatments (adjunctive medical therapy) is advised.

101–400 There is moderate plaquing present and the patient is likely to have plaque blocking an artery. The chance of having a heart attack is moderate to high.

400+ There is a very good chance that there is a large amount of plaque blocking at least one artery. The likelihood of having a heart attack in the near future is over 90%. The chance of having a heart attack is very high and prompt action should be taken to address the seriousness of the situation. Cardiac catheterization amongst other interventions should be involved.

The calcium score can be used as a guide to determine which patients should undergo a coronary angiography and, potentially, an angioplasty.

CONTRAINDICATIONS

Abnormal cardiac rhythms, such as atrial fibrillation, make cardiac CT difficult to perform. Due to the movement of the heart over the cardiac cycle, image acquisition must be synchronized to the heartbeat. This requires an accurate estimation of when the next heartbeat will occur.

If the patient's pulse cannot be brought below 65 beats per minute or they are unable to tolerate beta blockers, the patient may not be able to have a cardiac CT unless the equipment is dual-source CT.

People experiencing an acute myocardial infarct (AMI) need a timely percutaneous coronary intervention to salvage the infarcting muscle, not a diagnostic CT procedure. These patients should go straight to the cath lab.

People who are allergic to contrast media should make their physician aware of the allergy. However, an allergy is not a contraindication to the procedure, because the patient can be premedicated with antihistamines and steroids to avoid a reaction to the contrast.

Women who are pregnant should not undergo a CT procedure due to the effects of radiation on the fetus. Women who may be pregnant or are able to have children should have a beta Hcg measurement performed to determine the likelihood of pregnancy.

IMAGE QUALITY

High-quality images are of the utmost importance for this procedure and there are several steps to ensure good imaging. Patient preparation, the CT procedure itself, and the ECG timing are all crucially important to the success of the procedure.

Gating

The best pictures are taken when the heart is at rest, so the scanner can be programmed such that it films with high energy only during diastole. To achieve this, the image acquisition is linked to the patient's ECG (Figure 6-3).

Respiratory Artifact

It is crucial that patients hold their breath during the exam or there with be a motion artifact all through the collected data.

Beam-Hardening Artifact

X-ray beams are composed of individual photons with a broad range of energies. As a beam passes through the object being imaged, the beam becomes more intense. When a patient has surgical clips or stents, the resulting image is a blur or artifact on the final picture, making it difficult or impossible for the physician to read.

Stents

The best scanners currently available (64 slice) can diagnose in-stent restenosis in vessels with diameters greater than 3 mm. With smaller ves-

Figure 6-3. Gating.

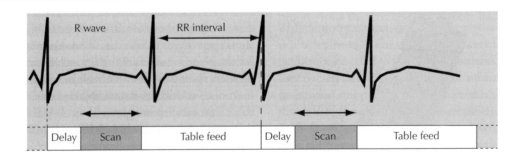

sels, the metallic artifact makes the images difficult to read.[2]

RISKS OF CARDIAC CT

The risks of the cardiac CT procedure are low. Occasionally, a patient will have an allergic reaction to a contrast agent, but this can be treated pharmacologically. This allergy should be noted on the records so the patient can be treated appropriately should he or she have to have another procedure using a contrast medium.

RADIATION EXPOSURE

The average patient radiation dose with MSCT is 6.7–8.1 mSv, but can be as high as 13.0 mSv, whereas the radiation dose with EBCT angiography is 1.5–2.0 mSv. The dosage is less with EBCT angiography because MSCT applies radiation throughout the cardiac cycle and is capable of a higher tube current. These values for a standard coronary angiography protocol are about 2.1–2.5 mSv (mean fluoroscopy time: 2.4 min without left ventriculography).[3]

PATIENT PREPARATION

The patient should be fasting for several hours before the procedure, because the contrast medium may make the patient nauseous and cause vomiting. The patient may also be asked to avoid caffeine, because a slower heart rate is necessary for good-quality images.

A functioning intravenous line will be necessary to allow the injection of contrast medium. A power injector is primed with contrast medium, flushed to remove any air from the system, and connected to the patient's IV line.

The patient should be warned about the warm feeling they may experience after the injection of the contrast media. As with cardiac catheterization, patients are asked to hold their breath briefly during this procedure. They should know why this is and why they must lie still during the procedure.

Figure 6-4. An enhanced, three-dimensional CT image of a heart and major vessels. *Source:* Image courtesy of Siemens Medical.

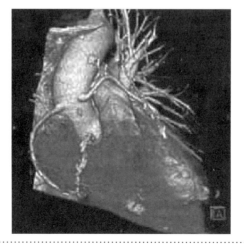

It is important to position and prepare the patient exactly according to protocol. Patients are placed in a supine position on the table. A three-lead ECG is attached so that the software can synchronize the image-taking with the patient's heartbeat. A noise-free ECG is the best way to ensure sharp images.

Inform the patient that the procedure can take about 15 minutes, and it will be necessary for him or her to remain still during the image-acquisition sequences.

PREMEDICATION

To achieve good images, a patient's heart rate should be less than 65 beats per minute. Faster heart rates have been shown to produce artifacts that make the images difficult or impossible to interpret. The most common approach to reducing the heart rate is to administer oral beta blockers an hour before the procedure to people who are not already on beta blocker therapy. An intravenous beta blocker can also be administered immediately before the scan to achieve an immediate, short-acting effect. If a patient is unable to take beta blockers, calcium channel blockers may be used instead.

Nitroglycerine capsules or sublingual spray given immediately before the scan dilates the arteries, improving the image quality. Nitroglycerine can increase the lumen of healthy arteries 20%–40% and 5%–10% in diseased arteries,[4] however by dilating the artery, it may cause the software to overestimate the degree of stenosis.[5]

PROCEDURE

The first-image acquisition run is usually performed at a low radiation level without contrast medium. These images are used to define the position of the heart for the next run and can be used to determine the patient's calcium score.

The second run is made with a short contrast medium injection to film the heart in detail. This run accurately determines the position of the heart so the equipment can be programmed for the following, more detailed runs.

There are two methods of acquiring images during the following high-detail, but high-radiation, runs: spiral or "step and shoot." Spiral runs take a continuous sequence of images throughout the cardiac cycle, over a number of heartbeats. This gives images of the heart in all phases, giving information on wall motion, ejection fraction, and valve function. The equipment can be programmed such that more energy is used (and therefore more detailed images generated) during diastole than systole.

Step and shoot involves timing the image acquisition such that it films only when the heart is in diastole. This is ideal when only the patient's coronary arteries need to be imaged. Whereas a spiral CT gives much more information about the heart, it also gives the patient a higher radiation dose.

Contrast Medium Injection

The injection of contrast medium is triggered from the control room. About 90 ml is injected at a rate of about 4.5 ml/sec. This gives about 20 heartbeats for image acquisition. The start of the acquisition run can be triggered automatically by the appearance of contrast medium in the ascending aorta.

POSTPROCEDURE

The power injector is disconnected from the patient's IV line, and the patient is helped from the CT apparatus onto his or her bed. Unless there is a contraindication, the patient's IV infusion is opened to encourage the contrast medium to be washed out. If the procedure is performed on an outpatient basis, the IV line can be removed and the patient discharged.

SUMMARY

Cardiac CT is a rapidly improving technology, producing increasingly clearer pictures. It is, and will continue to be, a powerful noninvasive imaging tool to diagnose cardiac and coronary disease. Proper patient selection will always be important, because this procedure is not for all patients; patients with acute MIs and other signs of obvious coronary disease should go directly to cardiac catheterization.

REFERENCES

1. Grube E, Silber S, Hauptmann KE, et al. TAXUS I: six- and twelve-month results from a randomized, double-blind trial on a slow-release paclitaxel-eluting stent for de novo coronary lesions. *Circulation* 2003;107:38–42.

2. Holmes DR Jr, Leon MB, Moses JW, et al. Analysis of 1-year clinical outcomes in the SIRIUS trial: a randomized trial of a sirolimus-eluting stent versus a standard stent in patients at high risk for coronary restenosis. *Circulation* 2004;109:634–640.

3. Hunold P, Vogt FM, Schmermund A, et al. Radiation exposure during cardiac CT: effective doses at multi-detector row CT and electronbeam CT. *Radiology* 2003;226(1):145–152.

4. Asselbergs W, Monnink S H J, Veeger N J G M, et al. TIO angiographic extent of coronary sclerosis in patients with stable angina pectoris. *Biochemical Society Clinical Sci* 2004;106:115–120.

5. Hoffman U, Ferenick M, Curry R C, Pena A J. Coronary CT Angiography *J Nucl Med* 2006 47: 797–806.

Chapter 7

CARDIAC MAGNETIC RESONANCE IMAGING

Jane M. Kasper, RN, BSN
Sandy Watson, RN, BN, NFESC

The use of cardiac magnetic resonance imaging (MRI) has increased rapidly over the last decade because of dramatic improvements in image quality and the speed of image acquisition. MRI has several advantages over other imaging modalities, such as computed tomography (CT) and angiography. MRI does not expose the patient (or staff) to ionizing radiation or require the use of nephrotoxic intravascular contrast agents, so it is not associated with any short- or long-term side effects.

MRI images are closer to those of echocardiography than CT, but with more detailed images, available in any plane. It also has excellent soft-tissue contrast, permitting accurate tracing of tissue edges, and providing information on tissue composition

The use of a contrast medium, injected intravenously, can provide information on blood-flow velocity, allowing flow quantification of cardiac output and shunt quantification. The way in which the myocardium takes up the contrast medium also gives information on tissue viability and necrosis.

MAGNETIC RESONANCE IMAGING

Magnetic resonance imaging (MRI) is a non-invasive, two- or three-dimensional imaging technique that differentiates tissue structures on the basis of their proton magnetic properties.[1]

During an MRI, a patient is placed in a strong electromagnetic field, made by a large superconducting magnet in the form of a tube. The patient's hydrogen atoms naturally align themselves parallel with the magnetic field, either in the same direction, or in the opposite direction. A powerful radio signal (at the same frequency as the hydrogen atoms) is sent through the patient, which pushes the hydrogen atoms out of alignment. When these atoms return to their previous alignment, they give off energy. This energy is sensed and digitalized. A computer analyzes this data and creates a composite image of the tissues.

There are subtle differences in the hydrogen atoms in various body tissues and differences in blood flow, or the viability of the tissue, causes the protons to emit different amounts of energy. These energy differences show up as different shades of gray on the MRI. Thus, the MRI offers a means of detecting areas of cardiac tissue that have poor blood flow (as in CAD) or that have been damaged (as after a heart attack).

With modern MRI equipment, these images can be shown in two or three spatial dimensions, in either static or dynamic cine mode. Once a 3-D MRI image has been obtained, it can be "sliced" and examined in detail and in any plane, offering precise, detailed information to the clinician. Specifically, cardiac MRI accurately depicts cardiac structure, function, perfusion, and myocardial viability (Figure 7-1).

The heart is in constant motion, making image acquisition problematic. To minimize the influence of respiration on the position of the heart, the patient holds his or her breath for the duration of the acquisition run. Image-sequence acquisition is also triggered to correlate with the R wave on the patient's ECG to reduce the influence of the beating heart.

Contrast Media-Enhanced MRI

With MRI, it is possible to differentiate between different tissues, but it cannot accurately show blood flow within small vessels nor tissue perfusion. For many cardiac studies, it is therefore necessary to inject a small bolus of contrast media into the patient's venous system.

The contrast media used in conventional angiography and CT contain iodine, which absorbs X-rays. In MRI, a paramagnetic contrast media, containing gandolinium, is commonly used. In general, these media have proven to be safer than angiographic contrast media.

The usual dosage of contrast media is 0.1 mmol/kg. The contrast media comes in prepared vials of 1 mmol/ml or 0.5 mmol/ml concentrations. The bolus can be injected by hand or with a power injector.

Figure 7-1. Short-axis MRI images: Cine images (a) diastole, (b) systole used to identify wall motion, LV mass, and LV volume. (c): Perfusion image used to identify areas of ischemic myocardium (arrow). (d, e): Grid tag images used to evaluate intramyocardial function by measuring deformation within the tagged images of the ventricular wall (d) diastole, (e) systole. (f): Delayed-enhancement used to evaluate areas of hyper-enhanced scarred myocardium (arrow).

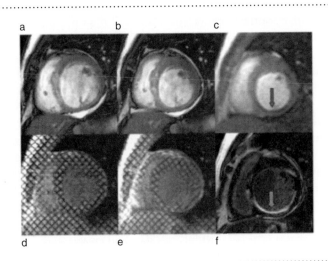

MRI contrast media diffuses quickly into the extracellular space, providing quantifiable images of what tissue is receiving blood and which is not. The contrast medium accumulates in areas with an increased extracellular space, as is the case in myocardial oedema or necrosis. Contrast media administration is, therefore, necessary for viability studies. Myocardial scar tissue is easily identified by high-intensity enhancement, because it dramatically contrasts the viable myocardium (Figure 7-2). As a result, MRI has an important role in the evaluation of myocardial viability versus necrosis in patients with ischemic heart disease.

Although gadolinium-based contrast agents are considered to be benign, they may have some impact on patients with impaired renal function. Hemodialysis may be ordered for renally impaired patients following a contrast medium-enhanced MRI.

MRI Perfusion Imaging

Vasodilating agents (adenosine or dipyridamole) are used to unmask cardiac perfusion defects, by inducing a so-called intracoronary steal phenomenon. After inducing maximal vasodilation, a small contrast bolus is quickly injected in a peripheral vein, and myocardial perfusion is assessed (stress perfusion). After 10 minutes, the contrast medium injection is repeated, and the images are compared. A perfusion defect detected under pharmacological stress, but absent in the resting images, represents myocardial ischemia. A fixed defect, which is unchanged on rest and stress images, represents a myocardial scar.

MRI Stress Testing

Making the heart work hard during an MRI examination can provide information related to cardiac structure, function, and perfusion, providing additional information beyond the scope of traditional stress testing or transthoracic

Figure 7-2. Two-chamber (left atrium and left ventricle seen) delayed-enhancement MRI image to delineate myocardial necrosis. Arrows indicate left ventricular anterior wall and apical scarring.

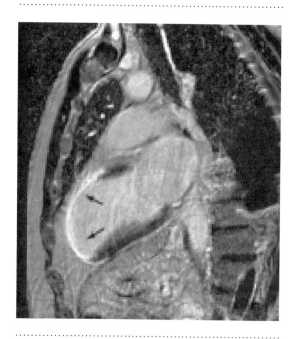

echocardiography alone. Pharmacological agents (e.g., dobutamine, dipyridamole, or adenosine) may be administered intravenously, or exercise-induced stress testing (using MRI-compatible exercise equipment) may be used to induce high heartbeat rates.

Once the myocardial contractility and heart rate are increased to the recommended level (85% of the maximum predicted heart rate response) for the patient's age, the images are recorded to assess the heart muscle contraction or perfusion while the drug is infused. Once these images have been obtained, or at the earliest sign of inducible ischemia, the medication or exercise protocol is terminated.

MRI stress testing has the advantage of relying on the measurable assessment of wall motion to determine ischemia rather than relying on subjective evaluations (e.g., patient complaints of chest pain or shortness of breath). MRI stress testing is considered to be as accurate as other noninvasive stress testing that incorporates radionuclide or ultrasound techniques.[2]

MRI AND CORONARY ARTERY DISEASE

Coronary artery imaging by MRI has presented a great challenge to investigators because of the arteries' small caliber (less than 4 mm), their continual displacement by respiratory and cardiac motion, their complex 3-D anatomy and tortuosity (especially among patients with ventricular hypertrophy), the surrounding signal from adjacent epicardial fat and myocardium, and cyclic variations in flow. Because of these challenges, CT imaging of the coronary arteries is easier, faster, more accurate, and is the preferred noninvasive imaging modality. MRI is, however, widely accepted in the assessment of larger arteries and veins, including the aorta (Figure 7-3) and the carotid and renal arteries, as well as peripheral vessels.

Magnetic resonance angiography (MRA) is an imaging technique that images flowing blood, either with or without contrast administration (Figure 7-4). It has been used to identify the course of anomalous coronary arteries and has proven effective in the assessment of coronary artery bypass graft (CABG) patency. Saphenous vein grafts and internal mammary grafts are relatively easier to image because they have a larger diameter and are less affected by cardiac and respiratory motion. Additionally, their course is relatively predictable and less tortuous than coronary arteries. However, MRI demonstrates some limitations in the assessment of graft patency of distal sequential grafts due to the signal loss created by metallic artifact from the surgical clips, sterna wires, prosthetic valves, and the like.

INDICATIONS

Cardiac MRI clearly shows not only the structure, but also the function of the heart muscle

Figure 7-3. MRA of the aorta to identify (a): coarctation and (b): ascending aortic aneurysm.

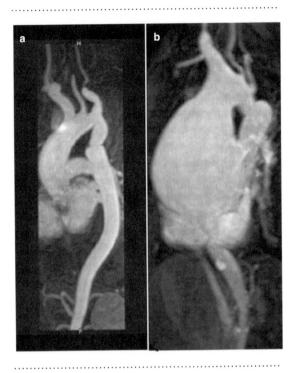

Figure 7-4. Coronary artery MRA.

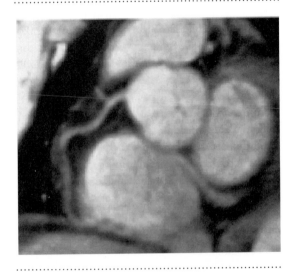

and valves. MRI can produce movie-like images of the beating heart that can be used to diagnose a variety of cardiovascular problems; the size and thickness of the heart chambers also can be accurately measured with MRI. After a heart attack, for example, an MRI examination can determine how well the heart is pumping, whether thrombus is present, what part the heart muscle is damaged, and whether the lining of the heart is swollen.

Cardiovascular MRI has many evolving roles, including the assessment of:

- Congenital heart disease
- Left and right ventricle function assessment
- Assessment of ischemic heart disease
- Assessment of cardiac viability
- Aortic disease (e.g., aortic dissection, aneurysm)
- Diseases of the myocardium (e.g., right ventricular cardiomyopathy)
- Diseases of the pericardium (e.g., constrictive pericarditis)
- Thrombi and masses
- Valvular disease
- Pulmonary artery disease

CONTRAINDICATIONS

Nevertheless, there are some contraindications that preclude its use. These include the presence in the patients of non-MRI-compatible metallic implants, such as:

- Cardiac pacemaker
- Implantable cardioverter defibrillator
- Electronic implant
- Aneurysm clip
- Intraocular metal fragment
- Cochlear implants

Cardiac valve implants and surgical aneurysm clips implanted since the early 1980s should pose no problems for an MRI examination. Coronary

stents produce image artifacts, but are not a contraindication for an MRI procedure.

There are also some conditions that limit its use in the clinical setting:[3]

- Patient's size
- Patient claustrophobia
- High cost of equipment and procedure
- Scarcity of dedicated cardiovascular MRI services
- Stationary nature of the equipment
- Inability to use equipment for ill patients

PATIENT PREPARATION

There is minimal preparation necessary for patients undergoing MRI, and it is commonly performed in an outpatient setting. Because the contrast agent rarely causes nausea, patients may eat and take their medications prior to the exam. However, if they are claustrophobic (approximately 5% of the patient population) and require sedation in order to complete the study, they may need to remain NPO (nil by mouth) to prevent nausea, vomiting, and potential aspiration resulting from adverse effects of the sedative.

Before the patient arrives in the MRI suite, she or he should be fully informed about the procedure—in particular, its benefits and risks. The patient should be aware of the length of the procedure (30–90 minutes, depending on the type of examination being undertaken) and about the enclosed space that he or she must lie in for this period.

Before entering the MRI suite, the patient is thoroughly screened for the presence of any metal or contraindications to MRI. The patient changes into a hospital gown and receives an IV line in case of complications and for contrast media administration.

Once the patient has been made comfortable on the table, ECG leads are attached for monitoring and gating purposes. Gating describes the timing of the MRI sequence acquisition to correlate with the R wave on the ECG.

Because of the high noise level during the scan, (MRI-compatible) headphones are supplied to lessen the noise irritation. The headphones also ensure that the patient hears commands from the control room. For many patients, guided imagery or listening to music through the headphones helps to prevent claustrophobia.

A radio energy receiver coil in the form of a moveable plastic grid is placed on the patient's chest. The coil weighs about 1 Kg (2 lb) and may be uncomfortable for frail or young patients. Although there are receiver coils within the MRI tube, much better images are provided by receivers directly touching the patient's body; there are also receiver coils directly under the patient.

All patients are provided with a "call light" in the event that they feel that they need to be removed from the scanner before the exam has been completed.

PROCEDURE

A first run (a so-called localizer with poor spatial resolution), is made to identify the position and orientation of the heart. Two more localizers are performed to determine the true long axis of the heart. These images form the basis of the following, more-detailed, studies.

The heart is then typically imaged by a series of short-axis slices, typically 8–14 slices, 6–10 mm thick, and some long-axis slices, typically several four-chamber, three-chamber, and two-chamber views. Other imaging planes are prescribed as required, such as to image the large vessels, conduits, or paracardiac structures.

During each image acquisition run, the patient is asked to hold his or her breath, eliminating the movement of the heart due to respiration. The patient is given instructions in the same way as with angiography.

PATIENT CARE POSTPROCEDURE

When the last run has been performed, the patient is rolled out of the MRI tube, and the coil is removed from his or her chest. A bed-bound patient will be transferred to bed, and an ambulant patient assisted to stand. Outpatients will change back into their street clothes and their cannula removed and dressed.

MRI RISKS AND SAFETY

Because MRI does not expose the patient to ionizing radiation and uses noniodine-based contrast media (which causes only rare allergic reactions or adverse effects), MRI poses virtually no health risks to the patient as long as certain critical safety policies are followed. Because the magnetic field generated by the MRIs is always on (even when not actively scanning a patient), it will attract ferromagnetic objects with significant force, possibly injuring the patient or personnel or damaging the equipment. Therefore, several safety measures must be in place in order to avoid the inadvertent introduction of non-MRI compatible metallic parts into the MRI suite.

- Provide all MRI staff, along with other staff that may have an opportunity to enter the MRI setting (nurses, doctors, environmental service, security, equipment engineers, etc.) with formal training on MRI safety.
- Post large red warning signs on the doors and walls in conspicuous locations outside the MRI suite indicating that the magnet is always on. Include warning against entering if the person has any MRI-contraindicated device or possessions. Include instructions to check with an MRI tech prior to entering the MRI environment.
- Carefully screen each person entering the MRI setting for magnetic objects in their

body (e.g., bullets, shrapnel, pacemaker/defibrillator, metallic implants), on their body (e.g., hair clips, underwire bras, zippers, jewelry), or brought with them (e.g., credit/bank cards with magnetic strips, wheelchair, oxygen tank, cart, tools).

- Have patients wear hospital gowns (without metallic snaps) during the scan.
- Maintain specialized MRI-compatible equipment including wheelchairs, monitors, carts, and IV supplies in the department to ensure safe patient care and prevent interference with the operation of the scanner.
- Allow only properly trained individuals to operate devices and monitoring equipment and to be responsible for the patient in the MRI environment.

Even devices that appear safe have become projectiles in the MRI environment. For example, sandbags, often used in the catheterization lab or angiography suites to promote hemostasis following a procedure, may contain ferromagnetic pellets that can be attracted by the MRI system and become a safety hazard. In addition to the risk of injury related to projectile force, there is a risk of heat injury to patients in contact with electrically conductive materials (e.g., ECG leads, cables, wires). Because the patient's tissue is conductive and may contribute to the formation of the conductive loop, it is imperative to prevent any of these materials from forming large-diameter conductive loops within the bore of the magnet.

NEPHROGENIC SYSTEMIC FIBROSIS

Nephrogenic systemic fibrosis (NSF) or nephrogenic fibrosing dermopathy is a rare but serious disease that appears to be associated with exposure to gadolinium in patients with renal failure. NSF involves fibrosis of skin, joints, eyes, and internal organs. Patients develop large areas of hardened skin with fibrotic nodules and plaques. There is no specific treatment for this ailment.

SUMMARY

MRI provides important diagnostic information and is considered to be a very safe procedure as long as safety measures are strictly followed. Medical practitioners and patients should be aware of the potential hazards associated with MRI prior to ordering or undergoing the procedure.

REFERENCES

1. Schoenhagen P, Halliburton S, White R, et al. Characterization of coronary atherosclerotic plaques and the significance of vessel calcification. *Appl Radiol 2001*;30:40–46.
2. Stillman AE. MR of acquired heart disease: ischemic heart disease. *Int J Cardiovasc Imaging* 2001;17:461–465.
3. Schvartzman PR, White RD. Magnetic resonance imaging. In: Topol EJ, ed. *Textbook of Cardiovascular Medicine*, 2nd ed. Philadelphia: Lippincott-Williams and Wilkins; 2002:1213–1256.

Chapter 8

Asepsis in the Cardiovascular Catheterization Laboratory

Rachael Ramsamujh, RN
Brenda Ridley, RN, BScN, MA Ed(C), CCN(C)

Maintaining asepsis within the CCL is essential if procedures are to be carried out safely and without the extra costs incurred by postprocedural infections or complications. The aseptic technique is a set of practices designed to prevent nosocomial infection by providing a clean, safe surgical environment.[1] This technique is multifaceted and spans many disciplines. Asepsis involves the preparation of equipment and patient site, sterilization methods, and the maintenance of aseptic techniques by all personnel involved in procedural care. It is a much-overlooked aspect of CCL procedures.

Sterilization is the complete destruction of all living organisms. For an item to be sterile, it must be free of all living organisms, including bacterial spores and viruses. Any breach in preparation, storage, or aseptic technique renders articles, equipment, or personnel contaminated and unusable. Disposable, single-use equipment is sterile only if aseptic techniques are maintained. In a situation where sterility is breached,

equipment must be disposed of and a new sterile field established.

CCL practice standards do not need to match operating room (OR) standards when percutaneous coronary interventions, diagnostic procedures, or straightforward electrophysiologic studies are being carried out, but they absolutely must meet OR standards for implanting permanent devices such as pacemakers.

This chapter will review these main areas as they relate to coronary procedures, both diagnostic and interventional, and the surgical implantation of permanent pacemakers and defibrillators.

HISTORICAL PERSPECTIVE

Hand washing with soap and water was the first measure of personal hygiene. In the 1800s, however, developments in surgery were being hampered by a postsurgery mortality rate as high as 90%.[2] In the 1840s, Simmelweis and Holmes concluded that the death of mothers from puerperal fever was reduced by the use of antiseptic hand cleansing rather than soap and water washing. Since then, hand washing with an antiseptic solution has been accepted as the most important method for preventing the spread of pathogens.

In the 1870s, Dr. Robert Koch recognized that pathogens could not be completely destroyed with water and carbolic acid, so he turned to the use of heat for disinfecting surgical instruments. However, this did not completely destroy spores, so heat was combined with water vapor, and this combination completely eradicated all pathogens and spores from instruments. Today, steam sterilization is still a frequently chosen method in health care.

In 1887, Lister introduced the use of carbolic acid as an antiseptic agent. Soon afterward, the staff at the Johns Hopkins Hospital in Baltimore began wearing gloves to protect their hands from the harsh, damaging effects of carbolic acid. When the patient infection rates fell, staff connected the use of gloves with the decrease in infection rates.

In 1892, Dr. Kurt Schimmelbusch supported Koch's research. He published findings that sepsis could be almost eradicated with antiseptic wound care. By 1910, sterile equipment, gowns, and gloves were being used during surgery, and nosocomial infection rates sank to manageable levels. This allowed surgeons to be more daring in their procedures, which spurred a great developmental phase, leading to surgery as it is known today.

EQUIPMENT STORAGE

Equipment in the CCL originates from various locations: External equipment is shipped in and reusable sterilized equipment comes from the central processing department (CPD) or from storage areas in the CCL. This equipment can be single use, reusable, and disposable. Packaging of the equipment will generally determine its use

and handling. All equipment in the CCL setting should be inspected for failure of barriers and potential contamination.[3]

Safe handling and storage of equipment is essential to ensure that its sterility is not compromised. Nursing and technical personnel should adhere to the Association of Operating Room Nurses (AORN) Recommended Practices for Aseptic Technique III: "All items presented to the sterile field should be checked for proper packaging, processing, moisture, seal integrity, package integrity, and the appearance of the sterilization indicator."[4]

Equipment should be stored in cupboards or metal racks that can be covered to keep the equipment free of dust. Equipment should never be stored on the floor or anywhere near potential liquid contamination. Wherever possible, equipment should be stored to provide enough for current use only. Stockpiling of supplies can lead to potential contamination from exposure, traffic movement, and dust. Rotation of stock will ensure items are used before their expiration dates.

Dust control is important, because sterile equipment can be contaminated by collected dust. Dust-free barriers and minimal traffic in storage areas are key requirements. Bacteria counts rise sharply as air travels through the clinical setting of the CCL. Currents pick up contaminated particles shed from patients, personnel, drapes, and other stationary equipment. The greater the activity, the greater the shedding and contamination risk.[5] Movement and storage in the CPD requires restricted traffic to minimize levels of dust contamination and the overhandling of supplies.

STERILIZATION OF EQUIPMENT

Equipment comes either in single-use, presterilized packages from the manufacturer or in multiuse forms that can be sterilized by steam, chemicals, or gas. Departments that provide the sterilization are responsible for ensuring that equipment is sterilized following stringent guidelines and are monitored for quality. Sterility assurance markers must be clearly visible on all packaging.[6]

STANDARDS FOR STERILIZATION

The Association for the Advancement of Medical Instrumentation (AAMI) produces recommended practices for sterilization that dictate the work standards of the central service or sterile processing department. Effective Sterilization in Health Care Facilities by the Steam Process emphasizes a systems approach that recognizes the importance of pre- and poststerilization practices as well as reliable sterilizer operation.

Recommended standard practices for emergency (Flash) sterilization provides requirements, including quality assurance criteria, for emergency steam sterilization carried out in such locations as ORs. Dry Heat, which is a tabletop dryer using heated air, is used in dentistry.

Radiation Sterilization covers radiation sterilization of healthcare products. This is used exclusively in industry, however, and not in hospitals.[7]

STEAM (AUTOCLAVE)

Steam provides the most economical method for sterilizing surgical steel instruments, basins, bowls, glassware, rubber, textiles, rubber products, and heat-resistant plastics.[8] Items need to be wrapped correctly to allow the entire item to receive the steam process equally.[9] Water quality is important for steam sterilization, so desalinated water is most often used. Fractionated, prevacuum sterilization is used most often in hospitals and is considered to be the safest method. It is a cost-effective, nontoxic, environmentally friendly, easy-to-manage procedure. The steam process can be broken down into four stages.

Stage 1

The type of sterilization is determined.

- Gravity (heavy air is displaced downwards from the sterilization chamber).
- Prevacuum (the chamber is evacuated once).
- Fractionated prevacuum (the air in the chamber is evacuated repeatedly, alternating with steam intake in a fractionated flow process that involves repeatedly filling the chamber until a required operating pressure is reached).

Articles should be cleaned prior to sterilization and materials wrapped in the appropriate format.

Stage 2

The material is heated with steam.

Temperatures will influence the time required for sterilization. The higher the temperature, the shorter the time required for sterilization. The exception is dry heat sterilization which requires a long time period for sterilization and is only used for equipment that will not tolerate moisture autoclave.

Ideally, similar articles are batched together to process at the same temperature and time intervals (Table 8-1).

Table 8-1. Batching of Materials for Sterilization

Temperature	Time	Method
270°F (132°C)	3 minutes	Flash sterilization
257°F (125°C)	8 minutes	Autoclave sterilization
245°F (118°C)	18 minutes	Downward displacement autoclave
320°F (160°C)	2 hours	Dry heat

Stage 3

The materials are dried.

The moisture that builds up must be allowed to drain properly during the sterilization process, and items must be placed to ensure adequate air movement during the sterilization process.

Stage 4

Articles are removed from chamber.

Items are now sterile and should be handled by appropriately gowned and gloved personnel. Equipment is stored per institutional recommendations.

FLASH STERILIZATION

If a gravity-displacement sterilizer is being used (where displaced air flows through a steam-activated exhaust valve), the correct cycle is 10 minutes at 270–272°F (132–133°C). If a prevacuum sterilizer is being used, the cycle is 4 minutes at 270–272°F (132–133°C) unless otherwise validated by both the sterilizer manufacturer and the tape manufacturer. In either situation, a drying cycle is not necessary unless a single wrapper is being used in a sterilizer specifically designed to flash sterilize at that particular configuration. Manufacturers' recommendations should be followed carefully to determine the correct cycle, including drying time, for each load.[10] Flash sterilization should only be used in an operating or sterile procedural area for items that will be used immediately. Items sterilized with this method cannot be wrapped and stored for future use unless they undergo longer, conventional sterilization methods.

CHEMICAL STERILIZATION

Chemical sterilization can be performed using a glutaraldehyde solution (a water-soluble oil used as a disinfectant) or a chemical in the form of a gas. Glutaraldehyde is caustic to skin, mucous membranes, and tissues, so caution must be taken when handling items for sterilization.

Items must be fully cleaned and rinsed in sterile saline or sterile water before undergoing chemical sterilization. Instruments must also be inspected for cracks, defects, or any damage prior to and after sterilization. Visual inspection is the key to ensuring that reusable instruments can indeed be reused. Cost constraints in the current healthcare environment come into play when looking at the time, labor, and financial resources required for sterilizing reusable equipment.

GAS STERILIZATION

The use of toxic gases to kill germs allows thermolabile materials to be sterilized at fairly low temperatures. Gas sterilization should be used only for material and supplies that will not withstand sterilization by steam under pressure. It is presently available with ethylene oxide (ETO) gas and with formaldehyde (FA). ETO is a colorless, extremely flammable gas with a sweet odor and is a colorless liquid below 10°C. The gas is slightly heavier than air and may spread over long distances. The metabolism of pathogens is blocked using this gas, which leads to their death.

The concentration of the gas and the temperature and humidity inside the sterilizer are vital factors that affect the gas-sterilization process. ETO gas-sterilization periods range from 3–7 hours, and all items must be allowed an aeration (airing out) period during which the ETO gas is expelled from the items' surface. Despite this, there is still potential for toxic residues to be left in products and materials that have been ETO gas sterilized.

ETO toxicity is similar to that of ammonia; however, its additional reactivity and mutagenecity require that elaborate safety precautions be taken with the use of this sterilizing agent. ETO gas sterilization can cause acute pulmonary edema in high concentrations. It has been associated with adverse reproductive and trans-placental effects, and it can also contribute to chromosomal damage and cancer incidence.[9,10] Using an ETO gas-sterilizer requires caution, and the manufacturer's instructions must be carefully followed.

FA alkalizes proteins. Pathogens are damaged so they can no longer proliferate. FA is highly toxic and can cause severe irritation to the eyes and mucous membranes.

OTHER STERILIZATION METHODS

Hydrogen peroxide gas plasma sterilization is a low-temperature, low-moisture sterilization process that is rapid enough to provide high through-put. There are no toxic residuals; therefore, no aeration is required. The primary by-products of the process are water vapor and oxygen. As a consequence, the cycle time for processing can be relatively short. Several recent improvements in hydrogen peroxide gas plasma sterilization technology have reduced cycle times from 74–55 minutes.[11]

Plasma sterilization is considered to be a useful alternative to gas sterilization, but it is not suitable for highly absorbent materials such as paper, linen, and textiles. It is suitable for sterilizing heat- and moisture-sensitive items, delicate instruments, and instruments with sharp edges.

ENVIRONMENT

Activity and attire separate the different areas of the CCL. A well-thought-out geographical setup of the procedural areas and the flow of personnel are the keys to maintaining asepsis in the CCL.

In an unrestricted area or control station, the ward clerk, manager, consulting physicians, and external personnel can enter, and street clothes are permitted. Nonclinical administrative activities take place in this area.

In the semirestricted areas which include sterile storage and access corridors, personnel are required to wear scrub attire. The scrub areas are located outside the procedure room and are considered a part of the semirestricted area. The sinks are usually ceramic or stainless steel with foot, elbow, or automatic controls for antiseptic solution and water.

In the restricted areas where cardiac procedures are performed, scrub attire is mandatory. Masks should be worn when implanting devices or foreign materials.

Three parameters of the CCL environment are controlled to inhibit the growth of microorganisms:

1. Humidity is maintained at 30%–60%.
2. The rooms are kept cool, at 68–73°F.
3. The room is ventilated through high-efficiency filters at a rate of 20–25 total room air exchanges per hour. A filter system is used to allow for maximum entrapment of microorganisms.

MAINTENANCE OF A STERILE FIELD

A sterile field is an area free of harmful micro-organisms. It is created by placing sterile towels or sterile surgical drapes around the procedure site and on the stand or table that will hold sterile instruments and other equipment to be used for the procedure. The edges of a sterile field are deemed unsterile. If a sterile field or item is left unattended, it is considered to be no longer sterile, because the integrity of that sterility cannot be guaranteed.

Scrubbed personnel should consider themselves sterile in front from waist to chest and from elbow to fingertips only. Hands should be held at chest level when not performing a task and should not touch an unsterile object. Non-scrubbed personnel should not lean or reach over the sterile field and should keep at least 12 inches away from it. Nonscrubbed personnel should not pass between two sterile fields. Sterile packets should be opened onto the sterile field away from the body. A sterile item that touches an unsterile area must be discarded and replaced. Wiping the item with a disinfectant is not sufficient to restore it to a sterile state. If sterility is in doubt, throw it out.

IMPLANTABLE DEVICES IN THE CCL SETTING

Permanent device implantation has the same risk of infection as any other surgical procedure. The procedure to implant a permanent pacemaker or implantable cardioverter defibrillator device involves an incision and the creation of a pocket to accommodate the device and its leads. Introducing any foreign material into an artificial opening in the body poses a risk of infection. Practices for implantation of pacemakers in the CCL requires adherence to OR standards.[12]

The current standard of care for pacemaker implantation is to perform the procedure under strict OR conditions (such as AORN, ORNAC, APIC, and Health Canada guidelines).[13] These include:

- The use of barriers at all times—sterile gowns, gloves, and masks.
- Staff trained in surgical asepsis and aseptic techniques.
- No eating or drinking in the restricted area.
- Movement of personnel in and out of the operating room or procedural room should be kept to a minimum during the procedure. This includes minimizing the number of people in the OR, the movement of those in the OR, and excessive talking during surgery.
- The air filter system should provide appropriate air exchanges and pressure relationship as per Canadian Standards Association (CSA) standards. A minimum of 20 air exchanges per hour is required, with positive pressure in the OR.

- The HVAC system should provide appropriate air exchanges and pressure relationship as per CSA standards:
  ○ total air changes per hour: 20
  ○ outdoor air changes per hour: 6
  ○ temperature range: 20–26°C
  ○ relative humidity range : 50%–60%
- Operating rooms shall be under positive pressure relative to the surrounding corridors.
- The ventilation system shall assure a controlled, filtered air supply.
- The ventilation system shall provide a separate supply, return, and/or exhaust.
- Air quality should be maintained through proper operation and maintenance of the air-handling system.
- Temperature, relative humidity, and pressure should be monitored continuously and include alarm systems.
- Thermostatic controls should be present.
- High-efficiency particulate-air (HEPA) filtration systems should be used. Recommended filter efficiency is 95% and prefilter efficiency 30%.
- The room setup should allow ease of movement without compromising the sterile field.
- Required supplies are enclosed, covered, and stored in cabinets to reduce the accumulation of dust and so that they can be easily cleaned.
- Time and/or distance separate traffic routes for clean and sterile supplies and equipment from those for soiled equipment and waste.

Many cath labs now have hybrid capacity, meaning that they can perform surgical procedures as well as diagnostic and interventional cardiac and peripheral vascular procedures. Percutaneous valve repair and replacement in cath labs, using large-bore catheters and requiring cutdown procedures, has meant that an OR standard of sterile technique has to be adopted in the cath lab; endocarditis in a prosthetic stent valve can have devastating sequelae for patients.[14]

CLEANING IN THE CCL

Cleaning between cases involves the removal of all equipment and linens soiled with body fluids. Spills should be cleaned from the floor, and the procedure table should be cleaned with a disinfectant. All equipment should be spot cleansed if soiled with body fluids. Patient stretchers, including any straps or attached equipment, are considered contaminated through patient contact and should be cleaned between patients. Refillable liquid soap dispensers should be disassembled and cleaned before refilling with fresh soap solutions.

When cleaning, personnel must wear appropriate attire and nonsterile rubber gloves to protect them from contamination. The cleaning of the CCL after patients infected with transmissible organisms will be determined by each center's policies and procedures as defined by infection control practices. Patients infected with transmissible organisms should ideally be done as the last procedure of the day.

Terminal Daily Cleaning

This should be the final activity in the CCL at the end of each procedural day. It involves cleaning the entire floor with disinfectant and washing all surfaces to remove contaminants and dust. All soiled equipment must be removed. Terminal cleaning is performed in the CCL procedure rooms, scrub areas, and utility areas. Surgical lights, tracks, fixed and ceiling-mounted equipment, all furniture, handles of cabinets and push plates, ventilation faceplates, horizontal surfaces and counters, tables, prep areas, and scrub sinks should all be cleaned.

Any material left in the room must be clean and free from any contamination. All biohazardous material should be removed to the dirty-utility area. Garbage is removed and any open, unused equipment should either be disposed of or sent for resterilization.

The procedure table is completely wiped down—mattress and frame—and cleaned with Virrox, as are the armrests, cables, and overhead equipment. In some labs, new transducers are used for each patient. In labs that use multiuse transducers, the used transducers should be discarded at the end of the day; a new one should be used each day.

Personnel

The strict sterile techniques used in the OR are not necessary for most CCL procedures, because infection is rare after invasive cardiovascular procedures. In a retrospective study of 385 laboratories, an infection rate of 0.35% was noted, with the incidence for cutdowns 10 times higher than that for percutaneous sites.[12]

The operator should use appropriate hand-washing technique and wear a sterile gown and gloves. Masks, eye shields, and protective caps are more important for keeping the patient's blood from splattering onto the operator than for protecting the patient from infection.[15,16] In cases where greater wound exposure is necessary such as pacemaker implantation or brachial cutdowns, full surgical-sterile technique should be adhered to.

Clothing change should involve scrub suit or greens for staff in the CCL area. Street clothes or shoes should not be permitted in the CCL area.

All personnel assigned to the CCL must practice good personal hygiene. Nails should be kept short and free from chipping nail polish. Long nails may cause tearing in sterile gloves worn for procedures, allowing for a break in asepsis, a potential risk of exposure to body substances for the healthcare worker or contamination of the sterile field. It is recommended that artificial nails not be worn due to the risk of fungal infections under or at the base of them.[13,17]

The wearing of jewelry by scrubbed personnel is a debated subject. In nursing, the traditional practice is to wear no jewelry; if timepieces are worn, they are fob watches pinned to the uniform. Current practice differs between institutions, but has become more lenient over the years. It is still recommended that clinicians in the surgical suite remove rings, watches, and bracelets before beginning the surgical hand scrub. Because these jewelry items can potentially act as hiding places for organisms, removal will allow for full skin contact with the surgical scrub product.[18]

Personnel with colds, sore throats, open sores, or other infections should not be permitted in the CCL procedure rooms.

If attire for the CCL procedure area includes head coverings, facemasks, and booties, these should not be worn outside the procedure area. They should be removed upon leaving and replaced before reentering the restricted area. This applies to sterile gowns and gloves worn during the procedure as well.

Scrubbing

Healthcare workers (HCWs) are guided to wash their hands before performing invasive procedures, between contact with high-risk patients, and after touching objects that could be potentially contaminated with pathogens.[14] The purpose of surgical scrubbing is to remove debris and transient microorganisms from nails, hands, and forearms. This reduces the resident microbial count to a minimum and also inhibits the rapid rebound growth of microorganisms.

Surgical hand scrub is an antiseptic preparation that reduces the number of microorganisms on intact skin; it is broad-spectrum, fast acting, and persistent. For aseptic procedures, hands and forearms should be scrubbed for 2–5 minutes (depending on manufacturer recommendation); longer scrubs are unnecessary.[17]

Hands should be considered to have five planes for cleansing: two sides, back, front, and finger tips. Forearms should be considered to have two planes: top and bottom. Each plane should be scrubbed individually.

When scrubbing, hands should be held above the elbows so that water drips from the hands to the elbows. It is recommended that hard brushes not be used to scrub because they may cause damage to the skin and promote sores or dermatitis, thus leading to possible infection. Hands should be dried with a sterile towel from fingers to elbows. One side of the towel should be used for each arm. Drying the hands well prior to gloving is important because organisms are transferred in much larger numbers from wet hands than dry hands.[13]

Waterless Scrub

A waterless antiseptic agent does not require use of exogenous water. Before applying the alcohol solution, prewash hands and forearms with a non-antimicrobial soap, and dry completely. After application of the alcohol-based product as recommended, rub hands together until the agent has dried[19] before donning sterile gloves.

The recommended practice is to start with a formal water-based scrub, followed by a waterless scrub for each subsequent procedure over the course of the day. Leaving the procedural area for breaks, or travel off the unit requires a water-based scrub before coming back to the scrub position for procedures.

Gowning

Gowning requires the assistance of an unsterile person. It is essential to check the surroundings to ensure adequate space for outstretched arms.

1. Hold the folded sterile gown away from the body by the collar.
2. Allow the gown to drop open, making sure that the gown does not touch the floor or any other object.
3. Slide the arms into the sleeves, keeping them above the waist at all times. Flex the elbows and abduct the arms.
4. The circulating nurse will grasp the collar of the gown, pull it over the shoulders, and fasten it at the back of the neck.
5. The gown can be tied at the waist after gloving.

Gloving

There are two ways to don gloves: the closed method and the open method. Using the closed method, the hands remain covered by cuffs of the sterile gown.

1. The arms are pushed only so far into the sleeve of the sterile gown that the hands are still covered by the cuff.
2. The nondominant hand (covered completely by the cuff) is used to pull the sterile glove onto the dominant hand.
3. The gloved hand then applies the remaining glove to the other hand.
4. Gloves are adjusted once both hands are covered.

The open method involves applying gloves with bare hands and pulling them over the gown sleeves.

1. The sterile gown is donned.
2. Using the nondominant hand, pick up the glove for the dominant hand at the cuff, using just the fingertips.
3. Slide this hand into the glove until a snug fit over the thumb joint and knuckles is achieved. The ungloved hand should only touch the folded cuff.

4. Slide the gloved fingertips into the folded cuff of the remaining glove. Slide the ungloved hand into the glove until achieving a snug fit.
5. Unfold the cuffs of both gloves down over the gown cuffs and up the sleeves as far as they will go.

Whichever gloving method is used, rinse the gloved hands with sterile solution to remove residual powder prior to starting the procedure. To maintain sterility, gloved hands must remain above waist level and may not touch any unsterile objects.

THE PATIENT

As with all procedures, it is essential to have a fully informed patient. It is especially important to explain the concept of a sterile field (i.e., what it is, where it is, why it is necessary, and the importance of not touching it).

Most institutions allow patients to wear their rings, chains, and earrings during the procedure. Even if your institution does not mandate the removal of dentures, it is important to know if your patient has them in the case of any emergency when airway patency may become an issue.

Site Preparation

Sterile preparation is mandatory for all vascular access sites. The site should be prepared using aseptic technique by the scrub nurse, technician, or physician.

Hair removal prior to the procedure should be performed using a clipper rather than a razor blade, and it should not be performed in the procedure area.[15,16] Shaving with a razor blade is no longer performed in the OR and CCL, because it was found to cause microbreaks in the skin integrity, which is a potential source for infection.

When the shaved patient is lying comfortably on the stretcher, the circulating nurse uncovers the patient's groin. Sterile towels and drapes are then used to cover the rest of the patient and any potential sources of contamination in the procedural field. The circulating nurse should also "police" traffic during the draping and skin preparation, because these are crucial times to prevent any break in asepsis or to prevent any movement that will create dust.[16]

Insertion sites should be prepared with an antiseptic of proven efficacy (Table 8-2). Most infections come from the patient's endogenous flora on the skin, mucous membranes, or hollow viscera. Chlorhexidine gluconate preparations (2% aqueous or 0.5% in 70% isopropyl or ethyl alcohol) may provide an advantage. The efficacy of 0.5% alcoholic chlorhexidine gluconate preparations has not yet been confirmed by prospective randomized trials, but in vitro and observational studies suggest that they may be superior to iodophors. Other suitable agents include 10% povidone-iodine, 1% tincture of iodine, and 70% isopropyl alcohol. It is advisable to check the manufacturers' recommendations, because some products may be incompatible with alcohol preparations.

The site should be swabbed using a circular motion from the center of the puncture site to the outside. The antiseptic solution should remain on the site for at least 30 seconds before being swabbed dry.

Table 8-2. Skin Preparation Solutions

70% Isopropyl alcohol
• Denatures protein, but is short acting.
• Effective against gram-positive and gram-negative organisms.
• Also a fungicidal and virucidal.

0.5% Chlorhexidine
• An ammonium compound that disrupts bacterial cell walls.
• Bactericidal but does not kill spore-forming organisms
• It is persistent and has a long duration of action (up to 6 hours)
• More effective against gram-positive organisms

70% Povidone-iodine
• Acts by oxidation/substitution of free iodine
• Bactericidal and active against spore-forming organisms
• Effective against both gram-positive and gram-negative organisms
• Rapidly inactivated by organic material such as blood
• Patient skin sensitivity can be a problem.

SUMMARY

All members of the healthcare team have a role in providing optimal care for the patient. Awareness of the principles of asepsis is only the first step in providing a cath lab environment that is safe for the patient and the staff.

Adherence to professional regulatory standards covers all facets of the aseptic process, from preparation of equipment to the nurse's or physician's role in care of the patient. Application of standards and quality assurance programs play a role in ensuring that aseptic techniques are maintained throughout the course of the patient's stay in the CCL.

Nursing can look to Florence Nightingale as a pioneer in infection control along with her medical counterparts: Lister, Simmelweis, Holmes, and Koch. Each made unique contributions to the understanding of asepsis and sterility, permitting the performance of the great range of invasive procedures seen today with such low infection rates.

REFERENCES

1. Association of Operating Room Nurses. Recommended practices for environmental cleaning in the surgical practice setting. *AORN J* 2002;76(6):1071–1078.
2. Rotter M. Hand washing and hand disinfection. In: Mayhall CG, ed. *Hospital Epidemiology and Infection Control*, 2nd ed. Philadelphia: Lippincott; 1999.
3. Chadwick S. Event related outdating: a fairy tale comes true. *Can Oper Room Nurse J* 1994; 12:22–26.
4. Association of Operating Room Nurses. *ORN Standards, Recommended Practices, and Guidelines*. Denver, CO: Association of Operating Room Nurses, Inc.; 1997.
5. Pearson ML. Guidelines for prevention of intravascular device-related infections. Part I. Intravascular device-related infections: an overview. The Hospital Infection Control Practices Advisory Committee. *Am J Infect Control* 1996; 24:262–277.
6. Surgical aseptic techniques. Available at: http://www.tpub.com
7. Association for the Advancement of Medical Instrumentation. *Recommended Practices: Sterilization in Health Care Facilities*. Arlington, VA: AAMI; 2003.
8. Mangram AJ, Horan TC, Pearson ML, et al. Guidelines for prevention of surgical site infection, 1999. *Infect Control Hosp Epidemiol* 1999;20(4):250–279.
9. Kumar P. ETO sterilization and the role of packaging materials. In: Medical Plastics Data Service website. Available at: http://www.medicalplasticsindia.com/mpds/2003/sept. Accessed December 12, 2004.
10. Miller D. Ethylene oxide sterilizers in health care facilities: engineering controls and work practices. Available at: http://www.cdc.gov/niosh/89115_52. Accessed December 12, 2004.
11. Spry C. Sterilization: low-temperature sterilization. Available at: http://www.infectioncontroltoday. com/articles/151steriliz.html?wts=2004121210 0224&hc=7&req=Spry. Accessed December 12, 2004.
12. Steelman VM. [Commentary on] Analysis of charges and complications of permanent pacemaker implantation in the cardiac catheterization laboratory versus the operating room. Yamamura KH et al. *Pacing & Clinical Electrophysiology* (22): 1820–1824.
13. Boyce J, Pittet D. Guideline for hand hygiene in health-care settings. Recommendations of the Healthcare Infection Control Practices Advisory Committee and the HICPAC/ SHEA/APIC/ IDSA Hand Hygiene Task Force. *MMWR Recomm Rep* 2002;51:1–45.
14. Lurz P, Coats L, Khambadkone S, et al. Percutaneous pulmonary valve implantation: impact of evolving technology and learning curve on clinical outcome circulation. *Journal* 2008;117: 1964–1972.
15. Infection Control Guidelines. Health Canada Communicable Disease Report. Circulation-Supplement Volume: 23S8. 1997.
16. Pryor F, Messmer P. The effect of traffic patterns in OR on surgical site infections. *AORN J* 1998;68(4):649–660.
17. Dharan S, Pittet D. Environmental controls in operating theatres. *J Hosp Infect* 2002;51:79-84. *AORN J* 2001;74(2):1820-1824.
18. Myers F, Parini S. Hand hygiene: understanding and implementing the CDC's new guideline. *Nurs Manage* 2003;34(4):1–14.
19. Centers for Disease Control and Prevention. Guideline for hand hygiene in health-care settings: recommendations of the Healthcare Infection Control Practices Advisory Committee and the HICPAC/SHEA/APIC/IDSA Hand Hygiene Task Force. *MMWR* 2002;51(No. RR-16).

SUGGESTED READING

Bashore T, Bates E, Kern M, et al. American College of Cardiology/Society for Cardiac Angiography and Interventions Clinical Expert Consensus Document on cardiac catheterization laboratory standards. A report of the American College of Cardiology Task Force on clinical expert consensus documents. *J Am Coll Cardiol* 2001;37(8):2170–2214.

Chambers CE, Eisenhauer D, McNicol LB, et al. Infection control guidelines for the cardiac catheterization laboratory: society guidelines for the Society for Cardiovascular Angiography and Interventions. *Catheterization and Cardiovascular Interventions* 2006;67:78–86.

Chapter 9

CATH LAB STAFF DUTIES

Sandy Watson, RN, BN, NFESC
Jeff Hunter, RTR, BS

OVERVIEW

This chapter is an overview of the responsibilities of the staff who assist physicians with procedures in a cardiovascular catheterization laboratory (CCL). All support staff members should hold certifications in basic life support (BLS), advanced cardiac life support (ACLS), and pediatric advanced life support (PALS), if pediatric cardiac studies are performed. All members of the team (cardiologists, nurses, technologists, and advanced-level practitioners) must understand the roles of the other members of the support team.

There are three broad categories of tasks performed by the CCL staff in every facility: scrub, circulator, and monitor.

SCRUB

The scrub nurse, or scrub assistant, stands at the table with the cardiologist, assisting with the instrumental side of the procedure. He or she must have a thorough knowledge of sterile surgical technique to reduce possible infectious processes. They must wash their hands to the elbows before each procedure, dress in a surgical gown, and wear sterile gloves.

Scrub assistants flush catheters, guide wires, and other invasive equipment that may be used inside the circulatory system. They also help with catheter exchanges, wires, and other devices. The scrub may also inject medications such as nitroglycerin, heparin, IIB-IIIA platelet inhibitors, and other medication through the catheters.

CIRCULATOR

This person is responsible for the room preparation before the arrival of the patient and to see that it is cleaned and reprepared afterward. The word "turnover" is often used to describe the process of taking the patient off the table after a procedure, removing the dirty equipment and supplies and disposing of them, and then preparing the lab for the next patient.

The circulator helps transfer the patient to the table, attaches the ECG electrodes, and inserts a peripheral IV line, if necessary. The circulating nurse hands or "drops" additional supplies to the scrub team as needed. This staff member handles the nonsterile equipment, administers the necessary medications, and keeps a personal watch on the patient's condition.

MONITOR

The monitor is responsible for recording the patient's vital signs, any procedural measurements needed to complete the study, and reproducing and storing the procedure event log and CD. This staff member is specifically responsible for monitoring the patient's vital signs during the procedure, spending the bulk of the procedure behind the computer, taking pressure measurements, making printouts, and providing other information as needed.

In centers with many laboratories, there may also be an X-ray technologist (or technician) who oversees the maintenance and smooth running of the X-ray equipment. Some centers have anesthetists who attach and monitor the ECG and monitor the patient's condition. Anesthetists are not widely used, however, except in the case of pediatric catheterization.

In some laboratories, each job (scrub, circulator, monitor) is quite distinct and is carried out by specific team members. In other labs, the roles overlap, and one person may carry out many, or even all, of the jobs. It has been learned that the best patient care is given when staff members cross-train; that is, they are trained and able to work comfortably in each job area in the lab. In addition to better patient care, when staff have cross-trained within the limits of their specific licensure or registry, they can fill in wherever they are needed in busy interventional laboratories, making staffing needs easier to meet. The greatest benefit is to the staff members themselves. Cumulative or overuse injuries caused by repeatedly using the same group of muscles for the same job are diminished when the roles during the day are rotated. For example, if scrub staff switch positions with the monitoring staff, both parties benefit. The monitor gets away from the computer and rests tired eyes; the scrub nurse can use different muscles and relax from standing in the same position for hours.

PROCEDURE PREPARATION

The number and types of equipment differ between countries and labs, but in general, the first steps of the day in a CCL are as follows:

The X-ray apparatus and recording system are switched on and warmed up. The computer has to be logged on. The printer paper supply should be checked.

Material should be constantly checked and restocked during the day as time allows, but the morning is a good time for a thorough review of what is on hand and which supplies are low.

The patient list for the day should be checked. The interventionalists should be questioned about whether there are old films/videos/CDs of the patients and what procedures they are expecting to perform. Patients at high risk should be identified. If a patient has renal insufficiency, they should be premedicated or prehydrated and a postprocedure hydration scheme agreed on to ensure adequate elimination of the contrast medium.

The procedure table on which the patient will lie is prepared, and the sterile equipment table arranged. The cart or table used for the equipment is cleaned with disinfectant at the start of the day and between each procedure. The defibrillator should be tested and left ready to go. Emergency medication should be drawn up and reserve stocks checked. The pressure injector must be warmed up and loaded.

Before entering the lab itself, the scrub should wash and scrub their hands for 3–5 minutes, covering fingers, hands, and arms (up to the elbow) in approved surgical antibacteriostatic cleaning solution.

As much water as possible should be allowed to drain into the sink before the scrub starts the trek into the lab. The less water that is dripped, the less chance there is of someone slipping on it. Newer surgical scrub solutions require no additional water and are considerably easier and actually cleaner to use.

Depending on the institution, gowns can be paper or cloth. Gowns should be donned using standard sterile technique; the outside of the gown should never be touched. The gown should be picked up by the inside at the top, and each arm is slipped into a sleeve. This can be done one arm at a time or both arms at the same time. With a paper gown, the scrub hands off the tie holder to the circulator and turns around, removing the tie from the holder, then tying themselves up. With a cloth gown, the assistant should let someone hold the tie with a sterile clamp as he or she turns. The assistant nurse then takes the tie back and does the tying.

The scrub nurse then turns to the table set. On the top should lay the scrub's sterile gloves, which are put on with the help of the gown's sterile cuffs. Once gowned and gloved, the scrub nurse's hands should never go beyond the sterile field.

The table set is usually a fully disposable, all-in-one, sterile package (although reuseable, resterilized material, or a combination of this and disposable material can also be used). The scrub nurse opens the table set and lays out the contents. The following is a list of basic equipment for the table:

- Two containers, one containing 500 ml of saline solution to which 5000 units of heparin have been added.
- A bowl for 1% or 2% lidocaine solution.

- A bowl for Betadine solution for cleaning the puncture site.
- Sterile swabs or prep sticks to do the cleaning.
- Syringes and needles.
- Sterile drapes to cover the patient to maintain a sterile area.
- An 11- or 15-mm blade.
- A needle for cannulating the artery.
- A two, three, or four-outlet manifold with attached lines for pressure, waste, contrast medium, or whatever is used in the clinic.
- Sheaths and catheters (these will vary and can be added to the table by the circulator once the patient is on the table and draped).

The circulating nurse should fill beakers as required, and then open the diagnostic catheter set. It is common to have the puncture needle, sheath, exchange wire, and diagnostic catheters packaged together. Each piece is flushed, removed from the package, wiped, and placed on the table. To ensure an uncluttered working space, it is best to loop all catheters and wires three or four times. A wet 4×4 can be placed on each.

In most cases, it is appropriate to prepare the sterile trolley in advance, and cover it with a drape until the patient is ready to begin the procedure.

PATIENT PREPARATION

The first exchange between the patient and the nurse should involve a greeting and an introduction. The patient should be properly identified by checking their wristband with their documents and the name on the CCL's program. During the identification process, the patient may be asked their name, date of birth, and the reason that they have come to the hospital. The patient should be able to describe what procedure will be performed in their own language. If necessary, a translator should be present from the very beginning of the procedure.

The staff member should ask patients how they slept, when they last ate, and whether they took any medication that morning. The best time to ask patients if they need to urinate is before they enter the laboratory. If the consent form has not yet been signed, it is best to do this before the patient moves to the X-ray table.

While the circulator and scrub are preparing the patient and the lab for the procedure, the monitor reads through the patient's notes, paying close attention to lab results. These are covered in detail in Chapter 10. Any abnormal values or findings should be discussed with the attending cardiologist and other team members.

As the patient is helped onto the X-ray table, a quick description of the X-ray tubes, monitors, and procedure tables is helpful in decreasing the anxiety some patients may feel. The procedure room is filled with many pieces of equipment and can be quite overwhelming.

By this stage, the nurse will have obtained a fairly good picture of the patient's state of mind. A nervous patient is often very talkative. In this case, the nurse should listen as much as time allows. The nurse should also try to steer the conversation back to the matter at hand and try to learn if the patient has any specific worries that can be cleared up.

An anxious patient tends not to talk and gives only the shortest possible answer to any question. It is important that the patient receive adequate reassurance from the nurse, both in manner and words. The staff should make sure that anxious patients are informed about their procedure and the reasons for it, even if they have heard the explanation before. The nurse's manner should show that the nurse is both competent and confident, that the procedure is routine, and that all possible care will be taken. Very nervous or anxious patients may require an additional dose of conscious sedation, and after baseline vital signs are obtained, orders to administer may be obtained.

One of the best elixirs for patient confidence is a lab that is run by friendly, positive personnel. Patients get the impression that the staff is competent and that they like to work there. This allows them to relax enough to confidently place themselves in the hands of the staff for the duration of the procedure.

The staff should try to see the procedure and the cath lab from the patients' perspective. They have just entered a room that looks like something out of a science fiction movie. Someone is about to remove their last article of clothing, shave and disinfect the most intimate part of their body, and start playing around with the inside of their heart. It is natural that patients will be apprehensive. Tell them something funny about the CCL, or about one of the staff members, to make it feel less threatening. This will help the patient see that the staff members are normal people, too, and they are there to help.

Pleasant music playing quietly in the background will also help put most patients at ease and give them something to listen to during a long procedure. A wide selection of music should be available to cater to each patient's taste.

The circulator is usually responsible for positioning the patient on the table. Each table and X-ray setup has a different optimal position for the patient, but because most tables can be freely moved by the operator, the important thing to check is that the patient is centered and close enough to the cranial end of the table to allow filming of the groin should problems arise during sheath insertion.

The concepts of neutral body alignment and positioning are helpful in decreasing the patient's discomfort from lying on a cold, hard table for an extended period of time. Start at the patients head. Support the back of the neck with a pillow, and perhaps place a towel at the nape to support the head, neck, and shoulders. This will decrease the incidence of shoulder spasms. Then look at the space at the back of the knee. If the knee is allowed to hyperflex, the stress of this unsupported position will lead to strain on the hamstrings, then to the gluteals, then to the lower back. This back pain can be decreased with the simple addition of a soft towel or blanket placed under the back of the knees, separating the patient's feet a few inches. As the patients' body is aligned in a neutral pose, the overall result is a more relaxed body to work with and a decrease in anxiety and the need for additional pain medication. If the nurse noticed that the patient walked with a limp or saw in the notes that he or she has back or hip problems, some form of special support may be necessary. The procedure tables are quite hard and must be narrow to allow free movement of the X-ray tubes. Remember, the patient must lie relatively still for over an hour; a small bit of comfort can make a big difference in how the procedure is experienced.

The circulator should check that the patient has a working IV line. If not, it should be explained to the patient that IV access is necessary should an emergency arise, and a cannula should be inserted. If the patient has no line because he or she has been rushed in as an emergency, the circulator can insert one if qualified to do so. Alternatively, the physician may choose to insert a venous sheath in the groin for access if needed. IV fluids may be necessary to maintain hydration unless the patient has a history of CHF or pulmonary edema.

During the preprocedure evaluation, diabetic patients should have blood glucose levels measured. If the blood sugar readings are over 200, one unit per 50 points of short-acting insulin should be given. If hypoglycemia is evident, an IV infusion of D5W may be warranted. If a sudden change in consciousness occurs, then D50 should be administered intravenously. If the schedule of the day delays the procedure, then blood glucose levels should be repeated prior to procedure.

The patient's medication, and when they were last taken, should be reviewed with the patient and discussed with the physician if anticoagulation or antihypertensives are taken regularly.

The patient should also be asked if they have ever had allergic reactions to anything, particularly to shellfish, because shellfish contains iodine as does the contrast medium. The patient should be asked this even if it is written in their notes that they have no allergies.

If the patient is receiving nasal oxygen, it is good to use an oxygen-saturation monitor. It may even be necessary for the patient to be monitored for the duration of the procedure if the saturation levels are not constant. In most institutions, conscious sedation requires the administration of oxygen and pulse oximetry monitoring during the procedure.

Catheterization laboratories are cold places; they have to be to prevent overheating of the X-ray equipment. The patient, who is almost naked on the table, feels this more than the staff does. The circulator should have a warming cupboard filled with sheets to offer the patient some warmth until the procedure is over.

During the preparation time, the scrub and circulator work together to get the patient to the point at which the procedure itself can begin. It is a good time to talk to the patient, to determine what they know about the procedure, to answer any outstanding questions, and to set them at ease. This is also a good time to prepare patients for the procedure in other ways. They should be told that during most of the procedure they will have to keep their hands behind their head. The nurse should find out if this is problematic for any reason.

During the procedure, and particularly during filming, patients should move as little as possible. As long as patients remain still, the only movements that are displayed are those necessary to breathe and those of the beating heart. The physician will prompt patients to breathe in deeply and then hold their breath for filming. The staff should tell patients about this at the start so they will be ready. The nurse should also explain to patients how to tell when filming is finished so they can breathe normally again. Taking a moment to explain to patients that a clearer picture will be obtained if the diaphragm is outside the frame encourages their cooperation.

During a normal shift in which staff may prepare as many as eight patients, it may be difficult, if not impossible, to approach each one with enthusiasm, explaining everything as if it were the first time. However, nothing is worse than subjecting the patient to a boring drone of information that has obviously been churned out the same way for years. That is where rotation of the jobs within the laboratory is important. The empathy and compassion that are so useful on the nursing unit are also the foundations of effective communication in the CCL.

ECG Electrodes

Although some labs place a full set of 12 leads, for the majority of interventions this is unnecessary, and the electrodes themselves often get in the way of a clear X-ray picture. Four electrodes should be placed on a relatively hairless (for better contact and for painless removal) and muscular (for optimal signal transmission) part of the body. In some cases, this area will have to be shaved, and in others, it will have to be cleaned with benzene to ensure effective electrode adhesion, because they tend not to stick well to fatty or dirty skin. The electrodes can be safely placed on the calf or thigh muscles, and on the shoulders or upper arms. Carbon cables, which do not show up under X-ray, can be helpful.

Once the ECG is connected and running, the nurse should check it before leaving the patient's side. The nurse should answer the following questions:

Are the connections good?
Is it as expected in terms of extra systoles and wave forms?
What is the heart rate?
Does the patient need comforting or additional medication?

At this point, a baseline recording of the ECG should be made.

Puncture Site

The area around the puncture site is to be shaved, disinfected, anaesthetized, and then punctured. Explain these steps to the patient before beginning.

The size of the area to be shaved depends on lab protocol and the choice of site, but a radius of at least 5 cm from the intended point of insertion is considered to be the minimum in terms of antisepsis. A much larger area is required if the sheath will be covered by plastic foil immediately after the procedure and removed later in the nursing unit. This will prevent the painful tearing out of the hair when the foil is removed. In some labs, the entire genital area is shaved to the knees, but this is usually restricted to high-risk patients because it adds otherwise unnecessary discomfort for the patient afterward.

In some high-risk cases, both sides may be prepped in case an intra-aortic balloon pump is needed.

The disinfection begins where the puncture site will be, and spirals outwards with a minimum of overlap. This is done twice with Betadine, and then the area is wiped off with a third swab. Some centers use prep sticks that do not require drying.

When the puncture site has been prepared, the scrub takes the sterile drape from the table, and places it over the patient with the opening in the center of the cleaned area. With one hand holding the drape in place, the other hand spreads out the rest of the drape with the help of the circulator.

The table controls and the lead shield should be covered with plastic covers. In some labs, the X-ray tubes are also covered.

The manifold is then plugged in, flushed, and zeroed. Manifolds usually have two or three ports. A three-port manifold has one port for pressure measurement, one for contrast medium, and one for heparinized saline. This setup makes it easy to flush the manifold. All the air must be taken out of the lines and replaced with saline at the beginning of the procedure and kept that way.

As the draping continues, X-ray tubes will be brought into position. They can be quite intimidating from the patient perspective, so taking a moment to explain the need for "close-up" pictures can do much to decrease any anxiety patients may feel from having such a big piece of machinery over their body.

PROCEDURE

When the physician arrives, he or she is assisted into the gown and gloves as necessary. The doctor will inject a local anesthetic into the area around the intended puncture site and give it a few minutes to begin working. The physician will then make the arterial puncture. There are a few cardiac catheter laboratories in which this task is performed by the nursing staff, but it is usually considered to be the physician's domain. See Chapter 11 for more details on puncture site access.

When the artery has been punctured, the wire is fed through the needle into the artery and the needle is removed. The sheath is then fed over the wire, placed into the artery, and the introducer (the internal part of the sheath) is removed. The wire may then be removed, first making sure that the sheath is firmly in place. Some operators prefer to leave the wire in place for catheter insertion.

When the wire is removed from the patient, it must be wiped and rolled together. The scrub nurse should use a wet swab in the left hand, squeezing it around the wire to assure a good wire wipe. Pulling the wire out at a steady pace using the right hand, the scrub nurse wraps it around on itself three or four times.

The flushing, wiping, and rolling that was performed when the catheters and the wires were first taken from their package is repeated every time they are removed from the patient. This should be done carefully and slowly to minimize the potential for spattering blood. Most splashes are caused by something that could have been prevented (distractions, hurrying, etc.). The scrub nurse should be aware of what he or she is doing, be methodical, and wear personal protection.

Guiding catheters are flushed in the same manner, with care being taken not to kink or bend them. Be aware of side holes when inserting guiding catheters into the sheath. It is good practice to aim the side holes away or cover them with something until they are inside the sheath.

The following must be monitored more or less continuously during the procedure:

- Blood pressure
- ECG
- Oxygen saturation
- Contrast medium
- Heparinized saline
- Patient
- Run of the procedure

All of these components are the combined responsibility of all members of the CCL staff. A good team will work as a unit, not only acting on these monitored signals, but also anticipating any changes in the patient's condition before they occur.

Blood Pressure

After the diagnostic catheter has been placed in the aorta and the proximal end connected to the manifold, a pressure tracing and digitalized values of the systolic, diastolic, and mean pressures will appear on the monitor. This value should immediately be checked and treated as one would treat any blood pressure measurement. If it is too low, it may indicate a vasovagal reaction, or a technical problem such as a loose connection. Once possible technical sources of the problem have been ruled out, the staff should ask the patient if he or she is feeling faint or nauseated. An injection of atropine, administration of IV fluids, or both may be warranted.

A low pressure may also be due to the patient being dehydrated. A patient who has been fasting since the previous evening and does not come onto the table until the afternoon will most probably be dehydrated, especially if it is a warm day. This can be corrected promptly with a saline or glucose and saline solution. This hypovolemia can be a great hindrance in invasive cardiology, because it can make it difficult to access the artery and can even be responsible for acute artery closures.

If an unusually high blood pressure is seen, ask the patient what his or her pressure normally is and if he or she has taken any medication that morning. Administration of a drug such as nifedipine or nitroglycerine may be necessary.

Hypertension may also indicate that the patient is anxious or nervous. If so, soothing talk may be enough to bring the pressure down. As time is usually of the essence once the patient's artery has been punctured, some form of sedative may be administered for a quicker and more certain result.

High blood pressure can also be an indicator of pain. This can be dealt with relative to the source of the pain. If it is the groin, more local anesthetic can be injected. For lower back pain, the patient's position and supports can be adjusted. If the pain has a cardiac source, it can be dealt with pharmacologically with some sort of analgesia.

Another cause of a high or low blood pressure reading is a full bladder. Contrast media is usually metabolized efficiently, and this, added to an IV infusion that may be running, can mean that the patient's bladder can fill quite quickly. A bedpan or bottle can usually be put in place without much difficulty, and the procedure can continue. If this fails to work, and the procedure still has quite awhile to run, a transuretheral catheter may have to be inserted.

A break in the pressure signal usually means that the doctor or assistant has disengaged the system, probably to inject contrast. It is also pos-

sible that a connection in the system has become loose. It is important for the staff to be familiar with the system, from catheter to the computer monitor, to isolate such problems should they arise.

ECG

The ECG should be monitored continuously during the procedure. Extra systolic beats can be expected when a catheter makes contact with the heart muscle, especially when entering the ventricle. Extra systoles occurring without manual stimulation should be recorded when possible and brought to the attention of the physician.

If the ECG suddenly goes flat, there are two possible explanations. The first is that the patient is in asystole. The pressure curve should be checked immediately. If the pressure reading is continuing normally and the patient is displaying signs of life, then you can assume that the problem lies within the ECG system rather than the patient. In most cases, the problem will be due to one or more of the ECG electrodes or leads becoming disengaged. Each one should be checked and replaced as necessary. Faulty connections or old cables can also be responsible for a break in the ECG signal. The staff should be familiar with the ECG's workings, from the electrodes to the computer monitor, and spare leads and connectors should always be on hand.

Cardiac catheterization cannot be safely carried out without a reliable, continuously monitored ECG. If a fault cannot be remedied with the staff and equipment at hand, another ECG monitor, even that in the defibrillator, can be used until that procedure is finished and a technician can repair it.

A shaky ECG can be due to the patient shivering. If the patient is cold, the nurse can place a prewarmed sheet under the one he or she is covered with or cover the arms with one. The electrodes can also be placed over muscles less susceptible to shivering.

Contrast Medium

There are two main methods of using the contrast medium. The first is the "open" system in which a bowl containing the liquid is placed on the table. The scrub nurse fills a syringe with this liquid and then connects it to the catheter, either directly or through a three-way tap or manifold bank. In a "closed" system, the bottle of contrast is connected to the three-way tap or manifold bank by an infusion line. The assistant can fill the syringe and inject it by simply turning the tap. The closed system cuts down on bubbles and makes it easier to estimate the amount of contrast that has been used during a procedure. It is important, though, that the bottle of contrast is changed before it is empty, otherwise air will be drawn into the line and may cause air emboli.

It is becoming more common for angiography contrast medium injections to be performed by a power injector. These ensure that the amount of contrast given is of a constant pressure and volume. The power injector can also be connected to the protocol, so that every injection is automatically recorded, and the total calculated.

To inject contrast medium during ventriculography and aortography, a power injector is always used. The scrub nurse should ensure that the syringe and line from the power injector are completely free of air. A tap with the knuckles or an instrument on the connection while it is held vertically, syringe end upwards, should be enough to dislodge and reveal any bubbles caught there. A small amount of contrast should be released while the line is being connected to the catheter, also to prevent bubble formation. During injection, the head of the power injector syringe is positioned downward so that any small bubbles that may be present in the syringe are kept away from the exit and will not be injected.

The scrub nurse should make sure the tubing is properly connected to the pigtail catheter before the ventriculogram is performed. That quantity of contrast medium can cover a great deal of

the lab in a very few seconds if the connection is not tight.

Before the injection, patients should be told that they will be experiencing warmth all over their body and that this sensation (caused by contrast medium being squirted into one of the chambers of the heart) will pass very quickly.

The circulating nurse should ask the doctor before each injection if the volume and speed are correct for that patient. When all is ready, the circulator should stand where the monitors are easily visible, but as far as possible from the X-ray tubes to lessen radiation exposure during filming. The pump should be fired shortly after filming has begun. If the filming stops suddenly due to some technical problem, stop the injection immediately.

The staff should be familiar with the power injector's settings and operation to make problem isolation more efficient if it does not function correctly. It is important to know where to begin when the machine will not work properly

Heparinized Saline

This solution is used throughout the procedure for many purposes. The catheters must be first flushed with it; gloves and the working area should be periodically cleaned with it to lessen the sticky effect of blood and contrast medium; contrast medium must be mixed with it in the inflator to blow up the balloon, and the catheters and the rest of the system must be periodically flushed to deter thrombus formation. It is a simple task to ensure that heparinized saline is always available to those working at the table.

The Patient

The circulator should talk to the patient as often as is practical (though preferably not during filming). Patients should be asked if they are in pain, if they are too hot or cold or uncomfortable, if they have any questions, or if they need to urinate. In addition to benefiting patients by relieving any discomfort they may have, this also helps to relax them and distract them from the procedure for a few minutes. Talking occasionally to the patient during the procedure has the added benefit of reminding the physician that the patient is actually present and taking part in it.

If the patient preparation has been thorough, there should be little that has to be done for him or her during a procedure of normal duration. If the procedure goes longer than expected, the staff will have to check the patient's well-being more frequently.

Run of Procedure

Watching the results of the angiogram is the best way to judge whether new material will be needed. If the diagnostic shows diseased vessels amendable to percutaneous intervention, the circulator can already begin to open the interventional material. Alternatively, healthy vessels should trigger a call to the ward for the next patient to be prepared.

PROCEDURE COMPLETION

Once the procedure is finished, it is up to the laboratory staff to get that patient off the table and the next patient onto it as quickly as possible. Just how this is best done is up to each team, and it depends a great deal on just how the various tasks are divided in the first place. Some rules, however, should be applied in every lab. The staff should always wear gloves while packing up the table and the room after each patient, and everyone should be aware of sharps. If the scrub nurse or physicians tend to leave needles or blades lying around, they should be told of the danger and the correct form of disposal should be pointed out.

At the end of the procedure, the physician should inform the patient of the results and display them on the monitor if this is warranted. The physician should also explain to the patient

what to expect for the next 24 hours or so. The staff can continue to clean up around them while this is going on, but they should do so in a manner that shows respect for the discussion.

If the sheath is not to be removed immediately following the procedure, the area should be cleaned with saline, dried, and covered with a sterile dressing. The nurse should inform the patient when the sheath will be removed and, in the meantime, which body parts can and cannot be moved. The nurse must make sure that the patient knows that it is very important to observe these motion restrictions and should explain to the patient what will happen if they are ignored. The patient can be responsible for observing signs of bleeding at the puncture site, such as wetness or stickiness between the legs. They should know to inform a staff member immediately if this occurs.

Before the patient leaves the CCL's observation area, they should be told how important it is to rehydrate to help flush the contrast media out of the body. Patients should drink as much as they can for the rest of the day and should urinate as soon as they experience any pressure on the bladder. They should also be informed of the possibility of chest pain over the next few hours and instructed to inform the nursing staff immediately.

The patient can be taught how to apply external pressure over the access site when they need to use the bathroom for the first 12 hours after the procedure. The patient should be told to refrain from driving for at least 72 hours.

Whenever practical, the nurse should shake the patient's hand and formally say good-bye as the patient leaves. Well-treated patients are satisfied customers.

SUGGESTED READING

Apple S, Lindsay J. *Principles and Practice of Interventional Cardiology.* Baltimore, MD; Lippincott Williams & Wilkins, 2000.

Baim DS. *Grossman's Cardiac Catheterization, Angiography, and Intervention*, 7th ed. Philadelphia: Lippincott Williams & Wilkins; 2006.

Fuster A, O'Rourke RA, Walsh R, et al. *Hurst's The Heart*, 12th ed. New York: McGraw-Hill; 2007.

Gibbons RJ, Chatterjee K, Daley J, et al. ACC/AHA/ACP-ASIM Guidelines for the Management of Patients with Chronic Stable Angina: a report of the American College of Cardiology/American Heart Association Task Force on practice guidelines (Committee on Management of Patients with Chronic Stable Angina). *J Am Coll Cardiol* 1999;33(7):2092–2197.

Kern MJ. *The Interventional Cardiac Catheterization Handbook*, 2nd ed. Philadelphia: Mosby; 2003.

King SB III, Yeung AC. *Interventional Cardiology*. New York: McGraw Hill; 2007.

Chapter 10

NURSING CARE OF THE INTERVENTIONAL CARDIAC PROCEDURE PATIENT

Marsha Holton, CCRN, RCIS, FSICP

First and foremost, everything a medical professional does is about the care of the patients. In order to give good patient care, the medical professional must be able to do a basic history and physical examination of the patients to identify what each specific patient needs. In order to get the information needed, the professional must develop good interviewing skills—then every patient, every skill, every piece of information gets well documented. Learn to practice and prioritize skills; become adept in the care of the interventional cardiac procedure patient.

PREADMISSION COMMUNICATION

It is easy to understand the fear and anxiety patients present with. The cath lab performs tests and interventions on their hearts, and any other vital organ that can be reached with a catheter. This is not something patients experience every day. In fact, it is likely something they would rather never experience at all. The best time to reassure, relax, and assess these patients is during introductions. First impressions really do count, especially with a worried patient.

Some institutions have a system whereby the patient is interviewed before he or she actually comes into the hospital for the procedure. It is not unusual for a staff member to call patients' homes and introduce themselves as part of the team who will be taking care of them during their tests. This time is well spent, both for information gathering (using the institutions' forms for data collection) and for providing the patient a chance to talk to someone about their concerns and physical needs. This is also the best time to ask what medications patients are taking because they have all of them at hand. Occasionally this vital piece of the history is incomplete simply because patients forget to bring a complete list of all their medications with them on admission.

Even if a preprocedure telephone call is made, patients should receive any necessary information in a written format. This information will vary among institutions and doctors, but it will include the following:

- The name of the procedure
- The date of the procedure
- What time they are supposed to arrive
- Where they are supposed to go in the hospital to be admitted for the procedure
- How long they can expect to be in the hospital

Patients should be informed not to eat or drink after midnight the evening before the test. They should, however, drink plenty of fluids up until bedtime. On the morning of the procedure, they should drink just enough water needed to take any medications. The patients should be informed which medications they may have and which they are not permitted to take that morning. This is especially important for diabetics, and care must be taken to ensure that the physician's orders concerning all medications taken preoperatively are followed.

Patients will not be allowed to drive themselves home afterward because most procedures are performed using the artery in the right groin, and driving increases the chance of bleeding from that incision. They should, therefore, arrange for transport from the hospital after the procedure has been completed.

PREPROCEDURE ASSESSMENT AND CARE

Each hospital has its own history and physical forms for patient admissions. The staff should look over their institution's format and learn to organize their thinking to follow it systematically. As simple as this sounds, it is a timesaving organizational skill that will reduce the possibility of missing important information. How to physically assess the patient, what questions to ask, and how to document and relay the pertinent information will all become second nature with practice. The trick is to assess each patient the

same way, every time; this decreases the chance of forgetting to ask a question or perform an assessment.

BASIC PREPROCEDURAL WORK-UP

As you learn to organize your unit area, these items can be organized into a small tray, trolley, or bag. When the patient has changed into his or hospital gown and has settled his or her belongings, equipment can be brought to the bedside to begin the work-up.

The necessary equipment includes the following:

- Patient history and physical assessment forms.
- Patient-informed consent forms for the procedure and, if needed, conscious sedation and anesthesia forms.
- Requisition forms for a chest X-ray, ECG, and any other preprocedural tests.
- All information required by the institution for a cardiac admission, such as the physician order for the examination, and the personal and insurance demographics for the record.
- An IV tray, complete with all tubing, solutions, and dressings.
- Laboratory tubes for complete blood count, blood chemistry, coagulopathy, urinalysis, and blood bank for type and screen.
- A sphygmomanometer, penlight, and thermometer.
- A razor to shave areas needed for electrodes, cannula placement, and the groin
- A security envelope for the patient's valuables.
- A key or system to secure the patient's clothes.

The order in which the work-up is carried out is up to each nurse. If time is short, it may be better to place the venous cannula and draw blood first so that the results will be available before the patient goes to the lab.

Another advantage to inserting the cannula after the vital signs are taken is that this time can also be used to talk to the patient, assessing the anxiety level and obtaining information for the history form. However, many prefer to begin with the history and other questions. They prefer to begin softly and work up to the physical assessment and cannula insertion.

The following breakdown of the preprocedural work-up follows the latter method, which assumes that time and staffing are optimal.

INITIAL CONTACT

After the patient has been received on the unit, he or she is instructed to change from his or her clothes into a hospital gown, and all personal belongings should be secured in a locker.

The patient is allowed to void, and if female, the decision will be made as to whether a pregnancy test is done at that time. All females who may be pregnant must be cleared before the procedure.

After voiding, height and weight are measured and recorded.

Patient History

A good assessment always begins with the same questions. Ask patients why they are in the hospital and what, specifically, is their chief complaint. These simple questions can focus patients and tune the staff into the problems that might surface during the procedure. It also reassures patients that the staff are on the same page with them. This is where trust is established between the cath lab staff and patients, so make a point of really listening to each patient's answers. Pay attention, not just to the words, but also to the underlying feelings that are also being communicated.

Chief Complaint

What is wrong? Why is the patient in the hospital? The reasons can range from chest pain to positive noninvasive diagnostic results such as stress tests, dizzy spells, decreasing stamina, or preoperative clearance for a surgical procedure. Once the chief complaint is identified, find out how long any complaints have persisted.

The patient who failed a stress test may have no pain to report, but is just as potentially unstable as the patient who had a recent heart attack. The timing of symptoms, severity of symptoms, and any activities that trigger the symptoms should be included in the opening area of the forms.

Allergies

Allergies are noted and highlighted. It is good practice to inform the patient that he or she will be questioned many times during the hospital stay about known allergies. This repetition allows all staff members to reinforce that vital piece of information before any medications are given.

Medication

List every drug—even the alternative or complementary vitamins and teas that the patient takes. Some herbal teas have potent stimulants or sedatives; some even interfere with normal clotting mechanisms. Many patients take a myriad of medications—some prescribed, some bought at health-store kiosks. A complete medicine history is vital.

Medical History

Ask about previous hospitalizations and any current medical problems including asthma, emphysema, diabetes mellitus, hypertension, cholesterol elevations, kidney problems, diagnosis of renal insufficiency, and gastrointestinal problems such as ulcers or history of hepatitis. As the nurse proceeds to the head-to-toe assessment, he or she should tie in the specific history to the specific system.

Family History

If there is a history of cardiac disease of any blood relative before the age of 60, this should be noted. When documenting, note who had the disease and what it was. All other medical family history is noted as well; however, the history of early cardiac disease should be most pertinent.

Social History

Ask how much alcohol the patient drinks and if he or she has a smoking history or a high-risk lifestyle. High-risk lifestyles include drug use and abuse and activities that raise the risk of HIV or hepatitis infection. Learn to ask these sensitive questions with the same manner as any other medical question. The answers are important to patient care.

Prioritize

The patient history is obtained systematically unless the patient comes directly to the cath lab, as is the case with patients having a myocardial infarction. Then, of course, all forms and paperwork are secondary to getting the patient onto the cardiac catheterization table.

Physical Assessment

Take the patient's temperature, blood pressure, pulse, and respiration rate. This is the baseline—and the first safety net. Abnormal vital signs need to be reported and treated. This sounds basic, but that is why they are called "vital" signs; they reflect potential or actual hemodynamic instability.

Neurological Assessment

Throughout the interview, watch the patient's face and listen to his or her speech. Ask him or her to frown, smile, stick out the tongue, and swallow. Check for pupil reactions and accommodation with the penlight. Ask the patient to move each extremity, noting if movement and strength are equal. Specifically, ask if the patient has a history of transient ischemic attack (TIA), cerebral vascular assault (CVA), or dizzy spells. An example of neurological charting would be:

> NEURO: Awake, alert, and oriented ×3. Cranial nerves II–XII grossly intact. Moves all extremities equally. Afebrile. No history of dizzy spells, TIAs, or CVAs. Occasional headache, relieved with aspirin.

Cardiovascular Assessment

Look at the patient's skin; feel and note the temperature and whether it is dry or moist. Normal is pink, warm, and dry. Locate and mark all pulses according to the documentation forms, noting the strength. This is usually graded 1+ (thready), 2+ (normal), and 3+ (visible pulsations). Marking these down will provide a quickly accessed baseline for the postprocedure observations.

Listen to the heart sounds, noting any unusual rhythms or sounds. Normal heart sounds are crisp S1 and S2, or the lub-dub, lub-dub. Listen just for the rhythm and then note any unusual sounds. Clicks sound like clicks; murmurs sound like whooshing or rumbling, and rubs can be heard either in the pericardial or pleural spaces. A rub sounds much like rubbing a few hair strands together back and forth over the ear. That scratchy sound heard over the heartbeat is indicative of pericarditis. It is the sound the body makes when the pleural layers are irritated. Patients with myocardial infarctions can develop a pericardial rub 2–3 days post attack. It is a painful condition, needing medication for relief.

The heart valves are auscultated independently: aortic—pulmonic, tricuspid—mitral. The sounds of murmurs and the timing of the murmurs (when they were heard) during systole or diastole are important diagnostic tools used to assess the status and integrity of the valves. The skill of locating and describing heart sounds becomes second nature with practice.

Take the time to find someone who is good at teaching this and learn from that source. Do not be intimidated by learning heart sounds. The body is full of noises; the fun comes in being able to diagnose from the sound and then get appropriate treatment and relief for the patient.

Repeat the history your patient gave you during your physical examination. Note again any pertinent cardiac history, both the patient's and the family cardiac history. An example of cardiovascular charting is:

> CARDIO: Normal heart sounds, no murmurs, rubs, or clicks. All pulses, radials, pedals, and posterior tibial are present and are Graded 2+. BP is 130/70, HR 77, RR 16, and regular. Skin is warm, pink, and dry. Both mother and maternal grandfather have history of heart attacks at age 50 and 57. No chest pain at present. Presents to the CCL for pre-op work-up for elective surgery next week.

Respiratory Assessment

The lungs have five lobes, three on the right, and two on the left. Listen to all five fields, noting equal and normally decreasing breath sounds top to bottom. Note any use of oxygen and any pulmonary history pertinent to the patient. Adventitious or extra sounds are always abnormal, and the crackles of air popping through fluid in the lungs are not to be overlooked once heard. Fluid-filled lungs can be differentiated from "smokers' lungs" by asking the patient to cough strongly a few times. If the sound is generated from "junk" from smoking, the rales or crackles will diminish after coughing.

The fluid that builds up in the lungs when the heart is not pumping effectively will not clear and will increase as the heart weakens. That is

why it is called *congestive heart failure*. The heart is failing, and it can decompensate quickly. Document the level of the rales from the base of the lungs to the top. The lungs fill up from the bottom because of gravity. This is why people with failure have coughing spells at night after they lie down, because the fluid spreads all through the lung fields. These spells are called paroxysmal nocturnal dyspnea because the coughing spells happen sporadically and at night. An example of respiratory assessment is:

> RESP: Bilateral breath sounds are heard over all lung fields. No rales or wheezing noted. No oxygen needed at this time. No history of asthma; however, did smoke 20–30 cigarettes daily for 10 years. Quit smoking 15 years ago.

Renal Assessment

Ask about a history of repeated urinary infections, kidney stones, or other abnormal problems. Some patients have only one kidney, having lost the other to trauma, cancer, or birth defect. These patients have less reserve than patients with two normal kidneys do, and because kidneys metabolize the X-ray contrast, this history is vital. An example of urinary assessment is:

> RENAL: BUN and creatinine are within normal limits, urinalysis is within normal limits. Patient is postmenopausal, and pregnancy test not done. No history of kidney stones or frequent urinary infections.

Gastrointestinal Assessment

Evaluating this system involves questions about ulcers and bleeding; liver disorders or history of hepatitis; pancreatic disorders (specifically diabetes mellitus); and any history of colon disease, bleeding, or cancers. The normal stomach and abdomen should be soft, not distended, and the bowel sounds should be audible over all four quadrants. Ask about bowel habits, noting any unusual diarrhea or constipation history, such as seen in patients with colitis. Ask also about eating and drinking habits, noting anything unusual. A normal example follows:

> GI: Abdomen is soft and nontender. Bowel sounds are present in all quadrants. No history of colitis, ulcers, or bleeding. Normal bowel movements, usually once daily. Family history is positive for adult-onset diabetes, mother. Social drinking only 1–2 glasses red wine daily.

Importance of Assessment

Taking a complete patient history and assessment is important. Many patients have been saved from unnecessary cardiac catheterization or potentially disastrous tests by accurate and thorough history taking. With experience, assessment skills become streamlined, and a comprehensive history and physical assessment can be performed within 30 minutes.

VENOUS CANNULATION

The venous cannula is usually placed in the left forearm if access can be obtained there. This is because it is easier to administer medications without being in the way of the cardiologist who routinely works from the right femoral assess. The right arm, or the back of either hand can be used, but extension tubing may be needed to facilitate IV administration. Mark the date and size of the cannula. Because many cardiac patients also have some level of vascular disease, venous access may be difficult.

The basic principles of cannula insertion apply here: The nurse should not insert a cannula into an arm if the patient has had a mastectomy on that side. For that matter, blood pressures are not done on that arm for the same reason. Severe lymphadema may result; a painful and avoidable complication from decreased lymph drainage after surgery.

Do not insert or obtain blood pressures on any arm that has a dialysis access placed, because the access can be damaged from those procedures, and blood flow altered.

Every person has a day when he or she just cannot get the vessel. Most of the time there is another person who can lend a hand and get access for you. Be considerate of the patient. In the rare cases where no venous access can be obtained, notify the lab staff. It is possible to obtain venous access in the groin when the patient is on the table. Again extension tubing may be needed, and after the procedure, the need for peripheral IVs will have to be addressed again for the recovery of the patient.

BLOOD TESTS

Blood tests include, but are not limited to, the following. Remember that all lab tests are absolutely useless if the blood tubes do not get to the lab to be run, and the results are not available before the procedure begins.

Complete Blood Count

The complete blood count (CBC), including a differential white blood count, is necessary to identify and establish baseline hematology. More than one patient has been saved from an unsafe catheter procedure when the admission CBC indicated that the patient had severe anemia or an infection. The platelet count is also necessary because antiplatelet drugs are routinely administered. A special note is made here as to the increase of heparin-induced thrombocytopenia. This complication is rare but can be deadly. Be alert for patients who have been on a heparin infusion for 24 hours; their platelet count drops by more than 50%. The standard procedure is for all patients who are on intravenous antiplatelet therapy to have repeat CBCs drawn every 6 hours to monitor for changes.

Chemistry

This must include a basic electrolyte panel, blood urea nitrogen (BUN), and creatinine. Lipid profiles, cardiac enzymes, and markers are occasionally included in admission blood tests. The body basically has three systems:, chemical, electrical, and mechanical. Chemistry makes electricity, which makes a mechanical event or electrolytes create a charge that is passed cell to cell; those charges work together to make a heartbeat, trigger a response. This is why the chemistry panel is necessary. Any deviation from a normal level changes the electricity in the body. Because small variances in these electrolytes can cause arrhythmias, they can be life threatening.

Coagulopathy

Coagulopathy tests include the PT/INR, PTT, or both. If the PT/INR is elevated, the procedure may be postponed to decrease the potential of postprocedural bleeding. Patients with mechanical valves or atrial fibrillation who are taking warfarin are in this high-risk group. Rechecking these values pre-op may save the patient from a serious complication.

Blood Bank

Not every institution has a type and screen drawn preprocedure. However, it is very useful in case the patient requires a transfusion or an emergency operation.

COMPLICATIONS

Complications are rarely encountered during patient preparation, but it is important to be ready in the event that they occur. The following are the most commonly encountered problems and the most appropriate interventions to rectify them.

Vasovagal Reactions

The body occasionally overreacts to changes in the blood vessels. In some patients, when a needle is inserted into a vessel, vein, or artery, the body acknowledges only that the blood flow has been changed and responds with a vasodilatation of the entire body's vascular system. This translates to a drop in blood pressure, then a drop in heart rate and the "faraway stare" these patients get, usually just before they pass out, throw up, or both.

A bolus of normal saline, and occasionally a dose of atropine, to block the vagus nerve is needed. The body responds quickly to these measures.

If the patient has a vagal reaction to cannula insertion, make sure that the lab staff are notified that this reaction occurred, because it might also happen when they insert the arterial sheath.

Vasovagal reactions are a common occurrence. Patients are dry (having been NPO all night) and usually a bit anxious (especially about being stuck with needles); some are sensitive to manipulation of their baroreceptors. These baroreceptors are areas within the body that autoregulate the vasoconstriction and vasodilatation of blood vessels according to changes in blood flow.

The staff prepare for these occurrences by having an organized approach to patient admission—by making up the admission tray in advance and keeping each tray restocked for the next person. Nothing is worse than reaching for a bottle of IV fluids to run wide open when the patient has a sudden drop in BP, only to find that the person before took the last one and did not replace it. This is a why being part of a good team and working together is vital to maintain a safe environment for both the patients and the staff. What healthcare providers do is take care of patient needs; what excellent healthcare providers do is work together to provide the best patient care available.

POSTPROCEDURE ASSESSMENT AND CARE

The postprocedure assessment begins with patient teaching. Make sure that the patient knows in what ways—and for how long—his or her mobility is restricted. Instruct the patient to tell his or her nurse immediately if he or she has increased pain in the groin or if he or she feels anything warm or wet at the insertion site. Instruct the patient to let the nurse know immediately if he or she experiences chest pain or becomes short of breath. The patient is the best source of this information, so bring him or her into the team, and give the patient the responsibility of calling when help is needed. This inclusion will reassure everyone that the goal is good patient care.

As soon as the patient arrives on the ward after the procedure, he or she needs to have another quick head-to-toe assessment. The assessment does not have to go into to the depth of the preprocedural assessment, but a quick, 90-second, head-to-toe evaluation is vital to establish a baseline before the patient is settled in again. Things do change in the procedure lab.

The post-op instructions now focus on keeping the access site free from complications and notifying the staff immediately if chest pain, nausea, or dizziness occurs.

The patient should know about the importance of keeping his or her head on the pillow and not bending the leg where vascular access was performed. Both of these restrictions decrease the chance of bleeding at the site postoperatively. Additional positional restrictions include keeping the patient supine and not raising the head of the bed more than 30°. Care is needed to decrease the potential trauma caused by increasing pressure at the groin site.

Post-op ECGs are standard for all patients after an intervention and usually unnecessary for those undergoing diagnostic studies. Usually all patients are monitored during recovery with consideration for the administration of any drugs used in conscious sedation; supplemental oxygen may be administered.

The minimum basic neurovascular and vital sign monitoring may include visual and palpable inspection of the access site and distal pulse. These are done in conjunction with the vital signs, which are taken every 15 minutes $\times$ 4, every 30 minutes $\times$ 2, then every hour $\times$ 2. The frequency of recording of vital signs depends on the invasive or interventional procedure.

Puncture Site Assessment

This first assessment should include the size and location of all arterial and venous access sites and a notation if any closure devices were deployed or attempted. Note the character of the site(s); any hematoma, swelling, or oozing. Check the patient's chart to see whether any medications have been ordered, and if there are any special tests that have to be done while the patient is on bed rest.

Look at the puncture site; touch it and ask how it feels. The site should be soft, relatively nontender, and, though there may be some normal tenderness, it should not be extreme. Remember the vascular plexus contains nerves, arteries, and veins, all in close proximity, so if a single vessel is damaged, there might be pressure on the nerve or bleeding at the site.

Any swelling is abnormal. Arterial bleeds may be external with pulsatile flow or internal into the site; a hematoma can grow very quickly from an arterial bleed. Managing access complications quickly is a learned skill.

It is important to know where the femoral artery and pulse can be palpated. To practice, a nurse can find the pulse on her- or himself. She or he can lie down; palpate the hipbone and pubic bone. The inguinal ligament is the rubber band-like tissue that connects the two points. The femoral pulse can be felt between these two bones.

The puncture site on the skin is about one fingerbreadth below the actual vascular puncture. Thus, if the nurse places one finger over the skin opening, the adjacent finger is then over the arterial puncture. Then, simply compress until the distal pulse is obliterated. The need for occlusive pressure is different for each patient, but averages only a few minutes, and then the pressure is lessened slightly to allow for the hemostatic process to begin. The complete hemostasis process can take 10–20 minutes, depending on the procedure and the patient condition. The management of access sites is a learned competency, and one learned with direct teaching and mentoring.

Pseudoaneurysm

The arterial puncture weakens the vessel wall, and blood can sometimes flow between layers of the wall, making a blood-filled pouch. This complication, which presents as a large, pulsatile mass, can be identified by palpation. When listening to the site with a stethoscope, a bruit may be heard, similar in sound to an arterio-venous graft seen in dialysis patients. The definitive diagnosis of a pseudoaneurysm is made with a color Doppler ultrasound. It is treated with Doppler-guided compression; surgical vascular repair is rarely necessary.

Retroperitoneal Bleed

This complication is caused by blood flowing from the arterial puncture into the body's cavities and is potentially life threatening. The diagnosis is usually made clinically; the patient becomes unstable with decreased blood pressure and an increased heart rate, a pasty color, and pain at the site, back, or rectum. This rectal pain is triggered by the pressure of the blood on the colon, giving the feeling of having to move the bowels. An emergency CT scan of the abdomen will make the definite diagnosis of a bleed.

The retroperitoneal bleed can result from a stick too high to be compressed or a stick that went right through the artery into the underlying tissue. If the patient has had anticoagulation or any combination of antiplatelet medication, the bleed can be potentiated.

Treatment of this life-threatening complication depends on the availability of the interventionalist to bring the patient back to the lab for access on the contralateral groin and the placement of a covered stent over the bleeding puncture site. If it is treated surgically, the patient should be transfused to maintain hemodynamic stability.

Embolus

A thrombus is a solid, fixed clot; an embolus is a moving clot. Coronary emboli can be seen radiographically by the development of the "slow or no-flow" phenomena. Subjective indications are pain and altered hemodynamics. Radiological evidence of ischemia causing angina shows up as decreased TIMI flow. An embolus that has become dislodged by catheter manipulation will not necessarily find its way to the coronary system, but will seek the distal arterial branch that is most direct in the flow.

With that in mind, the need for documenting the pulses and neurological status pre-op becomes clear. In order to know if there has been a change, the patient's preprocedure neurovascular status must be known. TIAs are possible; cold feet are possible (though infrequent, less than 1:1000), but the nurse needs to be prepared to identify and compare patient status pre- and post-op.

Hydration

By the time the procedure is over, the patient will have been NPO for a long time; he or she will need both fluids and mouth care. Usually patients are kept NPO until the sheath is removed and the site recovered. Check if sips of water can be offered during this post-op time period. Your patient will be more comfortable if he or she can drink even small amounts of water. The X-ray contrast medium is an osmotic diuretic and will further dehydrate the patient; the best protection from contrast-induced nephrotoxity is good hydration.

Blood Tests

There may be repeat blood coagulation tests ordered, such as an activated clotting time, which identifies how long it takes until the blood clots. Usually, when the number is below 180 seconds, it is safe to remove the sheath. The nurse may also have to repeat fasting blood sugars and electrolytes; hematology may have to be repeated and compared to the preprocedure values.

Pain Management

Any patient who is in pain, or who fears that his pain will not be relieved, has hormone and endocrine systems that are on full alert. This starts biofeedback mechanisms, and the body regulatory force starts looking for the reason for the unease. Pain is a powerful mechanism; keep your patient comfortable to decrease the risk of this response.

Patient Anxiety

Anxiety is usually diminished postprocedure but if it is not, find out what the source of the anxiety is. It could be the patient needs pain medication or has just been told he or she needs surgery or has experienced a stressful morning and needs to rest. It could be a simple as the doctor just said something he or she did not understand. This is where an ability to evaluate and treat the nursing problems really benefits the patient. If patients have pain, treat it; if they are thirsty, give them a drink; if they are confused, explain things. Then,

they really need to rest. Do all the things that need to be done, and then let patients relax or sleep until the sheaths are removed.

DISCHARGE INSTRUCTIONS

These instructions should be clearly printed on a form in a language the patient can understand. It is advantageous to give this information to patients to read long before the actual discharge. In this way, they have a chance to ask any questions when the nurse goes over the form with them. The form should cover the issues discussed here.

Medication

List all new drugs that the patient must now take; note when and for how long they are to be taken. Potential side effects should be included with instructions for what patients should do if they notice any reactions.

Activity

Note when patients can bathe or shower after returning home. List any activity limitations, such as not lifting anything over 10 pounds for several days, and not driving themselves home. Note when patients can return to work and when they may resume sexual activity.

Things to Watch

Let patients know that occasionally the groin site may rebleed. Show them how to evaluate the site; how to look for swelling, pain, or overt bleeding; and where to compress the artery if it is bleeding. If there is a serious bleed, patients should know to call 911 so they can be attend to. The puncture site may also display signs of infection in the form of redness or pain at the site or, in more serious cases, a feeling of malaise or fever. Information should be given regarding what to do if this occurs. Usually a temperature over 100.2°F needs to be reported.

Chest Pain

Angina is frightening. If patients are sent home with antiangina medication, they should be taught how to use them and what to do if the medication does not reduce their symptoms.

SUMMARY

The care and assessment of CCL patients on the ward is as comprehensive and thorough as the care of any patient on any critical care unit. These patients present with the same basic needs as any other critical care patient: alterations in comfort, actual or potential alterations in hemodynamic status, anxiety, and lack of knowledge. As the nurse's assessment skills and interventional

practices become fine tuned, he or she will be comfortable in his or her ability to be a part of a team working at the cutting edge of modern patient care.

SUGGESTED READING

Lynn-McHale DJ, Carlson KK, eds. *AACN Procedure Manuel for Critical Care*, 4th ed. Philadelphia: WB Saunders; 2001.

Black JM, Matassarin-Jacobs E, eds. *Medical-Surgical Nursing: Clinical Management for Continuity of Care*, 5th ed. Philadelphia: WB Saunders; 1997.

Urban N, Greenlee KK, Krumberger J, Winkelman C. *Guidelines for Critical Care Nursing*. St. Louis, MO: Mosby; 1995.

Urden LD, Stacey KM, Lough ME. *Thelan's Critical Care Nursing, Diagnosis and Management*, 4th ed. St. Louis, MO: Mosby; 2002.

Chapter 11

DIAGNOSTIC CATHETERIZATION

Darren Powell, RCIS, FSICP
Carl F. Moxey, PhD

INTRODUCTION

A diagnostic cardiac catheterization procedure is made up of a left heart catheterization (LHC), a right heart catheterization (RHC), or both. In many cases, an interventional procedure follows immediately afterward.

In RHC, the right heart and pulmonary system are accessed via the body's venous system, usually through the femoral vein. In the 1970s, Drs. Swan and Ganz developed the catheter that bears their names, the Swan-Ganz catheter. It facilitates passage through the anatomy of the right side of the heart by balloon flotation and is today the most commonly used diagnostic pressure and volume measurement catheter. An RHC usually entails just pressure measurements, but cardiac and pulmonary structures can also be visualized by using angiography.

An LHC is accomplished by accessing the arterial system and navigating in a retrograde fashion to the heart. An LHC is used to visualize

the coronary arteries and the pumping action of the left ventricle (LV). The primary indications for LHC include defining the presence of flow-limiting coronary atherosclerosis and evaluating LV function.

The practical application of coronary angiography was developed in the late 1950s by Dr. F. Mason Sones, a pediatric cardiologist at the Cleveland Clinic Foundation. He used a surgical cutdown technique to directly expose and access the brachial artery. This procedure became known as the Sones technique. Dr. Sones used a single, side-hole woven-Dacron catheter for selective right and left coronary arteriography, as well as left ventriculography. Today, the most commonly used technique for percutaneous vascular access is called the Seldinger technique. It uses a needle, a wire, and a sheath. It is named after Dr. Sven Seldinger, a Swedish radiologist.

Coronary angiography was refined by Dr. Melvin Judkins, a radiologist from Portland, Oregon, in the early 1960s. He invented the Judkins curves for femoral access coronary angiography commonly in use today. Using a heat gun or boiling water, Dr. Judkins bent and shaped catheters around copper pipes to get smooth curves. Two of Dr. Judkin's basic catheter curves, the Judkins left 4 (JL4) and Judkins right 4 (JR4), have remained essentially unchanged from their original design and remain in use today.[1]

Over the years, equipment has become disposable, refined, and miniaturized. The imaging equipment has been developed to improve visualization and reliability and to reduce patient and operator radiation exposure. Catheter-based interventional procedures for the treatment of cardiovascular disease continue to improve and are expanding beyond coronary arterial disease, treating hypetrophic obstructive cardiomyopathies, atrial and ventricular septal defects, patent foramen ovales, and vascular disease in the carotid, renal, and subclavian arteries. No interventional procedure can be carried out, however, until an accurate diagnosis has been achieved, and the new interventional procedures necessitate even more intricate and accurate diagnostic components.

INDICATIONS

Cardiovascular disease is the number one killer in the United States, and most of the patients referred to the cardiovascular catheterization laboratory (CCL) are there to assess coronary artery disease. Table 11-1 shows the different indications associated with various cardiac diseases.

CONTRAINDICATIONS

By definition, a contraindication means that a procedure should not be performed. Many relative contraindications can be overcome, however, by managing patients medically before they are brought to the lab; otherwise, these patients are at a higher risk of complications.

Table 11-1. Table of Indications *Source:* From Kern M. *The Cardiac Catheterization Handbook*, 4th ed. St. Louis: Mosby; Copyright © Elsevier 2003.

1. Suspected or known coronary artery disease
   a. New-onset angina
   b. Unstable angina
   c. Evaluation before a major surgical procedure
   d. Silent ischemia
   e. Positive exercise tolerance test
   f. Atypical chest pain or coronary spasm
2. Myocardial infarction
   a. Unstable angina postinfarction
   b. Failed thrombolysis
   c. Shock
   d. Mechanical complications (ventricular septal defect, rupture of wall, or papillary muscle)
3. Sudden cardiovascular arrest
4. Valvular heart disease
5. Congenital heart disease
6. Aortic dissection
7. Aortic Aneurysm
8. Pericardial constriction or tamponade
9. Cardiomyopathy
10. Initial and follow-up assessment for heart transplantation

Absolute Contraindications

- Inadequate equipment or catheterization facility
- Patient refusal

Relative Contraindications

- Acute gastrointestinal bleeding or anemia
- Electrolyte imbalance
- Infection and fever
- Medication toxicity
- Pregnancy
- Recent cerebrovascular accident (<1 month)

- Renal failure
- Uncontrolled CHF, hypertension, arrhythmias
- Uncooperative patient
- Unknown, uncontrolled bleeding diathesis

MAJOR COMPLICATIONS

Many factors contribute to complications, including procedural length, contrast dose, equipment available, radiation exposure, extent of cardiovascular disease, and comorbidities.[2] They also include operator and facility case volume. The American College of Cardiology/American Heart Association have guidelines[3] for cath lab and physician caseload minimum safe volume (Table 11-2).

Major Complications

- Cardiac arrest
- Cardiogenic shock
- Cerebrovascular accident
- Congestive heart failure
- Contrast reaction—major (analphylaxis)
- Death
- Myocardial infarction
- Respiratory arrest
- Ventricular tachycardia, fibrillation, or serious arrhythmia

Table 11-2. American College of Cardiology/American Heart Association Minimum Volume Guidelines

Minimum Lab Caseload
Adult catheterization laboratories, at least 300 cases/year.
Pediatric catheterization laboratories, at least 150 cases/year.
Minimum Individual Physician caseload:
Adult diagnostic catheterizations, at least 150 cases/year
Adult interventional procedures, at least 50 cases/year
Pediatric catheterizations, at least 50 cases/year
Electrophysiology procedures at least 100 cases/year

Other Complications

- Air embolus
- Aortic (Ao) dissection
- Cardiac dissection/perforation
- Contrast reaction—minor (hives)
- Heart block/asystole
- Hematoma
- Hemorrhage (local, retroperitoneal, pelvic)
- Hypotension
- Infection
- Loss of distal pulse
- Peripheral vascular dissection/perforation
- Pseudoaneurysm
- Renal failure
- Retroperitoneal bleed
- Supraventricular tachyarrhythmia, atrial fibrillation
- Tamponade
- Vascular injury, pseudoaneurysm
- Vasovagal reaction

CCL STAFFING

The optimum CCL team is multidisciplinary and includes members with various skill mixes. Members include nurses and radiology and cardiovascular technologists whose credentials may include RN, RCIS, RT(R), or LPN. Other allied health professionals such as EMTs, respiratory therapists, operating room scrub techs, physician assistants, and noncredentialed cardiovascular technologists are also valuable members of the team.

Minimum staffing levels are determined by hospital or cath lab policy and may be dependent on the type of procedure. Local laws or administrative codes may dictate that team members with specific credentials be present, such as having a radiological technologist present to change fluoroscopic programs or having registered nurses to administer all medications. Optimally, there will be three team members in addition to the staff physician, enough members of the CCL team to fill each of the primary roles of monitor, circulator, and scrub assistant. In academic facilities, where there may be cardiology fellows in training, there may be no need for a scrub assistant. A fully cross-trained team, where each individual is capable of stepping into a given role competently and confidently, is the most functional and efficient.

Monitor

The monitor must document all pertinent data from the procedure in the catheterization laboratory computer database. This should include, but not be limited to:

- Patient demographic information
- Date, time, and type of procedure
- Attending and referring physicians, fellows, recorder, and patient
- All hemodynamic data
- All medications administered (this information must also be documented on the appropriate medication sheets)
- Any changes in patient status
- All catheters and other equipment used
- Angiographic views
- Preliminary impression of the diagnostic procedure
- Complications
- IV infusion volume
- Contrast dose administered to the patient
- Fluoroscopy time/cumulative patient exposure (if available) for the procedure
- Disposition of the patient

All events that occur during a catheterization procedure are documented in the procedure log. The recorder, whether a nurse or technologist, is responsible for accurate, comprehensive documentation of the proceedings; handwritten logs must be legible. Any event that may directly affect the present or future care of the patient must

be noted. Examples of such events can include bleeding or hematoma at the access site, changes in heart rhythm/rate, hemodynamic instability, and medication reactions. Furthermore, all interventions that result from such events should be documented with a note in the progress section of the patient's medical record.

The findings of all diagnostic procedures and relevant hemodynamic values are recorded on a preprinted progress form or electronic medical record. This form is completed by the interventional attending physician or a designee.

The recorder may also be responsible for documenting all billable equipment and procedures. Many labs use an inventory control system, using a scanner with manufacturer barcodes. As the product is scanned, it is added to the patient bill and simultaneously removed from inventory for easy tracking and reordering.

All hemodynamic measurements may also be recorded by strip-chart recorder. These strips will be filed with the physician's report or a digital copy from the waveform file in the computer record will be generated

The recorder must document all pertinent data from the procedure in the catheterization laboratory computer database. This includes the material outlined for the LHC. All O_2 saturation and Fick measurements should be entered into the computer, and printouts from the oximeter will be filed with the physician's report.

Monitoring the patient's vital signs during the procedure is the monitor's primary objective. There are key moments in the procedure when total attention must be paid to the monitor:

- During vascular access, the patient may develop vasovagal reactions due to the puncture and manipulation of the vessels. This will manifest as a profound bradycardia and associated hypotension. Atropine IV, elevation of the patient's legs, a saline bolus at high speed, and oxygen should be implemented immediately.

- During navigation and vessel cannulation of any catheter, it is possible to disrupt or dislocate some plaque from the aorta or a vessel's ostium. While a catheter is being placed, the patient's vital signs should be monitored closely.
- During the first injection of each coronary artery, it is important to observe the ECG and hemodynamics. Watch especially for bradydysrhythmias/blocks when injecting the right coronary artery (which feeds the sinoatrial and atrioventricular node branches). Nonionic, low osmolar contrast media is better tolerated than older, high osmolar contrast agents.
- During high-volume bolus injections, such as for LV angiography, injections of large amounts of contrast media can cause various arrhythmias.

A tool to help increase patient awareness is the audible ECG signal. Generally, this can be set so it will only be heard within the control room, because many physicians may find the sound distracting. This will allow the monitoring personnel to notice rate and rhythm changes, even while typing into the procedure log or tracking the inventory for billing purposes. Although these are important, the patient must be continuously monitored and assessed.

Circulator

The circulator assists the flow of the procedure from outside the sterile field. Circulators are responsible for the direct assessment of the patient, the administration of procedural sedation and other medications, and the opening of sterile equipment for the scrub staff as needed. They may also control the contrast power injector, run the C-Arm and perform whole-blood oximetry and other blood analysis such as the activated clotting time (ACT). General tasks performed by the circulator include:

- Helping the monitor by being aware of the patient's vital signs at all times.
- Talking to the patient periodically and asking if the patient is experiencing discomfort or pain. If the patient is in pain, the circulator should ask the patient to rank it on a scale of 0 to10 (0 being no pain, 10 being intense pain). The circulator should remember that pain is subjective to each individual. If the patient is unconscious, observe the face and body movement for signs of increased discomfort.
- Keeping an eye on the operators' aseptic technique.
- Verifying any devices requested to be brought into the sterile field. If the operator asks for a piece of equipment, and the circulator believes that may not be the equipment intended, he or she should show the package or device first. This can save both time and money.
- Making sure each device is compatible with the procedure set. A circulator should not supply a 6F catheter if the access sheath is only 5F.
- Wearing mask and eye protection until the scrub nurse has disposed of all bloody equipment. Blood and body fluids can be splashed into the eyes of staff as the sterile field is broken down and disposed of.
- Verifying that the injector is loaded with contrast and free of bubbles before injection. The tip should always be pointed downward. As a safety measure, decals on many injector cylinders appear oval until the syringe is filled with fluid; then light defraction makes them appear circular.
- Verifying the site of any blood samples from the field before accepting it.
- Monitoring the patient's O_2 saturation continually so that appropriate oxygen therapy can be administered as needed.

Scrub Assistant

A cardiac catheterization requires too many complex psychomotor demands for one set of hands, and scrub assistants are the physician's right hand. They must anticipate the physician's needs and be prepared to change course rapidly. The scrub assistant maintains a strict sterile field and properly prepares all of the equipment per manufacturer and hospital protocol. The scrub assistant should:

- Properly identify all drugs on the table, preferably with a sterile label, though colored needles, type/color of syringe, or table location can be used. When in doubt regarding identification of a medication, dispose of it.
- Never force equipment into the patient. There should be little resistance. If resistance is ever met, stop; evaluate the situation, and assess the patient. Careful progress is paramount.
- Always preflush catheters and store them lengthwise on the table. The manufacturers have gone to considerable trouble and expense to package and deliver the catheter in a straight fashion. Coiling the catheter for an extended period will alter the shape of the shaft, making it more difficult to manipulate.
- Always read manufacturer inserts (but not in front of the patient). Inserts include facts about the inner diameter, rated burst pressures, and other important specifications.
- Never thread a needle over a guide wire because this may "shave" the outer layer off the guide wire.
- Always prep the manifold with the lights on, allowing any trapped bubbles, particularly near the stopcocks, to become visible.
- Always hold syringes with the tip pointed down, and aspirate a small amount of blood immediately prior to flushing or contrast or medication injection. Lightly tap the syringe so that any bubbles will rise, reducing the chance of air embolisms.
- Flush indwelling arterial lines every 3 minutes unless the line is attached to a pressurized drip.
- Carefully inspect equipment for damage before handing it to the physician or inserting it into the patient. Quality control by the manufacturers may be excellent, however, one last check is important because the equipment may have been damaged during shipping or unpacking.
- Save or retrieve the original packaging if there is equipment failure or if the equipment is defective in some way. This will allow the manufacturer to track down the source of the problem.
- Make sure that the wire is longer than the catheter. Use exchange-length ($\geq$260 cm) guide wires when the patient has a peripheral vessel disease or torturous vessels.
- Make sure that a sterile sleeve is in place over the exposed section of the catheter to allow for manipulation when the patient is on the ward when inserting a Swan-Ganz catheter that will be left in the patient after the procedure.
- Anticipate the procedure two steps ahead of the physician.
- Maintain aseptic technique and pay attention to instincts.

PATIENT PREPARATION

Premedication

In many institutions, it is common practice to give no premedication unless the patient demonstrates the need for it. In other institutions, all patients may be premedicated an hour before their procedure; for example with Valium (diazepam), 10mg p.o., and Benadryl (diphenhydramine), 25mg p.o.

If the patient has a known allergy to the contrast medium, he or she can be given prednisone, 60 mg p.o. every 8 hours for 2 days prior to the procedure. Alternatively, hydrocortisone, 100 mg IV can be given in the lab prior to the procedure, followed by prednisone 60 mg p.o. every 8 hours for 2 days. The physician may order an alternative protocol. These patients must be monitored closely for early signs of reaction including itchy skin, stuffy noses, hives on the chest, or signs of respiratory distress.

Conscious Sedation

To alleviate anxiety, conscious (also known as procedural) sedation is an important component of patient care in the cath lab. The patient should be monitored by fingertip pulse oximeter and auto blood pressure cuff for depression of the patient's respiratory drive, which can occur with most conscious sedation agents. Each patient must be assessed before, during, and after sedation. A common example of conscious sedation is fentanyl 100 µg and Versed 2 mg. These agents will be titrated to the patient's level of consciousness. Narcan reverses fentanyl, and Romazicon is the antidote for Versed. Both should be readily available.

Local Anesthesia

Prior to administering local anesthesia, the site chosen is prepped using strict aseptic technique. Local analgesia of the access site is accomplished by first injecting a small amount of 1%–2% lidocaine (or other local analgesic) subcutaneously with a short 25-gauge needle. The skin and subcutaneous tissues around the site vessels are then fully anesthetized with deeper injections of the local, using a longer 22-gauge needle. Care must be taken to ensure that an artery or vein is not inadvertently entered. For full effect, the local anesthetic should be administered 2–3 minutes prior to sheath insertion. This may be

accomplished by administering the anesthetic, then setting up the manifold or flushing/prepping catheters and equipment.

Access Sites

The choice of vascular access is dependent on the patient's anatomy. If there are no other considerations, the most often preferred access site for cardiac catheterization is the right groin. The following locations, in descending order of preference, can also be used: left groin, left arm, and right arm. Radial artery access (either right or left) has also been developed as an option. If only an RHC or myocardial biopsy is being performed, the right or left internal jugular or subclavian vein can be used.

Femoral Access

If the right groin has been chosen for percutaneous access, the femoral artery is palpated. Once the artery is located, the femoral vein will be found just medial to the artery (Figure 11-1). A small skin incision (2–4 mm) is made with a #11 scalpel blade about 2 cm below the

Figure 11-1. Landmarks for groin vascular access.

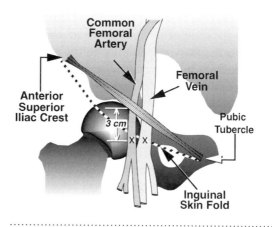

expected point of vascular entry, and a tunnel may be made through the superficial fascia with a straight hemostat.

For femoral arterial access, the vessel is entered with an 18-gauge, 7 cm vascular access needle. The needle is inserted at a 30°–45° angle. A pulse may be felt as the needle tip comes into contact with the arterial wall. Pulsating blood indicates a successful arterial puncture. With the needle located in the arterial lumen, a short guide wire is passed through the needle. The needle is removed, leaving the wire within the vein, and an introducer sheath with its dilator is passed over the wire (Figure 11-2). The dilator and wire are then removed from the sheath, and the sheath is aspirated and flushed through the side arm.

The procedure for venous access is similar, but a 10 mL syringe half filled with saline may be attached to the needle. As the needle is advanced into the skin at a 30°–45° angle, the syringe is gently aspirated. If arterial pulsation is felt, the needle is pulled back and redirected more medially. As the vein is entered, dark, nonpulsatile blood should enter the syringe.

Brachial Access

In patients with severe iliac disease or femoral artery bypasses, it may be necessary to use a brachial or radial approach. The method of choice is usually percutaneous, which eliminates the complications and difficulties of a direct brachial cutdown. It will be necessary to add an arm-board attachment to the procedure table. Generally, the right arm is placed on the arm board with a towel as a pad, then the antecubital fossa is prepped and draped. It may be somewhat awkward to work in this space if the team is accustomed to the femoral approach and using the patient's lap for equipment. The sterile procedure table can be brought closer to the patient field to work from.

For percutaneous access of the brachial artery, a technique similar to that described for the femoral approach is used. The staff physician may opt to use a shorter, 5 cm long sheath or a pediatric sheath with a longer dilator taper.

Radial Access

Recently, many physicians have been trained to use the radial artery for access which involves the

Figure 11-2. Vascular access: single-wall technique.

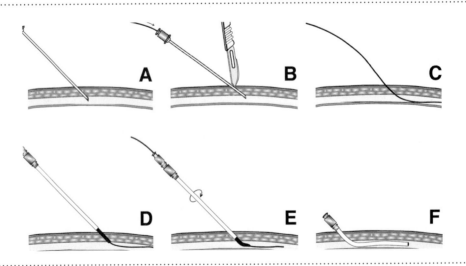

more common Seldinger percutaneous approach. Before proceeding, an Allen test is administered (Figure 11-3) to ensure that the perfusion to the hand could be satisfied by the ulnar artery alone in the event of radial complications. This is accomplished by occluding both radial and ulnar arteries simultaneously and having the patient pump their fist to blanch the hand. Release of the ulnar artery should allow for brisk return of color to the hand.[4]

For radial access, the arm board is used as just described. A rolled towel is placed under it to facilitate exposure, and the wrist is hyperextended. The vessels accessed are a smaller caliber than the femoral artery, so distal heparin, verapamil, and nitrates are often injected to reduce vasospasm and thrombotic complications. A two-stage sheath is often used. It has a .018-inch ID in the first stage, and .035 inch in the second. The right arm is most commonly used. If there is to be visualization of the left internal mammary artery (IMA), the left arm is strongly recommended because navigation from the right subclavian artery into the Ao root and up into

Figure 11-3. The Allen test.

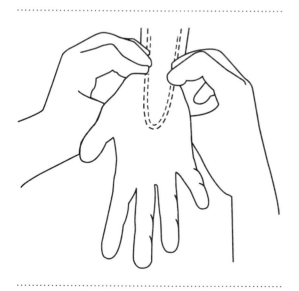

the left subclavian artery is most difficult. Another caveat of radial cases is the size limitation of the equipment. Usually, 6F is the maximum size that can be safely placed, which would exclude large-caliber interventional devices or intra-aortic balloon (IAB) placement.

EQUIPMENT

Needles

Vascular access can be obtained using a number of different one- or two-piece needles. Two-piece needles may have a blunt, tapered external cannula with a sharp, inner obturator or a sharp, external cannula with a blunt inner obturator. Most operators today prefer to use a single-piece, thin-wall 18-gauge needle.

In cases in which the vessel is very difficult to locate, the "Smart needle" (from Cardiovascular Dynamics, Inc., of Irvine, California) can be used. This is an 18-gauge thin-wall needle with an integrated Doppler crystal insert that is attached to a waterproof, hand-held Doppler monitor. It produces an audio signal (sort of a "swish" sound) when the needle is pointing toward a blood vessel. This signal becomes louder and more distinct the nearer the needle comes to the vessel. When the vessel has been breached, the insert is removed and the guide wire inserted.

Guide Wires

There are literally hundreds of different types of guide wires in different lengths, diameters, tips, or core stiffnesses, distal curves, coatings, and materials available for vascular procedures. The initial guide wire of choice is generally a 0.035-inch diameter wire with a 3 mm J-tip. Tortuous vessels may require a wire with a soft, floppy tip wire such as a Wholey Wire, or a slippery hydrophilic coating, such as a Terumo Glidewire (from Terumo Inc., of Japan). A caveat of the glide wire is that it must not be used through a needle because it is not made of metal and could shear. To cross a stenotic Ao valve, either a 0.035-inch movable-core straight wire or a 0.035-inch Amplatz stiff or super-stiff 3mm J-tip wire may be chosen.

Sheaths

An 11-cm introducer sheath is used for the bulk of diagnostic left heart cases, usually 4F, 5F, or 6F, depending on the clinic's or physician's preference. Many facilities that perform coronary interventions may choose to perform the bulk of their cases with a 6F sheath, switching from the diagnostic catheters to an interventional guiding catheter if a percutaneous coronary intervention is to be undertaken. Larger gauge diagnostic catheters make an unnecessarily large hole in the patient and may lead to more local vascular problems. They also require more time to reach hemostasis when the sheath is being removed. However, if a stenotic Ao valve is to be assessed, a sheath one French size larger than the catheters can enable simultaneous measurement of femoral and Ao pressures without damping.

A number of different specialty sheaths are available as well. Some of these are specifically designed for various types of diagnostic and therapeutic procedures, with sizes ranging from 3F to 24F and lengths from 5 cm to 120 cm. Long, 24-cm sheaths or Arrow Flexsheaths (from Arrow Critical Care) are commonly used when there is a lot of vessel tortuosity or femoro-iliac disease.

A larger gauge introducer may be placed in the access vein for RHCs, usually 6F to 8F, depending on what sort of measurements are to be taken. Tortuous iliac vessels may require the use of a 23-cm or longer sheath.

Catheters

The most commonly used coronary angiography catheters are end-hole JL4 and JR4 (Figure 11-4). Many other curves are available for a variety of anatomic differences (Figure 11-5). The choice of

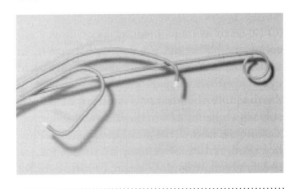

Figure 11-4. From L to R: Standard Judkins left, right, and pigtail catheters. *Source:* Courtesy of Boston Scientific Inc.

catheters should take into consideration whether the Ao should be larger or smaller because of the size of the patient or chronic Ao valve stenosis. The curve of the catheter must approximate the anatomy being cannulated. If difficulty is encountered in engaging the Judkins catheters, the Amplatz varieties are a frequent second resort. These come in Amplatz left (AL) and Amplatz right (AR) designs and different sizes (Figure 11-6).

The internal mammary has an extreme 90° takeoff from the subclavian artery, so the IMA catheter has an extreme curve on the tip (Figure 11-7). Although AR or JR catheters can usually be used to engage saphenous vein bypass grafts, some operators prefer (or the anatomy may dictate) the use of coronary bypass catheters.

For ventriculography and aortography, the catheter of choice is the side-hole pigtail catheter. Some operators feel that an angled pigtail catheter sits better within the LV than the straight version and leads to less catheter-induced ventricular ectopy.

Diagnostic multipacks containing a JR4, JL4, pigtail, sheath, and guide wire are now widely available. They save on both packaging and storage space.

RHC is usually performed with a balloon-tipped Swan-Ganz catheter. These come in a variety of types: monitoring, TD (for thermodi-

Figure 11-5. The range of Judkins left and Judkins right catheters. *Source:* Courtesy of Boston Scientific Inc.

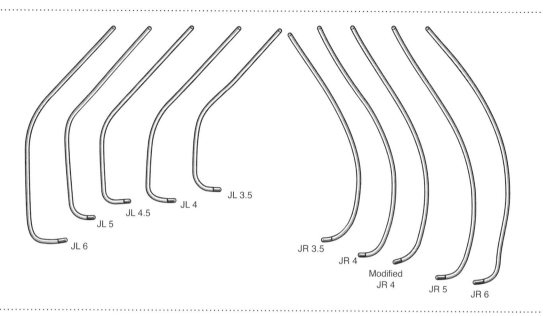

Figure 11-6. The range of Amplatz left and Amplatz right catheters. *Source:* Courtesy of Boston Scientific Inc.

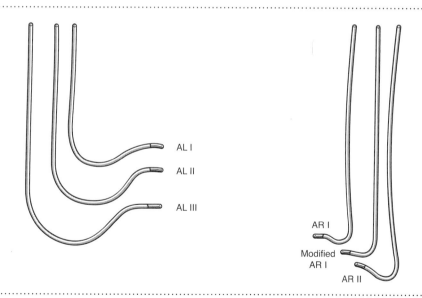

lution measurements), VIP, femoral S-tipped, and balloon-tipped pacing catheters. If cardiac outputs (COs) do not need to be measured, then the monitoring Swan-Ganz catheter is the best choice. A woven Dacron-pacing catheter, similar in design to a Cournand, the Zucker bipolar pacing catheter (from Medtronic AVE of Billerica, Massachusetts) is also available.

Figure 11-7. Bypass and Internal Mammary catheters. *Source:* Courtesy of Boston Scientific Inc.

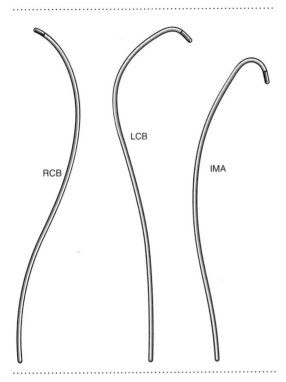

Figure 11-8. The range of multipurpose catheters. *Source:* Courtesy of Boston Scientific Inc.

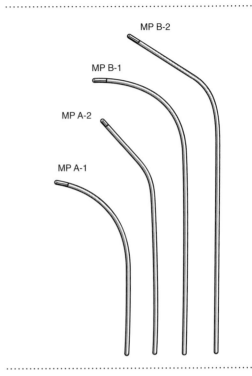

If a balloon-tipped catheter is not needed, then an end-hole Cournand or multipurpose (MP) catheter (Figure 11-8) is a good choice, especially if the patient has pulmonary hypertension or a severe tricuspid valve insufficiency where floating balloon-tipped catheters become a difficult challenge. Their main advantages over the Swan-Ganz catheters are significant cost savings and their smaller gauge sheath, which results in a smaller hole in the patient. One disadvantage is that it can be difficult to obtain a good wedge pressure with them, so valuable procedural time may be lost.

ANGIOGRAPHY

Angiography is an imaging technique that uses X-rays to take pictures of blood vessels and chambers of the heart. A small amount of contrast media is squirted through a catheter into the vessel or chamber of interest, while a series of pictures is taken. These can be assessed individually, or run as a film, providing accurate images of the inner lumen of vessels and chambers of the heart.

Every patient needs to be prepared for the case that the diagnostic procedure becomes interventional immediately afterwards. This makes contrast medium management a crucial part of monitoring and means that angiography should be performed using as little contrast media as possible. For a patient with a normal renal profile, a procedural limit of 3 ml/kg to 4 ml/kg of contrast medium is a good benchmark to use.

Coronary Angiography

When working on a coronary angiogram, it is important to look at the coronary branches to make sure that all of the vessels, including the origin of each, are clearly shown without overlap. Lesions can be missed unless each segment is shown in more than one plane. There are good starter angles for angiography, but they must often be customized somewhat for each patient.

It is important to see whether vessel branches are missing. This requires experience and is especially important when the patient has had CABG surgery. Which vessel portions perfuse which part of the myocardium need to be kept in mind because the two-dimensional pictures on the monitors need to be understood in three-dimensional context.

It is important to inject the contrast medium with enough pressure to fill the vessel and cause slight overflow into the aortic root. This avoids the error of underfill, which can lead to a false-positive diagnosis caused by the "streaming" of blood and contrast in the vessel. Another technique is to inject for three beats of the patient's heart, then stop. This will generally allow for enough contrast for complete vessel visualization and runoff of blood replaces contrast, helping to avoid excessive contrast dose. Do not initiate the injection until the image acquisition has started. The operator of the cine/acquisition pedal should be aware of the need to image longer if collateral vessel filling is noted.

Mechanical contrast medium management systems (Figure 11-9) can inject with programmable flow rate algorithms for the various vascular beds. They can be used for coronary angiography and left ventriculography.

Many labs use a one-way check valve in the contrast line between the bottle and the manifold. This prevents patient-contaminated contrast from being returned to the bottle and allows for the remaining contrast to be used on the next patient.

Precautions

If the patient has a significant lesion on the left main coronary artery (LMCA), there is a

Figure 11-9. Either a manifold or a contrast delivery system can be used to manage pressure, flush, and contrast delivery. *Upper panel:* three-port manifold. *Lower panel:* Acist injection controller. *Source:* Courtesy of Acist Medical Systems.

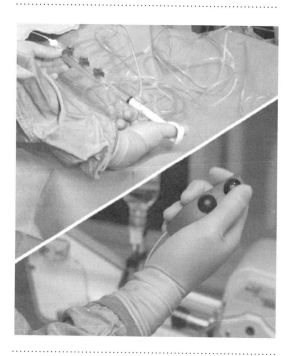

greater risk of complications occurring during the procedure, so it is important that it is spotted early. The patient's notes may reveal ominous signs such as a pressure drop during an exercise treadmill or large areas of ischemia on the nuclear study or ECG. Cannulation of the LMCA may give a damped or ventricularized pressure waveform as the catheter partially occludes the ostium. The monitor technician should be watching the physiologic monitor at the time of cannulation and should notify the physician of the damping immediately. A left coronary injection taken in a slight right anterior oblique or anteroposterior with cranial can lay out the LMCA and is a good first shot. The physician will limit the number of injections and most likely omit the LV angiogram if significant LMCA disease is found.

Left Ventricular Angiography

The left ventriculogram provides important information about the functioning of the LV, including whether the aortic and mitral valves are competent, the presence of a ventricular septal defect, and the presence and location of a ventricular aneurysm. Wall-motion abnormalities can indicate areas of previous infarction.

Calculation of end diastolic volume (EDV) and end systolic volume (ESV) are usually done by software incorporated into the imaging review station. By subtracting EDV from ESV, the stroke volume (SV) in ml can be calculated. Dividing the SV by the EDV yields the ejection fraction (EF). The EF is an important indicator of the heart's efficiency. A normal EF is about 50%–65%.

The catheter of choice for LV angiography is the pigtail catheter, either straight or angled. The two main advantages of the pigtail catheter are that it sits well within the ventricle and that the multiple side holes reduce catheter recoil and practically eliminate the possibility of wall perforation. The positioning of the catheter within the ventricle is important. If the catheter is too high, then the Ao valve may appear falsely regurgitant. Placing the catheter at the apex may result in arrhythmias.

The injection rate, using a power injector, is usually about 15 ml/sec with 0 sec linear rise. The total volume injected is 45 ml. These parameters are variable, depending on ventricular size, SV, hemodynamics, and operator preference. Many labs report adequate visualization with 12 ml/sec and 35 ml (with 5F catheters) or 8 ml/sec and 30 ml with smaller patients. Using digital subtraction angiography, ventriculography may be adequately performed with a 50% contrast/saline dilution or lower volumes of straight contrast.

Aortography

Aortography is the injection of a large bolus of contrast medium into the aortic root. This is usually a 50 ml bolus at 25 ml/sec with a 0.5 sec linear rise. This technique is used principally to assess aortic regurgitation (AR) or to find the origin of saphenous vein grafts.

The catheter of choice should be one with multiple side holes, usually a pigtail catheter. For AR, with best angle is 45° LAO. Coarctation of the aorta is best seen with 20° LAO, and a patent ductus arteriosus needs a very steep LAO.

AR severity is assigned a number on a scale from 1 to 4 (Table 11-3).

Other Angiographic Examinations

Right ventriculography can be performed in a manner very similar to left ventriculography. The key to successful right ventricular (RV) imaging is the placement of the catheter tip in the direction of the RV apex, not the outflow tract. Right ventriculograms may be performed with a variety of different catheters, including pigtail, MP, NIH, and Berman balloon-tipped angiographic catheters.

Iliac angiography is performed to assess the "quality" of the iliac arteries for IAB placement or to better assess them when difficult sheath placement is experienced. Typically, this is done with

Table 11-3. Aortic Regurgitation Severity

1+	Mild AR of no clinical significance.
2+	Moderate AR, in which contrast enters the LV outflow tract during each diastole and fails to clear with each systole.
3+	Moderately severe AR, in which there is filling of the entire LV, the contrast density in the LV and Ao being equal.
4+	Severe AR, in which most of the contrast enters the LV during diastole, and the density in the LV is greater than in the Ao.

Ao = aorta, AR = aortic regurgitation, LV = left ventricular/left ventricle.

an injection of 10 ml of contrast medium, either by hand or with a power injector.

Pulmonary angiography can be used to verify pulmonary hypertension, pulmonary emboli, arterio-venous fistulas, and other pathologic states. Pulmonary artery (PA) wedge arteriography, using a hand injection of a small amount of contrast through the end hole of the wedged catheter, can demonstrate the distal pulmonary vasculature and any intraluminal mass.

PROCEDURAL PROTOCOLS

Left Heart Catheterization

In most clinics, positive diagnostic LHC procedures lead directly to percutaneous revascularization achieved in the same setting. An advantage of this is that the patient only has to deal with one hospital stay and only has to prepare for one procedure psychologically, even though two procedures are being performed. One of the challenges is regulating the amount of contrast medium received by the patient in this double procedure.

The diagnostic LHC provides physiologic information by recording hemodynamic data from the Ao and LV and anatomic information from cineangiography of the coronary arteries, LV, and Ao root.

Procedure

1. *Arterial/Ao pressure.* A baseline pressure measurement (phasic and mean, scale 200) is taken prior to beginning angiography.
2. *Coronary angiogram.* This is usually performed before the left ventriculogram. If the patient has a previously unknown contrast media allergy, he or she will receive a smaller dose than if the ventriculography was performed first. The LMCA is usually visualized initially in a shallow RAO or RAO with cranial angle to examine the left main trunk. This establishes the presence or absence of the worst-case disease scenario.

3. *LV pressure.* Phasic-only, usually scale 200 LV pressure measurements (systolic, diastolic, and end-diastolic) are taken. Some institutions will also measure the LV pressure on 40 scale, 200 mm/sec paper speed as an additional means to measure the left ventricle end-diastolic pressure (LVEDP) and diastolic filling period.
4. *Left ventriculogram.*
5. *LV pressure.* Phasic only, usually scale 200 LV pressure measurements (systolic, diastolic, and end-diastolic) are retaken. A short period of time should be allowed for the patient's pressure to recuperate post angiogram prior to taking this measurement. It is important to measure the LVEDP post ventriculography, because at times, some patients have a substantial increase and may need to be observed for signs of acute CHF or pulmonary edema.
6. *LV-to-Ao pullback.* Phasic LV-to-Ao pullback pressures will provide an LV-Ao gradient if one is present.
7. *Ao pressure.* Phasic and mean systolic and diastolic Ao pressures should be recorded.

Additionally, as the situation may warrant, coronary artery bypass grafts (whether saphenous vein or IMA), Ao root, and renal and iliac arteries may be visualized.

Right Heart Catheterization

The diagnostic RHC provides physiologic information by recording hemodynamic data from the right atrium (RA), RV, PA, and pulmonary capillary wedge.

Procedure

1. *Superior vena cava (SVC).* Perform an O_2 saturation measurement.
2. *Inferior vena cava (IVC).* Perform an O_2 saturation measurement.

3. *RA.* Perform an O_2 saturation measurement.

4. *RA pressure.* Phasic and mean, scale 40 RA pressures (A wave, V wave) are measured.

5. *RV pressure.* Phasic only, scale 40 RV pressures (systolic, diastolic, and end-diastolic) are measured.

6. *Pulmonary capillary wedge (PCW) pressure.* Phasic and mean, scale 40 PCW prssures (A wave, V wave, and mean) are measured.

7. *PCW-to-PA pullback.* Mean PCW-to-PA pullback pressure is measured.

8. *PA pressure.* PA pressures (systolic, diastolic, and mean) are measured.

9. *PA.* PA O_2 saturation is measured. If a shunt is detected with these preliminary O_2 saturation measurements, the RHC procedure should be expanded to a shunt bilateral HC, as outlined later.

RECORDING AND DOCUMENTATION

The recorder must document all pertinent data from the procedure in the catheterization laboratory computer database. This includes, but is not limited to, the material outlined for the LHC and RHC just listed. All O_2 saturation measurements are entered into the computer, and printouts from the oximeter are filed with the physician's report.

Pressure Measurement

The different pressure waveforms that are met during catheterization are covered in depth in Chapter 3. They are the pressures measured in the various cardiac chambers and vessels, giving valuable diagnostic information on the condition of the heart. When recording tracings of the pressure waveforms, it is important to choose a scale with which the whole waveform is clearly displayed, both on the monitor and on the readout.

Cardiac Output Measurement

There are two commonly used methods to calculate CO: thermodilution and oxygen saturations. The oxygen saturations are analyzed using the Fick method.

Thermodilution

The Baxter CO machine senses temperature differences in the blood. These temperature measurements are made using Swan-Ganz catheters with temperature-sensing capabilities. Both Baxter Swan-Ganz TD and Swan-Ganz VIP catheters have this capability. In order to perform the test, a set amount of fluid of a known temperature is injected through a proximal port in the catheter, and the temperature is then sensed by a thermistor near the catheter tip. The machine does the appropriate calculations to determine the amount of blood flow over a given time and translates this into CO.

In some labs, injection syringes are filled with 10 ml of D5W at room temperature. It is possible to use a smaller injection amount (5 ml) or a chilled injection (0°C). There appears to be no difference in results using the lower temperature, but accuracy may be compromised by using the smaller volume. For CO measurements, some labs use both complementary techniques.

Fick Cardiac Output/Oxygen Saturations

To obtain data to calculate the patient's Fick CO, a mixed venous sample from the PA and a sample from the LV or Ao are needed. The patient's hemoglobin and oxygen consumption must be known. The hemoglobin can be sent to the laboratory if a co-oximeter is not present in the lab. It should be run at least once on the blood taken for the case and should be taken the day of the procedure. With this information, the Fick formula can be used to calculate CO:

$$CO \; (L/min) = \frac{oxygen \; consumption}{10 \; (CaO_2 - CvO_2)}$$

CaO_2 stands for arterial oxygen content, and CvO_2 is the venous content. The oxygen consumption data can be measured or assumed using the patient's body surface area (BSA) and gender to estimate. The following formula can be used to calculate the oxygen consumption:

$$Adult \; oxygen \; consumption \; (ml/min) = 125 \; ml/min/m^2 \; squared \times BSA$$

The units for both content variables are volume percent (when blood is run through an oximeter, the saturation is expressed as a percentage). To get a content value for the Fick formula from a saturation, this formula yields the appropriate volume percent:

$$Content = Saturation \; \% \times hemoglobin \; (g/dl) \\ \times human \; oxygen\text{-}carrying \; capacity \\ (ml \; O_2/g \; of \; Hgb)$$

Here is an example with normal values:

Ao saturation (SaO_2): 98%
PA mixed venous saturation: 75%
Hemoglobin (Hgb): 14 g/dL
Human oxygen carrying
   capacity: 1.36 mL O_2/g of Hgb
BSA: 2.0 m²

CaO_2 = CaO_2 = 0.98 × 14 × 1.36 = 18.66 volume percent
CvO_2 = 0.75 × 14 × 1.36 = 14.28 volume percent
oxygen consumption = 125 mL/min/m² × 2.0 m² = 250 mL/min

So the data is ready to be plugged in to the formula:

$$CO = \frac{250}{10 \times (18.66 - 14.28)} = \frac{250}{43.8} \\ = 5.71 \; L/min$$

The physiologic monitor's computer computes Fick and many other calculations once the proper data sets are entered.

Diagnostic catheterizations that assess both right and left heart hemodynamics may also include a full set of measurements of oxygen saturations for a shunt screen. Typically, the screening saturations will be taken: RA (or SVC and IVC), PA, and Ao. If there is a "step-up" ≥7% from RA to PA, then a full saturation run should be performed to determine presence of a shunt.

Oxygen saturation measurements are taken in conjunction with a measurement of the patient's oxygen consumption. There are several methods of measuring the oxygen consumed by the patient at rest on the table, but the easiest currently available is the water metabolic rate meter. This consists of a hood that is placed over the patient's head, which is connected via a short tube to the measuring device. This is much easier to use than the older bag technique.

RIGHT AND LEFT (BILATERAL) HEART CATHETERIZATION

Bilateral heart catheterization (BHC) is accomplished by accessing the arterial and venous systems. The BHC yields the anatomic information of the LHC and the physiologic information obtained by recording all cardiac chamber pressures, CO, and blood saturations. This information can diagnose hemodynamic abnormalities such as valvular pathology, cardiomyopathies, and congenital anomalies.

The diagnostic BHC provides physiologic information by recording hemodynamic data from the RA, RV, PA, pulmonary capillary wedge, Ao, and LV and anatomic information from cineangiography of the coronary arteries, LV, and Ao root. It provides information on the patency of all the valves as well as CO.

A BHC is often performed on a patient who is admitted for purely a right-heart diagnostic procedure because the added left-heart catheterization may reveal undiagnosed coronary heart disease. The patient is prepped and on the table anyway, so the added expense is not great.

Procedure

1. *SVC.* Perform an O_2 saturation measurement.
2. *IVC.* Perform an O_2 saturation measurement.
3. *RA.* Perform an O_2 saturation measurement.
4. *RA pressure.* Phasic and mean, scale 40 RA pressures (A wave, V wave) are measured.
5. *RV pressure.* Phasic only, scale 40 RV pressures (systolic, diastolic, and end-diastolic) are measured.
6. *Simultaneous PCW and LV pressures.* Phasic only, scale 40 PCW and LV pressures (diastolic and end-diastolic) are measured.
7. *PCW pressure.* Phasic and mean, scale 40 PCW pressures (A wave, V wave, and mean) are measured.
8. *PCW-to-PA pullback.* The mean PCW-to-PA pullback is measured.
9. *PA pressure.* The PA pressures (systolic, diastolic, and mean) are measured.
10. *LV and PA.* Perform O_2 saturation measurements. If a shunt is detected with these preliminary O_2 saturation measurements, the RHC procedure should be expanded to a shunt bilateral HC, as outlined later.
11. *LV pressure.* Phasic only, scale 200 LV pressures (systolic, diastolic, and end-diastolic) are measured.
12. *Left ventriculogram.*
13. *LV-to-Ao pullback.* Phasic LV-to-Ao pressure provides an LV-Ao gradient if one is present.
14. *Ao pressure.* Phasic and mean Ao pressures (systolic and diastolic) are recorded.
15. *Coronary angiography.*

Additionally, as the situation may warrant, the RV, PA, and left atrium (LA) may be visualized.

If a "step up" of ≥7% between the saturations in RA and PA is detected, a shunt may be suspected.

Alternatively, the patient may be undergoing the diagnostic procedure to verify and quantify a shunt that has already been found in echocardiography. The shunt BHC procedure should follow the BHC outlined previously, but it should also include the following oxygen saturation measurements (though any of these measurements may be omitted for reasons of patient safety or physician direction):

- High SVC
- Low SVC
- High IVC
- Low IVC
- High RA
- Mid RA
- Low RA
- High RV
- Apical RV
- RV outflow tract
- Main PA
- Left PA
- Right PA
- Ao arch
- LA, if accessed

TRANSSEPTAL CATHETERIZATION

Transseptal access across the fossa ovalis may be performed for a variety of reasons. Operators may not be able to cross an Ao valve with standard retrograde technique because of a mechanical prosthesis. Direct LA pressure measurements may be required to assess mitral valve disease with simultaneous LA and LVEDP pressures, to perform mitral vulvoplasty, to rule out pulmonary venous occlusive disease, and for left-side arrhythmia ablations. Transseptal catheterizations are routinely performed in laboratories that treat pediatric and adult congenital cardiac disease patients. Transseptal catheterizations should generally be performed in a laboratory equipped with a biplane fluoroscopic system, allowing the operator to better visualize anatomical structures and equipment position.

The right femoral vein is used for access, and a wire is advanced into the SVC. Prior to insertion, the Brockenbrough needle and transseptal sheath should be assembled and the distance between the needle and dilator hub measured to ensure that the needle remains inside the dilator until ready to perform the transseptal puncture. Next, an 8F Mullins transseptal sheath and dilator assembly (from Medtronic AVE of Billerica, Massachusetts) is advanced over the wire. The wire is removed, and the Brockenbrough needle is inserted into the sheath. This assembly is withdrawn from the SVC, into the RA, and positioned into the fossa ovale. Biplane fluoroscopy can be helpful in localizing the exact point to perform the puncture.

After the operator feels contact with the interatrial septum and is confident of being properly positioned within the fossa ovalis, the Brockenbrough needle is advanced outside the dilator. The LA pressure is observed and measured. The dilator is then advanced over the needle with a counterclockwise rotation of the needle. This action will help point the transseptal sheath anteriorly toward the mitral valve. The Brockenbrough needle is carefully removed, and the Mullins sheath is aspirated and flushed. The operator can now attempt to cross the mitral valve to assess the LV or perform vulvoplasty.

Transseptal catheterizations are considered difficult and somewhat high-risk procedures. They should only be performed by experienced operators who perform the technique on a frequent basis.

PROCEDURE CONCLUSION

The order in which the procedure is concluded depends on what procedures were performed and the state of the patient. The goal is to get the patient safely into his or her bed where the sheath can be pulled or to wait until he or she is transferred to the ward.

- When the procedure has been completed, all catheters are removed from the patient's body, leaving just the sheath in place.

- The X-ray equipment and monitors are moved away from the patient.
- The contrast medium and the pressure monitoring lines are disconnected.
- Depending on the method being used to close the puncture site, the sterile drape is taken off the patient carefully.
- If the sheath is to remain in place, non-vented sterile caps should be placed on the sidearm and the sheath secured and covered in a dry sterile dressing. An obturator may be inserted and a pressure flush bag attached if the sheath is to remain in place for a period of time.
- The patient is helped into his or her hospital gown, paying careful attention to infusion lines.
- Using a transfer board or the patient helping by grasping the overhead handle on the bed, the patient is transferred into the bed, making sure that his or her body and legs remain straight.
- The bed is then taken to the waiting area, and the catheter lab is prepared for the next patient.
- Any needles or blades on the equipment table are carefully transferred to the sharps container.
- All disposable material is wrapped into the sterile drapes and placed in medical trash receptacles.

Following completion of the catheterization and angiography, the monitor provides a report to the nurse who will be with the patient during the recovery period. In institutions with small teams, the recorder monitors and cares for the patient until he or she can be returned to the ward.

HEMOSTASIS

Although complications from catheterization procedures are rare, those related to vascular access and hemostasis are the most common. Patients will not remember million-dollar imaging systems, high-tech gadgetry, and advanced stents masterfully placed deep into their coronary arteries if they have a vascular complication. Instead, they will surely tell their friends and family about the large hematoma that migrated down their leg and took a month to heal.

Several factors lead to a difficult hold: patient obesity, elevated blood pressure or clotting time, Ao insufficiency, large sheath size, multiple sticks to gain vascular access (the sewing machine technique), or patients who sneeze, laugh, or cough frequently or who can't lie still. Many new devices have been developed to facilitate hemostatic efforts, including external C clamps, collagen plugs, suture mediated, vascular clips, and topical hemostasis accelerators.

For information on sheath pulling and hemostasis, refer to Chapter 26.

REFERENCES

1. Kern M. *The Cardiac Catheterization Handbook*, 4th ed. St. Louis, MO: Mosby; 2003.
2. Baim DS, Grossman W. *Cardiac Catheterization, Angiography, and Intervention*, 5th ed. Baltimore: Williams & Wilkins; 1996.
3. Laskey W, Boyle J, Johnson LW, Registry Committee of the Society for Cardiac Angiography and Intervention. Multivariate model for prediction of risk of significant complication during diagnostic cardiac catheterization. *Cadet Cardiovasc Diagn* 1993;30:185–190.
4. Allen EV Thromboangiitis obliterans. Methods of diagnosis of chronic occlusive arterial lesions distal to the wrist with illustrative cases. *Am J Med Sci* 1929;178:237–244.

SUGGESTED READING

Applegate RJ, Sacrinty MT, Kutcher MA, et al. Trends in vascular complications after diagnostic cardiac catheterization and percutaneous coronary intervention via the femoral artery, 1998 to 2007. *J Am Coll Cardiol Intv* 2008;1:317–326.

Berne RM, Levy MN. *Cardiovascular Physiology*, 8th ed. St. Louis: Mosby; 2001.

Cardiac Catheterization (Left Heart) website. Available at: http://www.emedicine.com/MED/topic 2958.htm.

Cardiovascular Credentialing International website. Available at: http://www.cci-online.org.

Chabner DE. *The Language of Medicine*, 7th ed. Philadelphia: W.B. Saunders; 2004.

Kern MJ, Kern M. *The Cardiac Catheterization Handbook*, 4th ed. St. Louis, MO: Mosby; 2003.

Chambers CE, Eisenhauer MD, McNicol LB, et al. Infection control guidelines for the cardiac catheterization laboratory. *Catheter Cardiovasc Interv* 2005. Available at: http://www.cmhvi.org/pdf/ID%20guidelines.pdf.

Opie LH, Gersh BJ. *Drugs for the Heart*, 6th ed. Philadelphia: W.B. Saunders; 2005.

Peterson KL, Nicod P. *Cardiac Catheterization: Methods, Diagnosis, and Therapy*. Philadelphia: W.B. Saunders; 1997.

Topol EJ. *Textbook of Cardiovascular Medicine*. Philadelphia PA: Lippincott-Raven; 1998.

Zipes DP, Libby P, Bonow RO, Braunwald E. *Braunwald's Heart Disease*, 7th ed. Philadelphia: W.B. Saunders; 2005.

Chapter 12

HEMODYNAMICS

Sandy Watson, RN, BN, NFESC
Jeff Davis, RRT, RCIS, FSICP

INTRODUCTION

Hemodynamics may be defined as the study of the forces related to blood circulation in the body. The measurement of the pressures within blood vessels and the chambers of the heart was one of the first routine procedures conducted in CCLs and is still one of the standard procedures today. Any staff that will assist in the various cardiac pressure measurements should be familiar with the concept of invasive pressures and how they are measured.

In the CCL, blood pressure is recorded in various parts of the circulatory system, most notably in the chambers of the heart. What is actually measured is the pressure being exerted on the blood by the heart, and therefore, the force of the heart's pumping action. Hemodynamic pressure measurements are used to evaluate heart function, enabling the doctor to diagnose particular disease states.

PRESSURE MEASUREMENT SYSTEMS

Pressure itself is defined as force per area. This can be expressed in a variety of ways, such as pounds per square inch or kilograms per square centimeter. The standard international (SI) unit is the pascal (Pa). One Pa equals 1 newton per square meter. In the cardiac catheterization laboratory, millimeters (and medicine in general), millimeters of mercury (mmHg) is the most commonly used unit of measure for blood pressures. One mmHg is the pressure exerted by a column of mercury 1 mm high at 0°C at standard atmospheric pressure and equals 133.3 Pa.

It is possible to measure blood pressure in a number of ways. Perhaps the most simple measurement technique was the one first used by the Rev. Stephen Hales in 1773. He inserted a glass tube into an artery of a horse, held it vertically, and measured the level to which the column of blood climbed.

Less intrusive is the use of a mercury manometer and a stethoscope, which has become the measurement system of choice in most of the world. Due to environmental concerns, mercury manometers have all but been replaced by electronic digital manometers, which use mmHg as the standard unit of measure. In the CCL, medical professionals have access to the bloodstream and the chambers of the heart, allowing direct measurement of intravascular pressures.

Any pressure measurement system is made up of an input signal, which is the true pressure being measured, and an output signal. In the CCL, the output is usually a digital signal displayed on a computer screen or lines printed on paper. The pressure exerted on the blood is transmitted through the fluid in a catheter. Pascal's law states that pressure applied to a liquid at any point is transmitted equally in all directions, so the pressure exerted on the column of fluid at the catheter tip is the same as that at the proximal end of

the tubing. This fluid column is connected by a length of tubing to a transducer that converts this pressure into a readable signal. Early transducers were rubber diaphragms directly attached to drawing systems, but today the pressure signal is transformed into an electrical signal, which can be displayed as desired (Figure 12-1).

This transformation from pressure into an electrical impulse takes place with the use of an electrical strain gauge. This makes use of the phenomenon that when a wire is stretched, its electrical resistance increases. A small metal diaphragm is attached to a system of wires that are arranged in such a way that when force is directed on them from the direction of the diaphragm, it results in a current flowing across the system. If there is no force, no current flows. This arrangement is called a Wheatstone bridge. It allows an electrical input to be modified by force. The electrical output is an expression of the force, which can be amplified and displayed against time in

Figure 12-1. Diagrammatic overview of a cardiac catheterization laboratory's pressure monitoring system.

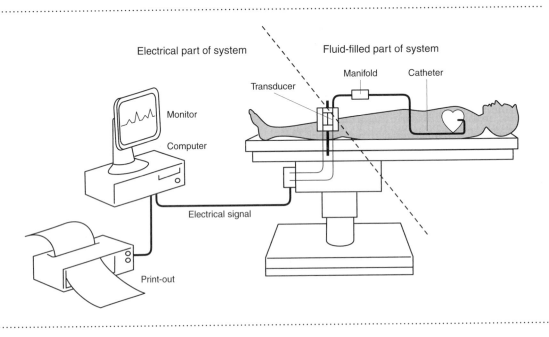

any number of forms to produce hemodynamic waveforms.

SOURCES OF ERROR AND ARTIFACTS

Along the pathway from the patient's vascular system to the eye of the person at the monitor, there are many possible sources of errors and distortions. To avoid them (or at least minimize their effect), it is important to know where they arise and why. The sources have been divided here into three groups: those arising in the fluid-filled part, those in the electronic part, and those that can be traced to the human portion of the system.

Fluid Artifacts

Intravascular pressure may be described simply as a "nudge" at the end of a path of water. Due to the dissipation of the pressure in the system, the longer the path of water, the longer it will take and the less forceful the nudge will be when it reaches the other end. This phenomenon is known as inertia; the shorter the connecting column of water, the less inertia, and the better the system will work.

These problems can be eliminated if the transducer is mounted right on the tip of the catheter. Such catheters are available (Millar Mikro-Tip catheters) as are guide wires that contain microtransducers at their tip (RADI PressureWire, Volcano SmartWire). With these systems there is no "overshoot" in the waveform and the frequency response is optimal (Figure 12-2). This makes transducer tip catheters or guide wires ideal for cases in which very accurate pressure measurements are necessary, such as in clinical research. Electronic micromanometer systems are relatively expensive for routine use in day-to-day practice. When the limitations of the system are known and accounted for, fluid-filled catheter systems are certainly adequate for most situations.

The intravascular pressure is transferred to the transducer by a column of liquid, usually 0.9%

Figure 12-2. Left ventricle-aorta pullback with fluid-filled and Millar catheter tip transducer systems recorded simultaneously.

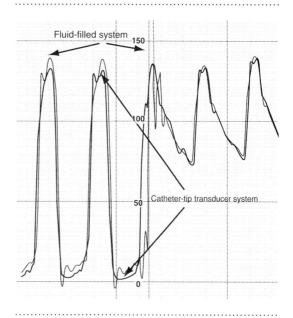

saline. The force exerted on this column is, as Pascal pointed out, exerted in all directions and that includes against the walls of the column. The column's container is fairly rigid tubing, but it must be reasonably flexible to be moved as needed by the operator. This means that it has a certain amount of elasticity and will tend to "bulge" somewhat under pressure from the fluid it contains. This dissipates some of the pressure before it gets to the transducer, making the pressure waveform "dampen" a little. When a waveform becomes dampened, it appears smoother with decreased amplitude.

Air bubbles within the system will also contribute to a damp pressure tracing. Pressure within the tubing can be dissipated internally by even tiny air bubbles, because the gases are highly compressible. When pressure is exerted at the catheter tip, some of this will be absorbed by the suspended gas, causing a damping of the curve.

It is therefore important to free the pressure lines of all bubbles when the system is flushed.

It is also important that the system be filled only with saline. Blood and contrast medium are more viscous, which also causes the transmitted wave to be slowed down. The pressure line should be well flushed between contrast injections and before every measurement. Due to the sensitivity of modern systems, a purely water-filled system will often be underdamped, causing "spikes" on the displayed waveform, making the pressure curve difficult to read. By artificially dampening the reading with a mixture of saline and a bit of contrast media, an accurate pressure can usually be obtained.

A loose or leaking connection will introduce air into the system and produce artificially low pressure readings. Connections to the manifold should be attached firmly during preparation and again with each change of catheter. The Tuohy-Borst adaptor ("Y-connector") used during interventional procedures is another common source of leaks. Similarly, the shape of the stopcocks and manifolds can cause resistance to the movement of fluid, particularly if the taps are not completely turned to the "on" or "off" position. They will also cause reverberations as the pressure waves bounce off them.

Another phenomenon that can cause some distortion of a hemodynamic waveform is the catheter "overfling" or "whip artifact." Movement of the catheter tip in response to the flow of blood or motion of the heart causes movement within the catheter. This movement is then interpreted at the transducer as a change in pressure. Catheter whip artifacts are often difficult to avoid, particularly in pulmonary arteries.

A phenomenon known as the Windkessel effect, a form of wave reflection is responsible for a higher pressure reading in the periphery than in the aorta. The walls of large arteries are muscular and contain elastic fibers. As blood is ejected from the heart during systole, the arteries (normally) increase their diameters to accommodate increased flow, and decrease their diameters when the blood pressure falls during diastole. The elastic recoil of the vessels helps to propagate blood flow through the body. Pressure measurements away from the heart measure not only the force of the heart's contraction, but also the waves of pressure that bounce off bifurcations and the walls of the narrowing arteries.

Also relevant is the phenomenon by which pressure waveforms taken peripherally occur later in the cardiac cycle in relation to the ECG. This is because the wave of pressure that is generated when the ventricle contracts must propagate outward and this takes time.

These differences in timing and pressure values between central and peripheral vessels are rarely of clinical importance except when two pressures measured at two different points are used to calculate a gradient. This occurs when the aortic pressure is taken via the sheath outlet and taken against the ventricular pressure measured through a catheter. In this case, care should be taken to synchronize the two curves, which can be done in real time on most modern hemodynamic systems.

During inspiration, the negative intrathoracic pressure is transmitted to the vascular bed, resulting in an increase in venous return to the right heart and lungs. This results in a slight decrease in arterial pressures. Although transmural pressures remain reasonably constant, respiratory artifacts do occur, most notably in the right heart and when the patient is dehydrated (Figure 12-3). This can be overcome in most cases by asking the patient to breathe superficially while the pressure is being recorded. By convention, hemodynamic measurements are typically recorded at end exhalation.

Conversely, artifacts can be produced by the Valsalva maneuver, which will reduce venous return and increase intrathoracic pressures. The Valsalva maneuver may be inadvertently performed by the patient under a number of common conditions, such as pain or a full bladder. These are

Figure 12-3. Pulmonary artery pressure at 5 mm/sec.

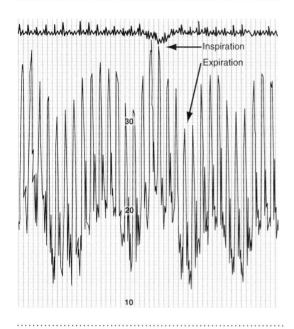

further exacerbated during deep breathing and may even produce an artificial gradient if release occurs during pull-back.

Electronic and Electrical Artifacts

An overresponsive system may cause ringing: multiple sharp upstrokes at the peaks of wave forms. This excessive oscillation is most evident just after large changes in pressure, such as the ventricular systolic peak in which a "spike" is usually apparent. This overshoot is, to a certain extent, due to the fact that moving particles (in this case, the column of water) tend to remain in motion, just as a car driven too quickly can miss a turnoff. This oscillation is also a natural part of the measurement system that occurs at a given frequency. A high frequency is necessary for a good frequency response.

Frequency response refers to the ability of the system to respond to changes in pressure at the measurement site. If the pressure at the catheter tip increases 100 mmHg in the space of 40 milliseconds (as occurs at left ventricular systole), how long does it take for this to be registered on the monitor? The frequency response of a system is determined by several factors, but with the accuracy of today's digital measurement systems, the inertia of the fluid-filled column is the single most important.

The extent to which a system is damped (its damping coefficient) is an important factor in obtaining an optimal signal. Too little damping will produce a wildly oscillating waveform that cannot be used for measurement purposes; too much damping will make the waveform sluggish and prevent it from reacting to sharp changes in pressure.

Cabling strung across floors can easily become damaged, cable connections that are not securely assembled, or fluid seeping onto plugs or connections can all cause artifacts whose source can be difficult to trace. If an unaccountable error arises, the culprit system's cabling should be exchanged with that of the other pressure system line (i.e., switching arterial with venous or vice versa) until the problem has been isolated and that cable replaced.

Electromagnetic noise can cause artifacts on the pressure curve to the point at which it is unusable. Poorly shielded devices and old X-ray equipment can produce strong electromagnetic fields, which will interfere with signal transmission in the same way that a car's engine can cause a car radio to crackle. Sometimes it is enough just to reroute some cables, but occasionally extensive shielding and grounding cables must be installed.

Human Error

Leveling and Balancing

It is important that the transducer is at the same level as the tip of the intravascular catheter. If the transducer lays lower than the tip, it is also measuring the force applied by the column of water within the pressure line, giving an inaccurately high measurement. If the transducer level is set too high, the force will be exerted in the other direction, making the measurement falsely low. Every 1 cm of difference relates to 0.735 mmHg. This may not seem to be a lot, but in right heart measurements, a few mmHg can be important and may be responsible for misdiagnosis, especially with children.

Leveling should be performed on each patient before balancing (zeroing) the transducer and should be left at that height for the duration of the procedure. To level, it is first necessary to find where the catheter tip will lay.

Most measurements are carried out in the left ventricle and the ascending aorta. These lay at the phlebostatic axis, which is midaxillary or midway between the patient's sternum and the tabletop when the patient is lying supine. Some laboratories use a point that is 5 cm below the level of the patient's sternum, which is also quite accurate. As a rule, there should always be a carpenter's level on hand to check the transducer's level before a right heart catheter procedure is performed. For left heart measurements, an eyeball estimate is usually adequate.

Proper balancing (zeroing) is as important as proper leveling. This involves the pressure measurement system between the transducer and the monitor, rather than the relation of the transducer to the heart. If a 0 mmHg reading is being displayed on the monitor, this means that no pressure is being exerted on the transducer. Technically, 0 mmHg means no pressure at sea level at 0°C. Because this is impractical in laboratories that are not on boats within the Arctic Circle, 0 mmHg is taken as equaling the equalizing to local atmospheric pressure at room temperature. This is achieved by opening a stopcock near the transducer to air to equalize to local atmospheric pressure (Figure 12-4). At the same time, the corresponding input channel on the hemodynamic

Figure 12-4. Manual calibration of pressure measurement system.

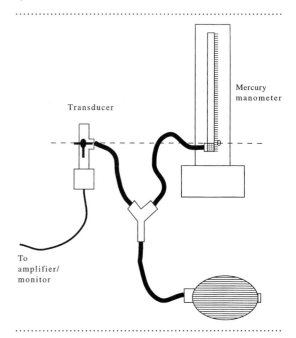

monitoring system is calibrated to "0" at the press of a button. When the stopcock is returned to measurement position, the system is measuring from an accepted zero point.

A system's zero may drift with time. The transducer(s) should be checked periodically and "rezeroed" during lengthy procedures. It is only necessary to turn the stopcock to atmospheric pressure. If the monitor reads "0," then the zero is still accurate and the stopcock can be returned to its operating position.

Slope Calibration

A slope error occurs when a system reads accurately at 0 mmHg, but its increase is inaccurate. The procedure to test this is quite simple and should only take a few minutes. Figure 12-4 shows how a mercury manometer is placed level with the transducer. The carpenter's level can be used here if necessary, because the zero point on the manometer must be exactly level with the transducer. The pressure measurement system is zeroed, and the two are then connected by tubing and a three-way connector to the manometer's pump. A stethoscope can easily be modified for this use. The manometer is then pumped up to 100 mmHg and then 200 mmHg, checking at each point that the monitor's readings agree. If there is some discrepancy, the amplifier's calibration will have to be modified. As discussed previously, mercury manometers are becoming difficult to obtain due to environmental concerns. Many manufacturers offer electronic devices designed to validate calibration.

HEMODYNAMIC WAVEFORMS

Now that the workings of the cardiac catheterization laboratory's pressure measurement system have been covered, the pressure waveforms themselves can be looked at in detail. Each chamber will be covered in the order that it is encountered by the circulating blood. The normal pressure values are shown in Table 12-1.

Central Venous Pressure/Right Atrium

Central venous pressure (CVP) is the pressure within the superior vena cava, directly outside the right atrium. CVP reflects the amount of venous blood returning to the heart, and the ability of the heart to pump the blood through the arterial system. A CVP pressure is generally measured by a catheter inserted into the subclavian vein, with the tip of the catheter resting in the lower third of the superior vena cava.

The right atrium is the chamber of the heart receiving venous blood from both the superior vena cava (which brings blood from the upper part of the body), and the inferior vena cava (which brings blood from the lower portion).

Both the right atrium and central venous pressure hemodynamic waveforms (Figure 12-5) consist of three positive deflections: the A, the C, and the V waves. The A wave is caused by a rise in pressure in the atrium during atrial contraction. The P wave of the ECG relates to the electrical stimulation of the atria and the mechanical atrial contraction occurs slightly after this. The A wave can therefore be found starting shortly after the peak of the P wave on the ECG. The V wave is the peak of passive filling of the right atrium when the tricuspid valve is closed.

During atrial contraction, blood is forced into the right ventricle and, as the atrium has

Table 12-1. Normal Supine Resting Pressure Values (in mmHg) in Humans

	Systolic	End diastolic	Mean	a-wave	v-wave
RA	–	–	0–8	2–10	2–10
RV	15–30	0–8	–	–	–
PA	15–30	3–12	9–16	–	–
PCW/LA	–	–	1–12	3–15	3–12
LV	100–140	3–12	–	–	–
Ao	100–140	60–90	70–105	–	–

Figure 12-5. Right atrium waveform.

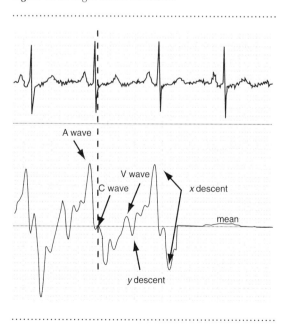

no valves between it and the vena cava, blood is also forced back into these. This free movement of blood ensures that the pressure in the right atrium never gets very high and that the upstroke of the A wave is relatively gradual. When atrial contraction is completed and ventricular contraction begins, the pressure in the atrium begins to fall. This causes a downstroke in the waveform called the *x* descent.

As the pressure in the ventricle increases, the tricuspid valve closes. The closing of the valve causes a small increase in pressure in the atrium (C wave), which looks like a bump on the *x* descent. The C wave is not always present on the waveform because the larger influence of the atrium can cover it up. The C wave, or where it should be if it is absent, can be found in line with the end of the QRS complex on the ECG.

When atrial contraction is finished and the tricuspid valve is closed, the movement of the ventricular contraction pulls it, and the tricuspid valve, downward. This has the effect of bringing the atrial pressure down, completing the *x* descent. The atrium then fills with blood again from the venous system. The blood entering the right atrium at this point is under very little pressure (usually between 2 and 8 mmHg), so once again there is only a gradual increase in pressure during this passive filling stage. This rise in pressure is shown on the waveform as the V wave, which is normally lower than the A wave.

When the V wave has peaked (meaning that the atrium is filled with blood at as much pressure as is present in the venous system), the right ventricle is in diastole. During this ventricular relaxation phase, when the pressure in the right ventricle falls below that of the right atrium, the tricuspid valve opens. The movement of blood from the atrium into the ventricle lowers the atrial pressure, causing a down stroke in the waveform, known as the *y* descent. When the pressures in the atrium and the ventricle equalize, the waveform bottoms out; it begins to rise again as the atrium contracts, forming the A wave again.

The mean pressure is a commonly measured parameter of the right atrium. The mean pressure is found by taking the peak value of the A and V waves, and the value in the following trough (*x* and *y* descent). The midpoint of these two values provides the mean. Modern equipment calculates the mean by averaging the pressure over the entire cardiac cycle. This value is important because it provides an estimate of the right ventricle's preload.

High CVP and right atrial A waves are found with:

- Tricuspid stenosis
- Pulmonic stenosis
- Right ventricular hypertrophy
- Pulmonary arterial hypertension

High CVP and right atrial V waves and no *x* descent are seen with:

- Tricuspid insufficiency

No A wave is present in atrial fibrillation.

Right Ventricle

The function of the right ventricle is to pump the venous blood into the pulmonary circulation. The peak of the right ventricular waveform is at the height of systole. This is when the ventricle is in full contraction, pushing the blood through the pulmonic valve into the pulmonary artery. The pressure generated by contraction of the right ventricle is much higher than that of the atrium. It is not transmitted into the atrium because the tricuspid valve is closed. The systolic pressure within a healthy right ventricle with healthy valves is around 25 mmHg at rest.

The mechanical systole begins at the end of the QRS complex on the ECG (Figure 12-6). The ventricle has received the electrical impulse and converts that into contractile force. The waveform rises rapidly, and the peak is reached

Figure 12-6. Right ventricle waveform.

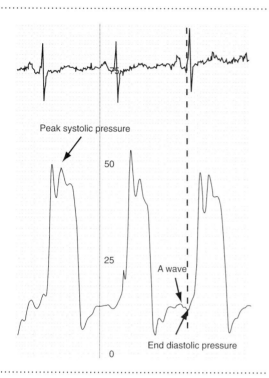

at the ECG's T wave. The ventricle then relaxes, exhibited by the rapid downstroke on the waveform. As the ventricular pressure falls below that of the pulmonary artery, the pulmonic valve closes. As it falls below the atrial pressure, the tricuspid valve opens, allowing the ventricle to be filled with blood from the right atrium. This refilling of the ventricle is shown as a rapid rise in pressure early in diastole (rapid filling phase) followed by a more gradual filling (diastolic), before filling is completed by atrial contraction. This takes place between the T and Q waves on the ECG.

One of the most important points on the right ventricular waveform is the right ventricular end diastolic pressure (RVEDP). This is the pressure in the ventricle when the atrium has finished its contraction and the tricuspid valve closes just as the ventricular contraction begins. This is usu-

ally present on the waveform as a small bump at the end of the diastole, known as the A wave. The end diastole pressure is taken in the trough after the A wave. If the A wave is not present, it can be found by drawing a vertical line from the R deflection of the QRS complex on the corresponding ECG.

The RVEDP is an indicator or how well the ventricle is filling, how well the patient is hydrated, and how elastic the myocardium is. The peak systolic pressure indicates whether the right ventricle has a normal contractility and whether it is pumping into a normal or an abnormal pulmonary artery bed.

High right ventricular peak systolic pressures are seen in:

- Pulmonary congestion due to left heart failure, mitral stenosis, etc.
- Primary pulmonary hypertension
- Pulmonic valve stenosis
- Left to right shunt
- COPD
- Peripheral PA stenosis

High right ventricular end diastolic pressures are seen in:

- Pulmonic valve insufficiency
- Restrictive myocardial disease (fibrosis)
- Endocardial fibrosis
- Constrictive pericarditis
- Cardiac tamponade

Pulmonary Artery

The pulmonary artery channels blood from the right heart into the lungs. During systole, when the pressure in the right ventricle exceeds that in the pulmonary artery, the pulmonic valve opens and there is a rapid rise in pressure. The systolic peak is reached early in the ECG's T wave. It has the same value as that of the right ventricular systole when the mitral valve is functioning correctly.

At the end of systole, and with the onset of ventricular relaxation, the pulmonic valve closes. This is reflected in the dicrotic notch, which is seen as a "bump" in the downstroke of the PA waveform (Figure 12-7). Instead of the rapid decrease in pressure at the beginning of diastole as exhibited in the ventricular waveform, the pressure in the pulmonary artery decreases more gradually. During diastole, the blood that was pushed into the artery during systole is distributed throughout the pulmonary tree. This equalizing of pressure over a large area and the elasticity of the arteries are the reasons for its gradual decrease.

The pressure in the pulmonary artery does not approach zero during diastole as it does in the ventricle. The pulmonic valve closes as the pressure in the ventricle falls below that in the artery. This prevents the blood from flowing back into the ventricle. This also provides enough continuous pressure to ensure that the blood is always being pushed through the arterioles of the lung.

Peak systolic pressure is an important value. When it is significantly lower than that of the right ventricle, it signifies a pulmonary valve stenosis.

Figure 12-7. Pulmonary artery waveform.

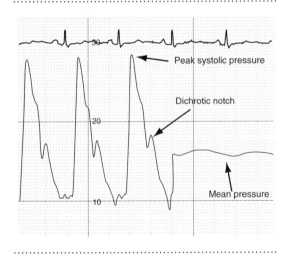

Mean pressure is not simply the midpoint between the systolic and diastolic pressures. Due to the fact that the waveform is not a perfect zigzag shape, more of the waveform is below the midpoint. Therefore the formula

$$\text{Mean} = \frac{\text{Systole} + (\text{Diastole} \times 2)}{3}$$

is used to calculate the mean pressure of the pulmonary artery.

High pulmonary artery pressures are seen with:

- Pulmonary emboli
- Mitral valve stenosis
- Chronic obstructive pulmonary disease
- Pulmonary hypertension
- Left ventricular failure
- Peripheral PA stenosis

Low pulmonary artery diastolic pressures are seen with:

- Pulmonic valve insufficiency

Left Atrium/Pulmonary Capillary Wedge Pressure

The pulmonary capillary wedge pressure (PCWP), sometimes referred to as pulmonary artery wedge pressure (PAWP), is obtained by inflating the balloon on a Swan-Ganz catheter in the pulmonary artery, allowing it to drift with the blood flow until it becomes lodged or "wedged" into a distal branch or carefully advancing an end-hole catheter (such as a Cournand) into a pulmonary arteriole. The objective is to position a catheter to measure the pressure on the left heart side of the pulmonary tree by temporarily obstructing proximal blood flow from the right heart.

The pressure distal to the arteriolar segment of the pulmonary circulation is equal to the left atrial pressure in the absence of an obstacle between the pulmonary arteriole and the left atrium (pulmonary vein stenosis, pulmonary emboli, etc.). There is a time delay and a degree of damping in the waveform when comparing a PCWP to that of a directly measured left atrium pressure. This is due to the transmission of the pressure through the pulmonary capillary beds. Therefore, the A wave is not found near the P-R interval in the ECG (as it is with the left atrium), but near the QRS complex (see Figure 12-8). Likewise, the rest of the components of the PCWP waveform occur later than with directly measured atrial waveforms. When these limitations are taken into account, the PCWP is a fairly good approximation of the left atrial pressure.

If the cardiologist is using an end-hole catheter to take the PCWP, it can be difficult to get a clean waveform without any pulmonary artery elements. The best way to ensure that the pressure tracing is that of the PCWP is to run

Figure 12-8. Pulmonary capillary wedge pressure waveform.

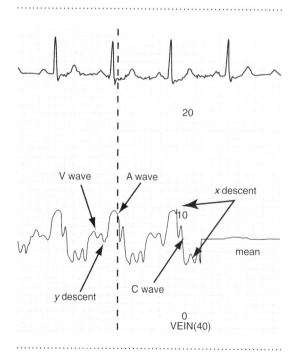

the LV pressure curve simultaneously on the same scale as that of the right heart curve and at a higher speed. The PCWP should demonstrate a rise (A wave) on the upstroke of the LV waveform as well as a rise (V wave) on the LV's downstroke. The PA waveform will have a rise only on the LV's upstroke. The other way to ensure that the tracing is a PCWP rather than a PA waveform is to do a pullback in mean. There will be a rise in the mean if the catheter was in the wedge position. Using an end-hole catheter instead of a balloon-tipped catheter also poses some risk, because the stiffer catheter tip may inadvertently dissect or perforate the pulmonary vasculature.

The atrial pressure itself is difficult to take directly. The shape of the left ventricle and the structure of the mitral valve make it difficult to safely approach it from the side of the left heart. It is possible to approach the left atrium via a transeptal puncture from the right atrium, but this procedure is not without risk, and so is not routinely undertaken.

The same nomenclature is used with the PCWP waveform as with that of the right atrium:

- The A wave is due to the contraction of the left atrium.
- The *x* descent shows the relaxation of the atrium and the downward movement of the mitral valve during left ventricular contraction.
- The C wave, caused by the closure of the mitral valve, is not always seen in the PCWP waveform due to the damping effect of the pulmonary capillary bed.

  The V wave is a rise in pressure brought on by the filling of the left atrium with oxygenated blood from the lungs.
- The *y* descent occurs as the pressure in the left atrium exceeds the left ventricle's diastolic pressure and the mitral valve opens. Blood then flows into the left ventricle, lowering the pressure in the atrium.

The values that are important with the PCWP are the peak of the V wave and the mean pressure.

The mean PCWP is derived from taking the point halfway between the peak of the A wave and the nadir (lowest point) of the x descent. The magnitude of the mean PCWP is related to the filling pressure of the left ventricle, which can be abnormal due to dysfunction of the mitral valve or left ventricle.

A low PCWP can be caused by:

- Hypovolemia

A high PCWP can be caused by:

- Left heart failure
- Mitral stenosis/insufficiency
- Tamponade
- Hypervolemia
- Ischemia
- Obstructive and restrictive cardiomyopathies
- Decompensated valve disease

A high PCWP V wave can be caused by:

- Mitral insufficiency

There are no A waves during atrial fibrillation. The PCWP will not reflect the left atrial pressure if there is pulmonary venous obstruction.

Left Ventricle

The left ventricle is responsible for generating enough contractile force to push the blood throughout the body. Its walls are thicker than those of the right ventricle and can therefore create a higher pressure. A healthy person's peak systolic pressure is around 120 mmHg, but in extreme cases, this can rise to 300 mmHg. Apart from the amplitude, the left ventricular waveform is similar to that of the right ventricle (see Figure 12-9). It is somewhat less "triangular" shaped with a steeper upstroke and downstroke due to its greater contractility.

Figure 12-9. Left ventricle waveform.

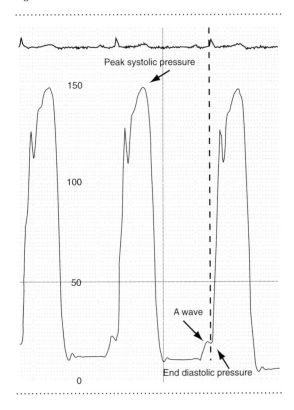

During systole, the aortic valve does not open until the ventricular pressure exceeds that of the aorta, so both valves are closed during the upstroke of systole. When the ventricular pressure equalizes, then exceeds aortic pressure, the aortic valve opens and the blood is pumped into the peripheral circulation. When the ventricular pressure falls once again below that of the aorta, the aortic valve closes. This is followed by the rapid downstroke as the ventricle relaxes.

At the end of this rapid downstroke, there is a slightly angled plateau as the relaxed ventricle fills with oxygenated blood from the left atrium. The end-diastolic pressure occurs when the ventricle is full of blood and its pressure is greater than that of the atrium. The mitral valve then closes, creating a small notch known as the A wave.

The end-diastolic pressure (LVEDP) is taken in the trough immediately after the A wave. If the A wave is absent, the end-diastolic pressure can be found in line with the R deflection of the QRS complex on the ECG.

Apart from the LVEDP, the other important value on the left ventricular waveform is the peak systolic pressure. This can be found in the same way as it was with the right ventricular waveform. Mechanical systole begins at the end of the QRS complex on the ECG. When the ventricle receives the electrical impulse, this causes depolarization, and this results in contractile force.

Low left ventricular pressure can be caused by:

- Left heart failure
- Inadequate LV filling (due to hypovolemia or mitral valve insufficiency)

High left ventricular systolic pressure can be caused by:

- Hypertension
- Aortic valve stenosis
- Peripheral arterial vascular disease

High left ventricular end-diastolic pressure can be caused by:

- Aortic valve insufficiency
- Diseases damaging LV compliance (hypertrophy, ischemia, etc.)

Aorta

The aortic pressure shows the amount of contractile force under which the blood has entered the systemic circulation. It is similar in shape to the pulmonary artery waveform with higher amplitude and no respiratory variance (normally). There is a rapid systolic upstroke as the blood from the contracting ventricle is pushed through the aortic valve into the aorta. With a high-fidelity transducer, an anacrotic notch is visible on the upstroke of the waveform as the aortic valve opens. The peak of the aortic waveform should correlate with that of the left ventricle because the valve is open at this time, allowing the pressures of the two to equalize. This is followed by a gradual downstroke as the blood flows distally through the aorta (see Figure 12-10). The peak systolic pressure is important, especially in relation to that of the LV. If it is significantly lower, an aortic stenosis may be present.

The dicrotic notch is usually apparent on the downstroke of the aortic waveform and is caused by the closing of the aortic valve. The valve closes as the ventricle relaxes and the pressure therein falls below that in the aorta. The dicrotic notch

Figure 12-10. Aorta waveform.

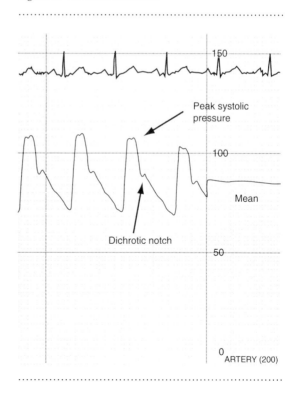

signifies the beginning of mechanical diastole, when the majority of coronary artery circulation occurs.

The values that are important with aortic pressure readings are the peak systolic, the diastolic, and the mean. In this case, the mean is calculated, as it is with the pulmonary artery, with the formula

$$\text{Mean} = \frac{\text{Systolic} + (2 \times \text{Diastolic})}{3}$$

Figure 12-11 shows how the aortic pressure is modified when the catheter tip is wedged into an artery occluding flow or up against the wall of the vessel. The waveform is a damped version of the aortic pressure and can be easily recognized by its lowered amplitude.

The operator's attention should be immediately called to such a waveform. Wedging, or deepthroating, the catheter in an artery is potentially dangerous. This effectively blocks blood flow to the vessel for a time, which may cause spasm or spontaneous closing of dilated or stented sections. A normal waveform also guarantees that a subsequent injection is not being made under a plaque, which can result in the immediate occlusion of the ostial segment. Injection of contrast medium in a wedged position is also the most common cause of ventricular fibrillation in the cardiac catheterization laboratory and must be avoided.

A significant left main trunk or right ostial coronary stenosis will produce another variation on the aortic waveform. Figure 12-12 shows a waveform with the catheter tip at the entrance to a right coronary artery with a 90% ostial stenosis. Notice the "AA wavelike" notch just prior to the upstroke. The appearance becomes elongated, resembling a ventricular waveform. This is why such an aortic waveform is said to be "ventricularized." The operator's attention should be called to this phenomenon immediately, because if ostial disease is suspected, angiography should be performed subselectively, with a minimum of ostium-catheter tip contact. This waveform can

Figure 12-11. "Wedged" aorta waveform.

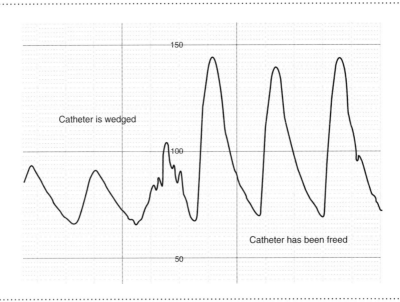

Figure 12-12. Ostial lesion aorta waveform.

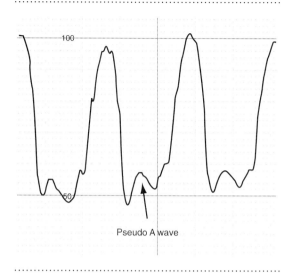

easily be distinguished from that of the ventricle due to its high diastolic pressure.

A high peak systolic pressure can be caused by:

• Peripheral arterial vascular disease

A low diastolic pressure can be caused by:

• Sepsis
• Aortic valve insufficiency

A low mean pressure can be caused by:

• Hypovolemia
• Insufficient left ventricular performance
• Decreased peripheral resistance

GRADIENTS

A pressure gradient is a difference in pressure caused by an obstruction. In the CCL, it usually refers to the functional capacity of a valve, although it can also be used to describe the physiologic effect of a stenosis. With the use of the hemodynamic wave-

forms, the gradient is given a numerical value that is a measure of the valve's efficacy:

$$\text{Gradient} = \text{Blood flow} \times \text{Resistance}$$

Thus an aortic stenosis may produce a deceivingly low gradient in the presence of left ventricle failure (see Figure 12-13).

Two measures of gradient severity are most commonly used. The peak-to-peak gradient is calculated by taking the peak systolic value (or the average of a series of peaks) of one waveform and subtracting it from the peak systolic (or average) of the other.

The mean gradient is the mathematical average value of the difference between the two waveforms. To calculate a mean gradient, a series of vertical lines are drawn in the area between the two waveforms, and the sum of these values is then divided by their number. The mean gradient is the more accurate of the two methods, and the more vertical lines used, the more accurate it is. LV/AO mean pressure gradients are calculated by hemodynamic computers by measuring the area between the two pressure curves and dividing

Figure 12-13. Aortic stenosis waveforms.

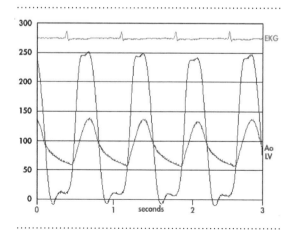

it by the systolic time interval. This is the most precise technique.

VALVE AREA CALCULATIONS

The extent to which a stenotic valve opens can be used to determine if it is the reason for the patient's symptoms and to determine how best to treat the patient. Aortic and mitral valve area calculations can be performed in the CCL using the Gorlin formula, specific for each valve. Basically, the Gorlin formula states that there is a relationship between the size of the opening of a valve, the flow rate across that valve, and the pressure gradient required to deliver that flow rate.

Aortic Valve

$$\text{Aortic valve area} = \frac{\text{cardiac output / sep} \times \text{HR}}{44.3 \times \text{square root of the mean pressure gradient}}$$

In the cath lab, determine the aortic valve flow rate by dividing the cardiac output (expressed in cc's per minute) by the amount of time the aortic valve was actually open in 1 minute.

The systolic ejection period (sep) per beat is the amount of time the aortic valve is open during each cardiac cycle. It can be determined by evaluating simultaneous LV and aortic (or a phase-shifted femoral artery) pressure waveforms. The sep begins when the aortic valve opens and is noted when LV pressure exceeds Ao pressure. The sep is over when the aortic valve closes and is noted when the LV pressure drops below AO pressure.

By multiplying the sep per beat by the heart rate, the staff can determine how long the aortic valve is open, and systolic ejection occurring, in 1 minute. The sep is usually less than 30 seconds.

The aortic valve flow rate can be calculated by dividing the cardiac output by the systolic ejection period per minute. For example, a patient with a cardiac output of 6 liters (6000 cc's) per minute, and a sep of 20 seconds per minute would have an aortic valve flow rate of 300 cc's per second.

The other variable in the Gorlin equation is the pressure gradient required to deliver that flow rate. By observing the simultaneous LV and AO (or phase-shifted FA) hemodynamic waveforms, the mean pressure gradient can be calculated manually or measured by the computer. The square root of the mean gradient is multiplied by 44.3 (the Gorlin constanant for the aortic valve). With the aortic valve flow rate and the mean aortic valve gradient, the opening area of the aortic valve can be calculated.

For example:

$$CO = 4.3 \text{ lpm, sep} = .22 \text{ sec/beat, HR} = 95,$$
$$\text{mean gradient} = 40 \text{ mmHg}$$

$$AVA = \frac{CO \times 1000/\text{sep} \times HR}{44.3 \times \text{sq. root pressure gradient}}$$

$$AVA = \frac{4.3 \times 1000/.22 \times 95}{44.3 \times \text{sq. root of } 40}$$

$$AVA = \frac{4300 \text{ cc's}/20.9 \text{ sec/min}}{44.3 \times 6.3}$$

$$AVA = \frac{205.7 \text{ cc's/sec}}{279.1}$$

$$AVA = 0.7 \text{ cm}^2$$

The Gorlin formula is considered to be the most accurate, but there is also a "shortcut" formula know as the Haaki formula:

$$AVA = \frac{\text{Cardiac output (in liters per minute)}}{\text{Square root of the pressure gradient}}$$

$$AVA = \frac{5}{6.3}$$

$$AVA = 0.8 \text{ cm}^2$$

Mitral Valve

The Gorlin formula for the mitral valve is similar, but the diastolic filling period is substituted for the systolic ejection period, and the Gorlin constanant is 37.7.

Mitral valve area =
$$\frac{\text{cardiac output (in cc's)/dfp} \times \text{HR}}{37.7 \times \text{square root of the mean pressure gradient}}$$

The diastolic filling period (dfp) per beat is the amount of time the mitral valve is open during each cardiac cycle. It can be determined by evaluating simultaneous LV and LA (or a phase-shifted PCWP) pressure waveforms. The dfp begins when the mitral valve opens and is noted when LA pressure exceeds LV pressure. The dfp is over when the mitral valve closes and is noted when the LV pressure exceeds LA pressure.

By multiplying the dfp per beat by the heart rate, the staff can determine how long the mitral valve is open and diastolic filling occurring in 1 minute. They then can divide the cardiac output by the dfp per minute and calculate the mitral valve flow rate.

For example, a patient with a cardiac output of 4 liters (4000 cc's) per minute and a dfp of 40 seconds per minute would have a mitral valve flow rate of 100 cc's per second. The dfp is usually greater than 30 seconds.

The other variable in the Gorlin equation is the pressure gradient required to deliver that flow rate. By observing the simultaneous LV and LA (or phase-shifted PCWP) hemodynamic waveforms, the mean pressure gradient can be calculated or measured by the computer. The square root of the mean gradient is multiplied by 37.7 (the Gorlin constant for the mitral valve). With the mitral valve flow rate and the mean mitral valve gradient, the opening area of the mitral valve can be calculated.

For example:

$$\text{CO} = 6.3 \text{ lpm, dfp} = .39 \text{ sec/beat, HR} = 98,$$
$$\text{mean gradient} = 15 \text{ mmHg}$$

$$\text{MVA} = \frac{\text{CO} \times 1000/\text{dfp} \times \text{HR}}{37.7 \times \text{sq. root pressure gradient}}$$

$$\text{MVA} = \frac{6.3 \times 1000/.39 \times 98}{37.7 \times \text{sq. root of } 15}$$

$$\text{MVA} = \frac{6300 \text{ cc's}/38.2 \text{ sec/min}}{37.7 \times 3.87}$$

$$\text{MVA} = \frac{164.8 \text{ cc's/sec}}{145.9}$$

$$\text{MVA} = 1.1 \text{ cm}^2$$

CARDIAC OUTPUT

The volume of blood delivered to the systemic circulation per unit of time is measured as the left ventricular cardiac output. Similarly, the volume of blood delivered to the pulmonic circulation per unit of time is the right ventricular cardiac output. Normally, the cardiac output of the left ventricle equals the cardiac output from the right ventricle.

Cardiac output is a function of stroke volume (the volume of blood ejected from the ventricle each beat) times the heart rate. Assuming a normal stroke volume of approximately 70 cc's, and a normal heart rate of 70 beats per minute, the staff can calculate a cardiac output of 4900 cc's or 4.9 liters per minute. The normal range for the cardiac output of an adult is 4.0 liters to 8.0 liters per minute.

Cardiac Index

Cardiac output is a very useful hemodynamic value; however, it does not take differences in body size into account. Cardiac index allows the medical team to normalize a patient's cardiac output, regardless of their size. If the cardiac output is divided by the patient's body surface area, they can calculate the cardiac index. For example, assuming a cardiac output of 5.4 liters per minute with a BSA of 2.0 meters^2, the CI = 5.4/2.0 or 2.7 liters per minute per meter^2.

Body surface area is a function of a patient's height and weight. BSAs are not normally measured, but can be calculated by several formulas. For example:

$$BSA\ (m^2) = 0.007184 \times weight\ in\ kg^{\,0.425} \times height\ in\ cm^{\,0.725}$$

The cath lab's computer will derive the patient's BSA based on the input of height and weight. A normal BSA for a 6-foot-tall male weighing 175 pounds would be approximately 2.0 meters^2.

Cardiac Output Formulas

Fick

Various methods to determine cardiac output are used in today's cath labs. The Fick equation of cardiac output is considered to be the "gold standard" and represents "forward" cardiac output.

The Fick equation states:

$$Cardiac\ output_{(Fick)} = \frac{VO_2}{(CaO_2 - CvO_2) \times 10}$$

where VO_2 is oxygen consumption per minute, CaO_2 is arterial oxygen content, and CvO_2 is venous oxygen content.

VO_2, oxygen consumption, is usually estimated rather than measured in most cath labs today. A patient's predicted oxygen consumption can be estimated based on an oxygen consumption index calculated from a patient's BSA and then be corrected for age and sex. Most labs assume a normal resting oxygen consumption index of

125 ml for oxygen per meter^2 BSA. If the team knows the predicted oxygen consumption index and the BSA, they can calculate the predicted oxygen consumption. For example, assuming an oxygen consumption index of 125 ml of oxygen per meter^2, and a BSA of 2.0 meter^2, they can multiply 125 × 2.0 and calculate a predicted oxygen consumption of 250 ml of oxygen per minute. A normal range for oxygen consumption is between 175 ml to 250 ml O_2 per minute.

The total oxygen content of arterial (CaO_2) and venous (CvO_2) blood can also be calculated by evaluating arterial blood and mixed venous blood. Arterial blood can be obtained from the aorta and mixed venous blood is usually obtained from the pulmonary artery. Oxygen is carried two ways in blood: bound to hemoglobin and dissolved as a gas in blood plasma. The great majority of oxygen is carried bound to hemoglobin in the form of oxyhemoglobin. The percent of hemoglobin saturated with oxygen can be measured with a pulse oximeter. Normal arterial oxygen saturation (SaO_2) is around 98% and normal mixed venous oxygen saturation (SvO_2) is around 75%.

The partial pressure of gaseous oxygen dissolved in blood plasma with a blood gas analyser. The normal partial pressure of oxygen in arterial blood (PaO_2) is around 80 to 100 mmHg, and the normal partial pressure of oxygen in venous blood (PvO_2) is around 40 mmHg.

When the amount of oxygen bound to hemoglobin is added to the amount dissolved in plasma, the total oxygen content of arterial (CaO_2) and venous (CvO_2) blood can be calculated. The formula is:

$$CaO_2 = (1.36^* \times Hgb \times SaO_2) + (0.003 \times PaO_2)$$

---

*1.36 is a constant; each gram of hemoglobin can carry 1.36 ml of oxygen. Some references use a constant of 1.34 or 1.39. The first part of the equation is the amount of oxygen bound to hemoglobin; the second part represents the amount dissolved in plasma.

For example, with Hgb of 14 grams/deciliter, SaO_2 of 98%, and PaO_2 of 90 mmHg:

$$CaO_2 = (1.36 \times 14 \times 98\%) + (0.003 \times 90)$$

$$CaO_2 = (18.7) + (0.3)$$

$CaO_2 = 19.0$ vol% (19 ml O_2 per 100 ml of blood or 190 ml O_2 per liter of blood)

Normal CaO_2 is around 19 to 20 vol%.
The calculation of the CvO_2 is similar.
A Hgb of 14 grams/deciliter, SvO_2 of 73%, and PvO_2 of 40 mmHg:

$$CvO_2 = (1.36 \times 14 \times 73\%) + (0.003 \times 40)$$

$$CvO_2 = (13.9) + (0.1)$$

$CvO_2 = 14.0$ vol% (14 ml O_2 per 100 ml of blood or 140ml O_2 per liter of blood)

Normal CvO_2 is around 14 to 15 vol%.
CaO_2 minus CvO_2 is also referred to as the a-v difference. It represents the oxygen content difference between arterial and venous blood. The difference is how much oxygen was given up by arterial blood to supply the metabolic needs of the tissues. There is an inverse relationship between the a-v difference and cardiac output. As cardiac output decreases, the tissues consume more oxygen. This will decrease the CvO_2 and increase the a-v difference.

Using the values in the previous examples, VO_2 of 250 ml per minute, CaO_2 of 19 vol%, and CvO_2 of 14 vol%, the Fick cardiac output can be calculated.

$$Cardiac\ output_{(Fick)} = \frac{VO_2}{(CaO_2 - CvO_2) \times 10}$$

$$Cardiac\ output_{(Fick)} = \frac{250}{(19 - 14) \times 10}$$

$$Cardiac\ output_{(Fick)} = \frac{250}{(5) \times 10}$$

$$Cardiac\ Output_{(Fick)} = \frac{250}{50}$$

$Cardiac\ output_{(Fick)} = 5$ liters per minute

In this example, if a patient consumes 250 ml of oxygen in 1 minute and each liter of arterial blood contributes 50 ml of oxygen, then the patient must have a cardiac output of 5 liters per minute.

Thermodilution

The thermodilution cardiac output can be determined in the cath lab. It is also a "forward" cardiac output. This method uses a 4 lumen pulmonary artery catheter.

The theory behind thermodilution is based on the principle that there is a relationship between the degree of temperature change and the cardiac output required to achieve that change in temperature. For example, assume two containers holding blood with a temperature of 98.6° F. One container holds 1 cup and the other 1 gallon. If a staff member injects 10 ml of 70 degree saline into both containers, the smaller one will have a larger change in temperature than the larger one. The temperature changes at the tip of the thermodilution catheter is a result of right heart cardiac output, so thermodilution is considered to measure the cardiac output of the right heart.

The procedure involves 5 ml or 10 ml of room temperature (or chilled) saline or D5W being injected into the catheter's CVP/RA proximal hub. This enters the right atrium to mix with the patient's blood. This saline/blood mixture then travels to the right ventricle and out into the pulmonary artery. A thermistor, located close to the tip of the pulmonary artery catheter, measures the temperature of the blood/mixture in the pulmonary artery. The change in temperature and the rate at which it occurs is then used to calculate the CO. Usually, three to five thermodilution measurements are performed, and the results are averaged after any outliers have been eliminated.

Thermodilution cardiac output may not be accurate in very low cardiac output states (less than 3 liters per minute), significant tricuspid or pulmonic valve regurgitation, and with atrial or ventricular septal defects.

Angiographic

The angiographic cardiac output measures the total volume of blood ejected from the left ventricle. Typically, a left ventriculogram is filmed in an RAO projection. The outermost visible margin of the left ventricle is traced to correspond with the end of diastole, and another tracing is made of the LV gram at the end of systole. The tracings can be done either manually or automatically with the computer software. The left ventricle is shaped like an ellipse, and a formula is used to estimate the left ventricular volume at the end of diastole and the end of systole from the LV lengths and areas. Modern cath lab computers will correct for magnification and make these calculations.

The left ventricular end-diastolic volume (LVEDV) and left ventricular end-systolic volume (LVESV) can be determined. Stroke volume, SV, is the difference between LVEDV and LVESV, so SV = LVEDV − LVESV.

For example: LVEDV of 130 ml, LVESV of 45 ml; SV = 130 − 45, SV = 85 ml. If this patient has a heart rate of 60, the angiographic cardiac output would be 85 × 60 = 5100 ml or 5.1 liters per minute.

The ejection fraction (EF) is the percent of blood ejected from the left ventricle each beat. The formula is: EF = SV/LVEDV. The EF of the previous example is 85/130 or 65%.

REGURGITANT FRACTION

Fick and thermodilution cardiac outputs are considered to represent forward cardiac outputs from the left and right hearts respectively, and angiographic cardiac output represents the total cardiac output of the left ventricle. This total flow may not all be moving forward, however. In mitral regurgitation, not all of the blood leaving the left ventricle goes forward into the aorta. Some will regurgitate across the mitral valve back into the left atrium. The regurgitant fraction (RF) can be calculated by comparing the total volume ejected from the left ventricle with the amount of ejected blood going forward.

The formula for regurgitant fraction is:

$$RF = \frac{\text{Stroke volume angiographic} - \text{stroke volume Fick or theromdilution}}{\text{Stroke volume angiographic}}$$

For example: a patient has an angiographic stroke volume of 80 ml and a forward stroke volume of 60 ml, as determined via Fick or thermodilution: 20 ml are regurgitating across the mitral valve with each beat.

The RF percentage can be calculated:

$$RF = \frac{80 - 60}{80}$$

$$RF = \frac{20}{80}$$

$$RF = 25\%$$

In this example, 25% of the left ventricular ejection regurgitates across the mitral valve and 75% moves forward into the aorta and systemic circulation

SHUNTS

Common shunts encountered in cath labs include atrial septal defects (ASD), patient foramen ovale (PFO), ventricular septal defects (VSD), patent ductus arteriosis (PDA), and anomalous pulmonary venous return. Shunts can be classified as being right to left, left to right, or bidirectional. In a right-to-left shunt, deoxygenated blood will shunt from the right heart or pulmonary artery to the left heart or aorta. The deoxygenated shunted blood bypasses the lungs and ultimately enters the systemic blood flow, lowering the overall systemic oxygen values. This may lead to cyanosis.

The cardiac output of the right and left ventricles are normally equal. Likewise, pulmonary blood flow (Qp, where Q symbolizes flow and p symbolizes pulmonary) equals systemic blood flow (Qs). Assuming that the cardiac output of both right and left ventricles equals 5 liters per minute, Qp and Qs both equal 5 liters per minute. This results in a normal Qp:Qs ratio of 5:5 or 1:1. However, intracardiac shunts will alter this normal ratio and blood flows.

In a right-to-left shunt, the systemic blood flow (Qs) will be greater than the pulmonary blood flow (Qp) because some of the venous blood is bypassing the lungs. This will result in a Qp:Qs ratio less than 1:1. In a left-to-right shunt, oxygenated blood will shunt from the left heart or aorta to the right heart, pulmonary artery, or vena cava. In this case, the oxygenated shunted blood bypasses the systemic circulation and makes an additional trip through the lungs. This causes the Qp to be greater than Qs, resulting in a Qp:Qs ratio greater than 1:1. The increase in pulmonary blood flow can ultimately result in an increase in pulmonary artery pressures and pulmonary edema. A bidirectional shunt will combine elements of both of these conditions.

For example: A patient having a LV Qs of 4 liters per minute, and a RV Qp of 12 liters per minute would have a Qp:Qs ratio of 12:4 or 3:1. This is greater than 1:1 and would imply a left-to-right shunt.

The absolute shunt is the total volume or amount of blood that shunts across a defect in 1 minute. The absolute shunt = Qp − Qs. In the previous example, Qp − Qs = 12 − 4 or 8 liters

per minute. In other words, there are 8 liters of blood per minute shunting across the defect.

The percent shunt shows the percent of the circulating blood that goes through the shunt. The formula for the percent shunt is:

$$\text{Shunt \%} = \frac{Qp - Qs}{Qp}$$

In the previous example,

$$\text{Shunt \%} = \frac{12 - 4}{12}$$

$$\text{Shunt \%} = \frac{8}{12} = 67\%$$

This means that 67% of the total pulmonary blood flow is comprised of shunted blood, making an additional trip through the lungs.

In the previous example, the pulmonic and systemic blood flows are 12 and 4 liters, respectively. The pulmonic and systemic blood flows can be calculated using a variation of the Fick cardiac output calculation. The formula for the Fick cardiac output uses the $CaO_2 - CvO_2$ difference as an indicator that reflects the oxygen content difference between the beginning and end of the systemic circulation.

$$\text{Cardiac output}_{(Fick)} = \frac{VO_2}{Q(CaO_2 - CvO_2) \times 10}$$

The beginning of the systemic circulation is the aorta, so the sample of arterial blood is taken from the aorta. Mixed venous blood is usually drawn from the pulmonary artery. In a left-to-right shunt, pulmonary artery blood no longer represents mixed venous blood because it also contains oxygenated shunted blood, so another source of venous blood is necessary. The Flamm formula uses a weighted average of superior vena cava and inferior vena cava blood saturations to calculate the SvO_2, and ultimately the CvO_2. Blood oxygen saturation measurements for the SVC and IVC are needed for this.

The Flamm formula for mixed venous saturation, $S_{mv}O_2$:

$$S_{mv}O_2 = \frac{(\text{Saturation SCV} \times 3) + (\text{Saturation IVC} \times 1)}{4}$$

The SCV saturation is weighted heaver to account for coronary blood flow that does not return through the vena cava but has a very low saturation.

Assuming a patient with a left-to-right shunt has a SCV saturation of 68% and IVC saturation of 75% the mixed venous saturation can be calculated as follows:

$$S_{mv}O_2 = \frac{(\text{Saturation SCV} \times 3) + (\text{Saturation IVC} \times 1)}{4}$$

$$S_{mv}O_2 = \frac{(68\% \times 3) + (75\% \times 1)}{4}$$

$$S_{mv}O_2 = \frac{(204\%) + (75\%)}{4}$$

$$S_{mv}O_2 = \frac{279\%}{4}$$

$$S_{mv}O_2 = 70\%$$

The systemic blood flow (Qs) can then be calculated using the Fick equation. To calculate the CaO_2, the patient's arterial saturation would be used to calculate mixed venous content ($CmvO_2$) using the 70% derived from the Flamm equation.

The calculation of pulmonary blood flow (Qp) is similar. The beginning of the pulmonary circulation is the pulmonary artery and the end is the pulmonary veins or left atrium. Blood is sampled from the pulmonary artery and left atrium or a pulmonary vein. Because left atrial saturation is usually equal to arterial saturation, arterial blood can be substituted for left atrial or pulmonary vein blood in a left-to-right shunt with an arterial saturation greater than 95%.

The following equations can be used to calculate systemic and pulmonary blood flows:

$$Qs\ (\text{systemic blood flow}) = \frac{VO_2}{(CaO_2 - CmvO_2) \times 10}$$

CaO2 = oxygen content of arterial blood
CmvO2 = oxygen content of mixed venous blood (derived from the Flamm equation)

$$Qp\ (\text{pulmonary blood flow}) = \frac{VO_2}{(CpvO_2 - CpaO_2) \times 10}$$

CpvO2 = oxygen content of pulmonary venous blood
CpaO2 = oxygen content of pulmonary artery blood

SUMMARY

Intravascular pressure measurements are easily obtained accurate diagnostic tools. Together with coronary angiography, they make up the bulk of the diagnostic procedures in today's cardiovascular catheter laboratories. These invasive pressure measurements can give valuable information on a disease state that cannot be obtained by noninvasive means. If a catheter laboratory's pressure measurement equipment is well-maintained and accurate, the staff can depend on it. It will not only detect and quantify illness and malformation, but it will give them important diagnostic information in an emergency.

Understanding of the theories behind (and the methods to calculate) hemodynamic measurements can help to understand the data and alert the team when the computer incorrectly interprets the collected information.

SUGGESTED READING

Aherns TS. *Hemodynamic Waveform Recognition*. Philadelphia: WB Saunders; 1993.

Dinnar U. *Cardiovascular Fluid Dynamics*. Boca Raton, FL: CRC Press; 1981.

Eisenhauser M, Kern M. *Invasive Hemodynamics in the Catheterization Laboratory: Self-Assessment and Review*. London: Remedica Pulishing; 2002.

Fowler NO. *Cardiac Diagnosis and Treatment*, 3rd ed. Hagerstown, MD: Harper & Row; 1980.

Grossman W. Pressure measurement. In Grossman W, Baim D. *Cardiac Catheterization, Angiography and Intervention*, 4th ed. Philadelphia: Lea & Febiger; 1991.

Kern MJ. *The Cardiac Catheterization Handbook*. Philadelphia: Mosby; 2003.

Kern MJ. *Haemodynamic Rounds: Interpretation of Cardiac Pathophysiology from Pressure Waveform Analysis*. New York: Wiley-Liss; 1993.

Lambert CR, Pepine CJ, Nichols WW. Pressure measurement. In Pepine CJ. *Diagnostic and Therapeutic Cardiac Catheterization*. Baltimore: Williams & Wilkins; 1989.

Rushner RF. *Cardiovascular Dynamics*, 4th ed. Philadelphia: WB Saunders; 1976.

Chapter 13

INVASIVE ULTRASOUND

Kenneth A. Gorski, RN, RCIS, RCSA, FSICP

Despite the universal acceptance of coronary angiography, it has limitations. Postmortem studies have shown major differences in the severity of lesions as compared to that demonstrated by angiography.[1] Angiography produces an X-ray roadmap of the coronary tree, however, it is limited by the fact that it produces only a silhouette of the arterial lumen. This restricts quantitative measurements to that of the vessel diameter only. An atherosclerotic lesion may be "foreshortened" if it is not filmed in a parallel plane of view or it may be misdiagnosed completely. For this reason, multiple contrast injections in multiple X-ray views must be performed to completely identify the coronary anatomy.

Intravascular ultrasound (IVUS) uses catheters with an array of transmitters and sensors around their distal tip, facing toward the vessel walls. Sound waves are bounced off the vessel walls, and their echo provides detailed images of the composition of lesions, and the vessels themselves. IVUS provides a safe and practical alternative to

coronary angiography and gives greater insight into the coronary artery disease process.

Ultrasound technology has also been modified to enable forward-oriented sensors to give accurate images of cardiac structures that cannot be accurately imaged from external echo sensors. Intracardiac echocardiography (ICE) is being used to guide radio frequency ablations and aid complex structural heart procedures.

IVUS AND CORONARY ARTERY DISEASE

With IVUS, a catheter with an ultrasound transducer mounted near the tip is placed directly into the coronary artery, producing a two-dimensional image from the inside out, and not confined to the lumen. The tomographic orientation of the ultrasound catheter within the artery allows for full 360° visualization of the vessel wall, permitting both direct measurement of diameter and cross-sectional area. In patients with localized angiographic coronary artery disease, IVUS

Figure 13-1. Schematic demonstrating the limitations of angiography.

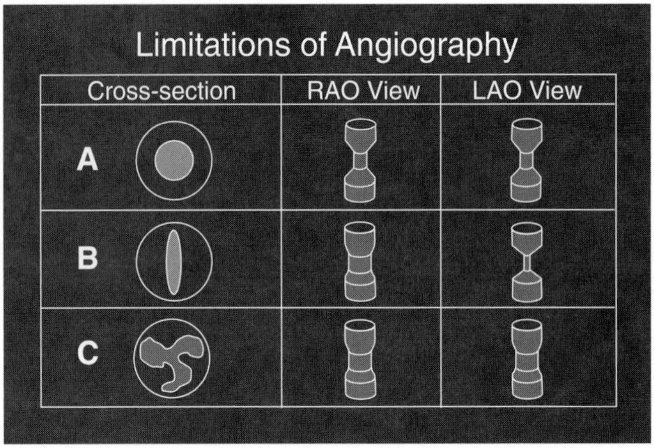

typically shows much greater deposits of plaque. IVUS also frequently reveals surprising plaque deposits in seemingly normal vessels, including concentric luminal narrowings, causing overall vessel shrinkage.[2]

With IVUS, it is possible to distinguish different plaque morphologies that may not be appreciated with angiography alone (see Figure 13-1).

HISTORY

Ultrasound was first developed during World War I (1917) for the detection of submarines and icebergs. In 1953, physicist Helmuth Hertz, working with the cardiologist Inge Edler, first de-

scribed echoes from the moving structures of the heart. The first catheter-based ultrasound system was utilized by Bom and associates in Rotterdam in 1971 for viewing cardiac chambers and valves. Through the early and mid-1980s, several groups tried to develop ultrasound catheters for intravascular use, and Paul Yock and colleagues reported the first human intracoronary images in 1988.[3]

Early applications of intracoronary ultrasound involved the use of very stiff 5F to 6F catheters. Cardiologists were limited to imaging proximal vessels, generally postintervention only. The large profile and rigidity of these early catheters were not favorable to the typically tortuous human

Table 13-1. Angiography vs. IVUS

Angiography	Intravascular Ultrasound
Planar imaging	Tomographic imaging
Periodic imaging with contrast injections	Continuous real time imaging
Shadow of lumen (lumenogram)	Direct lumen and wall visualization
Defines plaque location	Defines plaque morphology
Quantified vessel analysis adjusted for camera angle and magnification without magnification adjustments	Precise vessel diameter and cross sectional area

coronary anatomy. Advancements in micro-technology have allowed IVUS catheters to be miniaturized to 2.9F to 3.2F diameters. Newer catheters are much more flexible, allowing not only preintervention lesion imaging, but assessment of more distal vasculature as well. Despite this miniaturization, image quality has also improved greatly.

IVUS SYSTEMS

Currently, there are two distinct technologies available in catheter-based ultrasound imaging: mechanical transducers and electronic multielement phased-array transducers.

Mechanical IVUS catheters are designed with a moveable imaging core within an integrated sheath. Using sterile technique, the catheters are prepped with heparinized saline prior to use. The telescoping imaging core should be retracted to its most proximal position. A 6-inch (15-cm) extension tube is connected to the proximal hub of the catheter and a three-way stopcock is attached. A 3-cc and a 10-cc syringe, both filled with heparinized saline, are attached to the stopcock, and the imaging catheter is flushed with the 3-cc syringe. The 10-cc syringe is used as a fluid reservoir, and the catheter is flushed a second time to ensure that all air has been expelled. It has been the experience of some that with poor catheter prepping,

the IVUS image intermittently degrades, which may periodically require additional catheter flushing during imaging runs. The mechanical catheter designs also have short, monorail guide wire lumens, and catheter-handling characteristics remain inferior to the solid-state design.

Electronic, phased-array IVUS catheters require minimal preparation, involving only one step: handing off the electronic connection for imaging to a nonsterile circulator, who then plugs the catheter into the patient interface module (PIM9), which interfaces with the IVUS console.

The Volcano Therapeutics (San Diego, CA) phased-array IVUS catheters have 64 electronic elements mounted circumferentially near the catheters' distal tip. Microchips located proximal to the electronic transducer elements control transmission and reception of ultrasound signals. Echo signals are transmitted from the catheter tip to the image processor by seven hair-thin microcables. This solid-state design enables the catheters to have lower profiles, increased flexibility, and superior trackability and steerability without the nonuniform rotational distortion (NURD) artifact that commonly occurs with mechanical IVUS imaging catheters. A high-speed computer reconstructs the signals into an ultrasound image through a process of digital vector reconstruction, similar to that used for CT scanning (see Figure 13-2).

Figure 13-2. Volcano Therapeutics Eagle Eye IVUS Catheter.

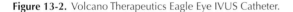
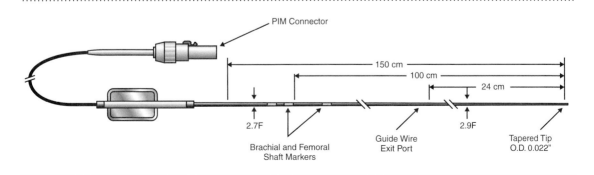

Current Volcano phased-array IVUS catheters operate at a frequency of 20 MHz. Additionally, the solid-state transducer produces a catheter "ring-down" artifact, which needs to be digitally subtracted (referenced) from the image. Newer Volcano consoles have an "auto-ring-down" function, which has greatly simplified this process for the console operator and improved imaging. For optimal imaging, it is recommended that the reference/ring down be performed with the catheter free in the aorta, in a position where tissue signals are not visible. The imaging elements are 10.5 mm proximal to the tip of the catheter, facilitating imaging of distal anatomy. The monorail guide wire lumen is 24 cm long, offering superior trackability through tortuous anatomy.

Volcano Corporation also offers catheters that utilize a mechanical transducer. Mechanical piezoelectric crystal transducers offer superior near-field resolution and gray scales compared to solid-state transducers. The ability to image at higher frequencies is of great benefit, particularly with the presence of fibrotic plaque morphology. These catheters are comprised of an imaging core within an integrated sheath. The catheter is inserted into the artery distal to the lesion prior to imaging. The imaging sheath remains stationary within the coronary artery, while the imaging core is advanced back and forth through the lesion. The distal end of the catheter body allows the imaging core wire to be advanced and retracted 15 cm without manipulating the catheter within the artery once the catheter is distal to the area of interest (see Figure 13-3).

The Boston Scientific Corporation catheters utilize a mechanical transducer, rotating a single piezoelectric crystal at 1800 rpm. The distal end of the catheter body allows the imaging core wire to be advanced and retracted 15 cm without manipulating the catheter within the artery once the catheter is distal to the area of interest. The catheters have a short monorail lumen with the proximal exit port 15 mm from the distal tip (see Figure 13-4).

Figure 13-3. Volcano s5 Imaging System and Track Back II Auto Pullback Device. *Source:* Courtesy of Volcano Therapeutics, Inc.

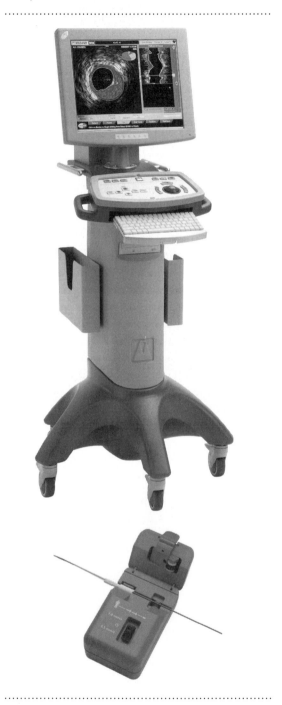

Figure 13-4. Boston Scientific Atlantis SR Pro IVUS Catheter: 1) 135 cm usable length; 2) Radiopaque marker band; 3) 1.5 cm guide wire rail length; 4) 2.1 cm marker band to transducer; 5) Imaging profile 3.2F; 6) 15 cm imaging core pullback. *Source:* Courtesy of Boston Scientific Inc.

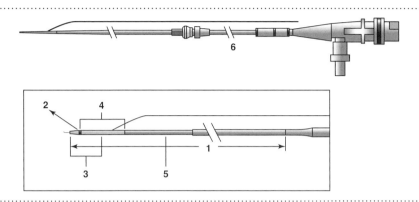

Pullback

Static IVUS images display a slice of the vessel, showing a two-dimensional view. It is possible to create a three-dimensional image of the section of the vessel by pulling back on the IVUS catheter during image acquisition. Mechanical pullback units can be used at a constant rate of 0.5 to 1.0 mm per second. Some systems have an integrated pullback system, which includes a digital display of pullback length and speed. The Volcano imaging systems are equipped with a longitudinal imaging function, stacking together and reconstructing hundreds of individual tomographic frames. Utilizing the mechanical pullback unit and the longitudinal function, the operator can accurately calculate lesion length. It is possible to create a three-dimensional image of the section of the vessel by pulling back on the IVUS catheter during image acquisition. (See Figure 13-3 and Figure 13-5.)

IVUS IMAGE INTERPRETATION

In the center of the screen is a black "dead zone" that is the space occupied by the IVUS catheter within the vessel (see Figure 13-6). With a 30–40 MHz catheter, the vessel lumen is "sonolucent," having

Figure 13-5. Galaxy Disposable Pullback Sled. *Source:* Courtesy of Boston Scientific Inc.

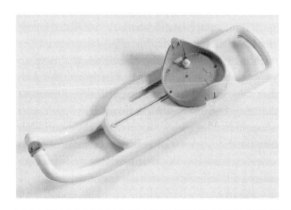

less gray due to the absence of tissue to reflect the sound waves. Blood appears as gray speckles that swirl or move about within the sonolucent lumen with active blood flow. The presence of blood speckles aid in determining where tissue ends and lumen begins, especially when there is a questionable vessel dissection. When in doubt, it is beneficial to inject a small amount of contrast medium, which appears as slightly brighter gray echoes than red blood cells, into the vessel, further helping in determining luminal borders.

Figure 13-6. iLab IVUS Console. *Source:* Courtesy of Boston Scientific, Inc.

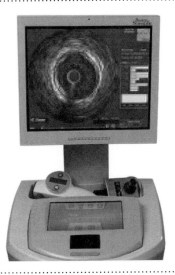

Figure 13-7. Normal coronary artery morphology. Single layered (left) and tri-laminar (right) appearance.

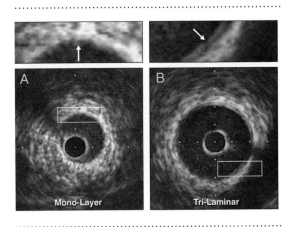

In vitro analysis of coronary anatomy demonstrates a typical trilaminar appearance of the intima, media, and adventitia, in addition to the external elastic lamina (EEL) and internal elastic lamina (IEL). The intima is composed of a single layer of endothelial cells; the media— smooth muscle; and the adventitia—collagen and elastin. In vivo imaging results differ from subject to subject. In some patients, a distinct ultrasound image of an intimal leading edge can be observed. With variations in transducers, instrumentation, and the age of the patient, "normal" arterial segments may exhibit either trilaminar or monolayered characteristics[4,5] (see Figure 13-7). Controversy surrounds whether the so-called sonolucent zone is always representative of normal vessel media. In all cases, the adventitia layer is the third, deepest layer and it varies widely from patient to patient.

With angiography alone, most lesions appear to be localized to a relatively small segment of the artery. Quantitative analysis of lesion severity assumes that the sites adjacent to the narrowing are normal and use measurements of these sites as references in their calculations. However,

IVUS demonstrates that these angiographic reference sites are rarely disease free. Many of these angiographic reference sites have plaque deposits that fill as much as 40% of their cross-sectional area.[4,6]

Plaque geometry, how the disease appears within the vessel, can be eccentric, concentric, or bicentric. Normally, there is a mild intimal layer thickening with age, uniform throughout the vessel segment. A truly eccentric plaque encompasses a segment within the vessel wall less than 360°. There is some segment of normal wall within the plaque area. Eccentric plaques are most often apparant at the ostial segments of sidebranches. Concentric plaques are distributed uniformly within the diseased segment, around the entire wall. Most atherosclerotic disease is bicentric; the plaque geometry changes, shifts between eccentric and concentric areas within the vessel segment.

Atherosclerotic lesions may be comprised of fatty lipid pools, fibrotic tissue, calcium deposits, or any combination of these. "Soft" refers to the characteristic of the IVUS image pattern, not necessarily the physical property of the disease. Lesions that are predominantly lipid produce echolucent (weakly reflective, dark gray echoes), with a homogenous pattern. There is full IVUS signal penetration producing a very clear image within this segment.

Fibrotic lesions are more echogenic (produce highly reflective, brighter, denser gray signals) when imaging than lipid. The IVUS signal may be attenuated, but without image fallout, by the denser property of the fibrotic tissue. These softer plaque morphologies typically respond more favorably to PTCA or primary stenting than calcified lesions.[7] Fibrotic disease is rarely seen alone, most often associated with mixed plaque morphologies. Cadaver studies have identified that unstable coronary lesions most often associated with acute myocardial infarctions have a thin, fibrotic cap overlying a soft, lipid-rich pool.

Hard, calcified lesions have a very characteristic appearance by IVUS, producing very bright white echoes (see Figure 13-8). Because the ultrasound beam is unable to penetrate the calcium deposits, there is shadowing or echo dropout of the deeper tissue structures beyond. IVUS has shown that calcium deposits are much more common in lesions than previously recognized with angiography alone. The presence of calcium within a lesion may be the most significant predictor of the success or failure of a percutaneous revascularization procedure. The presence of calcium within the vessel may be characterized by

depth (superficial, deep, or mixed) and quantified by measuring the arc in degrees. The greater the degree of the calcium arc, the greater the image drop out, shadowing, and signal reverberation. Artifacts related to signal reverberation may obscure information from less-diseased segments of the vessel wall. As the calcium arc approaches 360°, a characteristic white "napkin-ring" image is apparent. Lesions that exhibit superficial calcium may respond more favorably to debulking by rotational atherectomy than to conventional PTCA.[8]

Both Boston Scientific and Volcano Corporation IVUS consoles have software designed to aid in image interpretation. Computerized trace assist functions automatically detect both vessel and lumen borders to aid in analysis. Chroma-Flo, a color-enhanced display of the red blood cells as they move pass the catheter, is also available with Volcano IVUS. Boston Scientific's iSize software allows the user overlay area and length measurement graphics onto the image to aid in device-sizing decisions.

One major clinical limitation of current IVUS catheters is their inability to positively identify thrombus. Thrombus has been described as echolucent, similar in appearance to lipid or mildly fibrotic plaques. Thrombus overlies the intima,

Figure 13-8. Hard, calcified atheroma with acoustic shadowing.

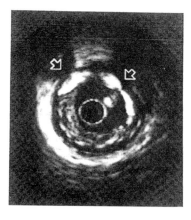 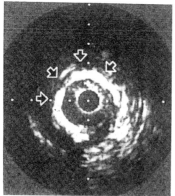

and small channels may be visible. Thrombus is best seen in a live image and may appear scintillating, mobile, or pedunculated similarly to cardiac myxomas viewed by transthoracic or transesophageal echocardiography. Higher frequency catheters and computer-based tissue characterization software show great promise in overcoming this limitation in the future.[4,9]

Virtual Histology Imaging

Easy, accurate, and reproducible IVUS tissue characterization greatly simplifies image interpretation, allow clinicians to identify high-risk atherosclerotic disease, and choose an appropriate method of intervention. Virtual histology IVUS uses spectral analysis of the radiofrequency ultrasound signals and tissue characterization software to correctly assess plaque components.[10] By analyzing the reflected ultrasound signal amplitude and eight spectral components, additional information about the plaque composition may be derived that otherwise would not be available without an autopsy.

VH IVUS converts raw radiofrequency data into color-coded images of the vessel wall, assigning different colors to each morphology. The colorized VH IVUS images show four basic plaque types: fibrous (green), fibro-fatty (green/yellow), calcific (white), and necrotic cores (red).

Boston Scientific iLab IVUS offers iColor designed to enhances image interpretation by adding color to the cross-sectional IVUS view, coloring the plaque and lumen based on the console's vessel Trace Assist software.

DIAGNOSTIC APPLICATIONS OF IVUS

Until fairly recently, atherosclerotic coronary disease was viewed analogous to a plumbing problem; through natural aging and/or a variety of risk factors such as smoking or diet, the vessel intima becomes damaged and debris is deposited, eventually forming flow-limiting plaques. A newer accepted model of plaque formation is vascular remodeling, first described by the pathologist Seymour Glagov in 1987.[11] Positive remodeling occurs when lipid-filled plaque deposits build up inside the vessel and the wall of the artery compensates by expanding outward to keep the lumen patent as long as possible. The vessel will continue to increase in size as disease progresses. Vessel compliance is reduced, and eventually plaque deposition overtakes remodeling, and the lumen area decreases. Negative/reverse remodeling occurs when there is vessel shrinkage in response to atherosclerosis.

IVUS has clearly demonstrated this phenomenon with serial studies of cardiac transplant patients. Despite the relatively young age of donors, significant atherosclerotic disease is detected by IVUS, despite normal angiograms.[12] Transplant patients often suffer from a condition referred to as transplant vasculopathy, which is characterized by an accelerated process of intimal thickening. The progressive nature of this disease is a major cause of retransplantation and death. Approximately 40% of patients have extensive intimal thickening just 1 year after transplantation. Theories regarding the nature of transplant vasculopathy center predominantly on rejection and/or antirejection therapies. IVUS now provides a way to serially assess the vascular remodeling and atherosclerotic progression, which in this patient population is asymptomatic. Ultimately, this may lead to different antirejection regimens to decrease or eliminate transplant vasculopathies.[4,6,13]

IVUS is an invaluable tool in assessing ambiguous angiographic lesions in symptomatic patients. Patients with atypical symptoms or who have experienced sudden cardiac arrest are commonly referred for angiography. When angiography is performed, there may not be a specific lesion to which the symptoms can be attributed. IVUS assessment frequently reveals significant segments of plaque not visualized with angiography. A 70% area of stenosis is considered to be hemodynamically significant. Even in some cases, however, it may be more appropriate to measure fractional flow reserve (FFR) or coronary flow reserve (CFR) for true physiologic assessment.

Left main trunk (LMT) disease may also be more appropriately assessed with IVUS. Even after taking multiple angiograms centering on the LMT (i.e., 40 LAO 30 Caudal), it still may be difficult to assess. Often, the distal segment of the LMT may be obscured angiographically by the LAD/LCX bifurcation, or the ostial LMT may be difficult to visualize because of contrast streaming. IVUS allows the clinician to overcome these limitations and should be routinely used in this situation, because the diagnosis of LMT disease often means the difference between medicine, Percutaneous Coronary Intervention (PCI), or open heart surgery.

IVUS can also detect atherosclerosis at sites within the vessel that are angiographically normal. These patients may or may not be symptomatic. Clinically, the value of detecting lesions unrecognized without IVUS in the asymptomatic patient is unclear, although early detection may assist in predicting and/or preventing future cardiac events.[2]

IVUS IN INTERVENTIONAL PROCEDURES

Until the development of IVUS, cardiologists could only guess at the composition of the atherosclerotic lesion, with the exception of fluoroscopically visible calcification. IVUS offers the operator the unique capability to directly examine the morphology of the atherosclerotic plaque. This gives the medical team the ability to practice a more "lesion-specific" approach to percutaneous coronary interventions.

IVUS is important for assessing the extent of lesion dissections, which can occur either spontaneously, or after mechanical trauma (PCI). Most commonly, dissections occur where there is a zone of transition, such as between fibrous and calcific, mixed morphology plaque or at the edge of stent struts and the vessel wall. Angiographically, the area may appear fuzzy or hazy. IVUS allows the clinician to ascertain the depth of the trauma; does it involve only the intima, or does it extend into the media, adventitia, or further? A classic IVUS dissection image will clearly show a flap, or dissection arm, extending away from the vessel wall into the lumen. Some plaques may separate away from the vessel at two points, giving a horseshoe appearance.

Intramural hematomas may also be diagnosed by IVUS. The ACC Clinical Expert Consensus Document on IVUS[14] defines intramural hematomas as an accumulation of blood within the media space that displaces the IEL inward and the EEL outward.

Figure 13-9. Complex Dissection after PTCA. A deep dissection (black arrow, left) is associated with a large intimal flap (black arrow, right).

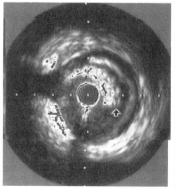
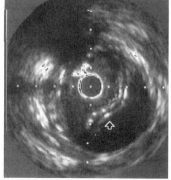

Figure 13-10. Pre- and post-rotoblator IVUS images.

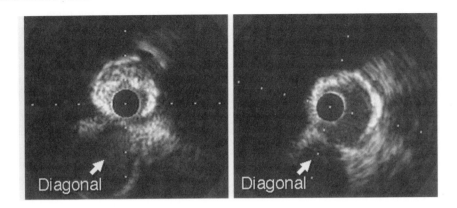

IVUS and Rotablator

The Rotablator rotational atherectomy device uses a diamond dust–tipped burr spinning at 150,000 to 200,000 rpm within the artery to pulverize calcified plaque. The device "selectively ablates" nonelastic diseased tissue, and normal elastic tissue or soft fatty plaques are pushed out of the way and left untouched. Calcium deposits within an artery can greatly influence procedural outcomes. Localized areas of calcium have been associated with large vascular dissections after balloon angioplasty;[8,15] extensive circumferential calcification may not yield to balloons, even at inflation pressures greater than 20 atmospheres. IVUS can correctly diagnose even superficially calcified lesions that may be invisible to angiography alone, thus identifying the patients who would be most benefited by rotational atherectomy therapy (see Figure 13-11).

IVUS and Stenting

In the early days of stenting, as many as 15%–20% of stent recipients experienced thrombotic occlusions of the treated vessels. IVUS studies identified two problems that predisposed stents to thrombosis: incomplete apposition of stent

Figure 13-11. Stent malapposition. After stent deployment in the proximal LAD, IVUS reveals malapposition of the stent (top left, white arrows) while angiography suggests a good result (bottom left, white arrow). After post deployment dilatation with a larger balloon inflated to 16 Atm, IVUS reveals complete apposition of the stent to the vessel wall (top right) while angiography shows no apparent change in vessel appearance or luminal dimension (bottom right).

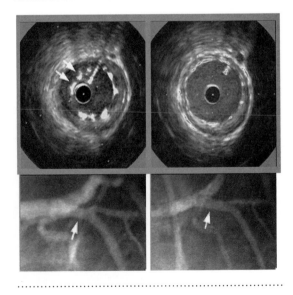

struts to the arterial wall and incomplete stent expansion within the lesion.[4] Incomplete apposition occurs when a part of the stent is not completely in contact with the arterial wall. As a result, blood flow in this area becomes turbulent. This also exposes sides of the stent's surface to blood flow. Both of these factors can significantly contribute to the formation of thrombus locally, resulting in arterial occlusion, generally within 7 days of the initial procedure. Incomplete expansion of stents may partially block blood flow or create turbulent flow within the artery. Incomplete expansion occurs within the stent where the plaque is most rigid, and in areas where some stents have flexible joints. IVUS recognition of incomplete apposition and incomplete expansion radically changed the way coronary stenting is performed. Poststent balloon inflation with high-pressure PTCA balloons with diameters 0.25 to 0.5 mm larger than the actual stent size are often performed to completely push the stent struts into the arterial wall. Serial IVUS imaging may be performed to determine the interventional end point. This has also reduced the need for aggressive poststent anticoagulation regimens. Patients are now discharged on clopidogrel (or ticlopidine) and aspirin, as opposed to warfarin therapy. This IVUS-guided strategy for stent deployment has effectively decreased the incidence of acute and subacute stent thrombosis and appears to have further decreased restenosis rates.[16]

IVUS COMPLICATIONS

Coronary vasospasm is the most common complication of IVUS, so patients often receive 100 to 200 μg of IC nitroglycerin prior to deployment of the IVUS catheter. This practice has nearly eliminated coronary vasospasm associated with intravascular imaging.

Other potential, but uncommon, complications of IVUS or ICE is coronary dissection or tamponade. Whenever a mechanical device is introduced into the heart, be it a guide wire, balloon, or any other device, there is a risk of disrupting the vessel intima or perforating a chamber. Great care needs to be taken when manipulating these catheters. It is also possible for the guide wire and catheter to separate and potentially hook an intimal flap. If this occurs as the catheter is withdrawn, the catheter may proliferate the dissection with an "intracoronary cheese-slicer" effect. If catheter-wire separation is visible under fluoroscopy, the catheter should be gently readvanced, then the catheter and guide wire withdrawn together as a unit. Other complications include ischemia due to the IVUS catheter obstructing distal blood flow with severe lesions, dysrhythmias, and myocardial infarction.

INTRACARDIAC ECHOCARDIOGRAPHY

ICE is a new invasive imaging modality. Lower frequency catheters allow for increased tissue depth penetration, providing superb anatomic detail and diagnosing complex cardiac abnormalities.

The transducer is contained within an enclosed acoustic housing at the distal segment of the catheter. The ultrasound imaging plane is a 360° cross-sectional scan with the catheter in the center. The Siemens ICE catheter also has the ability to deflect the catheter tip allows for easy manipulation inside the cardiac chambers. It also has full Doppler capabilities for blood flow, velocity, and myocardial wall motion measurements.

ICE has been used for electrophysiologic procedures, guiding radiofrequency ablations, transseptal punctures, evaluating aortic aneurysms, and aortic stent-graft procedures. Most recently, the technology has been applied to aiding complex pediatric, congenital, and structural heart procedures. These include repairs of atrial septal defects (ASDs), ventricular septal defects (VSDs), patent foramen ovales (PFOs), percutaneous mitral valve repairs, and percutaneous aortic valve replacements. ICE allows superior imaging to TEE by allowing a larger field of view, optimal soft-tissue contrast, and more precise evaluation of the anatomy and defects.[17]

OPTICAL COHERENCE TOMOGRAPHY

Optical coherence tomography (OCT) is a recently developed, catheter-based intravascular imaging technology that provides axial resolution in the range of in the range of 10 to 20 μm (compared to IVUS resolution of 150–μm). Instead of utilizing sound, OCT measures the intensity of back-scattered infrared light and translates the reflected light into an extremely high-resolution, two-dimensional image. The high-resolution OCT allows for better visualization of calcified areas without the problem of signal dropout/acoustic shadowing that occurs with IVUS. The superior near-field resolution of OCT will allow clinicians to easily identify the thin fibrous cap associated with vulnerable plaques and acute coronary syndromes. OCT may also allow researchers to detect and quantify the number of macrophages in plaques, furthering the knowledge of atherosclerotic disease.[18]

NURSING CARE OF IVUS AND ICE PATIENTS

The IVUS procedure can be easily and safely performed by a catheterization team experienced with percutaneous interventions.[19,20] Patients undergoing IVUS for diagnostic purposes receive 3000 to 5000 units of IV heparin prior to guide wire insertion to decrease the risk of thrombosis.

Otherwise, patients undergoing an IVUS or ICE procedure have the same needs as those undergoing any other invasive cardiac procedure. A common nursing diagnosis is anxiety related to catheterization results. Patients may need to verbalize their concerns prior to undergoing the procedure. Thorough patient teaching is necessary to increase patient knowledge and decrease the fear associated with the procedure. Other nursing diagnoses may include high risk for infection related to vascular access, high risk for altered tissue perfusion, and related limb ischemia secondary to arterial access, and others associated with routine catheterization or percutaneous interventional procedures.

SUMMARY

Although IVUS should be viewed as a complementary technology to angiography, not a replacement, IVUS and ICE have given the medical world a new outlook on the treatment of cardiac disease. The technology has experienced tremendous growth, and cost is the main factor limiting the use of this technology. In the era of drug-eluting stents, biventricular pacemakers and ICDs, ancillary procedural costs must be minimized. It has still to be clearly demonstrated that the ultrasound-driven diagnosis and procedural endpoints improve patient outcomes to justify the additional expense.

REFERENCES

1. Arnett EN, Isner JM, Redwood DR, et al. Coronary artery narrowing in coronary heart disease: comparison of cineangiographic and necropsy findings. *Ann Intern Med* 1979;91:350–356.
2. White CJ, Ramee SR, Collin TJ, et al. Ambiguous coronary angiography: clinical utility of intravascular ultrasound. *Cathet Cardiovasc Diagn* 1992;26:200–203.
3. Yock P, Fitzgerald P, Popp R. Intravascular ultrasound. *Sci Am Sci Med* 1995;2:68–77.
4. Nissen SE, Tuzcu EM, DeFranco AC. Coronary intravascular ultrasound: diagnostic and interventional applications. In: Topol EJ, ed. *Textbook of Interventional Cardiology*. Update 14. Philadelphia: WB Saunders; 1994:207–222.
5. Fitzgerald PJ, St. Goar FG, Connoly AJ, et al. Intravascular ultrasound imaging of coronary arteries: is three layers the norm? *Circulation* 1992;86:154–158.

6. Yock PG, Fitzgerald PJ. Intravascular ultrasound imaging. In: Baim DS, Grossman W, eds. *Cardiac Catheterization, Angiography, and Intervention*, 5th ed. Baltimore: Williams & Wilkins; 1996:391–405.

7. Popma JJ, Mintz GS, Satler LF. Coronary arteriography and intravascular ultrasound analysis of directional coronary atherectomy. *Am J Cardiol* 1993;72:55E–63E.

8. Whitlow PL, Buchbinder M, Kent K. Coronary rotational atherectomy: angiographic risk factors and their relation to success/complications. Abstract. *J Am Coll Cardiol* 1992;19:334A.

9. Moscucci M, Muller DWM. Restenosis. In: Freed M, Grines C, Safian RD, eds. *The New Manual of Interventional Cardiology.* Birmingham, MI: Physician's Press; 1996:432–438.

10. Nair A, Kuban BD, Tuzcu EM, et al. Coronary plaque classification with intravascular ultrasound radiofrequency data analysis. *Circulation* 2002;106:2200–2206.

11. Glagov S, Weisenberg E, Zarins C, et al. Compensatory enlargement of human atherosclerotic coronary arteries. *N Eng J Med* 1987;316:1371–1375.

12. Tuzcu EM, Hobbs RE, Rincon G, et al. Occult and frequent transmission of atherosclerotic coronary disease with cardiac transplantation: insights from intravascular ultrasound. *Circulation* 1995;91:1706–1713.

13. Fearon WF, Kern MJ, Litwinczuk J, Hodgson JM, et al. Nonangiographic coronary lesion assessment. In: Kern MJ, Ubeydullah D, eds. *The Interventional Cardiac Catheterization Handbook.* St. Louis, MO: Mosby Yearbook; 1996:349–368.

14. Mintz GS, Nissen SE, Anderson WD, et al. American College of Cardiology Clinical Expert Consensus Document on Standards for Acquisition, Measurement, and Reporting of Intravascular Ultrasound Studies (IVUS) *JACC* 37;2001:1478–1492.

15. Kovach JA, Mintz GS, Pichard AD, et al. Sequential intravascular ultrasound characterization of the mechanism of rotational atherectomy and adjunct balloon angioplasty. *J Am Coll Cardiol* 1993;22:1024–1032.

16. Colombo A, Hall P, Nakamura S, et al. Intracoronary stenting without anticoagulation accomplished with intravascular ultrasound guidance. *Circulation* 1995;91:1676–1687.

17. Koenig P, Cao Qi-Ling, Heitschmidt M, et al. Role of intracardiac echocardiographic guidance in transcatheter closure of atrial septal defects and patent foramen ovale using the amplatzer device. *J Inv Card* 2003;16:51–62.

18. Hoang KC, Kern, MJ. Lighting up the coronary: intracoronary imaging with optical coherence tomography. *Cath Lab Digest* 2008;16(10).

19. Hausman D. The safety of intravascular ultrasound: a multicenter survey of 2207 examinations. *Circulation* 1995;91:623–629.

20. Nissen SE, Gurley JC, Grines CL. Intravascular ultrasound assessment of lumen size and wall morphology in normal subjects and coronary artery disease patients. *Circulation* 1991;84:1087–1099.

SUGGESTED READING

Nissen SE, De Franco AC, Tuzcu EM. Coronary intravascular ultrasound. In: Freed M, Grines C, Safian RD, eds. *The New Manual of Interventional Cardiology.* Birmingham, MI: Physician's Press; 1996.

Strimike C. Understanding intravascular ultrasound. *Am J Nurs* 1996;96:40–44.

Tuzcu EM, De Franco AC, Nissen SE. Intravascular ultrasound imaging. In: Uretsky BF, ed. *Cardiac Catheterization: Concepts, Techniques, and Applications.* Malden, MA: Blackwell Science; 1997.

Yock PG, Fitzgerald PJ. Intravascular ultrasound imaging. In: Baim DS, Grossman W, ed. *Cardiac Catheterization, Angiography, and Intervention*, 5th ed. Baltimore: Williams & Wilkins; 1996.

Chapter 14

FUNCTIONAL ASSESSMENT OF CORONARY ARTERY DISEASE

Kenneth A. Gorski, RN, RCIS, RCSA, FSICP
Sandy Watson, RN, BN, NFESC

Angiography can provide the lumenal anatomy of the epicardial blood vessels, and intravascular ultrasound (IVUS) can differentiate the disease pathology, plaque burden, and true cross-sectional area, but neither method can adequately define the physiological impact of the diseased vessel or analyze how well that vessel is truly perfusing the myocardium. By inserting specialized 0.014-inch guide wires into the coronary artery, the pressure within the vessel can be accurately measured across a lesion. This information can be used to draw conclusions about the true functional severity of the diseased vessel.

HYPEREMIA

Myocardial blood flow is regulated by changes in vascular resistance at the level of the arterioles. As the oxygen demands of the myocardium increase, the arteriole beds dilate to increase blood flow to the region. At rest, the myocardium requires only a minimal blood supply, and the arterioles remain constricted. During exercise, however, these arterioles dilate; myocardial resistance is reduced to a minimum, and a greater volume of blood can reach the muscle. When a vessel is in a state of maximum dilation, it is said to be in a state of hyperemia.

If an artery is blocked by a stenosis, the myocardium receives less blood and, therefore, less oxygen than it requires. To compensate for this, the microvessels dilate as they do during exercise. When a flow-limiting stenosis is present, the distal microvasculature must compensate for this by being continuously dilated to preserve resting basal blood flow. In a vessel with a significant stenosis, the microvasculature is in a constant state of compensatory dilation.[1] As myocardial oxygen needs increase, the already-dilated microvasculature cannot supply greater blood flow to meet the demand.

Vascular resistance varies due to many factors such as exercise, ischemia, arterial blood pressure, vasomotion, and contrast medium injections.

Unless vascular resistance is constant, functional severity of a lesion cannot be accurately assessed. With maximum vasodilatation of the coronary vasculature, maximum flow is achieved, and the myocardial resistance is minimal and constant. Maximum dilatation occurs during physical exertion, but in the confines of a cardiac catheter laboratory, this can be achieved by administering a vasodilatory drug.

Several drugs produce a hyperemic response in the manner described. Nitroglycerine and other nitrates cause microvascular hyperemia, but their main effect is dilating the large epicardial vessels, increasing their cross-sectional area. This dilatory response reduces the speed of blood flow, negating the effect of any increased flow that may be related to microvascular hyperemia. Papaverine has also been used in many studies, with the most common side effect being prolongation of the Q-T interval. Rare cases of Torsade de Pointes have been reported with its use, and it is rarely used today. Adenosine, commonly used for breaking supraventricular tachycardia, has been found to be a fast-working hyperemic agent, and it has a short half-life, making it ideal for coronary hyperemic studies. One of the few side effects of adenosine is transient bradycardia and heart block, usually lasting only a few seconds.

Dosing and administration of hyperemic agents vary. Some practitioners prefer to administer the agents as a rapid intracoronary (IC) bolus, while others prefer to use an IV infusion to achieve a more prolonged, steady-state effect. At the Cleveland Clinic, the protocol for IC administration is to dilute 6 mg of adenosine into a 250 ml bag of D5W, providing a concentration of 24 µg/ml. The cardiologist administers initial doses of 36 µg to 48 µg IC for left coronary artery (LCA) branches, and 24 µg to 36 µg IC for the right coronary artery (RCA). If the injection is repeated, the dose is increased at the physician's discretion. For IV administration, the infusion is prepared by withdrawing 16 ml of fluid from a 50 ml bag of D5W, then adding 48 mg (16 ml of adenosine, at 3 mg/ml concentration). The infu-

sion is preferably administered through a central line; however, it is most often given through a 20 g (or larger) IV catheter located in the antecubital vein. The IV drip is very rapid, at a dose of 140 µg/kg/min.[2]

Due to the high cost of adenosine, some centers are reexamining the use of papaverine for inducing hyperemia. IC papaverine will produce hyperemia similar to that of IV adenosine. Papaverine is administered IC in dosages of 10 mg to 15 mg for the LCA, and 5 mg to 10 mg for the RCA. Peak hyperemic effects with IC papaverine occur about 30 seconds after administration and may last an additional 60 to 90 seconds. Additional considerations for the use of papaverine include its incompatibility with heparin, iodinated contrast agents, and Hexabrix. When papaverine is combined with one of these, the resulting solution is milky or opalescent. Nonheparinized flush solutions and nonionic contrast must be used.

INTRAVASCULAR PRESSURE MEASUREMENT

After the introduction of the first over-the-wire percutaneous transluminal coronary angioplasty (PTCA) balloon catheters, transstenotic pressure gradients were recorded to guide the progress of the dilatation. Aortic pressure was obtained from the guiding catheter and was used as the reference measurement. A pressure measurement was also obtained through the guide wire lumen of the balloon catheter, assessing the vessel distal to the lesion. Physicians typically used a postdilatation gradient of less than 15 mmHg to indicate a satisfactory result.

There were a number of limitations to this technique. The initial over-the-wire balloon catheters had shafts with diameters of 3.5F, and their large cross-sectional areas would often produce unpredictable pressures or even totally obstruct a stenosis. The original 9F guide catheters had inner diameters of .072 inches, and the balloon catheters would dampen the aortic pressures. Also, only low-frequency responses could be obtained with fluid-filled catheters and transducer systems.

Because of these limitations and the rapid development of online digital quantitative coronary analysis (QCA), interest in intraluminal pressure measurements waned. It was hoped that QCA alone would provide definitive diagnosis. QCA did live up to those expectations to some extent, but as cardiologists began to tackle more complex lesions and multivessel arterial disease, it became clear that there was a need for a reliable measurement of the functional significance of coronary lesions.

Coronary Pressures and Fractional Flow Reserve

Healthy coronary arteries and their associated microvessels dilate in response to exercise. When the coronary artery becomes diseased, there is a drop in pressure across the lesion and a compensatory dilatation of the microvasculature. As oxygen demands increase, the coronary artery constricts, and the pressure drop across the lesion increases. Since the microvessels are already in a dilated state, there is limited (or no) capacity left to meet the increased demands. This results in ischemia and chest pain.

Myocardial fractional flow reserve (FFR) can be defined as the maximal myocardial blood flow in the presence of a stenosis in the supplying coronary artery, divided by the normal blood flow. At maximum hyperemia:

$$FFR = Pd/Pa$$

where Pd equals mean distal pressure and Pa equals mean arterial pressure.

Two companies currently offer products for measuring FFR: RADI Medical (Upsalla, Sweden) and Volcano Corporation (Rancho Cordova, California).

Lesion Assessment

The most common indication for measuring coronary pressure and FFR is evaluating a mild-to-moderate stenosis to assess whether it is respon-sible for reversible ischemia. FFR measurements can save patients from undergoing unnecessary procedures. It can help to quantitatively assess the functional severity of the obstruction and, unlike Doppler assessment (CFR, coronary flow reserve), FFR is a lesion-specific index, with a clear normal value of 1.0 in every patient and every coronary artery. It has been repeatedly demonstrated that a FFR of < 0.75 confirms a functionally significant stenosis with a 95% diagnostic accuracy of predicting inducible ischemia.[3] Also, unlike Doppler, FFR is not influenced by heart rate, blood pressure, or microvascular disease. Since there is no need for a reference artery, FFR is also feasible in patients with multivessel coronary artery disease or serial lesions.

FFR can also determine the viability of myocardial tissue postmyocardial infarction. In patients with a recent MI, the occurrence of cardiac events is often related to coronary reocclusion, which cannot be predicted by angiography. The 0.75 threshold value of FFR is a surrogate for noninvasive stress testing to patients with a prior MI. If the coronary angiogram shows a mild-to-moderate lesion in the culprit vessel, performing FFR while the patient is in the laboratory eliminates the need for an expensive (though noninvasive) test after discharge.[4] FFR has shown to be not only a guide to successful intervention but also a strong predictor of 6-month outcome.[5]

FFR measurements can save patients from undergoing unnecessary procedures. In the DEFER Trial, 325 patients who were scheduled for angioplasty but presented without documented ischemia underwent FFR assessment of stenosis. If the FFR was > 0.75, they were randomized to either deferred angioplasty (91 patients) or performance of angioplasty (90 patients). If the FFR was found to be < 0.75, the angioplasty was performed as planned (144 patients). Event-free survival at 24 months was similar in the randomized group: 89% deferred versus 83% angioplasty. This shows that patients with a coronary stenosis and an FFR > 0.75 derive no clear-cut benefit from undergoing an intervention.[3]

The Fractional Flow Reserve Versus Angiography for Guiding PCI in Patients with Multivessel Coronary Artery Disease (FAME) study randomized 1005 patients with multivessel disease to angiography only or FFR-guided PCI. FAME showed that routine measurement of FFR during PCI in patients with multivessel disease significantly improves clinical outcomes when over angiography-only guided treatment. At 1 year follow-up, using FFR to guide PCI reduced the risk of death, MI, or repeat revascularization by 30% and death or MI by 35%, when compared to using angiography alone to guide interventional decisions.[6]

FFR may also be used to determine the viability of myocardial tissue post-MI. In patients with a recent MI, the occurrence of cardiac events is often related to coronary reocclusion, which cannot be predicted by angiography. The present data extends the validity of the 0.75 threshold value of FFR as a surrogate for noninvasive stress testing to patients with a prior MI. If the coronary angiogram shows a mild-to-moderate lesion in the culprit vessel, performing FFR while the patient is in the laboratory eliminates the need for an additional noninvasive test after discharge.[4]

FFR is proving to be useful during PCI in patients with multivessel disease. Routine measurement of FFR improves clinical outcomes when compared with traditional angiography-only guided treatment. FFR is proving itself to be a versatile and reliable modality that is relatively simple to use and gives reliable information on the functional assessment of CHD.[4]

System Components

Pressure guide wire units are comprised of a guide wire, a monitor, and connections. Unfortunately, the different units and their guide wires cannot be interchanged. For specific functions and operating techniques, consult a company representative or the unit's operator manual.

RADI Analyzer/PressureWire System

The guide wire is similar to a conventional interventional guide wire, with the exception of three microsensor elements 3 cm proximal to the distal tip at the transition of the radiopaque and radiolucent segments. Each of the three sensor elements has a specific function: one measures pressure/FFR, the second is designed to measure a thermodilution-derived CFR, and the third is a temperature sensor.

The pressure transducer is a silicon, piezoresistive microsensor coupled in a Wheatstone bridge with a working range of −30 to 300 mmHg. The RADI PressureWire is available in both 175 cm and 300 cm lengths. A 6-foot adapter/contact cable connects the PressureWire to the RADI Analyzer during pressure measurements and can be disengaged during wire placement and manipulation.

The RADI Analyzer is a portable computer system that is mounted on an IV pole and interfaces with the CCL hemodynamic system. It collects and interprets the signals sent by the guide wire micromanometer and allows the arterial waveform from the guide catheter and the PressureWire waveform to be simultaneously displayed on both the RADI Analyzer and the cath lab hemodynamic system. A remote control allows input of patient data and operation of the system. An optional thermal printer permits hard-copy measurements to be entered into the chart. The RADI Analyzer will store a number of patient recordings; optional RADI View software allows digital transfer of information to a personal computer for future reviewing, editing, reporting into spreadsheets and PowerPoint slide presentations.

Volcano ComboMap/SmartWire System

As with the RADI system, the distal, sterile component is the guide wire, which is similar to a conventional interventional guide wire with the exception of a micropressure transducer, 3 cm

Figure 14-1. The top figure shows a normal FFR (0.94) while the bottom figure shows an abnormal FFR (0.74).

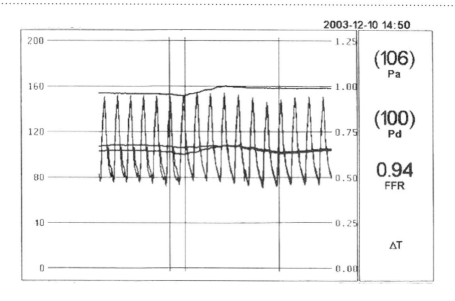

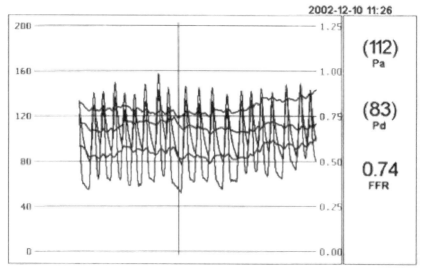

proximal to the distal tip at the transition of the radiopaque and radiolucent segments. An adapter cable connects the Volcano SmartWire to the ComboMap during pressure measurements and can be disengaged during wire placement and manipulation.

The ComboMap is a portable computer system that interfaces with the cath lab hemodynamic system (see Figure 14-3). The ComboMap collects and interprets the signals sent by the guide wire micromanometer and displays the numeric values of both the guide catheter and

Figure 14-2. RADI Analyzer. *Source:* Reprinted wth permission from St. Jude Medical™, © 2010 all rights reserved.

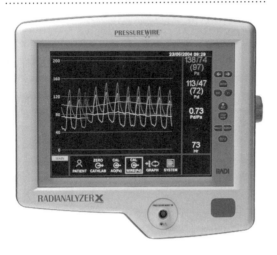

Figure 14-3. ComboMap. *Source:* Courtesy of Volcano Therapeutics, Inc.

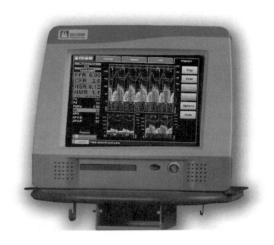

the SmartWire. Phasic and mean waveforms of both can be displayed on the cath lab hemodynamic system.

FFR Procedure

The patient should be heparinized per institutional protocol prior to inserting a FFR pressure wire. The guide wires need to be connected to their system and calibrated. A digital display will confirm that the FFR wire has calibrated correctly. The arterial transducer may now be closed to air and zeroed. Once confirmed, the transducer is opened to pressure.

Prior to crossing the lesion, with the entire radiopaque segment outside the distal tip of the guiding catheter, but inside the vessel, the FFR waveforms should be identical; this is accomplished electronically by pressing a button on the unit.

At this time, administer the hyperemic agent of choice. For IC injections, rapidly inject the medication through the guiding catheter and im-

mediately follow with a rapid injection of flush. Press the start or record key, and the FFR is automatically calculated and displayed continuously while recording. Press the stop key when the pressure values begin to rise. For IV administration, record the pressures for the entire duration of the infusion.

DOPPLER BLOOD-FLOW MEASUREMENT

The Doppler theory is named after the Austrian physicist who first described it, Christian Johann Doppler (1803–1853). Doppler works on the following principle: When an observer moves toward the source of a sound, the tone of the sound will be heard at a higher frequency than if the observer remains stationary. The same is also true if the observer remains stationary and the source of the sound moves. That is why when a car is driven toward you, the tone of the engine changes. It becomes higher pitched as it approaches and then lower pitched as it moves away from you. The alteration in tone can be measured as a change in frequency of the received sound waves, and with the Doppler formula, the speed of the object can be calculated. It is therefore possible to measure the speed of an approaching or receding object by bouncing a sound wave of known frequency off the object and accurately measuring the frequency of its returning echo.

In 1977, the first Doppler measurement was made inside a coronary artery using a modified 8F catheter, which had obvious restrictions due to its size. Technological advances have enabled the miniaturization of the necessary components so that they can be integrated into a 014-inch guide wire, making it more feasible for IC applications. A Doppler crystal in the tip of the guide wire sends out sound waves, which are returned as echoes reflected off circulating red blood cells. These echoes are captured and passed on to the monitor, which translates the signals it receives into a variety of readings. The velocity measurement of the cells is done in a sample area about 5 mm from the tip, so that the presence of the wire in the vessel does not affect the flow of the surrounding blood cells.

Lesion Assessment

There are several Doppler measurements that can be employed across a stenosis, but the coronary flow reserve (CFR) is the most commonly used. CFR measures the change in the velocity of the blood flow to determine the extent of microvascular dilation. When hyperemia is induced in a vessel with a significant stenosis (wherein the microvasculature is already in a permanently dilated state), the result will be less than a twofold increase in blood flow. In fact, when the CFR is greater than 2.5, the stenosis is not considered to be significant, and no intervention is indicated.

Another measurement method is to simply measure the speed of the blood flow proximal to the lesion and then directly distal to the stenosis. A proximal/distal (P/D) velocity ratio can be derived, which is considered significant if it is greater than 1.7.[7] One advantage of this method is that the hemodynamic effect of a stenosis can

be effectively isolated even in the presence of a series of obstructions.

Another method is the diastolic/systolic velocity ratio (DSVR). It has been found that a lesion will reduce diastolic blood flow and increase relative systolic flow.[8] The average diastolic and systolic peak velocities are measured and expressed as a ratio. The value can then be compared with a table of normal DSVRs, which are different for the different sections of each vessel.

Once the signal has been acquired, it becomes very important for the assistant to perform an accurate and rapid injection of adenosine (normally 18 µg into the left coronary or 12 µg into the right coronary), followed by a rapid injection of normal saline (2 to 3 ml). The Doppler system is then set to search for the maximal or peak flow velocity.

Evaluating Interventional Results

Generally, a CFR of 2.5 or more across a dilated lesion is an indicator of a successful intervention.[9] The Doppler guide wire can be left in position safely to perform the intervention, allowing for periodic CFR measurements to be obtained to assist in determining the therapeutic endpoint.

There are a few difficulties associated with the technique of measuring CFR. The Doppler wire must be positioned precisely in the vessel lumen to obtain a good signal and is very sensitive to motion. Also, blood velocity measurements are affected by changes in the large epicardial vessels as well as the microvasculature, making it difficult to assess the functional severity of an ambiguous lesion, particularly in diabetic patients. Because of these limitations, and the difficult reproducibility of CFR results, FFR is now the favored method for physiologic coronary disease assessment.

The Volcano ComboMap System can operate both the Doppler FloWire and the SmartWire. A ComboWire is also available that allows simultaneous measurements of Doppler CFR and pressure FFR. Volcano has integrated FFR assessment with the SmartWire into their IVUS system.

Other Considerations

Guide wire–based physiologic lesion assessment can be performed with relative ease in any CCL without adding significant time to the procedure. Although the transducer or crystal elements in the Doppler and pressure measurement systems are somewhat fragile and can be damaged with rough handling, patient complications are no different from those encountered using routine interventional guide wires.

The analyzer and monitor portion of the system is a capital equipment cost, but the expenses can be minimized through leasing or special contractual agreements for wires. Doppler wires and pressure wires may range in price from $400 to $600 each in the United States, depending on a hospital's purchase agreement.

The question really is: How necessary, or valuable, are physiologic measurements? FFR and CFR are tools with which the effectiveness of every interventional cardiology procedure can potentially be improved, but does that mean they should be used during every intervention?

Physiologic measurements can be most cost effective in the assessment of angiographically moderate lesions. As previously described, an artery that has a mid-grade lesion can be safely left alone without intervention. Ultimately, this translates into savings in materials and lab time and preventing subjecting patients to unnecessary cardiac interventions.

It is very difficult to put a figure to the cost of these possibilities and analyze whether they offset the cost of the systems and wires. Ongoing studies are trying to define under which circumstances physiologic assessment is best used and most cost effective. Until these many variables can be assessed, FFR and CFR measurements will probably remain a matter of preference to

a relatively small number of institutions. When the use of these systems becomes second nature in the cath lab and the hospital's administration recognizes the savings that their use can bring, IC pressure measurements can be a valued clinical tool.

REFERENCES

1. Wilson RF, Laxson DD. Caveat emptor: a clinician's guide to assessing the physiologic significance of arterial stenoses. *Cathet Cardiovasc Diagn* 1993;29:93–98.
2. Pijls NH, De Bruyne B, Peels K, et al. Measurement of fractional flow reserve to assess the functional severity of coronary artery stenoses. *N Engl J Med* 1996;334:1703–1708.
3. Bech GJ, De Bruyne B, Pijls NH, et al. Fractional flow reserve to determine the appropriateness of angioplasty in moderate coronary stenosis: a randomized trial. *Circulation* 2001;103:2928–2934.
4. De Bruyne B, Pijls NH, Bartunek J, et al. Fractional flow reserve in patients with prior myocardial infarction. *Circulation* 2001;104:157–162.
5. Pijls N, Klauss V, Siebert U, et al. Coronary pressure measurement after stenting predicts adverse events at follow-up: a multicenter registry. *Circulation* 2002;105:126–130.
6. O'Riordan M. FAME! FFR-guided PCI significantly reduces clinical events. October 14, 2008. Available at: www.theheart.org/article/911505.do. Accessed November 29, 2008.
7. Kern MJ, Aguirre FV, Bach RG, et al. Translesional pressure-flow velocity assessment in patients: Part 1. *Cathet Cardiovasc Diagn* 1994;31:49–60.
8. Kern MJ, Flynn MS, Aguirre FV, et al. Application of intracoronary flow velocity detection and management of ostial saphenous vein graft lesions. *Cathet Cardiovasc Diagn* 1993;30:5–10.
9. Sunamura M, Di Mario C, Piek J, et al. IC Doppler: guidance during angioplasty. The Doppler Endpoints Balloon Angioplasty Trial Europe (DEBATE) study: results of the second interim analysis. Presented at the 6th International

Symposium on Quantitative Imaging; June 19–20, 1995; Rotterdam, The Netherlands.

SUGGESTED READING

Freed M, Safian R. *The Device Guide*, 2nd ed. Royal Oak, MI: Physicians' Press; 1999.

Kern MJ. Intracoronary Doppler flow velocity in coronary interventions. In: Reiber JHC, Serruys PW. *Progress in Quantitative Coronary Arteriography*. Dordrecht, The Netherlands: Kluwer Academic Publishers; 1994.

Kern MJ, Flynn MS. Clinical applications of intracoronary Doppler flow velocity in interventional cardiology. In: White CJ, Ramee SR. *Interventional Cardiology: New Techniques and Strategies for Diagnosis and Treatment*. New York: Marcel Dekker; 1995.

Pijls NH, De Bruyne B. *Coronary Pressure*, 2nd ed. Dordrecht, The Netherlands: Kluwer Academic Publishers; 2000.

Chapter 15

PERCUTANEOUS CORONARY INTERVENTIONS

Rick Meece, CCT, RCS, RCIS, FSICP
Kenneth A. Gorski, RN, RCIS, RCSA, FSICP

INTRODUCTION

According to the American Heart Association, coronary artery disease caused 864,500 deaths in 2005 and is the single leading cause of death in the United States today. Also, 7,900,000 people in the United States have a history of heart attack, and each year about one million Americans have a new or recurrent coronary attack.[1]

Until the year 1977, patients diagnosed with significant coronary artery disease could be offered only two treatment options: medical therapy or high-risk coronary artery bypass graft surgery (CABG). Bypass surgery represented a quantum leap in the treatment of heart disease, increasing survival and improving the quality of life expectancy for these patients, however, mortality levels remained high. The underlying mechanisms of CAD were still poorly understood, leaving many cardiologists and surgeons frustrated with the ongoing progression of disease and death of their patients.

On September 16, 1977, after years of experimentation on canine and cadaverous vessels, Dr. Andreas Gruentzig dilated a proximal LAD lesion through a catheter, and so performed the first human percutaneous transluminal coronary angioplasty (PTCA). Since then, the number of people undergoing this procedure has grown dramatically. In the year 2006 alone, over 1,300,000 angioplasty procedures were performed on diseased coronary arteries in the United States, and the worldwide figure is about twice this, making it one of the most common therapeutic interventional procedures performed anywhere.[2]

In the early days of PTCA, treatable lesions were limited to proximal and large lumen coronary sites. Refinements and developments made over the intervening decades have freed the interventionalist to be both more creative and aggressive in their approach. Multivessel angioplasty has become commonplace, enabling cardiologists to reach even the most distal lesions, as well as difficult clinically significant chronic total occlusions (CTOs).

Mechanical debulking techniques and stenting have made significant improvements in the long-term benefits of angioplasty, in particular to nonsurgical and diabetic candidates. Drug-eluting stents are now the standard of care, having far-reaching benefits for patients with CAD. The term PTCA was originally coined for "plain old balloon angioplasty," and with the advent of atherectomy and stenting, the term evolved into percutaneous coronary intetervention (PCI). This covers the entire range of catheter-based interventions performed on coronary arteries.

INDICATIONS

Indications for PCI include, but are not limited to, the following:

- Acute myocardial infarction
- Unstable angina with single or double major vessel disease
- Acute coronary syndrome
- Nonsurgical candidates with multivessel disease

Indications for PCI in patients with angina pectoris (AP) are:[3]

- Severe stable AP resistant to medication
- Occlusion of left anterior descending artery (LAD) or a three-vessel disease is suspected on the basis of an exercise tolerance test (also when the symptoms are mild)
- Ischemic ST ($>$ 2 mm) with minimal load and low heart rate
- Deficient rise in blood pressure (BP) during exercise test
- Angina pectoris after acute myocardial infarction
- Pain at rest or when walking while the patient is still in the hospital
- AP and severe heart failure (myocardial stunning)

- ST-depression during exercise outside the infarction area
- Unstable angina resistant to medication
- In cases of rapidly recurring angina after CABG, PCI may be considered.

Indications in patients without AP are:

- Survivors of ventricular fibrillation without MI
- When the exercise ECG is clearly pathological
- In acute pulmonary edema without cause
- After a T wave (non-Q wave) infarction
- Management of acute imminent myocardial damage
- When thrombolysis is contraindicated because of the risk of bleeding or it is not effective

THE CARDIOVASCULAR CATHETER LABORATORY TEAM

Most CCL teams consist of a physician and three team members; circulator, scrub assistant, and recorder/monitor. Every CCL team member should possess comprehensive knowledge and competency in performing the procedure at hand, regardless of the mix of roles. The most important consideration of intraprocedural roles is the decision on what aspects each team member contributes to the procedure and for what they have ultimate responsibility for. Teams of excellence have the ability to change roles quickly as needed by the physician, yet maintain control of where their responsibility lies within that procedure.

Team members must meet specific state or national requirements for the administration of sedation and analgesics, the use of radiographic equipment, patient monitoring, and documentation. All team members should be certified in advanced cardiac life support (ACLS) and have yearly skill assessments reviewed by both physicians and peers. Major cardiovascular institutions should have definitive clinical achievement ladders for all CCL personnel to promote and reward the increase of knowledge sets and expansion of roles.

MONITORING

The recorder or monitoring personnel may be a technologist or nurse, dependent on regional or federal laws pertaining to the use of ionizing radiation in cardiovascular procedures. Regardless of their background, in areas where regulations are not compulsory, strict institutional guidelines for CCL personnel should be in place to ensure competence and patient safety. Hemodynamic assessments and calculations that are entered into permanent medical documents must be performed only by individuals with appropriate didactic education and/or credentialing to do so.

In most cases, the report generated during the procedure is the primary record of events and the procedures performed, and it will be archived as a permanent legal document. All events and equipment used must be documented accurately.

Baseline ECG, BP, O_2 saturation, and lab values should be recorded upon arrival into the procedure room. All events should be accurately recorded in the procedural notes. Close monitoring of the patient for ECG ST-segment changes, arrhythmias, and hemodynamic compromise is critical during PCI.

Engaging the guide catheter into the coronary ostium may cause arterial pressure damping at any time and left undetected, can lead to vessel spasm, closure, arrhythmia, and hemodynamic instability since they can be induced by balloon inflations and other factors. These can happen at any time during the procedure, but the most critical times include engaging the guide catheter, crossing the lesion with a wire, and inflating/deflating the balloon/engaging the PCI device.

The monitoring nurse or tech carries tremendous responsibility during interventions.

Radiation dose is continually monitored during all catheterization procedures, particularly interventions. Monitoring patient exposure and/or dose area product is particularly important in cases where a single imaging angle dominates the procedure. Each institution should have policies regarding maximum exposure time or dose in a single procedure for patients. Depending on the brand and age of the fluoroscopic unit, postprocedural radiation documentation should include total fluoro time (in minutes) and a measurement of patient dose or dose area product (i.e., Gys, $mGysCm^2$, $GysCm^2$).

MATERIAL

Although many PCI procedures are scheduled, all diagnostic cardiac procedures should be approached as "possible intervention" procedures. For most cases of scheduled PCI or postdiagnostic ad hoc interventions, patients are more stabile, with a lower risk of adverse cardiac events than patients presenting with an MI or acute coronary syndrome. In any case, interventional and reserve materials should always be close at hand.

When the angiography has been performed and the interventional physician decides to proceed to an intervention, the sterile procedural table should be prepared for the interventional phase. Additions to a standard diagnostic table will generally include:

- Guide catheter for delivering the PCI device
- Inflation device to inflate/deflate the balloon catheter
- Diluted contrast: 50% contrast/50% saline (or institutional preference) for inflation/deflation of balloon catheter
- Hemostasis valve (Y-adaptor, Tuohyborst): attaches to the proximal end of the guide catheter. The central lumen

with an o-ring allows manipulation of the guide wire and PCI device, while the side arm enables injections of contrast media through the guiding catheter.

- Guide wire, generally 0.014 inches diameter for crossing the lesion
- Steering device (torque tool) for guide wire manipulation.
- Intracoronary nitroglycerin Adenosine, Nitroprusside, and Verapamil should be available.
- Sterile cups
- Sterile syringes for intracoronary medication, ACTs, and lab tests

Additional sterile towels, clips, gauze, and stopcocks may be necessary. Intracoronary nitroglycerin should be ready for immediate administration. Wet gauze saturated in saline should be available to use for wiping and anchoring the wires and balloons as they are used and seated. The balloon/stent inflation device should be filled with the diluted contrast and purged of air.

The sterile field should be organized and uncluttered as possible to provide a clean work area for balloon and stent preparation.

The success of coronary interventions can be greatly affected by the choices made of the interventional equipment used. Having a solid understanding of how different materials work with and against each other in a myriad of situations is how the experienced interventionalist teams define their excellence. Although success is not guaranteed, the array of modern equipment offers every chance to obtain the best outcome possible.

Guiding Catheters

The guiding catheter may be the most important decision for a timely and successful intervention. The guiding catheter will provide the optimal support for the insertion of a guide wire and balloon catheter or device to the target lesion. The operator's assessment of aortic arch/root morphology and coronary artery ostial position during diagnostic imaging will assist in choosing the correct catheter. An important consideration is the relationship between the catheter French (F) size, curve, and potential damping of coronary blood flow.

Figure 15-1. Basic PTCA equipment and setup.

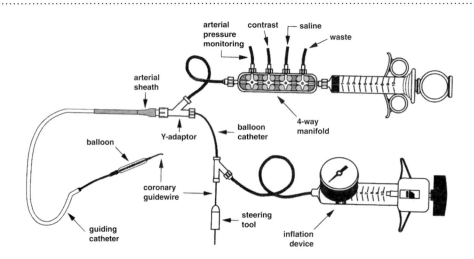

The majority of PCI cases currently performed use 6F equipment, thanks to the smaller, more flexible tools now available. Smaller, 5F guide catheters are also available in limited curves. 5F guides are rarely used today, with the exception of radial access interventions. The difficulty of maneuvering 5F PCI equipment to the lesion can be challenging, and the amount of back-up support required from the guiding system should be assessed carefully. Where maximum support is needed, physicians may choose a larger 7F- or 8F-sized system to keep the catheter comfortably seated. Larger lumen-guiding catheters have a tendency to be stiffer, which may aid in improving backup for inserting interventional equipment to the target area.

In some cases, where stiff backup plus a larger lumen is needed, some operators may choose a guiding catheter with factory-made side holes to allow distal coronary artery perfusion. Side-hole catheters give a false sense of security, however, the catheter tip may still be occluding flow into the vessel, while guide catheter side holes sit outside of the coronary ostium and reflect the aortic pressure on the hemodynamic monitors. The use of side-hole catheters may also increase the CM dose (spilling out of the side holes) and can reduce the ability to fill large lumen arteries/grafts in higher perfusion states.

Interventional guiding catheters offer variable construction designs to give the operator choices between flexibility and seating within the coronary ostium. Some manufacturers offer guiding catheters with both stiff and soft secondary curves to aid in manipulation. Almost all interventional guiding catheters have a soft, pliable tip to decrease the risk of damage or dissection of the coronary ostium.

Guide catheters come in traditional curves (Judkins, Amplatz, multipurpose; see Figure 15-2). Proprietary extra-support guide catheter curves (XB, Voda, GL) have a long terminal primary curve and a stiff secondary curve to seat the catheter firmly in the aortic root, much like an

Figure 15-2. Common guiding catheter configurations.

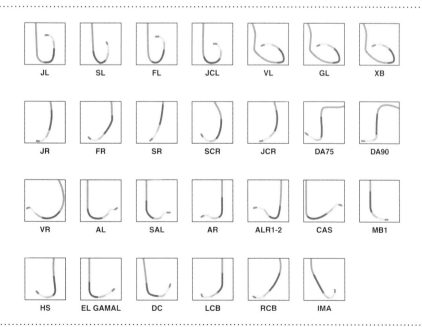

amplatz catheter but with more maneuverability. These shapes greatly improve the ability to firmly seat smaller French-size catheters in the coronary ostium and support delivery of the guide wire and PCI device.

Guide Wires

Guide wire choice will be the second critical element because of the relationship between guiding catheter and the trackability of the guide wire and device. The purpose of guide wire placement is to provide safe and stable access to the lesion for the balloon, stent, or other interventional device.

Guide wire lengths can vary according to application, but are primarily one of two lengths: approximately 145 cm and 300 cm (exchange length), depending on the manufacturer. The shorter guide wires are designed for rapid exchange/monorail systems and are controlled by the operator for most of the procedure. Exchange length guide wires are good for complex interventions where frequent device exchange is anticipated.

Interventional guide wires generally have a soft, atraumatic tip that may be shaped by the operator (see Figure 15-3). Shaping is performed to enhance the ability of the wire to pass through and around the curves of the target coronary artery. The transition point of a guide wire refers to how it is constructed between the microthin

tip and the 0.014-inch main body. The transition of the guide wire determines many of its properties and best applications. Most operators have a "workhorse" guide wire they turn to first, giving an edge in predictability of how it reacts as it is advanced. Most guide wire manufacturers will offer wall charts or pocket guides classifying their products and recommended applications; some include competitive products in their listings.

Traditionally, guide wires are primarily classified as floppy, intermediate, or standard (see Figure 15-4). Stiffer standard and intermediate wires have more pushability, whereas more flexible or floppy wires tend to track more easily through a tortuous artery.

There are literally hundreds of guide wires available, made of different materials and coated with a choice of agents. Each one has a unique property of use and technical applications. Many guide wires have coatings such as Teflon to aid in smooth tracking of the balloon over the wire. Hydrophilic-coated guide wires are an invaluable tool for crossing thrombosed coronary arteries because of their lubricious nature, but the hydrophilic agent also increases the chance of dissection and perforation with the guide wire tip.

Some guide wires are constructed of Nitinol rather than the more common stainless steel. Nitinol retains a "memory" of its original shape and can be helpful for use in certain conditions requiring a balance of pushability and tracking.

Figure 15-3. Guide wire construction.

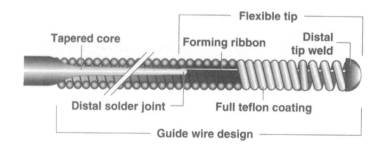

Figure 15-4. Guide wire core construction.

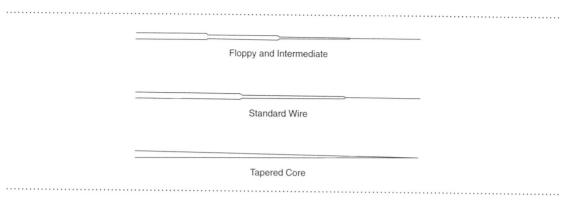

Floppy and Intermediate

Standard Wire

Tapered Core

Nitinol guide wires should be wiped frequently with heparinized solution gauze while exposed to air to promote smooth device movement.

Specialty guide wires are available with markers that aid in measuring target lesion length, taking away the guesswork in measuring around tortuous lesions.

A second guide wire is often used to protect side branch vessels when intervening on main artery. Many operators will choose this option so that in the event of acute closure of the side branch, there will still be access through the area, hopefully to enable PCI if necessary.

A second guide wire is also used when employing the "kissing balloon" technique, whereby, two guide wires and two balloons are advanced simultaneously down a main vessel and side branch (such as an LAD and a diagonal). The balloons are then positioned one against the other, and simultaneously inflated at low pressures to perform a bifurcation, or "kissing balloon" angiosplasty. One complication that can occur with this procedure is that the two guide wires can become wrapped or entwined together during positioning. When advancing the first balloon, if there is significant resistance to further advancement past the bifurcation without an obvious cause, pull back the remaining guide wire and readvance. This will usually remedy the situation and enable the other balloon to push forward.

Advancing any coronary guide wire should be done with extreme caution. Intimal staining with contrast dye indicates possible dissection and should be assessed before proceeding further.

Angioplasty Balloons

Balloon choices are made based on experience and preference by the physician. The primary differences between balloons that affect their performance are: material design, tracking ability, and length.

There are three main types of balloon catheter systems (see Figure 15-5):

Over the Wire

Over-the-wire balloons have a central guide wire lumen that runs from the proximal hub to the distal tip. These balloons can be loaded onto the guide wire from either the front or back after the lesion has been crossed. With guide wire support within the entire catheter body, these balloons may offer more flexibility and trackability than rapid-exchange balloons.

Single-Operator Exchange

Single-operator exchange, more often referred to as rapid-exchange (RX) or monorail balloons, are

Figure 15-5. Balloon catheter designs.

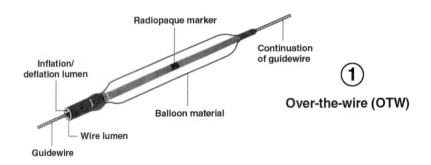

Radiopaque marker

Inflation/
deflation lumen

Continuation
of guidewire

Balloon material

Wire lumen

Guidewire

Over-the-wire (OTW)

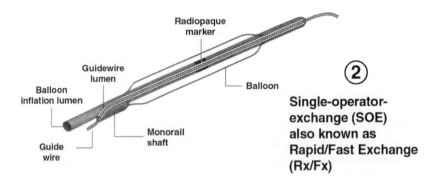

Radiopaque
marker

Guidewire
lumen

Balloon

Balloon
inflation lumen

Monorail
shaft

Guide
wire

**Single-operator-
exchange (SOE)
also known as
Rapid/Fast Exchange
(Rx/Fx)**

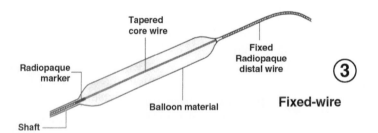

Tapered
core wire

Fixed
Radiopaque
distal wire

Radiopaque
marker

Balloon material

Shaft

Fixed-wire

designed to be more easily handled by one person. These balloons load only from the front end with the guide wire exiting approximately 30 cm from the tip. This enables the operator to control both the wire and balloon while crossing into and away from the coronary artery. This design also allows for balloon-catheter exchange without the use of a 300 cm wire, guide wire extension, or exchange assist device (such as the Boston Scientific Trapper or Magnet). The catheter body of single operator balloons tends to be stiffer for more pushability.

Fixed-Wire Balloons

The original balloon designed by Andreas Gruentzig was a fixed wire. The over-the-wire design of John Simpson quickly improved on Gruentzig's concept. Because of limitations in technology, fixed-wire designs resurfaced as a way to treat smaller distal vessels, side branch lesions, and some bypass graft lesions.

Advances in balloon design and materials have overcome earlier limitations. Today, the need for fixed-wire balloon catheters is not as common, and they are no longer available in the United States.

Perfusion Balloons

Perfusion balloons were designed to enable blood "flow" into the distal coronary artery when the balloon is inflated. It is necessary pull the guide wire back between the proximal and distal balloon ports. Commonly called the "bailout" balloon for spontaneous closure, perfusion balloons were an important development in early PTCA before stenting.

Like fixed-wire balloons, the onset of direct-stenting and use of newer antiplatelet agents have eliminated the need for perfusion balloons. These devices now are simply an interesting note in the annals of coronary intervention.

Balloon Compliance

Balloons are constructed of a variety of material to fit different applications. Most of the early-generation balloons were made of polymers like the outer wrap of a cigarette pack. Balloons were stiffer and had higher profiles, making distal and complex lesions difficult to reach because of limited flexibility. Later designs brought on the development of new polymer hybrids to meet specific anatomic and technical challenges.

Compliant Balloons

These polymers are more responsive to balloon inflation pressures, having a tendency to increase in diameter with each ATM applied. Balloons with materials are classified as compliant, because of their nature to predictably increase in diameter with increased pressures. Compliant balloons are flexible and trackable over guide wires through high-degree, tortuous coronary lesions. Compliant balloons also have a tendency to shape to the artery as they are inflated. Unfortunately, compliant balloons have the tendency to "dog-bone" over highly stenotic and/or calcific lesions, increasing the risk of intimal disruption and dissection with higher inflation pressures.

Noncompliant Balloons

The polyethyleneterphthalate (PET) balloons are suited to long inflation balloon angioplasty and coronary stenting. Good stent apposition requires firm deployment of higher pressures at the lesion site, and the noncompliant balloons serve well. Once inflated to their maximum designed diameter, PET balloons do not tend to comply with increased diameter under rising pressure. This noncompliance holds across the length of the balloon, minimizing the dog-bone effect. The nature of noncompliance makes these balloons ideal for unstable and calcified lesions where overinflation increases the risk of intimal dissection. Noncompliant balloons are also used for postdilatation after stent implantation. They provide firm apposition and remodeling. A technical issue with noncompliant balloons is their stiffer nature, and they may be less able to pass through tortuous anatomy. As balloon profiles (their preinflated diameter) become smaller, this is becoming less of an issue over time.

Cutting Balloons

Balloon dilatation of an atherosclerotic lesion not only stretches the vessel and partially compresses the lesion, it cracks and splits the plaque. Fissures and dissections occur, some of which may cause acute vessel closure.

The Flextome Balloon (from Boston Scientific of Maple Grove, Massachusetts) has three or four microtome blades embedded on a hard polymer inflation balloon. The microtomes are protected within the folds of the wrapped balloon, but as the balloon is inflated, the blades are exposed and pushed out, creating microsurgical incisions into both hard and softer plaque areas.

The AngioSculpt Scoring Balloon (from AngioScore of Fremont, California) has a Nitinol wire with three rectangular spiral struts wrapped on a semicompliant balloon. Inflation of the balloon focuses uniform radial force along the Nitinol elements, scoring the atherosclerotic plaque.

Cutting or scoring the plaque allows easier stent expansion than direct stenting or predilatation with a traditional balloon. Cutting balloons are valuable for PTCA of smaller diameter vessels and bifurcation side branches. Cutting balloon angioplasty is a favored dilatation approach for the treatment of in-stent restenosis.

Embolic Protection

Ulcerative lesions in saphenous vein bypass grafts (SVGs), native coronary arteries, and carotid and renal arteries can be highly unstable. When these lesions are compressed during PCI, the plaque can erupt, sending thromboembolic debris distally down the vessel. This can clog the distal vascular bed, leading to myocardial infarction, cerebrovascular accident, or renal infarction, depending on the vessels involved.

Embolic protection devices have been developed to protect the distal vessel from the embolic consequences of PCI. These are discussed in further detail in Chapter 17.

PATIENT PREPARATION

Before a patient undergoes a PCI, he or she must be assessed and a teaching plan initiated. This plan should be individually tailored to the patient's needs. Patient assessment and preprocedure evaluation are covered in depth in Chapter 10.

In scheduled and possible emergent cases, the patient should be visited by either the cardiologist nursing liaison or appropriate laboratory personnel. Along with an introduction and answering any patient and/or family inquiries, they will check the patient's chart for precath physician consultation and orders, advanced directives, allergies, appropriate permit, and establish the patient's understanding of what is to occur.

Patient demographics and medication allergies should be clearly noted, both on the identification arm band and the front of the chart. There should be documentation by the attending cardiologist in reference to discussion with the patient and/or the family regarding the risks, benefits, and alternatives to PCI and/or possible emergent bypass surgery. This should also include the risks of skin damage during prolonged interventional procedures associated with fluoroscopic radiation, and that the patient and/or the family understand and agree to proceed.

Conscious Sedation

Institutional and physician preference may vary regarding the use of conscious sedation for patients in the CCL for diagnostic and interventional procedures. The circulator, whether a registered nurse or otherwise, must be fully aware of, and work in compliance with, policies and procedures as directed by institutional, state, or federal requirements for administering such agents.

In many cases, the attending physician will document both the patient's status and eligibility for conscious sedation based on their history and physical assessment. All these facts should be checked by the circulator before initiating conscious sedation. Allergies should be reviewed carefully and a verbal acknowledgement from the patient (when possible) that the agents to be given are appropriate. Situations where the patient may not desire sedation should be immediately discussed with the attending physician.

Anticoagulation Therapy

Careful monitoring of anticoagulant therapy will be necessary during the entire PCI procedure. Recent Coumadin (warfarin) therapy warrants prothrombin/INR (International Normalized Ratio) assessment for bleeding risks.

In interventional cases where unfractionated heparin is administered for anticoagulation, weight-adjusted doses are often used to avoid excessive anticoagulation, and lower ACT levels can be expected. Lower weight-adjusted doses of heparin are used when adjunctive GP IIb/IIIa inhibitors are administered to minimize the incidence of serious bleeding.

Fixed standard dose bolus: 5000 to 10,000 units
Fixed low-dose bolus: 2500 to 5000 units
Weight-adjusted standard dose heparin bolus: 100 units/kg
Weight-adjusted low-dose heparin bolus: 50 to 70 units/kg

An activated clotting time (ACT) of between 250 and 350 seconds is necessary before a PCI can be safely carried out. The ACT should be checked within 5 minutes of the first dose, then every 30 minutes (or as directed) throughout the procedure. If the target ACT value is not reached after the heparin bolus has been given, additional boluses of 2000 to 5000 units can be administered until the target value has been reached. Higher ACT levels may increase the risk of bleeding.

In all situations involving anticoagulation, extreme caution must be exercised by the operator to gain clean arterial access to reduce the incidence of site hematoma/bleeding. IV access sites should be monitored closely. Recent surgery or history of internal bleeding represents a contraindication for thrombolytic and/or anticoagulant therapy as determined by the cardiologist and the institution's policy. The possibility of emergent bypass surgery is important to consider as well in decisions regarding anticoagulation. The patient is closely monitored for bleeding, neurological changes, unrelated pain, and distension from unusual source sites. A significant increase or decrease in blood pressure or heart rate should be given differential assessment as according to preprocedural status. In interventions conducted in the setting of acute myocardial infarction, patient hemodynamic stability is less predictable.

Use of specific anticoagulation, antiplatelet, and fibrinolytic agents are discussed in greater detail in Chapter 38.

PROCEDURE

In most cases, the PCI procedure is carried out immediately after a positive angiography procedure. The patient will be on the CCL table, covered with a sterile drape, with a sheath in an artery, usually the patient's right femoral or radial artery. It may be necessary to change the sheath, because interventional catheters are usually 6F or 7F and diagnostic catheters 5F.

With the help of the 0.035-inch exchange wire, the guiding catheter is pushed up the aorta to the mouth of the artery containing the lesion. The selected guide wire will then be passed through the catheter and into the artery. At this point, the torque device is attached to the proximal end of the guide wire.

The interventionalist then manipulates the guide wire until its distal end has passed through the lesion. It is then pushed further into the vessel and parked in a small branch. Once the guide wire access has been established, the scrub assistant will anchor the guide wire with wet gauze to prevent accidental movement or contamination. Guarding the guide wire should be continually performed by the assistant throughout any interventional procedure. Experienced operators never forget losing guide wire access after an hour was spent getting it!

The balloon catheter is then passed over the guide wire, through the catheter, to the artery. The interventionalist advances the balloon catheter until the balloon is within the lesion. Once the target lesion has been successfully crossed with the balloon, the inflation device is connected and set to negative pressure. This is important to ensure the balloon maintains the smallest possible profile and that air is not introduced into the inflation lumen after being prepped.

The balloon is gradually inflated until the desire pressure is reached. Lesion type and morphology will influence whether higher or lower pressures are tried first. A longer inflation time, while gradually increasing pressure until the lesion yields, may cause less vessel trauma. Another technique, useful in calcified lesions, involves multiple short inflations in rising increments of pressure. Noncompliant balloons may be helpful to prevent central balloon resistance, called "dog-boning," and enable higher pressure inflations.

When a satisfactory result has been obtained, the operator will remove the balloon, while leaving the guide wire in place to safeguard access through the lesion. It is critical that the interventionalist and assistant work in tandem to prevent losing guide wire placement while removing the balloon. With an over-the-wire system, it is im-portant to keep the right hand firmly on the table with each movement back along the table, while making sure that the balloon is sliding back easily with the left hand. Fluoroscopic imaging should be utilized to confirm guide wire position.

There is always the possibility that a negative result or inability to cross with a balloon may cause the interventionalist to proceed with a different therapeutic approach. Whether it involves stenting, atherectomy, thrombectomy, or some other device, the team must be flexible and ready for a quick change of equipment and direction from the operating physician.

Guide Wire Biasing Phenomenon

When a stiff guide wire is passed through a tortuous artery, the guide wire's resistance to bending tends to trap the walls of the intima against the wire as the artery is forcibly straightened. If the artery is relatively compliant or more flexible, this can sometimes aid in creating a straight path for the balloon to pass toward the target lesion. Calcified vessels are less compliant, and the resistance to the guide wire increases. This can create a situation where the wire is so tightly trapped against the vessel wall that nothing can pass over the guide wire at the turn. Aggressive attempts to pass balloons or stents beyond these areas can increase the risk of intimal dissection, if they pass at all.

At this point, a decision must be made whether to reattempt crossing with a more flexible and compliant balloon or a more flexible guide wire. If a balloon change proves unsuccessful, the interventionalist may choose to remove the current guide wire for a more compliant one that can more readily track through the tortuous artery.

No Reflow

No reflow occurs when the blood flow in the target artery ceases, usually just after the distal seating of the guide wire or immediately following the first or second balloon inflation. It manifests by the contrast media remaining static in the vessel during angiography and not washing out. It is believed to be a result of postdilatation microscopic intimal debris (microemboli) becoming lodged in the microvascular system.

No reflow can be reversed with a timely intracoronary bolus (through the guiding catheter) of nitroglycerin or Nitroprusside (100 mcg to 200 mcg), Verapamil (50 mcg to 100 mcg), or Adenosine (24 mcg to 48 mcg). These agents dilate the microvasculature, and (ideally) flush it clean over a period of seconds or minutes. Prophylactic intracoronary injection of Nitroprusside or Verapamil may be helpful in reducing the incidence of no-reflow in both native and vein graft PCI.

PCI of Saphenous Vein Bypass Grafts

Performing PCI on SVGs is commonplace, but can present technical difficulties. An important consideration with SVG intervention is the amount of relatively loose debris that lies along the inner wall, particularly in older venous graft vessels. This debris is easily disturbed and can move distally toward the anastomosis and beyond, as guide wires and catheters are inserted. This microvascular debris appears to contribute to no-reflow phenomenon.

Embolic protection devices are used in virtually all PCI procedures in an SVG. Originally designed for carotid artery interventions to reduce the incidence of stroke, these devices have proved invaluable in the technical success rates of SVG interventions. These devices are discussed in detail in Chapter 17.

Primary stent implantation without predilatation is commonly used to dilate main saphenous vein grafts. Trapping the debris with stent placement, along with distal protection devices when indicated, reduces the risk of no-reflow. In primary stenting only, one device is tracked across the debris-laden lesion before entrapment, increasing the likelihood of successful vein graft PCI.

Stent Implantation

Primary stent implantation has become the therapeutic standard of care. Ongoing data supports the use of both bare metal (BMS) and drug-eluting (DES) stents for long-term patient benefits.

Intracoronary stenting is discussed in Chapter 16.

Acute Myocardial Infarction

In the acute MI condition, with continued ST-elevation and unstable angina, emergent PCI is the treatment of choice where it is available. Studies showing reduced mortality and rebound of myocardial function have encouraged aggressive intervention in the early stages of MI, preferably within 2 hours of onset.[4–6]

Time is muscle; recognizing that injured myocardium may regain functionality with aggressive revascularization, every minute is critical getting the acute myocardial infarction (AMI) patient into the cardiovascular laboratory as soon as possible

Rapidly performed, prompt, expertly performed PCI in the setting of acute ST-elevation MI (STEMI) is not easy to obtain and maintain. The American College of Cardiology Door to Balloon (D2B) Initiative advocates six key (and one optional) strategies that practice-based evidence have shown to reduce door-to-balloon times:[7]

- Emergency department physician activation of the cath lab
- Single-call activation system activates the cath lab—#64 (MI), CODE STEMI
- Cath lab team available within 20–30 minutes
- Prompt data feedback
- Senior management commitment
- Team-based approach (ED, cardiology, cath lab, nursing, management, ancillary personnel)
- (Optional) Prehospital 12-lead ECG activates the cath lab

The fastest D2B times are achieved in communities where paramedics perform a 12-lead ECG in the field and are able to triage patients to the appropriate facility. Prior notification of a STEMI patient saves valuable time when the patient arrives at the hospital.

Assessment

Angiographic TIMI 3 flow and a symptom-free patient will generally signify procedural success in most cases.

IVUS, FFR (intracoronary pressure), or CFR (or Doppler flow) can be useful in assessing the result of PCI. Intracoronary ultrasound gives a physical view of the vessel lumen and composition of the target area in comparison to surrounding vasculature. FFR and CFR assess the physiologic significance of a lesion by measuring pressure or blood flow velocities across the target area. For further information on IVUS, CFR, and FFR, see Chapters 13 and 14.

POSTPROCEDURAL DUTIES

When the interventionalist is satisfied with the result of the intervention and the final diagnostic angiograms have been performed, all equipment except the arterial sheath may be removed from the patient. It is a good practice to safeguard or cover all equipment in a sterile fashion until the physician has left the procedure area.

In many cases, a device is used to close the hole in the artery made by the sheath after the sheath has been removed. These devices and manual hemostasis are discussed in Chapter 26. If no mechanical hemostasis device is to be used, the patient should remain draped until the sheath is properly sutured and anchored. In the event that something should happen to the patient in those first few minutes after PCI, it is a strategic advantage to have maintained a sterile field to facilitate access to the site or sheath exchange if necessary. The sheath should be secured with a quality suture. Caution must be exercised not to penetrate deep below the skin with the suture needle and risk a significant bleeding issue in the presence of anticoagulant therapy. Needleless devices for sheath anchoring are also available.

Once the sheath has been secured, aspirated and flushed, a 500 ml bag of pressurized heparinized saline can be hooked up and set to a slow KVO (Keep Vein Open) drip to prevent sheath and intraluminal thrombosis. This pressure line can also be set up to allow arterial monitoring. Pad and support the hub of the sheath with rolled up 4-inch × 4-inch gauze and covered with a paper tape or clear surgical dressing.

Any access site hematoma should be marked and documented appropriately. If there is swelling or bleeding around the sheath hub that will not relent after applied pressure, a topical hemostasis pad may be applied. Alternately, the physician may choose to exchange the sheath for a larger diameter one until it is to be removed. Applying a pressure dressing or device may help control the bleeding, however, it may also hide a growing hematoma.

The monitor and circulator make final notes and talk with the patient to assess his or her physical and neurological status. If the patient is awake and responds appropriately to questions, preprocedure teaching should be reinforced, particularly regarding movement and positioning with the arterial sheath in place.

If a urinary catheter was not in place, the patient should be asked if they have the urgency to void. A distended bladder can cause the sheath to be pushed to the side, increasing the possibility of a hematoma or even a retroperitoneal bleed. Hypertension secondary to hypervolemia or agitation from discomfort may lead to similar complications.

Once the postintervention orders have been written by the physician, a member of the team should give a report to the receiving nurse, giving information about the procedure, the patient's physical and neurological status, and the initial care plan.

POSTPROCEDURE PATIENT CARE

Patient stability should be assessed immediately by the receiving nurse. This will include, but is not limited to, ECG rate and rhythm with ST documentation, vital signs, oxygen saturation level, urine output, and cardiac, respiratory, pulmonary, and gastrointestinal status. If the patient arrives from the CCL with a sheath in the femoral artery site, the site and distal pulses should also be assessed immediately. Particular attention must be paid to the peripheral vascular assessment of the lower extremities at all times.

If a patient should become hypotensive with oxygen desaturation and increased respiration, a retroperitoneal bleed should be considered. The patient may or may not be experiencing pain in the lower back. The interventional cardiologist should be notified immediately, and the patient is watched closely until further orders can be carried out. Retroperitoneal bleeding in anticoagulated patients is very serious, and their condition can deteriorate rapidly without direct intervention. Immediate considerations will include volume and hyperoxygenation for hemodynamic support. Emergency vascular surgery may be required in more critical settings.

According to institutional policy, the nurse will check vital signs and distal pulses every 15 minutes × 4; then 30 minutes × 2; then hourly. ACT is checked according to written orders with a minimum of 180 seconds or less prior to sheath removal.

In most institutions, the physician or designated personnel remove the arterial sheath. Sheath removal is managed by ward nurses in some institutions; others have the cath lab or other specially trained personnel remove it. In all instances, institutional policies and procedures should be followed and accurately documented.

Any change in the patient's neurological or vascular status should be reported immediately to the attending physician. If the cardiac catheterization was performed under conscious sedation, the institutional policy for conscious sedation documentation should be followed.

If the patient is stable and awake, he or she will remain on strict bed rest with the head of the bed no higher than 30°. The leg of the sheath site must be kept straight for around 8 hours after the sheath is removed, and a pressure bandage applied.

Encourage the patient to drink at least 2 liters of fluid during the first 12 hours post if it is not contraindicated. The nurse should maintain the patient record on hourly fluid intake and output.

If the patient starts to bleed at the puncture site, notify the physician immediately and hold pressure just above the insertion site until the bleeding stops or the attending physician arrives. After hemostasis has been attained, recheck all peripheral pulses and document them.

FINAL NOTE

The best interventional institutions understand teamwork. What the medical team can accomplish together is not just for the moment, but forever in the fast-moving timeline of cardiology. Therefore, strive to be excellent; demand an institution that supports excellence, both psychologically and financially. Excellence in staffing lies in their diversity of knowledge and teamwork.

REFERENCES

1. American Heart Association Heart Disease and Stroke Statistics. Available at www.americanheart.org/down loadable/heart. Accessed September 1, 2009
2. American Heart Association Angioplasty and Cardiac Revascularization Statistics. Available at www. americanheart.org/presenter.jhtml?identifier= 4439. Accessed September 1, 2009
3. Braunwald E. Management of patients with unstable angina and non-ST segment elevation. Myocardial infarction update. *J Am Col Cardiol* 2002;40:1366–1374.

4. Cannon CP, Braunwald E, Hirudin L. Initial results in acute myocardial infarction, unstable angina and angioplasty. *J Am Col Cardiol* 1995;25(Supplement):30S–37S.

5. Sim I, Gupta M, McDonald K, et al. A meta-analysis of randomised trials comparing coronary artery bypass grafting with percutaneous transluminal coronary angioplasty in multivessel coronary artery disease. *Am J Col Cardiol* 1995;76: 1025–1029.

6. Vaitkus PT Percutaneous transluminal coronary angioplasty versus thrombolysis in acute myocardial infarction. *Clin Cardiol* 1995;18:35–38.

7. Available at: www.d2balliance.org/

SUGGESTED READING

Kern MJ, Kern M. *The Cardiac Catheterization Handbook*, 4th ed. St. Louis, MO: Mosby; 2003.

Peterson KL, Nicod P. *Cardiac Catheterization: Methods, Diagnosis, and Therapy*. Philadelphia: W.B. Saunders; 1997.

Topol EJ. *Textbook of Cardiovascular Medicine*. Philadelphia, PA: Lippincott-Raven; 1998.

Zipes DP, Libby P, Bonow RO, Braunwald E. *Braunwald's Heart Disease,* 7th ed. Philadelphia, PA: W.B. Saunders; 2005.

Chapter 16

INTRAVASCULAR STENTS

Sandy Watson, RN, BN, NFESC
Kenneth A. Gorski, RN, RCIS, RCSA, FSICP

A stent is a tiny, fine mesh cylinder. Stents act as scaffolding, giving vessels added structural support. They also reduce vascular recoil, tack up intimal dissections, and increase vessel lumen diameter. Initially, stents were used in "bailout" situations, when acute vessel closure was threatened, or as "backup" when suboptimal results had been achieved with angioplasty. Today, "primary stenting," in which the stent is implanted without first treating the vessel with balloon angioplasty, has become common practice.

Bare-metal stents (BMSs) have been associated with a decline in post-PCI (percutaneous coronary intervention) complication rates and reduced restenosis compared to balloon angioplasty. Although BMSs reduced the incidence of restenosis, they did not eliminate it. The introduction of drug-eluting stents (DES), designed to reduce inflammation and inhibit cellular proliferation, has lowered restenosis rates even further, and DESs have become the standard of care in many parts of the world.

HISTORY

In the first decade following the birth of angioplasty, the hazards of the procedure started to become apparent. The procedure often left intimal tears, called dissection flaps, in the walls of treated vessels. These flaps could protrude into the lumen, causing postangioplasty angina and sometimes causing acute vessel closure. Work was soon begun on the construction of mesh devices that could be implanted in the vessel at the point of injury to hold up the vessel wall, keeping the lumen open.

In 1986, in Toulouse, France, a coronary stent (the Wallstent, a self-expanding mesh stent) was placed in a human for the first time. By 1988, 117 of these had been placed in human coronary arteries, and the results, reported some years later, were quite sobering: Over 23% of the stents had occluded completely, and there was an additional restenosis rate of 14%.[1] The 1-year mortality rate was 8%. It must be kept in mind, however, that the early Wallstents were only used to salvage poor outcomes of a balloon angioplasty, which would probably have had worse outcomes if stents had not been used.

The Gianturco-Roubin was another early coronary stent. It was small, flexible, and constructed from stainless steel suture wire of 0.15 mm in diameter. This was the first balloon-expandable stent, and the coil design resembled that of an ink-pen spring. The design allowed for great flexibility, allowing it to be easily placed in most circumstances. It was the first stent to get FDA approval for use in acute "bailouts" during coronary angioplasty. The large spaces between the stent wires, however, allowed tissue prolapse, encouraging excessive neointimal growth that contributed to a relative high rate of restenosis.

The Wallstent provided sufficient vessel coverage, but lacked adequate radial strength; the Gianturco-Roubin coil stent had better radial strength, but failed when it came to adequate coverage. With these early failures, for a time it looked as if coronary stenting was to be locked away in the "good idea, but it doesn't work" drawer.

This was changed by two randomized trials using Palmaz-Schatz stents: BENESTENT[2,3] was carried out in Europe and STRESS in North America.[4] They showed that the use of Palmaz-Schatz stents in selected cases could benefit the patient's clinical outcome. These studies changed the way interventional cardiology is practiced. For the first time, patients with coronary artery disease had a truly effective alternative to coronary artery bypass surgery. It also created a multibillion-dollar medical business, almost overnight.

Stent placement has quickly become the standard of care, and they are being implanted in more than 80% of interventional procedures in most centers. The steep increase in the number of stent implants is due to two factors.

The first is pharmacologic. In the mid-1990s, the stent patient had to remain in the hospital for several days after a stent was placed. Because a permanent metallic device was being placed in arteries 3–4 mm in diameter, there was great fear of thrombotic events. It was felt that in-stent thrombosis had to be aggressively combated prophylactically. In the cath lab, ACTs for stent implantation were kept at above 350 seconds, and intravenous dextran was given for its antiplatelet effects. Postprocedure, heparin drips were initiated directly after sheath removal, and maintained parallel to warfarin therapy, until the patient's INR had reached an acceptable level. The patient was then released on oral anticoagulation, plus aspirin, for 6 months.

It was eventually found that a simpler anticoagulation regime, involving aspirin for life and thienopyradines (ticlopidine or now clopidigrel) for several months, achieved a reduced rate of subacute thrombosis.[5,6] Thus, stent patients could leave the hospital as soon as if they had undergone a balloon angioplasty.

The second factor was intravascular ultrasound (IVUS). IVUS visualization revealed that many stents were not being fully expanded in the vessel.[7] Poor stent-strut apposition allows blood to flow between the stent struts and vessel wall and leads to increased rates of thrombosis and vessel closure. It was found that avoiding vessel trauma with aggressive predilatation, and complete stent expansion were vital in preventing thrombosis[8] and that fully expanded stents, with the struts nestling well against the endothelium, produced better long-term patency rates.

The quality of coronary stents has also improved markedly over time. They now have very low crossing profiles and are more flexible, permitting easier placement in complicated lesions. Their struts are finer, and they are shaped to protrude as little as possible into the bloodstream

INDICATIONS

As operator experience increases and stent materials and design improve, the indications for intracoronary stenting will, no doubt, continue to widen. The following are indications for which solid evidence has been gathered from randomized and observational studies.

- Treatment of abrupt and prevention of threatened coronary occlusion after PCI
- Primary treatment to reduce restenosis in de-novo focal lesions
- Saphenous vein graft disease
- Suboptimal results after PTCA
- Chronic total occlusions
- Restenotic lesions after PTCA
- Restenotic lesions after prior stent placement
- PCI for acute infarction

CONTRAINDICATIONS

Even though elective stenting in these patients significantly improves the overall outcome, stent placement may not be more beneficial than balloon angioplasty in every case. The challenge for the experienced interventionalist is to stent only when the case warrants it. All other situations should be considered to be relative contraindications.

Relative contraindications for stent placement are:

- Stenting will occlude a major side-branch.
- Patient cannot take clopidogrel.

STENT TYPES

Every type of stent has a unique design, and each has its own advantages and disadvantages. The major differences are in the materials used, the design of the stent itself, its level of radiopacity, and the method of expansion (see Table 16-1). Because of reliable delivery of newer stent designs, many operators now perform direct stenting without predilation (see Table 16-2).

Self-Expanding

The prototype of the self-expanding stent is the Wallstent, the first stent to be placed in a human being. It consists of a woven-wire mesh that is fused together to form a mesh tube of a specific size. This tube is then compressed and covered by a plastic membrane. When the plastic membrane is withdrawn, the mesh returns to the dimensions at which it was manufactured. The mesh design means that there is a great deal of metal in the vessel. It gives very good coverage, but does tend to block off side branches, so its recommended coronary applications have been limited to saphenous vein grafts and the right coronary artery.

The latest generation of self-expanding stents are often very flexible, usually made from nitinol. Today, self-expanding stents are most often utilized for treating saphenous vein grafts, peripheral vascular disease in the iliac and femoral vessels, and carotid artery stenting.

Balloon-Expandable

Balloon-expandable stents are mounted on a PTCA balloon catheter and are deployed in the vessel by inflating the balloon. When the balloon is deflated, the stent will remain in the vessel wall, and the balloon is withdrawn. Early Palmaz-Schatz stents had to be carefully hand crimped onto an angioplasty balloon before implantation. Today, coronary stents are almost always premounted on a balloon.

Balloon-expandable stents are made of surgical-grade stainless steel or cobalt chromium alloys. Stainless steel stents tend to give higher radial strength, but are less flexible than those made from cobalt chromium. Most balloon-expandable stents are of a slotted tube design, cut with laser from a fine metal tube, although the Driver from Medtronic is made up of crowns that are welded together.

IN-STENT RESTENOSIS

Although stenting produces very good short-term results, there is a phenomenon by which the vessel lumen narrows very slowly within the

Table 16-1. Stent Characteristics

Characteristic	Definition	Determinants
Biocompatibility	Resistance to corrosion, thrombosis	Material coatings, metal surface area
Conformability	Degree to which an expanded stent can bend around its longitudinal axis	Material, stent design
Deliverability	Ability to deliver stent to target lesion	Longitudinal flexibility, crossing profile, trackability, nesting
Expansion ratio	Degree of stent expansion when fully deployed (opposite of recoil)	Stent design, strut thickness, metal surface area, stent recoil
Flaring	Separation of the stent strut from the delivery balloon during insertion around bends	Stent design (bigger problem with open or coil designs)
Flexibility	Degree to which an unexpanded stent can bend around its longitudinal axis	Material, stent design
Metal surface area	Percent of surface area covered by metal after stent deployment	Stent design, strut thickness
Nesting	Security of stent attachment to delivery system	Stent design, profile
Radial strength	Resistance to vessel recoil	Stent design, strut thickness
Radiopacity	Ability to identify stent during fluoroscopy	Strut thickness, material (nitinol, steel)
Scaffolding	Ability of stent to completely cover and support the vessel	Material, stent design, strut thickness, metal surface, area, radial strength
Shortening	Decrease in stent length when fully deployed	Stent design
Trackability	Ease of movement over guide wire	Profile, shaft coating, stiffness, distal tapering

Table 16-2. Comparison of Direct Stenting to Conventional Stenting with Predilatation

Technique	Advantages	Disadvantages
Direct stent	• Less procedural time, radiation exposure, contrast volume, cost	• Not well-suited for complex anatomy
	• Theoretical benefit of less balloon injury and lower restenosis	• Rigid lesion maybe more difficult to treat after stent deployment
	• Theoretical benefit of less distal embolization in vein grafts	• Potential stent embolization if stent will not cross target lesion
Stent after predilation	• Ensures that lesion will "yield" prior to stent deployment	• More procedural time, radiation, exposure, contrast volume, cost
	• Well-suited for complex anatomy (calcification, angulation, ostial, or total occlusion)	

stent. This is caused by an exaggerated proliferative response by the vessel wall to the presence of the stent, which is a natural healing response to arterial injury. Growth within the stent is mostly due to smooth-muscle cells, which migrate from the vessel wall. This neointimal hyperplasia can occur to such a degree that the vessel can close completely, even though the original stenosis may have been only moderately severe. The incidence of in-stent restenosis after BMS placement differs between studies, but it is accepted to be 20%–30%,[9] and reaches its peak at about 6 months post stent implantation. Its incidence varies greatly between patient and lesion groups, being higher in diabetics, long lesions, and small vessels.

Treatment

Treatment of in-stent restenosis was traditionally redilatation with a balloon, but recurrent restenosis after balloon dilatation treatment ranges from 30%–57%.[10] The cutting balloon has been found to provide good initial patency, although long-term results have not been so positive. Debulking devices—laser and rotablator in particular—have been used with good initial results, but the long-term results have been mixed. Debulking has its own drawbacks in terms of costs and the level of experience that operators have to maintain.

Brachytherapy is the use of radiation within a vessel, and it has been shown to effectively reduce neointimal hyperplasia, working on the cellular level. Radiation cuts long-chain macromolecules such as DNA, leading to impairment of cellular function and cell death by preventing cell division and replication. The procedure requires additional, specialized personnel in attendance, as well as special storage facilities. Although initial and short-term results of brachytherapy to treat in-stent restenosis were positive, it was found that the use of DESs in restenosed lesions produced better results.

The most common treatment for in-stent restenosis is the placement of a DES within the old stent. If the original stent was a DES, a DES that carries a different drug could be beneficial.

Prevention

Many stents are coated with something that inhibits restenosis. These coatings are classified as being either passive or active. Passive coatings are substances that the vessel does not respond to with neointimal hyperplasia, and the active coatings release substances that disperse into the vessel wall and interfere with the neointimal hyperplasia process.

Passive-Coated Stents

Both stainless steel and cobalt chromium have been used in thousands of orthopedic operations with success and are generally considered to be treated as a neutral entity by the human body. The in-stent restenosis rates, however, show that this does not really apply to coronary vessels, so the possibility of coating the stents in another substance that is even less tissue reactive has been investigated widely. Ceramics, noble metals, titanium-nitride oxide, carbon, and silicon carbide are just a few of the coatings that are in use or are being investigated. The clinical process necessary to validate a stent coating is expensive and time consuming.

Active Coatings (Drug-Eluting Stents)

Active stent coatings are those that elute a medication into the vessel wall, known as DESs. DESs are made up of three elements: the stent, the drug, and (usually) a carrier. The carrier is often referred to as the polymer because they are made of large molecules with repeating structural units. It binds the drug to the stent, and then releases the drug over a prescribed time period. The drug and the polymer shouldn't trigger an inflammatory response by the body and they have to be able to undergo sterilization. Keeping in mind how miniscule these polymer layers are, their rapid development in such a short time is very impressive (see Figures 16-1 and 16-2).

The ideal drug must inhibit the restenotic process without interfering with stent endothelialization. In addition, it has to have a fairly wide therapeutic window, without unacceptable toxicity to the vessel's medial and adventitial layers. Many drugs, including immunosuppressants, anti-inflammatories, antineoplastics, antiproliferatives, antibiotics, and even sex hormones have made it to clinical trials, but few have made it onto the market.

Drug-Eluting Stents in the United States

Sirolimus (also known as Rapamycin) was first identified on Easter Island in the 1960s. It was initially classified as an antifungal antibiotic but was found to block the cell cycle of proliferating cells and was used extensively to treat transplant organ rejection. During the G1 phase of the cell cycle, the cell en-

Figure 16-1. Cypher Sirolimus-Eluting Coronary Stent. *Source:* Courtesy of Cordis Johnson & Johnson

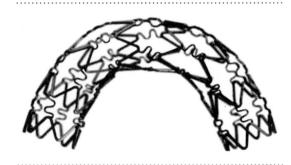

larges and begins to produce new proteins. Within this phase there is a checkpoint beyond which the cell commits to completing the cycle (see Figure 16-3). Sirolimus, a cytostatic agent, stops cellular proliferation just prior to this checkpoint, allowing viable cells to return to a resting state. This results in inhibition of exaggerated healing/cellular proliferation and "normal" reendothelialization of the stent. Sirolimus has a broad therapeutic window and is

Figure 16-2. Detail of Cypher Stent, showing polymer coats. *Source:* Courtesy of Cordis Johnson & Johnson

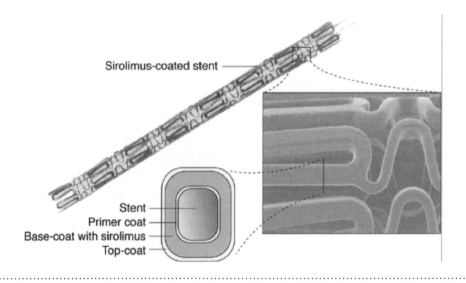

Figure 16-3. The Cell Cycle. Pharmacologic agents in drug eluting stents must inhibit the restenotic process without interfering with stent endothelialization or causing cellular death. *Source:* Courtesy of Cordis Johnson & Johnson.

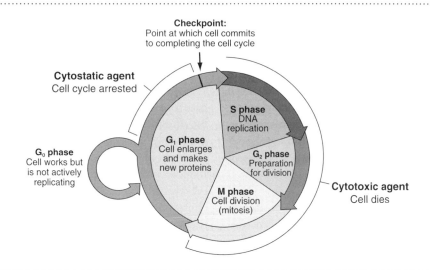

used in the Cypher Bx Velocity stent from Cordis, which was the first DES to be marketed.

Paclitaxel was originally derived from the Pacific yew tree. It is a potent antineoplastic drug that inhibits cell replication and has been used to treat certain tumors. For the treatment of atherosclerotic disease, paclitaxel has a narrower therapeutic window than sirolimus. At higher doses, paclitaxel affects the G1, G2, and M phases of the cell cycle, leading to cellular death (cytotoxicity). At low doses, however, it only affects the G1 and G2 phases, leading to cytostasis. Boston Scientific's Taxus Express 2 stents utilize paclitaxel as their active element.

Everolimus, used on the Endeavor stent from Medtronic, is a derivative of Rapamycin and works in the same way as sirolimus. It is used as an immunosuppressant to reduce the incidence of organ rejection following transplants.

Zotarolimus is also an immunosuppressant produced by semisynthesis from rapamycin. It is used on the Xience stent from Abbott Vascular and the Promus stent from Boston Scientific.

Drug-Eluting Stents Worldwide

The FDA has strict regulations on medical implantables commercially available in the United States, but scores of DES are available in other parts of the world. Sahajanand (Surat, India) produces relatively inexpensive sirolimus and paclitaxel-eluting stents that are popular in India. Widely implanted in Asia, the Excel from JWM (Weiheio, China) uses a biodegradeable polymer with sirolimus, and the Firebird from Microport (Shanghai, China) uses sirolimus on their Mustang BMS.

The BioMatrix from Biosensors International (Morges, Switzerland) and the Nobori from Terumo (Tokyo, Japan) stents elute an analog of Sirolimus, Biolimus A9. The drug is suspended in a biodegradeable polymer, which dissolves into carbon dioxide and water over 6 to 9 months. What's more, the drug/polymer matrix is only on the abluminal surface to the stent struts.

Another type of DES, the Yukon stent uses a stainless steel stent with a microporous "pearl" surface finish. When a lesion is to be treated, a stent of the appropriate size is placed in a stent-coating machine, which is about as big as a photocopy machine. The type and amount of drug that is coated onto the stent is programmed by the operator, and the drug-coating process takes place directly in the CCL. With this system, treatment can be modified to each patient's requirements, although it does take 15 minutes to coat each stent, and this can slow down the procedures significantly.

DES Complications

Although restenosis still occurs with DES, it is at much lower rates than with BMSs. DESs are not a cure-all; the same laws of anatomy and physics that apply to BMSs also apply to DESs. Thrombi still form within a DES if a dissection is not completely covered, and the same can occur if the stent struts are not well apposed into the vessel wall. DES usage is no excuse for sloppy angioplasty. In fact, it will tend to highlight it.

When predilating, it is prudent to choose a balloon shorter in length than the DES to be deployed to avoid trauma/dissection outside the stent. The DES should be long enough to cover proximal and distal ends of the lesion, reaching from healthy vessel to healthy vessel. Postdilatation balloons should be semi- or noncompliant and a little shorter in length than the stent. Inflating the balloon outside of the DES may result in trauma, increasing the chance of thrombosis. Using a noncompliant balloon with a diameter 0.25 to 0.5 mm larger than the deployed DES may be necessary to ensure complete apposition to the vessel wall.

Stent Thrombosis

Analysis of the early randomized studies comparing DES with BMS showed a substantial (three- to fourfold) reduction in restenosis at 12 months with DES, but no difference in the more important end points of myocardial infarction and death[11,12] nor was there any apparent increased risk of stent thrombosis with DES.

However, 4-year follow-up data released by the stent manufacturers indicates a higher rate of stent thrombosis with DES compared with BMS: 1.3% versus 0.8% for the Taxus and 1.2% versus 0.6% for the Cypher.[13] Nevertheless, this excess risk is not associated with an increased risk of MI or cardiovascular death. The increased risk of adverse consequences due to late-stent thrombosis is balanced by a reduction in risk due to reduced restenosis and a reduced need for repeat intervention.[13] Restenosis is a far less serious complication than stent thrombosis, but nevertheless, carries approximately a 10% risk of causing an MI.[14]

Patients in the early randomized studies had relatively simple lesions, whereas in the "real world," DESs are frequently used for more complex coronary lesions. It is estimated that "off-label" use accounts for at least 60% of DES usage in the United States.[15] The likelihood of stent thrombosis is higher in more complex coronary lesions and therefore any increased tendency toward stent thrombosis with DES will be accentuated.

Thrombus can appear in DESs even 3 years after implantation,[16] whereas they seldom form in BMSs after the first few months. A reason for this may be that DESs, while inhibiting neointimal hyperplasia, may also inhibit endolthelialization of the stent.[17] This phenomenon is known as delayed healing, and it may leave the stent struts exposed to the bloodstream indefinitely.

OTHER STENT TYPES

Bioabsorbable Stents

Neointimal hyperplasia is triggered by the presence of a foreign body (the stent) in the vessel. If the stent were to disappear over time, restenosis may be reduced. Using a magnesium alloy, Biotronik AG (Bulach, Switzerland) is developing an absorbable metal stent (AMS). The magnesium alloy apparently has an effect on smooth-muscle and endothelial cell proliferation. Company reports state that in animal models, the AMS gradually disappears within the vessel. Although the stent showed promising results in below-the-knee applications, it is being further modified for coronary applications.

Abbott Vascular is also developing a bioabsorbable stent that also elutes a drug. The stent itself is made of polylactic acid material, and it delivers everolimus. The stent is fully absorbed over time by the vascular tissue as part of the body's normal processes. If clinical results are positive, bioabsorbable drug-eluting stents could eventually offer an alternative to metallic drug-eluting stents.

Bioengineered Endothelialization

Orbus MT (Fort Lauderdale, Florida) has developed a process that allows for engineered endothelialization of the stent. The stent has a coating designed to attract endothelial progenitor cells (EPCs), which originate in bone marrow and circulate within the bloodstream. The EPCs are captured by the coating and immobilized on the surface of the stent struts, and endothelial encapsulation begins within 1 hour after implantation. This rapid endothelialization reduces the risk of acute thrombosis and may reduce the need for antiplatelet therapies. Orbus hopes that this process can be applied not only to endovascular stents, but to vascular grafts, cardiac valves, artificial organs, and a broad range of other surgical implants.

Side-Branch/Bifurcation Stents

The occlusion of vessel branches can be a problem with stent implantation. Side-branch lesions are coronary lesions that involve the ostium (at

least) of a branch of the main vessel. Bifurcation lesions (see Figure 16-4) are a version of the side-branch lesion, but where both branches are of a similar caliber. When a strut of the stent runs across the mouth of a side branch, it may close off that branch, and the patient will experience a small infarct. There is often a trade-off between the amount of myocardium at risk if the main vessel is not treated and amount of myocardium supplied by the side branch should it close. The struts of modern stents are relatively fine, and the spaces between them may allow for a guide wire to pass, depending on the vessel shape and operator experience. Balloon dilatation between the struts of a stent will produce a patent lumen into the side branch. The side branch can then

Figure 16-4. Bifurcation lesion.

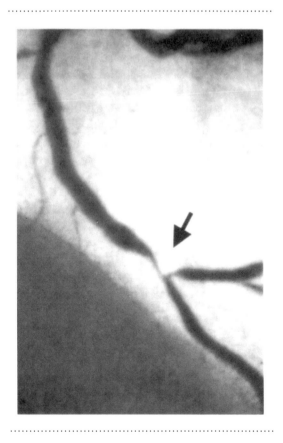

be stented, if necessary, and the procedure is usually completed by inflating balloons (kissing-balloons) in both vessels.

Several stent manufacturers have produced stents wherein the middle section has less struts, or a larger open cell, than the rest of the stent. When the middle section is correctly placed over the mouth of the side branch, occlusion of the side-branch is less likely and dilatation through the stent struts is easier.

Bifurcation stents are also under development by various manufacturers with a number of novel designs being tested. Some use several separate stents designed to fit into each other, and others use a "Y"-shaped stent mounted on two balloons, which are expanded simultaneously.

Experience, however, is showing that with careful PCI, accurate stent placement, and a planned approach to bifurcation lesions, the use of normal, single-vessel stents should be adequate. DESs placed in the main vessel may provide some benefits to inhibiting ostial disease of a side branch.

Covered Stents (Stent Grafts)

These stents have been covered with a material that becomes semi-impermeable when it is exposed to blood (see Figure 16-5), but porous enough to allow endothelialization. Similar, larger devices have been used in the aorta with success for many years. They have now been reduced to such a size that they can be placed in coronary arteries and coronary artery bypass vessels These covered stents are used to seal pseudoaneurysms and perforations in these vessels. Thankfully, it is rare that a vessel perforates during a procedure, but when it does, it can develop into an emergency situation very quickly. A selection of these stent grafts are good to have on hand, because the only alternatives for the patient are prolonged balloon inflations, surgery, or both.

Figure 16-5. Covered stent for coronary pseudoaneurysm.

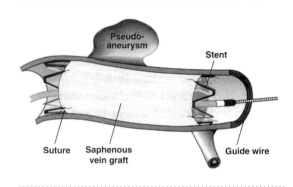

COST

The cost of conventional, bare-metal stents has decreased significantly over the years, especially following the introduction of DES. Healthy competition and wide usage has lowered them into a price range where the outlay for the stent is easily offset by reduced hospital stays. However, when the cost of the subsequent treatment for in-stent restenosis is added to the equation, the result becomes less clear. The introduction of DESs at a price about five times that of an uncoated stent has lead to a further adjustment to this equation. Hospital buyer groups, preferred vendor contracts, and increased competition has driven the prices down, however, the costs of DES are still a burden on the economics of the healthcare system.

SUMMARY

The world has experienced great technological advances in the area of coronary stents, and the developments will, no doubt, continue. Subacute thrombosis and in-stent restenosis are troublesome consequences of stenting, but good PCI technique and established antiplatelet regimes can bring in-stent thrombosis down to manageable levels. Coating stents with substances that discourage neointimal hyperplasia has decreased restenosis significantly. When the problems of neointimal hyperplasia have been solved comfortably, perhaps a fine coating of a platelet or thrombin inhibitor on the stent to discourage thrombus formation will be added. The medical world may yet see tailored DES, coated with special compounds targeted for saphenous vein grafts, diabetics, or specifically for in-stent restenosis. Now that coating stents is becoming accessible technology, medical professionals can expect advances and new trials to verify these advances. Hopefully the healthcare system can support these improvements.

It is important to remember that more than most bare-metal stents triggered no restenosis, and so placing a DES, in many cases, is a waste of hospital resources. Medical personnel have to learn how to safely identify patients who can receive just as much benefit from a less-expensive, bare-metal stent.

REFERENCES

1. Serruys PW, Strauss BH, Beatt KJ, et al. Angiographic follow-up after placement of a self-expanding coronary artery stent. *N Engl J Med* 1991;324:13–17.
2. Serruys PW, de Jaegere P, Kiemeneij F, et al., for the Benestent group. A comparison of balloon-expandable-stent implantation with balloon angioplasty in patients with coronary artery disease. *N Engl J Med* 1991;324:52–53.
3. Fischmann DL, Leon MB, Baim DS, et al., for the Stent Restenosis Study investigators. A randomized comparison of coronary-stent placement and balloon angioplasty in the treatment of coronary artery disease. *N Engl J Med* 1994;331:496–501.
4. Macaya C, Serruys PW, Ruygrok P, et al. Continued benefit of coronary stenting versus balloon angioplasty: one year follow-up of BENESTENT trial. *J Am Coll Cardiol* 1996;27:255–261.
5. Barragan P, Sainsous J, Silvestri M, et al. Ticlopidine and subcutaneous heparin as an alternative regimen following coronary stenting. *Cathet Cardiovasc Diag* 1994;32(2):133–8.
6. Gregorini L, Marco J, Fajadet J, et al. Ticlopidine and aspirin pretreatment reduces coagulation and platelet activation during coronary dilatation procedures. *J Am Coll Cardiol* 1997;29:69–77.
7. Goldberg SL, Colombo A, Nakamura S, et al. Benefit of intracoronary ultrasound in the deployment of Palmaz-Schatz stents. *J Am Coll Cardiol* 1994;24:996–1003.
8. Colombo A, Hall P, Nakamura S, et al. Intracoronary stenting without anticoagulation accomplished with intravascular ultrasound guidance. *Circulation* 1995;91:1676–1681.
9. Radke PW, Kaiser A, Frost C, Sigwart U. Outcome after treatment of coronary in-stent restenosis. *Eur Heart J* 2002;24:266–273.
10. Nairns CR, Holmes DR, Topol EJ. A call for provisional stenting: the balloon is back! *Circulation* 1998;97:1298–1305.
11. Hill RA, Dundar Y, Bakhai A, et al. Drug-eluting stents: an early systematic review to inform policy. *Eur Heart J* 2004;25:902–919.
12. Moreno R, Fernandez C, Hernandez R, et al. Drug-eluting stent thrombosis: results from a pooled analysis including 10 randomized studies. *J Am Coll Cardiol* 2005;45:954–959.
13. Boston Scientific. Resources for healthcare professionals. Data on the drug-eluting stent safety debate. Available at: www.taxus-stent.com. Accessed February 2007.
14. Chen MS, John JM, Chew DP, et al. Bare metal stent restenosis is not a benign clinical entity. *Am Heart J* 2006;151:1260–1264.
15. U.S. Food and Drug Administration. Update to FDA statement on coronary drug-eluting stents. January 4 2007. Available at: www.fda.gov/cdrh/news/010407.html. Accessed February 2007.

16. Daemen J, Wenaweser P, Tsuchida K, et al. Early and late coronary stent thrombosis of sirolimuseluting and paclitaxel-eluting stents in routine clinical practice: data from a large two-institutional cohort study *Lancet* 2007; 369(9575):1785–1786.

17. Joner M, Finn MAV, Farb A, et al. Pathology of drug-eluting stents in humans: delayed healing and late thrombotic risk. *J Am Coll Cardiol* 2006;48:193–202.

SUGGESTED READING

Drug Eluting Stent Center. Available at http://www.tctmd.com.

Kutryk MJB, Serruys PW. Stents: the menu. In: Topol EJ, ed. *Textbook of Interventional Cardiology*, 4th ed. Philadelphia: Saunders; 2003.

Smith S, Feldman TE. ACC/AHA/SCAI 2005 guideline update for percutaneous coronary intervention. *Circulation* 2006;113:156–175.

Chapter 17

DISTAL EMBOLIZATION PROTECTION

Brenda McCulloch, RN, MSN, CNS
Corissa Pederson, BS, RCIS

INTRODUCTION

Distal embolization of atheromatous debris has been increasingly recognized as a source of morbidity and mortality in patients undergoing percutaneous interventional procedures, especially when the intervention is being performed in a saphenous vein graft (SVG). SVG lesions are more friable, more diffuse, and progress more rapidly than atheroma in native vessels.[1] Old atherosclerotic disease of the native coronary arteries, carotid, and renal arterial systems can also create lesions that are highly friable. When these lesions are compressed with a balloon and/or a stent, the plaque can erupt, sending thromboembolic debris distally down the vessel. This can cause microvascular occlusion leading to acute myocardial infarction, evidenced by new Q waves on the 12-lead electrocardiogram and increases in CK-MB and troponin biomarkers.

Multiple randomized clinical trials have established the efficacy of distal protection devices in reducing major adverse cardiac events (MACE) during SVG intervention.[2–4] The 2005 ACC/AHA/SCAI practice guideline update for PCI encourages the use of distal embolic protection devices when technically feasible in patients undergoing SVG intervention.[4] Not all SVG lesions, however, lend themselves to the use of distal protection. Technical consideration for their use include the presence of an adequate "landing zone" distal to the lesion, inability to protect major side branches, a nontortuous graft, no aorto-ostial lesion, and a large enough vessel diameter.[3]

About 15% of SVGs occlude within 1 year of surgery, and up to 40% occlude 10 years after surgery. Because a reoperation carries higher risks of morbidity and mortality, PCI is an alternative that many patients and physicians choose for SVG disease. As SVGs age, they degenerate and they become ulcerative. The atheroma may be more widespread and more friable.[1] Plaques within the vessels are soft, being lipid-rich with little calcium content. There is a higher risk of major adverse

Figure 17-1. Friable sapheneous vein graft lesion.

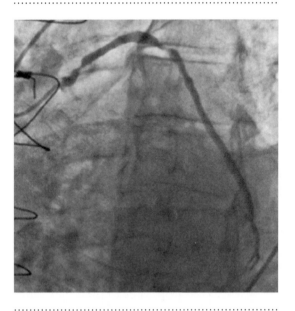

cardiac events in SVG interventions, predominately due to periprocedural MI from no-reflow and distal embolization.[2]

The use of distal protection devices in SVG PCI have been clinically shown to decrease the incidence of periprocedural complications, including no-reflow and embolization. Despite strong clinical data, distal protection devices are used less than half the time in SVG intervention.[5] They have been associated with an increase in procedural cost and risk. Their use may also slightly increase procedural time and patient exposure to radiation because of the time required to place the device.

Currently, there are three types of distal protection available: distal balloon occlusion devices, distal filter devices, and proximal occlusion/flow-reversal devices.

Distal Balloon Occlusion Devices

Balloon occlusion devices stop the flow of blood through the vessel during the ballooning and stenting. An aspiration catheter is then used to remove debris from the treated vessel, the balloon is deflated, and antegrade blood flow is restored. Examples of balloon occlusion devices include the GuardWire (from Medtronic, Inc., of Santa Rosa, California), the TriActive FX embolic protection system (from Kensey Nash of Exton, Pennsylvania), and the GuardDog (from Possis Medical Inc., of Minneapolis, Minnesota).

Balloon occlusion devices seal the vessel distal to the treatment segment to protect against embolic debris. Theoretically, there is no limit to the amount of debris that they can trap. A disadvantage of these systems is that as soon as the occlusion balloon has been inflated, there is no blood flow to the distal portion of the vessel until the balloon is deflated again. This can induce ischemia, chest pain, hypotension, and left ventricular dysfunction, depending on the length of the procedure and the presence of collateral vessels. This ischemia may not be well tolerated by the patient. Placement of the occlusion balloon can be difficult and it is not possible in every case. If the device is placed distal to a side branch, debris can flow freely down the side branch.

The following is a description of how to use a distal balloon occlusion device. Other balloon occlusion devices work in a similar fashion. See the specific device instructions for detailed directions.

1. A special guide wire with a distal balloon is placed into the vessel, beyond the lesion.
2. The distal occlusion balloon is then carefully inflated. CM should be injected through the guide catheter to verify that there is no flow beyond the occlusion balloon.
3. The balloon or stent is then loaded onto this guide wire, positioned within the lesion, and the vessel is treated.
4. The balloon is removed from the lesion.
5. An aspiration catheter is delivered over the occlusion balloon guide wire, and the thromboembolic debris is removed.*

---

*Some operators use mechanical thrombectomy devices in conjunction with the balloon occlusion device.

Figure 17-2. Distal balloon occlusion device. *Source*: Courtesy of Ev3.

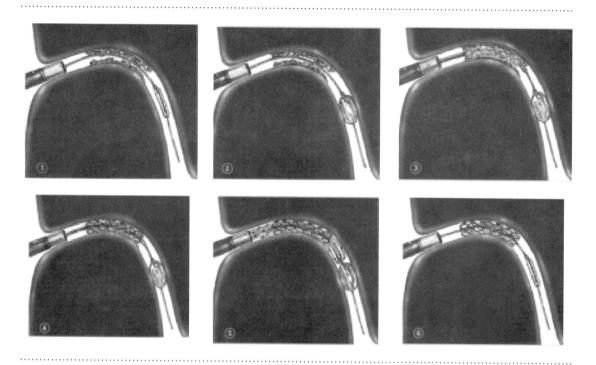

6. The aspiration catheter is removed and the occlusion balloon is deflated.

Distal Filter Devices

Filter devices incorporate a net or umbrella on the distal end of a guide wire (see Figure 17-3) that expands when it is distal to the lesion. The net allows blood to flow through it, while catching any emboli in the blood. The filter is designed to capture embolic material less than 100 μm. After the vessel has been treated, the filter is collapsed, and the embolic debris is retrieved from the vessel. Examples of filter devices include Filterwire EX and EZ (from Boston Scientific of Natick, Massachusetts), SpideRX (from ev3 of Minneapolis, Minnesota), AngioGuard (from Cordis Corporation of Miami, Florida), Accunet (from Abbott Vascular of Abbott Park, Illinois), and Emboshield and Emboshield Pro (from Mednova/Abbott of Galeway, Ireland).[6]

An advantage filter devices have over occlusion balloon devices is that they are easier to use and they allow antegrade blood flow continuously through the vessel during the procedure. Because blood continues to flow distally (unless the net becomes full of debris), vessel ischemia is not a concern as with balloon occlusion devices. The design of filter devices also permits contrast medium injections at any time.

There are some disadvantages to distal filter devices as well. Depending on the product and the shape of the vessel, the filter can have poor wall apposition. Unlike balloon devices that totally occlude the distal vasculature, some embolic debris may be permitted to flow around the filter. Filter devices may also cause some embolization while crossing the lesion.

Figure 17-3. FilterWire EZ. *Source:* Courtesy of Boston Scientific Inc.

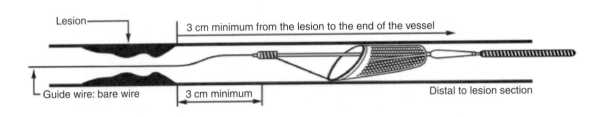

There is also a limit to the amount of debris that the filters can capture. After the limit has been reached, blood flow will become sluggish and eventually cease. When this occurs, the filter has to be removed.

The following is an example of how to use a distal embolic filter device. Most distal filter devices work in a similar fashion as described here. See the specific device instructions for detailed directions.

1. When unpacked, the filter is constrained inside a delivery sheath. This is passed through the catheter and into the vessel until the filter lies distal to the segment to be treated. Once in place, the delivery sheath is withdrawn a little, in order to make the filter open into position in a landing zone about 15 mm distal to the lesion.

2. The delivery catheter is retracted, and the self-expanding filter is exposed within the vessel. Depending on the device, the filter may be either concentrically or eccentrically attached to the guide wire shaft.

3. The balloon or stent delivery system (SDS) is loaded onto the filter guide wire, and the vessel is treated as in a normal PCI procedure. After the lesion has been treated, the balloon or SDS is removed.

4. The filter device delivery catheter is placed back on the wire and advanced into the vessel. As the delivery catheter is advanced to the filter device, the wire is retracted, partially collapsing the filter and trapping the thromboembolic debris. The filter is then withdrawn from the vessel, through the guide catheter, and a final angiogram is performed.

5. The basket can then be opened to flush with saline to clear the debris captured during the procedure.

Proximal Occlusion/Flow-Reversal Devices

Other embolic protection devices occlude the target vessel proximally before the device is placed. A sealing balloon is placed proximal to the lesion, temporarily suspending the blood flow. With the blood flow suspended, the intervention is performed on the diseased area. Once completed, fluid and debris are aspirated from the vessel prior to deflating the proximal occlusion balloon, eliminating distal embolization. Currently available proximal occlusion products include Proxis (from St. Jude Medical of Minneapolis, Minnesota) and the Gore Neuro Protection (from Gore & Associates of Flagstaff, Arizona).

Technically, this may be the most difficult method of providing embolic protection; however, this type of device may have an advantage in thrombotic lesions. Proximal embolic devices have an advantage over distal protection devices because they can evacuate embolic particles regardless of size. They can potentially capture an unlimited amount of vessel debris, because there is no distal filter basket that may become filled. Proximal occlusion devices protect the distal vasculature prior to crossing the lesion with a wire of device, which always poses potential embolic risk.

The following is an example of how to use a proximal occlusion embolic protection device. Other proximal occlusion/flow-reversal devices work in a similar method. See the specific device instructions for detailed directions.

1. A low pressure balloon is placed prior to the lesion, impeding antegrade flow of blood.
2. The balloon is inflated and a small amount of contrast is injected, enough to visualize the vascular bed.
3. Saline is infused and aspiration of debris is performed.
4. The lesion is crossed with a guide wire.
5. While maintaining suspended antegrade flow, the selected interventional device is advanced to the lesion. After the device is deployed, it is removed, and the vessel is aspirated to remove any suspended debris.

SUMMARY

Saphenous vein graft intervention is a relatively high-risk procedure. Whenever feasible, the use of distal protection devices should be employed to prevent no-reflow and myocardial infarction. Additional uses of distal protection devices include during acute myocardial infarction interventions, carotid and renal artery stenting, and femoropopliteal interventions.

REFERENCES

1. Akbar O, Bhindi R, McMahon C, et al. Distal protection in cardiovascular medicine: Current status. *Am Heart J* 2006;152:207–216.
2. Coolong A, Baim D, Kuntz R, et al. Saphenous vein grafting and major adverse cardiac events: A predictive model derived from a pooled analysis of 3958 patients. *Circulation* 2008;117:790–797.
3. Mehta SK, Frutkin AD, Milford-Beland S, et al. Utilization of distal embolic protection in saphenous vein graft interventions (An analysis of 19,546 patients in the American College of Cardiology—National Cardiovascular Data Registry). *Am J Cardiol* 2007;100:1114–1118.
4. Smith SC, Feldman TE, Hirshfeld JW, et al. ACC/AHA/SCAI 2005 guidelines for percutaneous coronary intervention—summary article: A report of the American College of Cardiology/American Heart Association task force on practice guidelines. *Circulation* 2005;113:156–175.
5. Rogers JH, Low RI. Embolic protection devices in aortocoronary saphenous vein graft intervention. *Endovascular Today* 2006,October:72–77.
6. Southard JA, Wong GB. Embolic protection device technology. *Endovascular Today* 2006, October:55–62.

Chapter 18

ATHERECTOMY AND THROMBECTOMY

Kenneth A. Gorski, RN, RCIS, RCSA, FSICP

Andreas Gruentzig originally theorized that the mechanism of PTCA (or "plain old balloon angioplasty"—POBA—as it is often referred to today) was to compress atherosclerotic plaque against the vessel wall, like "footprints in the snow."[1] However, intravascular ultrasound (IVUS) demonstrated that POBA increases a vessel lumen by stretching, shifting, splitting, and uncontrollably dissecting the plaque.[2] Atherosclerotic plaques are complex and often have mixed morphologies. Plaques may not only be soft, fluidic/fatty but also more solid, fibrotic/calcific. Atherosclerotic plaque is not removed by POBA, and acute reocclusion may occur through dissection and abrupt closure. Elastic recoil, vascular remodeling, and inflammatory responses lead to restenosis rates of 35%–50% with POBA, and lesions with a large plaque burden have higher rates of restenosis.[3] Even before IVUS studies showed the true mechanism of balloon angioplasty, some cardiologists began to theorize that removing the plaque from the vessel

wall would lead to increased vessel diameters, and subsequently better clinical results.

ATHERECTOMY DEVICES

Directional Coronary Atherectomy

Directional Coronary Atherectomy (DCA) was developed by Dr. John Simpson, who also designed the first over-the-wire balloon angioplasty catheter, as well as the Perclose and other devices commonly used in today's cath lab. The Simpson Atherocath for directional coronary atherectomy became the first FDA approved alternative to PTCA in 1991.

Directional coronary atherectomy (DCA) removes the plaque material by slicing it away from the vessel wall and collecting it for removal. Near the distal end of the catheter was a hollow metal housing with a window on one side. Inside the housing was a cup-shaped cutter attached to a drive cable. On the opposite side of this window, a small balloon was used to stabilize the DCA cutter during plaque removal. The distal end consisted of a flexible nose-cone with a chamber to collect the excised plaque material; the guide wire lumen accommodated a 0.014-inch guide wire (see Figure 18-1). The cutter drive shaft was activated by a hand-held, battery-operated motor drive unit (MDU), spinning the cutter at 2000 rpm. The cutter was slowly advanced, spinning at 2000 rpm, shaving away plaque, which was collected in the distal nose-cone chamber. After deflating the anchoring balloon, the catheter was rotated, repeating the process until a satisfactory angiographic result or the nose-cone was filled with excised plaque material.

Despite good acute angiographic results, DCA had a greater number of peri- and postprocedural complications (particularly non-Q wave MI), increased costs, and longer procedural length.[4]

DCA taught medical professionals much about the pathology of coronary artery disease. Pathologic examination of the excised plaque has shown unique differences in lesion subsets. It has been found that De Novo lesions are fatty, fibrotic, calcific, foam cells, thrombus, and necrotic cells; restenotic lesions are often mural thrombus and tissue hyperplasia, possibly related to an inflammatory response.[5]

The DCA device's main downfall was that it excised plaque blindly, running the risk of cutting too deeply, beyond the vessel media into the adventitia. Attempts were made by Guidant (now Abbott Vascular) and IVUS manufacturers to design a combination IVUS/DCA platform. DCA began to fall from favor as companies began to concentrate research and development on furthering stent technologies. The Guidant DCA products are no longer marketed. The concept of directional atherectomy has been revived with the peripheral SilverHawk device (ev3/Foxhollow, Plymouth, MN).

Rotational Atherectomy

Rotational atherectomy involves the use of a high-speed rotational device designed to pulverize plaque into minute particles. These particles, smaller than red blood cells, are washed distally through the coronary arteries, then removed from the body by way of the reticuloendothelial system (see Figure 18-2). The high-speed energy produced from the device selectively ablates atheromatous material in the walls of the diseased artery, while normal elastic vessel wall is pushed safely away from the device. Atheromatous tissue is more rigid than normal tissue and therefore offers resistance to the device, whereas the normal, nondiseased compliant vessel wall does not.[6,7]

Figure 18-1. AtheroCath and motor drive unit.

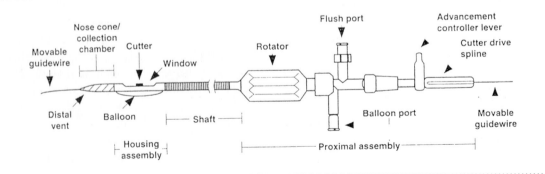

Figure 18-2. The minute particles produced by Rotablator therapy. *Source:* Courtesy of Boston Scientific Inc.

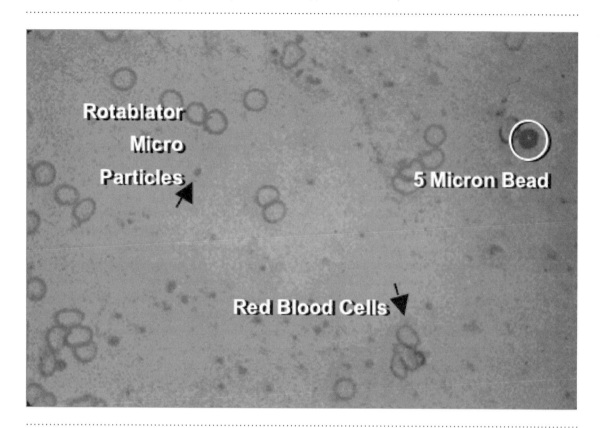

The Rotablator (from Boston Scientific Corporation of Natick, Massachusetts) was developed to tackle specific lesion subsets: long, rock-hard, diffusely diseased calcified lesions associated with a high rate of dissection and ostial-aortic lesions, which are often fibrotic, that POBA failed to effectively treat. Some physicians believe that the selective tissue ablation effect of the Rotablator is the best choice for calcified coronary lesions.[8]

Components

The Rotablator Rotational Angioplasty System is controlled by the Rotablator Advancer containing a fiberoptic tachometer cable, irrigation port, and a nitrogen gas delivery hose (see Figure 18-3).

Figure 18-3. Rotablator diamond coated burr. *Source:* Courtesy of Boston Scientific Inc.

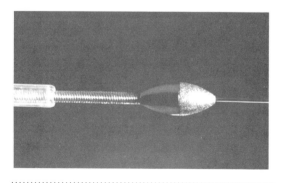

The system is powered by pressurized nitrogen and the rotational speed of the catheter and treatment time is monitored and digitally displayed on the drive console. The Rotablator RotaLink catheter consists of an oval-shaped, nickel-plated brass burr coated with diamond dust on the distal tip of the drive shaft. The drive shaft is covered with a 4F Teflon sheath that is continuously lubricated by a pressurized flush solution. The rotational speed of the burr is controlled by a foot pedal, attached to the console and activated by the physician or scrub assistant. The fiberoptic tachometer cable and nitrogen gas delivery hose are connected to the front of the console; the tachometer cable produces a digital readout of the speed, displayed on the front of the console revolutions per minute (rpm).

The nitrogen tank is hooked up to the back side of the console. The amount of gas available in the tank should always be checked prior to the procedure; 500 psi is the lowest acceptable range to begin a procedure. If the tank is at or slightly above 500 psi, the circulating nurse or technologist should pay special attention to make sure the tank does not run out.

Rotablator atherectomy requires the use of specially developed guide wires. The guide wire shafts are uncoated stainless steel. Any coating typically used on conventional PCI wires could be stripped off by the high-speed rotating burr, resulting in embolic debris. The shaft of the Rotablator guide wires is 0.009 inch; the tip diameter is .014 inch on the current Rota-Floppy wire family. Each of the Rota-Floppy guide wires comes packaged with a "guide wire clip" intended to be used as a torque device. The wire clip also acts as a secondary brake during burr exchanges.

Like other atherectomy devices, highly supportive guide catheters are essential to the success of the procedure. Required guide catheter sizes are dependent upon the size of the burr selected (see Table 18-1).

Depending on the catheter manufacturer, a 2.0 mm burr may safely fit through a 7F-guiding

Table 18-1. Appropriate Guide Catheter for Burr Selected

Burr Selected	Appropriate Catheter Guide Size
1.25–1.5 mm burrs	6F
1.75 mm burr	7F
2.0 mm burr	8F
2.25–2.38 mm burrs	9F
2.5 mm burr	10F

catheter and a 2.25 an 8F. An 0.04-inch clearance between the burr size and the inner lumen of the guiding catheter is necessary to ensure that the rotating burr does not shave debris off the guiding catheter's inner lumen. Currently, 10F-guide catheters are not readily available and 9F are also uncommon. This has meant that the larger burr sizes (2.38 and 2.5) are not commonly used.

Some cardiologists prefer to use a conservative, two-burr approach beginning with a device slightly larger than the minimal existing lumen diameter. Beginning the procedure with too large a burr may run the risk of large drops in rotational speed, increasing the odds of creating larger microparticulate debris, no-reflow, higher increases in cardiac enzymes, and MI. The second burr should have a burr/artery size ratio of 0.75–0.08. With the two-burr approach, it is wise to begin with a guiding catheter sized for the larger burr.

Another rotational atherectomy device, the Diamondback 360° Orbital Atherectomy System (from Cardiovascular Systems, Inc., of St. Paul, Minnesota), is currently approved for peripheral vascular disease. Similar in design and function of the Rotablator, the Diamondback differs by having an eccentric diamond-coated crown on the end of the drive shaft. As the eccentric crown rotates within the vessel. the debulking area grows larger as the speed of rotation is increased.

A pressure bag infuses the flush solution through the Rotablator device, allowing for lubrication to prevent the burr from overheating during its operation. Coronary vasospasm as a result of the high-speed burr spinning inside the artery has led to the development of specific "flush recipes" that may be added to the pressure bag. Medications included in such recipes are nitroglycerin, verapamil, and heparin. Some physicians believe that adding these medications may aid in the reduction of coronary vasospasm and reduce the incidence of no-reflow during the procedure.[9] Various doses can be used and may vary by institution or physician. One institution uses the following:

500 ml normal saline
1000 units heparin
4 mg nitroglycerin
5 mg verapamil
10 ml Rotaglide lubricant

The Rotaglide lubricant is a proprietary lipid-based emulsion added to reduce friction between the drive shaft and guide wire. The Rotaglide lubricant should not be used if a patient has an allergy to egg products or olive oil.

Procedure

After placement of the Rotablator wire distal to the stenosis, the Rotablator catheter speed is tested and adjusted outside of the body. Using the control knob on the front of the console, the circulating nurse or tech will adjust the burr speed until the digital display reads 160,000 to 200,000 rpm. Smaller burrs will be set at higher speeds. The burr is then advanced into the artery just proximal to the lesion. While infusing the pressurized flush solution, the foot pedal is activated, and the burr is advanced slowly with the control knob on the Advancer. Careful attention must be given to the burr speed while advancing through the lesion. A drop in speed of more

than 5000 rpm could potentially result in larger debris, increasing the risk of embolization and thrombus formation.

For catheter exchange, the burr is removed from the body, leaving the guide wire in place. The advancer knob on the housing of the unit is moved forward completely and locked into place. The catheter connector latch is depressed, and the burr detached from the advancer, exposing the driveshaft connection. The brown hypotube connection of the RotaLink catheter is slid forward gently, and the connections are carefully pulled apart. To attach the next catheter, the connections of the Rotablator Advancer and RotaLink catheter should be aligned, and the brown hypotube slid back and carefully pulled to assure a tight connection. At this point, the RotaLink catheter is ready to be connected to the Rotablator Advancer.[10]

IVUS has shown that rotational atherectomy leaves behind a smooth, cylindrical lumen (see Figure 18-4). Because the rotating burr selectively ablates harder plaque material, the instance of intimal dissection is significantly lower than balloon angioplasty in these lesions. Because the burr sizes are relatively small compared to the actual vessel size, adjunctive balloon and/or stent implantation generally occurs.

Complications

Intracoronary nitroglycerin injections of 100 μg to 200 μg are frequently given after each ablation run to reduce the risk of coronary vasospasm. Verapamil, adenosine, and diltiazem may also be injected, and they should be readily available. The monitoring nurse/technician should pay close attention to the ECG rhythm and blood pressure during each ablation run. Hypotension, bradycardia, asystole, and ventricular tachycardia are more commonly seen during rotational atherectomy than POBA. A temporary pacer, wire, and cable should be readily available. In high-risk patients, the physician may elect to

Figure 18-4. IVUS images of Rotablator therapy. *Source:* Courtesy of Boston Scientific Inc.

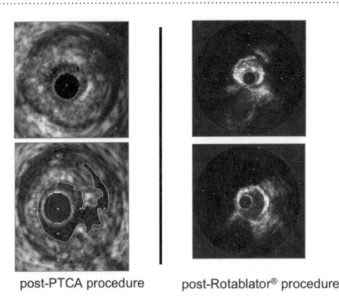

post-PTCA procedure   post-Rotablator® procedure

place a temporary pacer prior to initiating therapy, especially those patients undergoing a Rotablator procedure involving the right coronary artery.

Rotational atherectomy carries a higher risk of procedural-induced non-Q wave MI than balloon angioplasty. It is believed that the higher risk is due to the debulking of the plaque, producing small embolic particles. Most particles are smaller than red blood cells and pass harmlessly through the circulation. It has been reported that a CK-MB of greater than two times normal is seen in 6%–8% of Rotablator patients. Adjunctive pharmacotherapy with IIb/IIIa agents (ReoPro, Integrillin, Aggrastat) are associated with a 50% reduction in Creatinine Phospho-Kinase (CPK) elevation and decreased platelet aggregation.[11]

Perforation is another, but rare, complication associated with rotational atherectomy. Perforations are more likely to occur in lesions located on bends, near bifurcations, or in very tortuous vessel segments. Coronary artery perforation, depending upon its extent and location, may be successfully treated with long balloon inflations, or a Jograft Coronary Stent Graft (from Abbott Vascular). Heparin must be reversed with protamine sulfate. If a IIb/IIIa agent is infusing, it must also be discontinued. Some patients will require an emergency pericardiocentesis or surgery.

Rotational atherectomy is technically challenging. With the advent of the cutting balloon and the use of direct stenting, use of the Rotablator has dropped significantly. Studies have shown high acute success rates with rotational atherectomy, particularly in ostial, and heavily calcified lesions, although use in long (> 25 mm) lesions has been associated with increased postprocedural wall-motion abnormalities, restenosis, and mortality. Rotational atherectomy should be avoided in patients with severe LV dysfunction and when thrombus is suspected. In saphenous vein bypass grafts, the degenerating, friable vessel wall increases the risk of embolization and infarction.

Laser

Albert Einstein first proposed the principle of stimulated emission of radiation in 1917. *L*ight *a*mplification by *s*timulated *e*mission of *r*adiation, more commonly referred to as "laser", is used in a number of daily applications such as checkout scanners, presentation pointers, and CD players, as well as a multitude of medical applications.

The first laser systems used in interventional cardiology were continuous wave laser systems, but these produce heat and cause thermal damage. Some systems, such as the Spears Laser Balloon Angioplasty system, used laser energy in the near-infrared spectrum to heat a balloon to have a tissue-welding effect. Although the acute procedural outcomes were good, the resultant thermal damage to the adjacent tissue produced scarring and a high percentage of restenosis compared to balloon angioplasty alone. Because of the disappointing long-term results with hot laser, clinical trials with these and other thermal devices (microwave, radiofrequency) were quickly abandoned.

One laser system did receive FDA approval for coronary revascularization: the Excimer Laser System from Spectranetics. Excimer is an acronym for "excited dimer." The system uses high-voltage electricity to ionize xenon and chloride gases (XeCl) and emits energy in the ultraviolet spectrum at a wavelength of 308 nm. The laser beam is transmitted through a catheter by a series of bundled fiber optics. The laser energy is pulsed in brief bursts at controlled energy levels, measured in millijoules/mm2 (known as the Fluence), and frequency, measured in Hz.

Excimer laser catheters are available in sizes of 1.4 mm, 1.7 mm, and 2.0 mm. Although the catheters are more flexible than the DCA and Rotablator devices, extra support guide catheters (i.e., Amplatz, XB) and wires are recommended.

The catheters are energized by the Spectranetics CVX-300 laser system.

Procedure

Operators advance the catheter until it comes in contact with the lesion and flush the manifold and guide catheter with 20 to 30 ml of saline to clear the lasing field of blood and contrast. Without injecting contrast, the operator begins lasing while continuously injecting saline at a rate of 2 to 3 ml/second. This process is repeated for each successive laser ablation. The catheter should be advanced slowly, at a rate of 1 mm/second.

Initial settings should be at Fluence of 40 mj/mm2 and a frequency of 20 Hz; if the lesion does not yield, maximum settings are 60 mm/mmj2 and 30 Hz. A programmed lasing train of 5 seconds, followed by a pause of 5 seconds off between lasing decreases adverse acoustic shock effects generated in the artery. The Point 9 X-80 high-energy ELCA catheter allows for higher maximum settings of 80 mj/mm2 Fluence, 80 Hz pulse rate, and lasing trains of 10 seconds on, 5 seconds off.

Similar to DCA and the Rotablator, enthusiasm for laser intervention has fallen off significantly. Long-term results have shown no major benefit over POBA, although the lesions typically treated with ELCA are difficult. ELCA may still hold promise for ostial and long lesions, as well as subtotal to total obstructions. Excimer Laser has also found a niche in the treatment of lower extremity atherosclerosis. However, leasing or capital equipment costs for the laser generator, coupled with the catheter costs, are prohibitive for many institutions.

THROMBECTOMY DEVICES

Acute MIs, in both native vessels and bypass grafts, involve thrombus formation. Fibro-calcific plaques may ulcerate and rupture, activating the coagulation pathway and thrombus formation. Unstable angina in patients post-CABG, particularly in older degenerating saphenous vein grafts, often present to the cath lab with fuzzy, hazy appearing angiograms. These "hairball" clogs have always been a challenge for the interventional cardiologist to treat.

Although generally easy to traverse with a guide wire, balloon dilatation and/or stenting will only temporarily shift the clot material within the lumen and commonly sends a shower of embolic debris distally. Thrombotic lesions are considered high risk, associated with increased embolization, no-reflow, and acute occlusion.

A number of different approaches to treating clots in the coronary vasculature have been developed with varying degrees of success. If the patient is stable, a cardiologist may opt to pretreat the patient for a period of 2 to 14 days with heparin and aspirin in an attempt to reduce the clot burden. Patients may also receive a IIb/IIIa agent or prolonged intracoronary infusions of Urokinase or tPA.

AngioJet

The AngioJet (from Possis Medical, Inc./Medrad of Minneapolis, Minnesota) is a mechanical, rheolytic thrombectomy catheter. The catheter is combined with a pump and drive system to create a low-pressure zone within the artery, effectively removing thrombus.

Components

The AngioJet system has three primary components: the drive unit, the disposable pump set, and the AngioJet catheter. The drive unit is the nonsterile component; a mobile cart that controls the catheter and pump set, monitors the system performance and operating pressure, and regulates infused saline volume and fluid outflow to assure patient safety. The system is activated by a foot pedal.

The AngioJet pump set is sterile and consists of a bulbous, piston-driven pump, a saline spike, inflow and outflow tubing, a double-lumen paratube, and a collection bag. The pump pressurizes heparinized saline through the supply lumen of the paratube, which has a high-pressure, elliptical-shaped hub that attaches to the AngioJet catheter. The outflow lumen of the paratube attaches to the luer lock connector of the catheter.

As the drive unit and pump set delivers pressurized saline through one lumen to the distal tip of the AngioJet catheter, it is directed backward through a second lumen at approximately 390 miles per hour, creating a low-pressure vacuum zone of about −600 mmHg (see Figure 18-5). Thrombus is drawn into the catheter through the Cross-stream windows, where it is entrapped, fragmented, and removed from the body and deposited in the pump set collection bag. A hemostasis valve on the proximal end of the catheter allows the thrombus evacuation lumen to be sealed around the guide wire.

The coronary AngioJet catheters, the rapid exchange R-XMI, and the over-the-wire XMI and XVG catheters are compatible with 0.014-inch interventional guide wires. As with other atherectomy/thrombectomy coronary devices, use of extra-support guide catheters and guide wires is recommended. The AngioJet XMI catheters have profiles of 4F, compatible with most 6F-guide catheters, and are recommended for vessels 2 mm to 5 mm in diameter.

The AngioJet XVG catheter has a profile of 5F, is compatible with most 7F-guide catheters, and is recommended for vessels 3 mm to 8 mm in diameter. A larger, peripheral catheter, the Xpeedior + 120, is also available; this catheter is compatible with 0.035-inch guide wires, has a shorter 120 cm shaft, and is recommended for vessels 4 mm to 12 mm in diameter.

Although the AngioJet device aspirates clot, it does not excise plaque or prevent distal embolization of thrombus. Embolization may be

Figure 18-5. Angiojet mechanism of action. *Source:* Courtesy of Possis.

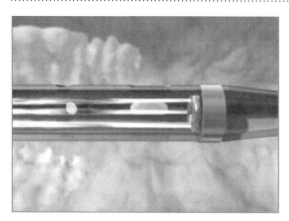
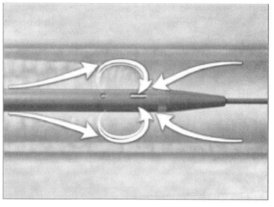

Saline jets travel backwards at 390 mph
to create a low pressure zone.

Cross-Stream windows optimize the drawing
action for more effective thrombus removal.

overcome by using the device in combination with a distal-embolic protection device.

Other Mechanical Devices

The X-Sizer, from ev3 (Plymouth, MN), is a combination atherectomy/thrombectomy device with a slow-rotating (2100 rpm), helical cutter and vacuum catheter powered by a 9-volt battery that simultaneously removes plaque and thrombus (see Figure 18-6).

The Rinspirator, also from ev3, has a hand-held mechanism controlling two syringes that the physician manually squeezes to simultaneously "rinse" the vessel walls with saline and aspirate soft thrombotic debris. The physician may choose to use a pharmaceutical agent (i.e., a fibrinolytic or glycoprotein IIb/IIIa inhibitor) instead of saline for the rinse solution.

The Jetstream Pathway PV (from Pathway Medical of Kirkland, Washington) is also a combination atherectomy/thrombectomy device approved for peripheral applications. The catheter is designed with a unique, expandable cutting tip that not only debulks, but has

multiple distal ports located at the catheter tip, designed for independent infusion and aspiration of tissue and thrombus. The blades fan open to expand from 2.1 mm to 3.0 mm in diameter.

Many other mechanical thrombectomy devices are available for use in the peripheral vasculature. However, these products are currently either not FDA approved or not suitable for use within the coronary arteries.

Manual Aspiration Devices

There are a number of catheters currently on the market for manual, aspiration of soft coronary and peripheral thrombus, including:

- Export, Medtronic Cardiovascular
- Pronto, Vascular Solutions
- Diver, ev3/Invatec
- Fetch, Possis
- QuickCat, Kensey-Nash

These products are simple catheters with a large inner lumen and a vacuum syringe for soft clot

Figure 18-6. Rotating Archimedes screw draws the thrombotic material into the catheter and shears it off, while the Vacuum Lumen aspirates debris. *Source:* Courtesy of Ev3.

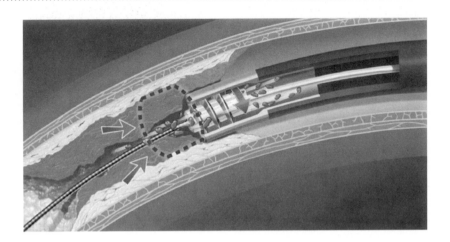

and emboli removal. Designs vary slightly; the catheters are rapid exchange, with either a distal, open end (Export, Diver, Fetch, and QuickCat) or an eccentric, large sidehole proximal to a tapered distal tip (Pronto).

POSTPROCEDURAL CARE

Care following atherectomy procedures differs little from that of post-PTCA care. The patient should be admitted to a cardiac telemetry step-down unit or intensive care unit per institution policy. A 12-lead ECG is performed after the procedure and the following morning to rule out silent ischemic events. Cardiac enzymes should also be ordered postprocedure to rule out a non-Q wave MI.

Frequent monitoring of vital signs, assessment of pedal pulses, and groin-site checks are a must for optimal patient care following any coronary intervention. Groin-site observation is especially important where larger sheaths (8F to 10F) have been used as may be necessary with some atherectomy procedures. Patient comfort must also be

considered. Many patients may receive an arterial closure device of some kind. However, if the access sheath remains in place after the procedure, current patient care protocols require patients to lie on their backs with the head of the bed no greater than 30° for several hours until the ACT drops below 175 secs or point of care aPTT is below 45. Oral pain medication such as acetaminophen with codeine or oxycodone may help relieve the back discomfort frequently experienced while on bed rest.

SUMMARY

In nearly all instances, atherectomy devices have failed to prove themselves superior to POBA or direct stenting, despite good acute results from the centers that use these devices frequently. This may be due to the selection of appropriate lesions for the procedure, as well as operator experience. Removal of existing thrombus prior to treating an underlying lesion may seem logical, but results from trials with thrombectomy devices have had mixed results as well.

These devices certainly have a place in the treatment of specific lesion subsets not initially treatable with balloon or direct stenting. It is worth noting, however, that adjunctive angioplasty and stenting is necessary in the vast majority of these cases to achieve acceptable clinical results.

REFERENCES

1. Gruentzig A. Transluminal dilatation of coronary artery stenosis. *Lancet* 1978;1:263.
2. Portkin BN, Keren G, Mintz GS, et al. Arterial responses to balloon coronary angioplasty: an intravascular ultrasound study. *J Am Coll Cardiol* 1992;20:942.
3. Ellis S, DeCesare N, Pinkerton C, Whitlow P. Relation of stenosis morphology and clinical presentation to the procedural results of directional coronary atherectomy. *Circulation* 1991;84:644–653.
4. Topol EJ, Leya F, Pinkerton CA, et al. A comparison of directional atherectomy with coronary angioplasty in patients with coronary artery disease (CAVEAT). *N Engl J Med* 1993;329:221–227.
5. Rosenchein U, Ellis S, Haudenschild C, et al. Comparison of histopathologic coronary lesions obtained from directional atherectomy in stable angina versus acute coronary syndromes. *Am J Cardiol* 1995;75:1015.
6. Holcomb-Simmons S. Atherectomy: A Different Way To Unblock Coronary Arteries. *Nursing* 1993;93(23):44–47.
7. O'Neill W, Niazi K. Rotational coronary atherectomy using the Rotablator atherectomy device. In: Holmes D, Garratt K, eds. *Atherectomy*. Cambridge, MA: Blackwell Scientific; 1992:43–59.
8. Safian R, Baim D, Kuntz R. Coronary atherectomy. In: Baum D, Grossman W, eds. *Cardiac Catheterization, Angiography, and Intervention*, 5th ed. Baltimore: Williams & Wilkins; 1996:581–611.
9. Coletti RH, Haik BJ, Wiederman JG, et al. Marked reduction in slow-reflow after rotational atherectomy through the use of a novel flushing solution. *TCT* 1996; Washington DC.
10. Boston Scientific Corporation Northwest Technology, Inc. *Rotablator Rotational Angioplasty System with Rotalink Exchangeable Catheter: Instructions for Use*. Redmond, WA: Boston Scientific; 1996.
11. Reisman M., Safian RD, Rotablator atherectomy. In: Safian R, Freed M, eds. *The Manual of Interventional Cardiology*, 3rd ed. Birmingham, MI: Physicians' Press; 2001:617–639.

SUGGESTED READING

Freed M, Safian RD. *The Device Guide*. Birmingham, MI: Physicians' Press; 1996.

Safian RD, Baim D, Kuntz RE. Coronary atherectomy. In: Baim D, Grossman W. *Cardiac Catheterization, Angiography, and Intervention*, 5th ed. Baltimore: Williams & Wilkins; 1996.

Chapter 19

CARDIAC DEFECT CLOSURE DEVICES

Sandy Watson RN, BN, NFESC

Small openings are sometimes present in the human cardiovascular system that can cause problems. Most of these, such as a patent foramen ovale (PFO), are birth defects, whereas ventricle septal defects can also be a consequence of a myocardial infarct. When these small passages are hemodynamically significant and cause symptoms, they usually have to be closed. Traditionally, only surgery (with all its associated drawbacks) was able to rectify this, but the development of miniaturized devices has meant that most can now be closed with catheter-based technology.

PATENT FORAMEN OVALE

Fetal blood flow relies on the patency of several openings in the heart and the great vessels that close soon after birth (in most cases). While in the womb, a neonate's blood is oxygenated in the placenta, and most of the blood bypasses the undeveloped pulmonary system by flowing directly from the right atrium into the left atrium

through an opening. It then moves into the head and upper extremities. The wall between the atria (the atrial septum) is made up of two structures: the fibrous septum premium coming from the direction of the ventricles and the muscular septum secundum coming from the direction of the aorta. These structures overlap, and this forms an effective one-way valve called the fossa ovalis or foramen ovale.

After birth, the pulmonary circulation develops very quickly, and the pressures in the left atrium become higher than those in the right. This pushes the thinner septum primium onto the septum secundum, closing the valve. In most people, the flaps fuse together, and the septum is formed. In about a quarter of the population,[1] the flaps don't fuse, and this is known as a PFO. Left atrial pressures are usually higher than the right atrium's, so the valve usually remains closed, and it has no clinical consequences. In some cases, however, the PFO remains open, and shunting continues between the two atria.

In some cases, there is also excess atrial tissue present, and this allows increased movement of the septum secundum. This is known as an atrial septal aneurysm (ASA) and is present in 2%–4% of the population.

About 80% of strokes are of ischemic origin, and about one-third of these are cryptogenic,[2] which means that the source of embolism causing the stroke cannot be detected. It has been theorized that a PFO could permit emboli to bypass the pulmonary system (where they would be filtered out) and enter the arterial circulation and the brain, causing a stroke. This hypothesis is supported by data which shows that a PFO is present in 46% of patients younger than 55 years old who have had a cryptogenic stroke, compared to 11% in matched controls.[3] Although still controversial, some studies have suggested that patients with PFO (especially younger patients with an ASA) have a higher risk of stroke than those with a patent septum.

Traditionally, treatment for cryptogenic stroke (with or without the presence of PFO) has been medical therapy with aspirin and oral anticoagulation, but this was shown to have a 1-year recurrence rate of up to 12%.[4] Developments in materials and production techniques have brought several devices onto the market that are capable of closing PFOs with a large-bore venous catheter.

Although the connections between PFO and cryptogenic stroke are theoretical and statistical, several international trials that randomize medical therapy against PFO closure are currently underway. If they show a significant reduction in subsequent stroke rates, percutaneous PFO closure will become a common procedure in most cath labs.

Percutaneous PFO closure has proved to be a safe and reliable procedure, providing complete PFO closure at 1 year in about 94% of cases.[5] The encouraging results over the last few years have led to the widening of indications for PFO closure. Studies performed on patients with mi-graine with aura, and on scuba divers indicate that they may also benefit from transluminal PFO closure.

Devices

During the 1990s, several PFO occluders were developed, including the Angel Wings and the Clamshell devices, but their technology was often relatively crude (some involved sewing). There are now several well-established PFO closure devices on the market: the PFO Star, Cardioseal/Starflex, BioSTAR, and the Amplatzer PFO occluder.

The Amplatzer PFO occluder (from AGA Medical of Plymouth, MN) is constructed from a Nitinol wire mesh that is woven into two discs connected at their centers, much like a squashed hourglass (see Figure 19-1). Nitinol has physical memory; it can be pulled into a linear shape to pass through a catheter, and it will always spring back to its manufactured state when released. The disc that sits in the right atrium is larger than that which sits in the left atrium, and it is available in sizes 18/18 mm, 25/18 mm, and 35/25 mm. The Amplatzer device is robust, and although it contains a great deal of metal, it has

Figure 19-1. Amplatzer PFO occluder. *Source:* Courtesy of AGA Medical Corporation.

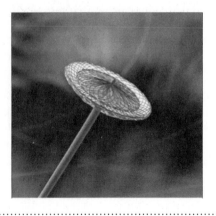

been shown that this does not encourage thrombus formation.[6]

The CardioSEAL/STARFlex (from NMT Medical of Boston, Massachusetts) devices (see Figure 19-2) are third and fourth generations of the clamshell-device technology. Each implant is comprised of two knitted surgical fabric "umbrellas": one in the left atrium and the other in the right atrium, which sandwich the PFO. The STARFlex differs from the CardioSEAL by the addition of a self-centering microspring that alternates between umbrella-arm tips to further improve conformability. Both are available in a variety of sizes ranging from 17 to 40 mm.

NMT also has the BIOStar septal repair, the only bioabsorbable septal repair implant. It has a bioabsorbable material on the STARFLex framework. The scaffold material is a tissue-engineered, highly purified acellular collagen matrix derived from the submucosal layer of the porcine small intestine. Also, an ionically bound heparin coating is added to decrease acute thrombogenicity while not adversely affecting the long-term healing response.

The intrasept PFO device (from Cardia, Inc. of Burnsville, Minnesota) is the fourth generation of the Cardia occluder (originally the PFO Star).

Six stranded/woven nitinol arms are connected to a dual-articulating center post (see Figure 19-3). This articulating center post allows the device to conform to any septum as well as provide a very flat, low profile within the atria.

The size of the device is an important consideration. Although it seems logical to place as large a device as possible, if a device is too large, it can rub against the walls of the atria, especially in the direction of the aorta. Over time, this can cause erosion of the atrial wall, so an 18 mm closure device is usually adequate.

Procedure

The patient is brought into the cath lab and prepared as if undergoing a coronary procedure. Depending on the institution's policy, a dose of IV antibiotics may be administered before the procedure begins. A venous sheath is placed, and a bolus of 5000 IU heparin is administered. A diagnostic multipurpose catheter is then passed through the PFO into the left atrium. Oximetry will verify its position if there is any doubt from the X-ray images. Using a standard exchange wire, the catheter is replaced with the transseptal sheath provided with the device. These differ a bit between

Figure 19-2. CardioSEAL/STARflex PFO occluder. *Source:* Courtesy of NMT Medical, Inc.

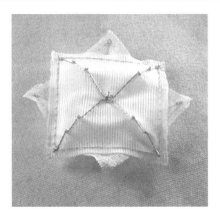

Figure 19-3. The PFO Star device. *Source:* Courtesy of Cardia, Inc.

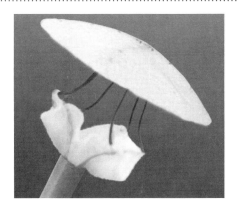

manufacturers, but they are basically tubes that take the device through the PFO. These sheaths are 8 to 12F; care must be taken to prevent air being taken into the sheath during the procedure.

The exchange wire is removed, and the device is fed into the sheath. The device is loaded into the sheath on the table next to the patient, rather than on his or her leg, to reduce the chance of air entering the system. The device is fed through the catheter until the distal part emerges into the left atrium under fluoroscopy. Whether it has arms that extend or a disc that forms, it should exhibit elastic resistance to a gentle pull, without falling through back into the right atrium. When the position of the distal part of the device has been established, the sheath is slowly withdrawn, and the rest of the device emerges from the sheath and extends in the right atrium. When a bolus of contrast medium through the sheath confirms that the device is firmly in place and patent, it is disengaged and the sheath is withdrawn.

The procedure can be performed with or without transthoracic echo guidance, and intracardiac ultrasound has proven a useful adjunct in many cases. Depending on the experience and confidence of the operator, PFO closure can be performed safely under fluoroscopy alone. Depending on the patient's age and risk-factor profile (and because the patient is already in the lab), an angiogram may be performed to check for coronary artery disease. Otherwise the procedure is now finished, and the patient can be returned to his or her bed. The patient will have an echocardiogram prior to discharge to ascertain good placement of the device and look for a residual leak (that may close completely during follow-up due to endothelial coverage of the device). In cases where a "leak" is still detected after several months, a second device can be placed in the remaining hole.

Patient Care

A complication-free PFO closure procedure can take as little as 15 minutes from when the patient leaves his or her bed until he or she is returned to it, so patient contact is often short. The patient will already have been informed about the procedure, but ask again if there are any questions.

The patient typically experiences no pain during the procedure, so no additional analgesia is necessary in most cases. Endocarditis prophylaxis is usually prescribed, as is aspirin for life and clopidogrel for 6 months. Patients should be observed postprocedure as with other coronary catheter patients. Their mobilization should follow hospital protocol for vessel puncture.

ATRIAL SEPTAL DEFECT

An atrial septal defect (ASD) is a congenital defect in which the atrial septum has a hole (or several holes) in it, which permits the flow of blood between the left and right atria. In adults, this defect is rarely produced by an MI affecting the septum, causing a rip in the tissue. An ASD can allow emboli to pass into the arterial bloodstream, causing MI, stroke, or peripheral embolization. Although an ASD can be closed surgically with a mortality of less than 1%,[7] the risk of complications associated with the general anesthetic, the sternotomy, a long hospital stay, and the resulting scar mean that this is usually performed transluminally.

Devices

ASD devices are very similar to PFO occlusion devices, differing in the range of sizes that are available. The most widely used is the Amplatzer device (from AGA Medical of Plymouth, MN), which is available in sizes ranging from 4 to 40 mm and can be used to close ASDs up to 38 mm in diameter.

Amplatzer has also developed a device for ASDs that are made up of multiple fenestrations. The Amplatzer Cribiform septal occluder has large discs (18–35 mm diameter) and a very narrow waist. It is placed in the most central fenestration and covers all of the surrounding holes.

The STARflex device has a microspring system that connects the distal tip of each arm to its opposing arm. This keeps the tips of each arm against the septum wall and centers the device in the ASD. These devices can be used to close ASDs with diameters up to 23 mm.

Procedure

ASD closure is carried out in a similar manner as a PFO closure. The patient is prepared as for a routine cath lab case. A femoral vein puncture is performed under local anesthetic, and a multipurpose catheter is steered through the ASD.

Because the size and shape of ASDs can vary greatly, measurement of the hole is usually necessary to determine what size device should be placed. This is performed with the use of a measurement balloon, a large highly compliant balloon that is placed through the ASD and then inflated with a mixture of contrast medium and saline. An angle directly perpendicular to the catheter is chosen, and an X-ray image is taken that shows the "waist" of the balloon where it is constrained by the rim of the ASD. Using quantitative coronary analysis (holding a ruler against the monitor also works), the waist of the measurement balloon is compared to the opaque markers on the shaft of the balloon catheter. Thus, the diameter of the ASD can be accurately calculated and an appropriate size device selected.

The same considerations on device size as with PFO occluders are also relevant here: The device must completely cover the ASD, but too large a device can rub against the walls of the atria, especially in the direction of the aorta, causing erosion of the atrial wall. A minimal distance of 5 mm between the margins of the ASD and the neighboring cardiac structures is necessary. Otherwise surgery is indicated.

Once the optimally sized device has been selected, it is positioned through the ASD as with PFO closure, and the delivery catheter is withdrawn.

Patient Care

The postprocedure patient care is similar to that of a PFO-closure patient.

VENTRICULAR SEPTAL DEFECT

A ventricular septal defect (VSD) is usually found as a form of congenital heart disease in 0.13 to 1.24% of live births.[8] The interventricular septum is formed by the fusion of several tissues: the muscular septum, the endocardial cushions, the bulbar ridges, and the aorticopulmonary system. A VSD can occur if any of these tissues fails to fuse with another, but the defect usually rectifies itself by about 7 weeks after birth.

It is very rare for a VSD to be caused by an infarct, but it does occur in about 0.2% of infarctions.[9] A transluminal procedure to close a VSD has several advantages over a surgical option: The patients are usually too unstable to undergo open heart surgery, and once on the cath lab table, the coronary cause of the infarct can also be treated.

Devices

ASD and PFO closure devices have been used to close VSDs in the past, but there is now a range of purpose-built devices for VSD closure. The Amplatzer devices that are designed for closing a VSD in an infant look very similar to their ASD and VSD devices; they are comprised of two nitanol mesh discs joined in a waist at their centers (see Figure 19-4). They are available in sizes from 4 to 18 mm. For adult patients, the muscular Amplatzer VSD occluders have a longer, thicker waist that takes into account the relative thickness of the ventricular septum. They are available in sizes from 16 to 24 mm.

NMT has a CardioSEAL for closure of VSDs in high-risk patients. It has a double umbrella implant, with a polyester tissue scaffold MRI-safe framework. It is available in sizes from 17 to 40 mm.

Figure 19-4. Amplatzer muscular VSD occluder. *Source: Courtesy of AGA Medical Corporation.*

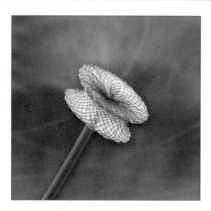

Procedure

VSD closure is also carried out in a similar manner as PFO closure. The patient is prepared as for a routine cath lab case. The VSD is usually crossed from the left side using a Judkins right catheter. It is often possible to cross from the venous side of the heart, but extra care must be taken not to go through the trabeculae in the right ventricle.[10] The delivery sheath is quite thin and navigating the curves necessary to get the device into position may cause kinking. In these cases, access via the internal jugular vein can be considered, so the patient must be prepared for jugular access in addition to the femoral sheaths already in place.

Patient Care

Postprocedure patient care depends on the age and condition of the patient. Continuous monitoring for arrhythmias may be maintained for several days, and a series of echocardiograms will confirm the device's position and patency. Complete patency can be difficult in post-MI patients, because the VSD is often a rip rather than a hole (as is the case with ASDs). When a VSD closure is per-

formed on a child, improvement in their hemodynamic status can be instant, and their observations must take into account the adjustments that their cardiovascular systems must now make to compensate for the lack of interventricular shunt.

PATENT DUCTUS ARTERIOSUS

The ductus arteriosus is a channel that runs between the pulmonary artery and the aortic arch in the neonate. Its purpose is to shunt blood away from the undeveloped fetal lungs into the systemic circulation. It usually closes off soon after birth, leaving a fibrous band that helps maintain the position of the aortic arch relative to the pulmonary arteries. The incidence of patent ductus arteriosus (PDA) is inversely proportional to the gestational age at birth: It is evident in about 20% of premature infants with greater than 32 weeks' gestation, and in 60% of those with less than 28 weeks'.[11] A PDA can be long and thin, or so short that it is little more than a window between the two vessels;[12] determination of the size and shape of a PDA is important in determining which type and size of occluder is to be used.

Devices

Because many PDAs are effectively just long tubes, it has been common practice to close these using embolization coils. These come in a number of loops and lengths and are basically spiraling wire springs that have dacron feathers attached. These feathers encourage embolization, which will block the PDA passage.

Amplatz also produces a closure device specifically designed for PDA closure. They range in size from 5/4 mm to 16/14 mm.

Procedure

The patient is prepared as for a routine cath lab case. A femoral vein and a femoral artery puncture are performed under local anesthetic. A

Figure 19-5. Amplatzer PDA closure device. *Source:* Courtesy of AGA Medical Corporation.

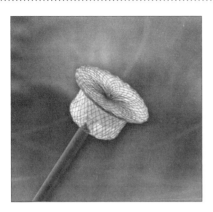

left- and right-catheter procedure is performed to rule out other cardiac defects. A descending aortogram is performed to provide a roadmap for the procedure and to measure the size and shape of the PDA. The delivery catheter brings the selected device in a retrograde fashion to the mouth of the PDA. The coil or occlusion device is delivered into the body of the PDA, and an aortogram is performed to verify positioning. The device is disengaged, and the delivery catheter is withdrawn.

Patient Care

The postprocedure patient care is similar to that of a PFO-closure patient.

LEFT ATRIAL APPENDAGE

The trabeculated left atrial appendage (LAA) is another remnant of neonate cardiovascular pathology. It has the shape of a windsock and lies between the pulmonary veins and the mitral valve. Although usually of no significance, it has been found that 90% of thrombi related to stroke in patients with atrial fibrillation (AF)

originate from the LAA.[13] Chronic AF not only affects the shape of the left atrium, but also the LAA, making it more voluminous and giving it a larger mouth, which encourages thrombus formation. The traditional treatment for chronic AF is oral anticoagulation, but there has recently been development of devices that are designed to occlude the LAA.

Devices

The percutaneous LAA occlude (PLAATO) (from EV3 of Plymouth, MN) is a ball-shaped nitinol cage covered by a trafluouoethylene membrane (see Figure 19-6). The nitinol frame contains three rows of small spikes that anchor the device in the LAA once it has been positioned. It is available in sizes from 15 to 32 mm.

The WATCHMAN LAA filter system (from Atritech of Minneapolis, MN) is a filter device that is placed in the LAA (see Figure 19-7). Its frame is made of nitinol and incorporates a row of fixation barbs around the mid-perimeter. It has a 160 μm PET filter on the proximal face of the device that allows only blood to pass through until full healing has occurred. It is available in sizes 21, 24, 27, and 30 mm.

Some success has also been had with placement of Amplatz occluders in the LAA.[14] The mouth

Figure 19-6. The PLAATO device. *Source:* Courtesy of Ev3.

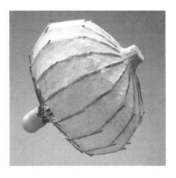

Figure 19-7. The Watchman filter device. *Source:* Courtesy of Atritech.

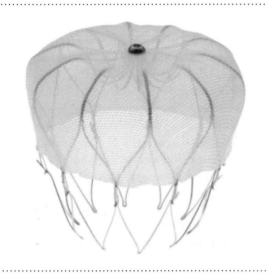

and initial section of the LAA are quite membraneous, and the Amplatz occluders grasp these structures when positioned. Although the use of ASD occluders has proven successful, Amplatzer are currently designing a purpose-built LAA occluder that is not yet ready for market release.

Procedure

The patient is prepared as for a routine cath lab case. A femoral vein puncture is performed under local anesthetic, and a multipurpose catheter is steered transseptally to the mouth of the LAA. If a PFO is present, this can be used; otherwise a transseptal puncture should be performed using a Brochenbrough needle, as described in Chapter 21 for mitral valvuloplasty. After transseptal access has been verified, a bolus of heparin is administered. A left atriography is performed to assess the size of the appendage and the diameter of its orifice.

The multipurpose catheter is replaced by the product's delivery sheath, and this is positioned at the mouth of the LAA. The device is then deployed in the LAA in a fashion similar to the other closure devices. A contrast media injection distal to the device through a special lumen in the device, and one from the side of the left atrium, will verify its patency.

Patient Care

The patient should experience no pain during the procedure, so neither additional anesthesia nor analgesia should be necessary. Their mobilization should follow hospital protocol for vessel puncture. The patient will have several postprocedure echocardiographies to verify the device's position and patency. Aspirin for life, clopidogrel for 6 months, and endocarditis prophylaxis will be prescribed. Although initial results have been encouraging, at this stage, patients are considered for this procedure if they are not suitable for oral anticoagulation therapy. Randomized trials are necessary to determine whether LAA closure is as effective as oral anticoagulation therapy in preventing strokes.

REFERENCES

1. Hagen PT, Scholz DG, Edwards WD. Incidence and size of patent foramen ovale during the first 10 decades of life: an autopsy study of 965 normal hearts. *Mayo Clin Proc* 1984;59:17–20.
2. Schwerzmann M, Windecker S, Meier B. In: Meier B. *Interventional Cardiology: An Atlas of Investigation and Therapy.* Oxford: Clinical Publishing; 2004.
3. Lechat P, Mas JL, Lascault G, at al. Prevalence of patent foramen ovale in patients with stroke. *N Engl J Med* 1988;318:1148–1152.
4. Khairy P, O'Donnell CP, Landzberg MJ. Transcatheter closure versus medical therapy of patent foramen ovale and presumed paradoxical thromboemboli: a systematic review. *Ann Intern Med* 2003;139:753–760.

5. Braun M, Gliech V, Boscheri A, et al. Transcatheter closure of patent foramen ovale (PFO) in patients with paradoxical emboloism. *Eur Heart J* 2004:25;424–430.

6. Krumsdorf U, Ostermayer S, Billinger K, et al. Incidence and clinical course of thrombus formation on atrial septel defect and patent foramen ovale closure devices in 1,000 consecutive patients. *J Am Coll Cardiol* 2004;43,2:302–309.

7. Hijazi ZM. Catheter closure of atrial septal and ventricular septal defects using the Amplatzer devices. *Heart Lung* 2003;12:S63–72.

8. Kieth JD, Rowe RD, Vlad P. eds. Heart Disease in Infancy and Childhood. 3rd ed. New York: MacMillan; 1978.

9. Holzer R, Balzer D, Amin Z, et al. Transcatheter closure of postinfarction ventricular septal defects using the new Amplatzer muscular VSC occluder: results of a U.S. registry. *Catheter Cardiovasc Interv* 2004;61(2):196–201.

10. Hijazi ZM. Device closure of ventricular septal defects. *Catheter Cardiovasc Interv* 2003;60:107–114.

11. Wyllie J. Treatment of patent ductus arteriosus. *Semin Neonatol* 2003;8:425–432.

12. Sims SL. Alterations of cardiovascular function in children. In: McCance KL, Huether SE. *Pathophysiology: The Biologic Basis for Disease in Adults and Children*. St. Louis, MO: CV Mosby; 1990.

13. Windecker S, Meier B. Percutaneous obliteration of left atrial appendage in atrial fibrillation. In: Meier B. *Interventional Cardiology: An Atlas of Investigation and Therapy*. Oxford: Clinical Publishing; 2004.

14. Meier B, Palacios I, Windecker S, et al. Transcatheter left atrial appendage occlusion with Amplatzer devices to obviate anticoagulation in patients with atrial fibrillation. *Catheter Cardiovasc Interv* 3003;60(3):417–422.

Chapter 20

SEPTAL ALCOHOL ABLATION

Sandy Watson RN, BN, NFESC

HYPERTROPHIC OBSTRUCTIVE CARDIOMYOPATHY

Hypertrophic cardiomyopathy (HCM) is characterized by a thickening of the ventricle, often involving the septum. It is capable of obstructing the left ventricular outflow tract (LVOT), producing a left ventricular-aortic gradient. When it becomes obstructive, it is referred to as hypertrophic obstructive cardiomyopathy (HCM). The obstruction of the LVOT is caused by the systolic anterior motion (SAM) of the mitral valve leaflet where it hits the hypertrophied septum, causing obstruction and turbulent flow (see Figure 20-1).

HOCM can be responsible for dyspnea, angina pectoris, palpations, syncope, and sudden cardiac death. Although it was once thought to be very rare, HCM has been found to some extent in 1 in 500 people.[1] Twenty-five percent of patients with HCM have HOCM, and 10% of those have severe symptoms despite maximum medical therapy.

The treatment options for HOCM include medical therapy, atrioventricular (AV) pacing, surgical myectomy, or alcohol ablation for patients refractory to medical therapy. The surgical option, a myectomy, involves physically removing hypertrophied muscle from the wall of the heart. It remains the treatment of choice for these patients, but enthusiasm for this approach has been tempered by a relatively high operative mortality rate (1%–8%), and by a significant risk for postoperative morbidity (8%–10%).[2]

Septal alcohol ablation (SAA)—also called percutaneous transluminal septal myocardial ablation (PTSMA), transcoronary ablation of septal hypertrophy (TASH), or alcohol septal ablation (ASA)—was performed after it had been noted that some patients with HOCM lost their symptoms, and their gradient, after having an anterior MI.[3] The previously hypertrophied myocardium became necrotic, shrank, and no longer obstructed the LVOT.

Figure 20-1. Hypertrophic obstructive cardiomyopathy.

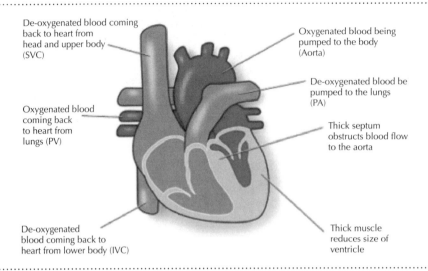

De-oxygenated blood coming back to heart from head and upper body (SVC)

Oxygenated blood being pumped to the body (Aorta)

De-oxygenated blood be pumped to the lungs (PA)

Oxygenated blood coming back to heart from lungs (PV)

Thick septum obstructs blood flow to the aorta

De-oxygenated blood coming back to heart from lower body (IVC)

Thick muscle reduces size of ventricle

In 1995, Ulrich Sigwart transferred that effect into the cath lab by injecting pure alcohol into a septal branch of the left anterior descending artery. The patients' symptoms improved, and their LVOT obstruction was reduced to a degree similar to surgery.[4]

Necrosis of the anterior basal septum is caused by introducing absolute alcohol directly into a proximal septal perforator artery, producing a myocardial infarction within the proximal ventricular septum. This ultimately reduces LV wall thickness, enlarging the outflow tract, and reducing the impedance to LV ejection. Although immediate rapid reduction of the resting outflow gradient may occur, more frequently a progressive decrease occurs after 6 to 12 months.

PROCEDURE

The patient is prepared at the groin as for an angiography or angioplasty procedure. One venous sheath (generally 6F to 8F), and two arterial sheaths (one 4F and one 6F) are placed. Because of the 50% risk of intraprocedure AV block, a temporary pacemaker is placed in the right ven-

tricle of all patients via a 6F venous sheath at the beginning of the procedure. A bolus of heparin, heparin infusion, or both, should be administered once the temporary pacemaker catheter is in place.

A ventriculography is performed, and then the catheter remains in the left ventricle during the procedure to enable continuous pressure monitoring. Using a diagnostic catheter through the 6F sheath, simultaneous pressure measurements are obtained from the left ventricular apex and the proximal aorta at rest and during provocation with the Valsalva maneuver or a catheter-induced extra systole. An angiography is then performed to rule out multivessel disease or a proximal LAD lesion and to get a map of the septal vascular bed.

A large septal branch of at least 1.5 mm in diameter is located, although it may be a diagonal branch or ramus that supplies this septal area, rather than a septal branch. An appropriate guiding catheter is placed, and a guide wire is passed into the vessel. An over-the-wire balloon is passed over the guide wire, then inflated at low pressure (3 to 4 Bar) in its proximal section.

There are no balloons available that are made specifically for septal ablation, so regular angioplasty balloons are used. The balloon should be short, and it should not disintegrate in alcohol. A 2 mm balloon is commonly used, although this depends on the size of the septal branch to be obstructed.

The guide wire is removed from the balloon catheter, and contrast medium is injected through the catheter's guide wire lumen to check for collateral circulation, and to ensure that the balloon is fully obstructing the vessel. Myocardial contrast echo (MCE) may be performed, either with a transesophageal probe or with an intracardiac echocardiography catheter. This enables localization of the septal branch supplying the critical septal segment (i.e., the point of SAM of the mitral valve and maximum ventricular outflow tract turbulence). MCE helps avoid an injection of alcohol too close to the right ventricle, apex, or papillary muscle, reducing the risk of inducing complete heart block and the need for a permanent pacemaker.

When vessel appropriateness and effective balloon obstruction have been confirmed, a small amount of alcohol is then injected through the lumen of the balloon catheter. Usually 1 ml of alcohol per artery is enough; small amounts of alcohol have been associated with a lesser incidence of AV block.[5] The alcohol should be injected slowly, and the ECG monitored carefully. After the alcohol has been injected, the balloon must be kept inflated for at least 10 minutes, and the catheter flushed with normal saline to prevent leakage of alcohol back into the LAD.

Once the balloon has been deflated, it should be removed carefully so that no alcohol that may be remaining in the catheter lumen leaks into coronary arteries.

The gradient is then measured again, and a second branch may be ablated if necessary, but the ablation of one major septal artery is usually enough.

PATIENT CARE

When the alcohol reaches the myocardium, the patient will experience a localized myocardial infarction, and this usually causes pain. The patient should be prepared for this, and a decision be made on pain relief medication before the procedure begins. A bolus of 5–10 mg of morphine IV shortly before ablation is usually adequate, and the pain resolves by itself in a few minutes due to necrosis.

The temporary pacemaker is kept in place for about 12 hours, and the patient should remain monitored for at least 36 hours after the procedure.[6] Some clinics leave the temporary pacemaker in for 24 hours, then in-hospital monitoring for 4 days because of the risk of late heart block.

An echocardiograph is performed shortly after the procedure and again before discharge to assess the extent of the necrosis and to assess the LVOT gradient.

Alcohol ablation of the septum to treat HOCM is an effective and safe procedure. The recovery is rapid, and the procedure involves very little pain. The hospital stay is around 5 to 6 days, depending on the patient's need for a permanent pacemaker implantation. About 10% of patients have nonsustained ventricular tachycardia or fibrillation, and permanent pacemaker implantation is necessary in about one-third of cases.[7]

REFERENCES

1 Maron BJ, Gardin JM, Flack JM, et al. Prevalence of hypertrophic cardiomyopathy in a general population of young adults. *Circulation* 1995;92:785–789.

2. Glower DD. Acquired aortic valvular disease. In: Sabiston DC, Spencer FC, eds. *Surgery of the Chest*, 6th ed. Philadelphia: W B Saunders Co., 1995;1755–1756.

3 Sigwart U. Non-surgical myocardial reduction for hypertrophic obstructive cardiomyopathy. *Lancet* 1995;346:211–214.

4. Sigwart U. Non-surgical myocardial reduction for hypertrophic obstructive cardiomyopathy. *Lancet* 1995;346:211–214.

5 Faber L, Seggewiss H, Gleichmann U. Percutaneous transluminal septal myocardial ablation in hypertrophic obstructive cardiomyopathy: Results with respect to intraprocedural myocardial contrast echocardiography. *Circulation* 1998;98:2415–2421.

6 Hess O, Como F, Wolber T. Alcohol ablation of septal hypertrophy. In: Meier B. *Interventional Cardiology: An Atlas of Investigation and Therapy*. Oxford: Clinical Publishing; 2004.

7 Sigwart U, Asher CR, Lever HM. In: Topol EJ. *Textbook of Interventional Cardiology*, 4th ed. Philadelphia: Saunders; 2003.

Chapter 21

PERCUTANEOUS VALVE COMMISSUROTOMY, REPAIR, AND REPLACEMENT

Sharon Holloway, RN, MSN, ACNP-CS, CCRN
Rena L. Silver, RN, MSN, ACNP-C

For the heart to effectively pump blood through the circulatory system, the heart's valves must operate correctly. A normal valve provides unidirectional flow, neither impeding forward flow nor allowing backward flow. The valvular condition that impedes forward flow is known as stenosis, and the condition resulting in backward flow is known as regurgitation.

Valvular heart disease is classified as being either congenital or acquired. It is estimated that valvular dysfunction occurs in 1.8% of the westernized population with rates increasing as patients age.[1] Generally, symptoms do not develop acutely; instead, they progress over time due to the high degree of adaptability the heart possesses. Once the adaptive capabilities of the heart have been exhausted, however, symptoms occur, and various treatment modalities must be evaluated.

In the following sections, the percutaneous management of each valvular condition will be detailed including a review of the pertinent patient-care considerations. The valves, their pathologies, and treatment will be discussed from the left to the right; the mitral, then the aortic valve, followed by the pumonic, and the tricuspid valves.

MITRAL VALVE

The mitral valve is a bicuspid valve located between the left atrium and the left ventricle. In adults, the mitral valve measures 4–6 cm2. The mitral valve apparatus is composed of two leaflets (the larger anterior and the smaller posterior), the chordae tendineae, and the papillary muscles. Together, the chordae tendineae and the papillary muscles provide the pulling mechanism necessary to hold the valve in place. The mitral valve allows oxygenated blood coming from the lungs to leave the left atrium and enter the left ventricle in preparation for distribution throughout the circulatory system.

Mitral Stenosis

Mitral stenosis is a valvular lesion that primarily affects adults, with two-thirds of cases occurring in women. The etiology is usually rheumatic, resulting from an episode of childhood rheumatic fever. Mitral stenosis results in several changes to the integrity of the valve: the valve cusps thicken; the edges or commissures of the leaflets become stuck together; the chordae tendineae become thickened and shortened; and calcium deposits form.

The first symptom of mitral stenosis is usually the hallmark clinical sign of dyspnea on exertion. The symptoms of mitral stenosis are the result of the increase in the pressure needed to propel blood from the left atrium into the left ventricle through the stenotic mitral valve. This increase in pressure produces a measurable pressure gradient across the mitral valve. As the stenosis increases in severity, left atrial dilatation occurs as a compensatory mechanism. During this period, the patients are often asymptomatic.

Once the heart's compensatory abilities have been exhausted, atrial dilatation leads to a backward flow of blood, causing an increase in pulmonary venous and capillary pressures, a decrease in pulmonary compliance, and pulmonary congestion. This increased pulmonary congestion results in further symptoms of fatigue, orthopnea, paroxysmal nocturnal dyspnea, peripheral and pulmonary edema, and hemoptysis. Often, patients complain of palpitations as a result of atrial fibrillation, which is a common arrhythmia due to the left atrial enlargement. These effects are reflected in the hemodynamic signs of mitral stenosis: an elevated left atrial pressure (LAP), an elevation in pulmonary artery pressure (PAP), a decrease in cardiac output (CO), and a transvalvular pressure gradient between the left atrium and left ventricle.

Physical examination of these patients reveals a loud S1 (due to abrupt leaflet closure), a loud S2 (due to the elevation in PAP), an opening snap (OS) (due to tension on the valve leaflet), and a diastolic rumble (due to turbulent blood flow across the stenotic valve). A mitral regurgitation murmur may also be detected.

Clinical evaluation of mitral stenosis begins with an in-depth history and physical examination. The diagnostic testing used to evaluate the presence and severity of mitral stenosis includes an M-mode and 2-D echocardiogram with a Doppler study, a chest radiograph, and a transesophageal echocardiogram (TEE).

The M-mode echocardiographic data may show evidence of an enlarged left atrium, thickened or calcified mitral valve leaflets with reduced excursion, and concordant leaflet motion. The Doppler study will allow for evaluation of the pressure gradient across the mitral valve and an estimation of the degree of mitral regurgitation. A transmitral pressure gradient is the hemodynamic hallmark of mitral stenosis, indicating obstruction to flow between the two chambers. A gradient as high as 20 mmHg is needed to maintain blood flow when the mitral valve area is < 1cm2. The echocardiographic data can also be used to generate an echo score, another tool in evaluating the degree of valve deformity and the potential success of percutaneous balloon dilatation.[2] The echo score evaluates leaflet thickening, subvalvular deformity, calcification, and leaflet mobility. Each area is scored on a maximal scale of 4, and the scores are added together.

The chest X-ray may reveal an enlarged left atrium, cardiomegaly, and valvular calcification. The TEE is used to rule out the presence of a left atrial thrombus. Atrial fibrillation due to left atrial enlargement causes blood to stagnate within the left atrium, predisposing the patient to thrombus formation.

Once the clinical diagnosis has been confirmed, left and right heart catheterizations are performed to both further support the diagnosis and lay the foundation for percutaneous therapy.

Percutaneous Mitral Commissurotomy

The treatment options for mitral valve disease have been under investigation since the beginning of the 20th century. On February 8, 1902, Sir Lauder Brunton speculated about the possibility of performing mitral commissurotomy.[3] Using autopsy hearts, he observed that fused mitral commissures could be dilated with a finger, prompting him to question the potential for surgical therapy.

In the 1920s, Cutler used a valvotome to attempt a partial valve excision,[4] and Souttar, using a finger, performed a transauricular dilatation,[5] both with poor results. The closed surgical treatment for mitral stenosis was first reported in 1948.[6]

Inoue Technique

Percutaneous therapy for mitral commissurotomy was innovated by Inoue in 1982. He developed a unique balloon catheter system for dilatation of the fused mitral valve commissures. Although the statistical success of surgical mitral commissurotomy and valve replacement are well documented, comparable results have been achieved using the Inoue device.[7–13] The ease and atraumatic nature of the procedure and the shortened hospital stays have meant that patients not considered to be surgical candidates can be treated percutaneously. The majority of patients, even those who are considered poor surgical candidates, can expect a successful immediate and long-term result. Over two-thirds of patients do not require additional procedures for more than 5 years.[14]

The Inoue balloon is constructed of a nylon mesh sandwiched between two layers of latex. The balloon is available in three sizes: 26, 28, and 30 mm. The appropriate balloon size is selected based on the patient's height. For instance, a 26 mm balloon is used for patients < 160 cm tall; a 28 mm balloon is used for those who are 160–180 cm tall, and a 30 mm balloon is selected for patients > 180 cm tall.[15]

A left heart catheterization is performed to rule out, or delineate, the presence of coronary artery disease. A left ventriculogram is performed to directly measure the left ventricular end diastolic pressure (LVEDP) and to assess the amount of mitral regurgitation present. The diagnosis of coronary artery disease may necessitate postponement of the mitral valve procedure until the coronary blockage can be effectively treated. Both procedures may be performed percutaneously during the same hospitalization or the severity of the coronary artery disease may indicate that a surgical procedure is preferable.

Procedure

The ventriculogram should be performed in the right anterior oblique projection to best visualize and assess the degree of mitral regurgitation (see Figure 21-a). The presence of severe regurgitation is a definitive contraindication to the procedure. This is due to the potential for causing the existing regurgitation to worsen, as well as the limited effect opening the valve will have clinically for the patient whose symptoms may be primarily the result of regurgitation and not valve stenosis. A right heart catheterization is performed to measure the hemodynamic effects of the mitral stenosis—for example, the right atrial pressure (RAP), PAP, pulmonary capillary wedge pressure (PCWP) and cardiac output (CO). These measurements are also performed postprocedure to measure procedure success.

An 8F Mullins sheath is inserted into the right femoral vein. A transseptal needle is inserted via the sheath into the right atrium (see Figure 21-b). Successful performance of the transseptal needle puncture, in order to gain antegrade access to the mitral valve, is the most critical part of the procedure. Presently, some operators are foregoing use of the Mullins sheath apparatus and simply using the dilator to perform the transseptal technique.

Figure 21-1a–b. Transseptal technique. *Top:* catheters used to complete transseptal puncture. *Top left to right:* Mullins sheath and dilator; Brockenbrough needle and stylet; position of needle within the dilator; orientation of the needle hub. *Bottom:* schematic of transseptal puncture technique. *Bottom left:* the heart in right anterior oblique. The transseptal catheter passes through the fossa ovalis into the left atrium above the mitral valve. *Bottom right:* the heart in left anterior oblique. The transseptal catheter is crossing the fossa ovalis, pointing posteriorly. *Source:* Bottom portion: Reprinted from Roelke M, Smith AJ, Palacois IF. The technique and safety of transseptal left heart catheterization: the Massachusetts General Hospital experience with 1,279 procedures. Cathet Cardiovasc Diagn 1994;32(4):332–339.

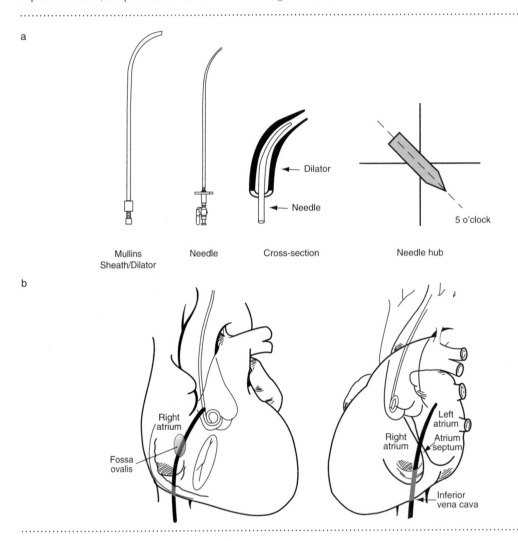

A change in pressure can be seen between the right and LAP measurements, indicating a successful puncture. If there is any doubt, oxygen saturations can be measured on a blood sample drawn from the transseptal needle.

A 0.025-inch spring coil wire is inserted via the Mullins sheath after the transseptal needle has been removed, and the wire is passed into the left atrium. The coiled end of the wire has a soft spring tip that protects the left atrium during passage of the balloon.

The balloon is readied by passing the rigid metal stretching tube through its central lumen, which is then locked into place. This causes the balloon to narrow in its uninflated form to allow passage of the balloon through the transseptal puncture site. The balloon is inserted through the skin without use of a femoral sheath, directly into the right atrium, on through the interatrial septum, into the left atrium. The balloon is unstretched in the left atrium, and continues to track over the wire until the mitral valve is reached.

Once the balloon is in place, the wire and stretching tube are removed. A steering stylette is inserted into the central balloon lumen and used to facilitate balloon movement into the left ventricle before the balloon is positioned across the mitral valve. A mixture of saline and contrast is used to inflate and visualize the balloon during the dilatations. The balloon can be sequentially increased in size in a step-wise fashion to match the increase in the mitral valve orifice achieved after each inflation. This is done without changing the initial balloon apparatus. As the balloon is deflated, it usually falls into the left atrium without the need for additional manipulation.

Initially, the proximal portion is inflated slightly to increase steerability, helping to position it in

Figure 21-2. *Panel 1:* Balloon in its elongated or "slenderized" configuration, with the rigid metal stretching tube inserted. *Panel 2:* Balloon in its "stubby", relaxed configuration, with the tube pulled back. *Panel 3:* Balloon inserted into the left atrium and partially inflated with saline. *Panel 4:* Further inflation causes the proximal part of the balloon to inflate. *Panel 5:* The distal part of the balloon inflates, creating a dogbone around the mitral valve. *Panel 6:* further inflation causes the center part of the balloon to expand. *Source:* From Toray Marketing & Sales, Inc., Houston, TX.

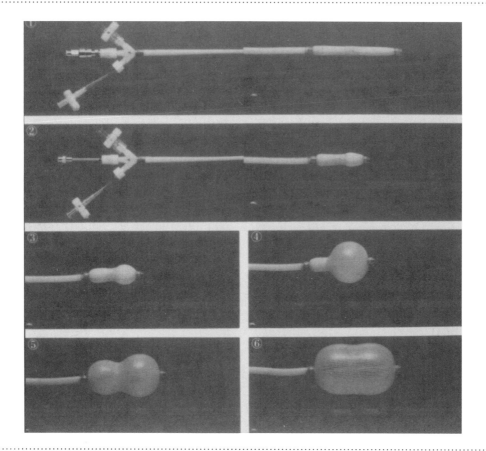

the left ventricle. Then the proximal portion of the balloon inflates. This results in locking the mitral valve between the proximal and distal portions of the balloon but allowing free movement of the balloon across the mitral valve. Finally, the middle portion of the balloon inflates, transferring the complete dilating force onto the fused mitral commissures, effectively splitting them. Often, the balloon's "waist" will open abruptly, which indicates that the commissures have split. The weave of nylon mesh in the latex of the balloon is loosest in the front, midrange in the rear part of the balloon, and tightest in the center,

accounting for the step-wise or sequential inflation of the balloon.

Once the inflations are complete, a direct measure of the left atrial pressure (LAP) can be made by using the central catheter lumen. First, the steering stylette must be removed, and then a transducer pressure connection is made to the catheter. With the pigtail in the left ventricle, the pressure gradient between the left atrium and left ventricle can be measured. A reduction in the mean LAP and reduction of the gradient signifies successful treatment of the stenosis. However, more inflations may be necessary after

Figure 21-3. Fluoroscopy of Inoue inflations. (A) Balloon catheter inserted through the mitral valve into the left atrium. (B) Further inflation of the distal end of the balloon. (C) The mitral valve is locked between the proximal and distal balloon ends. (D) The balloon is fully inflated, opening the fused mitral commissures. *Source:* From The University of Chicago Hospitals, Hans Hecht Cardiac Catheritization Laboratory, Chicago, IL.

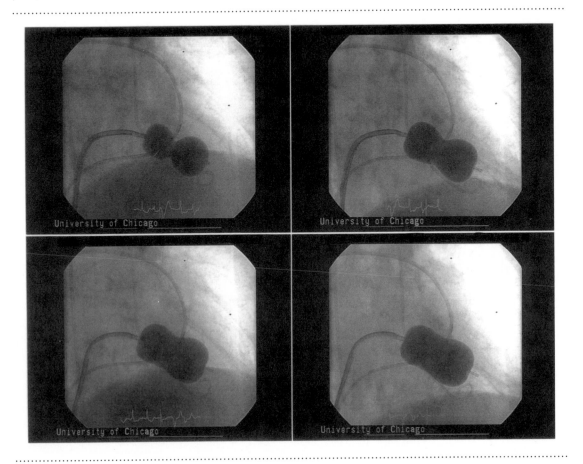

these measurements have been made. Also, results may reveal worsening of the pressures, and an increase of the V wave indicates an increase in mitral regurgitation, and the need to abort the procedure. In-lab echocardiography, a repeat left ventriculogram, or both can be used to measure the amount of mitral regurgitation.

Hemodynamically, after a successful procedure, there is a decline in LA pressure, the transmitral pressure gradient, and the PA pressure, while there is no change in the LV diastolic pressure; the patient's cardiac output rises accordingly. This dramatic improvement becomes clinically evident during the procedure, because the patients often comment on a sense of relief from their shortness of breath while still on the catheterization table.

Once the procedure is complete and all the measurements have been taken, the balloon is removed by reinserting the stretching tube over the guide wire within the left atrium. Once the balloon catheter has been removed, a pressure dressing may be applied or a venous sheath may be inserted for hemostasis until final removal.

Complications

The most significant risk of the procedure is damage to the mitral valve, resulting in an increase in mitral regurgitation. The balloon itself may also cause damage to the leaflets or chordae tendineae. An increase in mitral regurgitation may necessitate an emergency valve replacement during the same hospitalization or soon afterward. Patients may be stabilized in-lab with vasodilator therapy (i.e., a nitroprusside infusion or an angiotensin-converting enzyme inhibitor).[15] Fortunately, results show this to be an infrequent occurrence. Less than 3%[16] of patients within the Inoue North American registry underwent valve replacement during the procedural hospitalization.

Other complications include perforation, atrial septal defect, stroke or transient ischemic attack (TIA), and vascular compromise.[16] Use

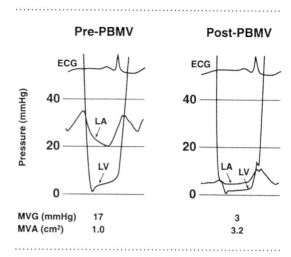

Figure 21-4. Hemodynamics of mitral stenosis, pre- and post-therapy. PBMV: Percutaneous balloon mitral valvuloplasty; LA: Left atrial pressure; LV: Left ventricular pressure; MVG: mitral valve gradient; MVA: mitral valve area.

of the double-balloon technique has resulted in ventricular perforation in 1%–2% of patients.[17,18] Perforation during the Inoue procedure is linked to the transseptal puncture being safely performed, which is basically operator dependent.[19]

With the consistent performance of TEE prior to the valve procedure, the occurrence of stroke and TIAs has been minimized. TEE can uncover a left atrial thrombus that may result in the catastrophic complication of stroke. The potential for stroke and TIAs, which is inherent to all percutaneous procedures, is still present due to the unavoidable use of wires and catheters, which may result in embolization. This risk can be minimized by the prophylactic use of heparin; 5000 IU given intravenously preprocedure.

A significant atrial septal defect caused by the procedure (shunt ratio greater than 1.5:1) is only 3%–5%,[16] despite the large puncture needed to deliver the catheter system to the mitral valve. Often, the presence of an atrial septal defect is related to an incomplete procedure, which leaves a pressure gradient between the left and right atrium. In the few months postprocedure, most shunts close. The persistent shunt seen with an incomplete dilatation causes left atrial hypertension, and this hypertension maintains the shunt over time. The need for catheter or surgical correction of the atrial septal defect is extremely rare.

Vascular complications can result from the trauma caused by the insertion of the sheath and devices needed for the procedure. Complications tend to occur in patients with a history of peripheral vascular disease or those in whom access is not easily achieved and for whom multiple punctures are necessary. Careful attention given to the postprocedure care by the nursing staff can mini-

mize groin complications, alerting the physician to complications before they become severe.

Other Techniques

Although the Inoue balloon is considered to be the best percutaneous treatment option, there are other modalities available. Single- and double-balloon techniques remain in use. Initially, single balloons, intended for peripheral dilatation were used to dilate stenosed mitral valves. The single- and double-balloon techniques require stiffer balloons with sharper tips, so the risk of ventricular perforation is significant. The double-balloon technique requires a larger atrial septal

Figure 21-5. Mitral valvuloplasty double balloon technique. (A) Transseptal puncture with the wire extending into the left atrium. (B) Advancement of the wire into the left ventricle. (C) Placement and partial inflation of a single balloon across the mitral valve. (D) Dilatation of the atrial septum with an Olbert catheter. (E) Placement of the two balloon catheters across the mitral valve. (F) Inflation of both balloons. *Source:* Adapted from Srebro J, Ports TA. Catheter balloon valvuloplasty. In: Chatterjee K, et al, eds. Cardiology: An Illustrated Text. Philadelphia: Lippincott-Raven; 1991:9.54.

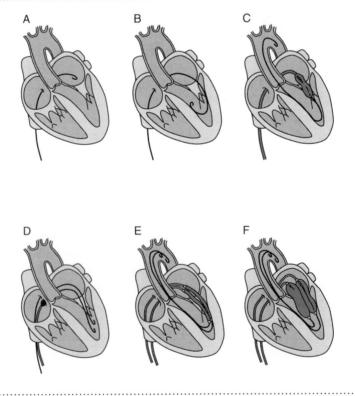

puncture, and the risk of an atrial septal defect is greater. Also, the stiffer, bulkier double balloons may cause an increase in ventricular ectopy.

There is a newer variation of the double-balloon technique called the multitrack system, which uses a monorail balloon system with the goal of decreasing procedure complications when compared to a traditional double-balloon technique.[20] Comparisons have been made between the Inoue balloon and the double-balloon technique.[21–23] The valve area achieved postprocedure is comparable between the two techniques; however, the risk of procedural complications is increased when the double-balloon technique is employed.

Mitral Regurgitation

Leakage of the mitral valve, known as mitral regurgitation, occurs in approximately 2% of the population, effecting men and women equally. This valvular incompetence causes the backward flow of blood from the left ventricle into the left atrium during systole. Mitral regurgitation results from several abnormalities described as either functional or anatomic. Most common mitral regurgitation is due to cardiomyopathy and/or myocardial infarction. In cardiomyopathy, the failing left ventricle enlarges and stretches the valve apparatus, preventing the leaflets from closing tightly. Myocardial infarction can result in rupture of the chordae tendinae or papillary muscle compromising the valve's function. Both cardiomyopathy and myocardial ischemia result in mitral regurgitation, with anatomically normal mitral leaflets, and are thus known as functional abnormalities.

Other causes of mitral regurgitation are due to degenerative changes, rheumatic inflammation or endocarditis resulting in anatomic deformity of the valve. The valve deformity results in the inability of the leaflets to co-apt or seal together during systole causing regurgitant blood flow.

The cardinal symptoms of mitral regurgitation are exertional dyspnea, orthopnea, paroxysmal nocturnal dyspnea, pulmonary edema, and congestion. These symptoms occur as a result of the pressure caused by the backward flow of blood into the pulmonary vascular bed. Some individuals have few symptoms, but still may have elevated pulmonary pressures. Once symptoms occur and ventricular function begins to decline, repairing or replacing the valve is indicated to avoid any further cardiac impairment.

Percutaneous Mitral Valve Repair

Surgical mitral valve repair or replacement has been a longstanding and successful treatment for symptomatic mitral valve regurgitation.[24] However, because patients are living longer and are often challenged by multiple comorbidities, the surgical approach is not without risk. Surgical repair requires a prolonged hospital stay with its risk of nosocomial infections, prolonged pain, and the possibility of needing repeat surgery at a later date.

Percutaneous mitral valve repair is an attractive treatment option in appropriately selected patients. A percutaneous approach has been developed for individuals with either functional mitral regurgitation (those lacking any anatomic deformity of the valve apparatus) or degenerative mitral regurgitation. The procedure was developed (based on a surgical procedure developed by the Italian surgeon Dr. Otavio Alfieri in 1991), whereby a stitch is applied to the "leaking" center of the mitral valve leaflets, approximating the leaflets' "edge to edge," creating a double orifice or figure-8 valve (see Figure 21-6). This diminishes the area of regurgitation, and allows the remainder of the valve to open and close normally.[25]

The MitraClip system (from Evalve Inc. of Menlo Park, CA) is a polyester-covered mechanical clip device that clips the flaps together, rather than sutures them. They are mounted on the end of a delivery catheter, with two arms that are opened and closed by a mechanism at the end of the delivery system (see Figure 21-7). There

Figure 21-6. The Alfieri stitch, surgical technique approximating the mitral valve leaflets "edge to edge" creating a double orifice to treat mitral regurgitation. *Source:* Adapted from Evalve, Inc.

Figure 21-7. The MitraClip. *Source:* Adapted from Evalve, Inc.

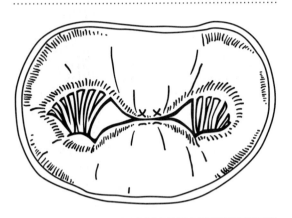

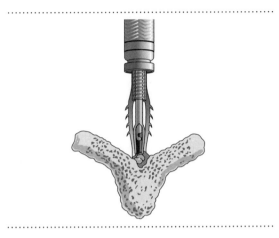

are grippers inside the device that aid in securing the valve leaflets. A steerable catheter system is used to apply the clip percutaneously to the mitral valve leaflets.[26] This device is still under investigation, but the initial results are encouraging. Importantly, surgical options are preserved for those receiving a clip percutaneously.

AORTIC VALVE

The aortic valve is a tricuspid valve located between the left ventricle and the aorta. In adults, the healthy aortic valve area is 2.6 to 3.5 cm2. The aortic valve apparatus is composed of three fibrous cusps and three connecting commissures. The three cusps have been named the left, right, and noncoronary cusps. The aortic valve is the doorway to the circulatory system, allowing the forward flow of blood into the aorta during ventricular systole and preventing regurgitation back into the left ventricle during diastole.

Aortic Stenosis

Aortic stenosis is a valvular lesion primarily affecting adults in the sixth and seventh decade of life. The etiology can be congenital, degenerative, and occasionally rheumatic. Congenital aortic stenosis can result from unicuspid, bicuspid, or even tricuspid valves. Unicuspid aortic valves are usually diagnosed in infancy, and they are often fatal. A bicuspid aortic valve is often undetected in childhood, because the valve is not usually stenotic at birth and the abnormality is not seriously restrictive. Progressive valvular narrowing occurs due to the architectural abnormality, leading to turbulent blood flow, commissural fusion, fibrosis, and calcification. Congenital tricuspid aortic stenosis is due to differences in size between the cusps that causes turbulent blood flow and subsequent commissural fusion and calcification.

Aortic stenosis acquired in adulthood is known as degenerative, or senile, aortic stenosis. The force required to eject blood through the aortic valve for distribution throughout the body causes a high degree of mechanical stress. This normal "wear and tear" results in calcium deposition along the base flexion lines of the valve cusps, effectively immobilizing them. This calcium deposition can extend to the mitral valve annulus and coronary arteries. Cusp calcification without commissural fusion in degenerative aortic stenosis prevents the normal opening of the valve during systole.

Rheumatic aortic stenosis results in a thickening of the cusps, fusion of the valve commissures, and calcium deposition; this usually occurs in patients under 40 years of age.[27] Rarely is rheumatic aortic stenosis an isolated disease. Generally, it occurs in combination with mitral and tricuspid valve disease. The aortic valve is usually not as significantly affected by the rheumatic process.

Symptoms of aortic stenosis begin subtly. Often, a routine physical examination reveals the characteristic murmur. An echocardiogram is then performed to complete the diagnosis. Patients with aortic valve areas greater than 1.5 cm2 and a pressure gradient less than 20 mmHg are usually asymptomatic.[28] In mild asymptomatic aortic stenosis, symptoms may take 5 to 15 years to develop before treatment is required. The principal signs and symptoms include fatigue, dyspnea on exertion, chest discomfort, and syncope.

Symptoms result from the compensatory attempts of the heart to maintain an adequate CO. These changes occur gradually. Initially, the left ventricle hypertrophies, which increases the pressure against the aortic valve, forcing it to open. As the narrowing continues, the pressure gradient between the aorta and the left ventricle increases. The aortic stenosis then leads to left ventricular dilatation, left atrial enlargement, an increase in pulmonary vascular pressures, and an increase in right-sided heart pressures culminating in left- and right-sided heart failure.

These hemodynamic findings are evidenced clinically by dyspnea on exertion and generalized fatigue. Syncope results from a fixed CO or dysrhythmia.[29] Left ventricular oxygen consumption is increased due to the increased contractile force and ventricular mass. This mismatch among the left ventricular mass, the oxygen it requires, and a fixed blood supply may lead to angina. On angiography, 50% of aortic stenosis patients experiencing angina have no evidence of significant coronary disease.[30] Usually, relief of anginal symptoms is gained with treatment of the valve disease.

The hemodynamic signs include elevated LVEDP, increased LAP, pulmonary capillary wedge pressure, right ventricular pressure and right atrial pressure, and a decrease in CO. Once a critical narrowing is reached (i.e., an aortic valve area of less than 0.75 cm2 and a pressure gradient of 50 mmHg or greater) without treatment, the survival period is estimated at 2–3 years.[28]

The physical examination findings develop as the degree of stenosis increases. In the beginning, a systolic ejection sound or "click" is heard as the valve attempts to open. As the stenosis increases, a harsh crescendo-decrescendo murmur is heard in mid-systole. As the narrowing becomes severe, the second heart sound may become inaudible. For mild aortic stenosis, the murmur is heard best at the apex or second right intercostal space. Once the aortic stenosis becomes severe, the murmur may be heard in the neck and shoulders.

The diagnostic tests used to confirm the diagnosis include an M-mode and 2-D echocardiogram with a Doppler study and a chest X-ray. The echocardiogram will differentiate the presence of a congenital abnormality, the degree of left ventricular hypertrophy and dilatation, and any additional chamber involvement. The degree of calcification will be seen and any supra- or subvalvular disease will be appreciated. Signs of rheumatic heart disease can also be assessed.

The aortic valve area can be measured using Doppler. The Doppler examination is also used to calculate the transaortic pressure gradient and the presence and severity of valvular regurgitation. The aortic valve is clearly visualized with the transthoracic echocardiogram, therefore, a TEE is not usually indicated. The chest X-ray may show chamber enlargement, valvular calcification, and pulmonary vascular congestion.

Once the clinical and diagnostic information has been evaluated, a decision is made regarding therapeutic treatment options. Presently, surgical aortic valve replacement is the mainstay of therapy.[31] However, percutaneous therapy is beneficial in certain situations.

Percutaneous Aortic Valvuloplasty

The first percutaneous treatment of aortic stenosis was performed on children in 1983.[32] Percutaneous balloon therapy for aortic stenosis results in an increase in valve area and CO, with a decrease in the transvalvular pressure gradient. Clinically, patients often obtain relief of symptoms, but the results are not long lasting. A procedure that began with great enthusiasm is now met with lukewarm regard as recurrent stenosis within 24 months after valvuloplasty has limited its use. However, for patients in cardiogenic shock, with severe left ventricular failure or who are considered high risk for surgery, balloon aortic valvuloplasty remains an important adjunct warranting consideration.

Technique

As with all interventional valve procedures, a left and right heart catheterization is first performed. Once the coronary anatomy has been assessed and the diagnostic pressure measurements have been obtained, the procedure can safely begin. A 0.035 inch or 0.038 inch extra-stiff wire is used to exchange the diagnostic sheath for a larger 12.5F sheath. Most patients are given 5000 IU of heparin at this stage. A balloon of about 20–25 mm in diameter is then used to cross the aortic valve in a retrograde fashion. A transeptal approach can be used, although generally the valve can be crossed without difficulty and transeptal puncture is not required.

It is important to cross the valve in a timely fashion, because most patients cannot tolerate the added procedure time when crossing is diffi-cult. There are various catheters designed to assist with crossing a stenotic aortic valve, and there is also a dedicated triple balloon (Trefoil) that has been designed specifically for valvuloplasty. It consists of three parallel-mounted balloons that form a triangle when viewed in cross-section. This design maintains blood flow even during inflation.

Due to the force of ventricular ejection during systole, maintaining the initial balloon position midway across the valve can be difficult. To correct for this, some operators are utilizing rapid right ventricular (RV) pacing during the critical seconds needed for device placement. Rapid RV pacing causes a decrease in cardiac output and blood pressure, which reduces the pulsatile flow against the aortic valve during balloon placement. This technique should be considered if difficulty is encountered while trying to successfully engage the aortic valve during valvuloplasty.

Diluted contrast medium administered via a large syringe is used to inflate the balloon. The syringe is connected to the balloon with a high-pressure stopcock. A smaller 10 cc syringe connected to the side arm of the stopcock is used to give a last thrust of pressure at the end of each inflation. This is how maximal inflation pressure is delivered to the balloon. Occasionally, two operators are necessary to time and deliver the inflation successfully. As an alternative, dedicated inflation devices for large balloons can be used.

Once the inflation is completed, the balloon is immediately withdrawn from the aortic valve before full deflation has occurred in an attempt to minimize the ventricular ectopy and hypotension caused by the inflation. Repeat inflations are performed until a successful result is achieved. Repeated inflations under high pressure may result in balloon rupture, which is not uncommon. If rupture occurs, the balloon and the sheath may have to be removed as a unit. Sometimes, a new sheath is required even without balloon rupture. The stretching and deformity of the balloon during the procedure may make it difficult to fully

Figure 21-8. Aortic valvuloplasty.

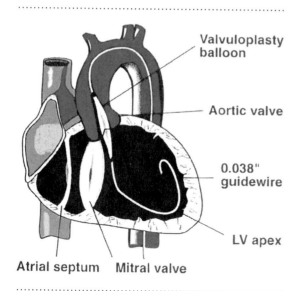

Valvuloplasty balloon

Aortic valve

0.038" guidewire

LV apex

Atrial septum   Mitral valve

withdraw it through the sheath after the procedure is completed. For safety reasons, it may be necessary to take out the whole system and replace the sheath.

Procedural success is achieved in almost all patients with percu taneous therapy and are comparable to valve replacement therapy, minus the risks of surgery.

The greatest limitation of aortic valvuloplasty is its lack of procedural durability. Most patients experience a return to the preprocedural valve area and clinical symptoms within hours or 6–18 months postprocedure.[33] The mechanism used to achieve valve opening (fracture of the calcific nodules) leads to fibrous tissue accumulating in the fissures produced by the balloon. The healing process results in scar tissue formation, which again produces a functionally stenotic aortic valve.

Complications

The potential risks of the procedure include perforation, arrhythmias, embolic events, damage to the valve itself, and femoral site complications.[34,35] The balloon used to perform the procedure is bulky and has a sharp tip. During manipulation, it is possible to perforate the ventricular wall with either the balloon itself, or the guide wire used to place the balloon catheter. Perforation occurs in 1%–3% of cases, with cardiac tamponade resulting from a perforation occurring in 1% of cases.[36]

The bundle of His and the atrioventricular node are located directly adjacent to the aortic valve annulus. As the balloon is inflated, it may impinge upon the conduction system, causing complete heart block.[37] Pacing may be required and should be anticipated with any preexisting bundle branch block. Permanent pacing is seldom required postprocedure.

Damage to the valve resulting in aortic regurgitation is rarely seen. TIA or stroke occur in 1%–3% of patients.[38] This is due to the use of guide wires and catheters, which can be thrombogenic.

The use of multiple catheters, wires, and large French sheaths may result in trauma to the femoral artery. Treatment of the access site may include additional bed-rest time to allow the groin to heal or surgical repair of the damaged artery. Hematomas and blood transfusions from arterial bleeding is reported in 10%–20% and 5%–15% of patients, respectively.[38] Careful attention to the site during sheath removal and postprocedure monitoring of the site by the nursing staff will minimize complications.

The in-laboratory mortality rate for the procedure is 1%.[38] The hospital mortality is higher and depends on the types of patients selected for therapy. Percutaneous balloon treatment is often performed as a bridge to surgical valve replacement. The procedure is performed to provide improvement in hemodynamic values, allowing a patient to undergo replacement therapy with less surgical risk. Also, patients who are deemed nonsurgical candidates may benefit from valvuloplasty by achieving an improved quality of life with little mortality risk from the procedure.[39]

Although percutaneous balloon aortic valvuloplasty for aortic stenosis is clearly not superior or equal to aortic valve replacement, there still remains a population of patients who benefit from the procedure.

Percutaneous Aortic Valve Replacement

The risk of cardiac surgery increases with advanced age and comorbidities such as kidney disease, diabetes, congestive heart failure, previous cardiac surgery, and/or previous stroke.[40] Prognosis with medical therapy alone is very poor, complicated by frequent hospitalizations for heart failure, and has a 30%–50% 1-year mortality rate. In addition, balloon valvuloplasty has not proven to have good long-term results and is appropriate in only a subset of patients. Therefore, the need for other percutaneous treatment options remains. Percutaneous aortic valve replacement is being developed to treat symptomatic, severe aortic stenosis in individuals who are considered high risk for surgery or are not candidates for traditional aortic valve replacement (AVR) surgery.

The first percutaneous valve implantation in a human was performed in 2000.[41] The device was a bovine jugular vein valve sewn onto a large metal stent and crimped onto a deflated 18 mm balloon catheter. The valve was delivered through the femoral vein of a 12-year-old boy with a stenotic prosthetic pulmonary conduit. Advanced through the venous circulation to the location of the right ventricle to pulmonary conduit, the balloon expandable stent valve device was implanted resulting in relief of the stenosis.

The first percutaneous aortic valve replacement was performed in 2002.[42] Percutaneous aortic valve replacement is currently investigational and is being developed to treat symptomatic, severe aortic stenosis in individuals who are considered high risk for surgery or are not candidates for traditional AVR surgery. This therapy may

prove to be a treatment option with less risk and a shorter recovery period than traditional valve surgery, with longer lasting results than aortic valvuloplasty.

Presently, there are two investigational devices that are currently in clinical trials, the Edwards Sapien (from Edwards, Inc. of Irvine, CA) in the United States, and CoreValve (from CoreValve of Paris, France) in Europe and Canada. The Edwards Sapien device is a trileaflet valve made from bovine pericardium, which is the same as the bioprosthetic leaflet material used in bioprosthetic surgical devices. The percutaneous valve leaflets are attached to a stainless steel stent, either 23 or 26 mm in diameter.

Procedure

The procedure is currently performed in the CCL under general anesthesia with the aid of fluoroscopy and transesophageal echocardiography. To minimize LV contraction and prevent ejection of the balloon-mounted device during the critical seconds needed for device placement, a short period of rapid burst RV pacing at a rate of 170–220 is performed. This technique mimics ventricular tachycardia and results in a temporary decrease in BP and cardiac output, thereby reducing pulsatile flow against the valve during device implantation. A short trial run of rapid RV pacing while monitoring arterial pressure should be performed in advance of actual device implantation.

Figure 21-9. Edwards Sapien valve. *Source:* Adapted from Edward Lifesciences.

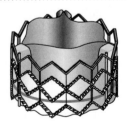
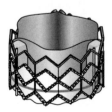

Figure 21-10. Rapid right ventricular pacing at 170–220 beats per minute. *Source:* Courtesy of T. Feldman, MD.

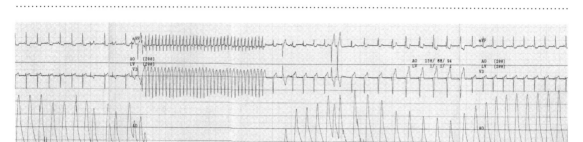

Valvuloplasty with rapid RV pacing is performed to predilatate the valve before device implantation. The valvuloplasty balloon is then removed, and the right femoral artery is dilated up to 22F or 24F to allow the passage of the large, long arterial sheath that is positioned beyond the iliac vessels into the distal aorta.

Immediately prior to insertion into the large arterial sheath, the valve device is crimped onto a deflated aortic valvuloplasty balloon catheter using a special crimping tool. The balloon-mounted device catheter is inserted into a specially designed delivery catheter. The catheter is large and stiff, but has active flexion of its tip, allowing for navigation around the aortic arch and into the valve. The delivery catheter is advanced through the aorta and the balloon and device are positioned above the valve.

To reduce the chance of device dislodgement, rapid pacing is not discontinued until the device has been expanded in the valve orifice and the balloon pulled back from within the device into the ascending aorta. Fluoroscopy, aortic root angiography, and transthoracic and transesophageal echocardiography are used to evaluate device placement, the amount of aortic valve regurgitation, and the existence of a paravalvular leak from gaps between the stent struts and the native aortic valve.

Following device placement, a pigtail catheter is advanced over a wire into the LV and peak and mean systolic pressure gradients between the AO and the LV are recorded to measure the reduction in gradient achieved by device implantation. Right heart hemodynamics and cardiac output are measured and compared to those preprocedure.

Figure 21-11. Fluoroscopy image of catheter and device.

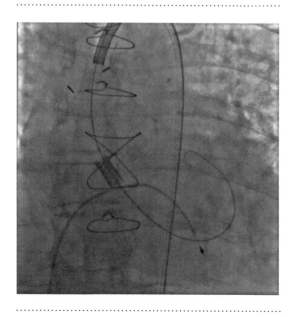

Figure 21-12. Hemodynamics of aortic stenosis, pre- and post-therapy. PBMV: Percutaneous balloon aortic valvuloplasty; Ao: Aortic pressure; LV: Left ventricular pressure; AVG: Aortic valve gradient; AVA: Aortic valve area.

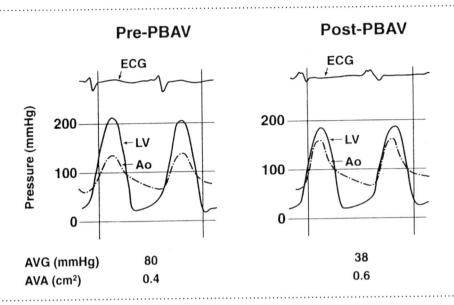

	Pre-PBAV	Post-PBAV
AVG (mmHg)	80	38
AVA (cm²)	0.4	0.6

Complications

The potential risks of this procedure are similar to those associated with aortic valvuloplasty and include cardiac perforation, arrhythmia or heart block, embolic events, damage to the valve and vascular complication, hypotension and LV failure related to aortic balloon inflation, and infection. Patients who become hemodynamically unstable require intravenous pressor support with phenylephrine infusion, epinephrine boluses, and/or dopamine infusion. Sustained ventricular arrythmias may require cardioversion and antiarrythmic administration. Device dislodgement or embolization can occur and may require surgical retrieval.

The most frequent complications are vascular, resulting from use of the large arterial sheaths. Consequently, covered stents, arterial occlusion balloons, and standby vascular surgery are all needed to support these procedures. Overnight bed rest is necessary for groin access site stabilization and patient safety postanesthesia. Groin access sites must be monitored for bleeding or hematoma forma-

tion. The right groin will have a dressing in place from surgical removal of the large arterial sheath.

PULMONIC VALVE

The pulmonic valve is a tricuspid valve located between the right ventricle and the pulmonary artery. In adults, the pulmonic valve is similar in size to the aortic valve and measures 2–4 cm2. The pulmonic valve is composed of three cusps and three connecting commissures. The pulmonic valve allows the return of unoxygenated blood from the circulatory system back to the lungs for reoxygenation.

Pulmonic Stenosis

Pulmonic stenosis is a congenital abnormality often diagnosed on physical examination immediately after birth or during early childhood. During this period, physical examination reveals the prominent systolic murmur and parasternal thrill. Congenital pulmonic stenosis is due to fusion of the valve cusps during development, resulting in doming of the valve and narrowing of the orifice, with the leaflets remaining thin and pliable.[43] In a small percentage of patients, pulmonic stenosis can be attributed to a carcinoid lesion or rheumatic heart disease. Malignant carcinomas may lodge into the right ventricular outflow tract, causing constriction of the valve ring and fusion of the valve cusps.[44] Although rare, rheumatic heart disease can lead to thickening of the valve cusps, fusion of the commissures, and calcium deposition.

Symptoms of pulmonic stenosis are due to restriction of the right ventricular outflow tract. In children, the initial symptoms are cyanosis and dyspnea on exertion.[43] Critical stenoses in children, causing right ventricular failure may necessitate early intervention. Otherwise, treatment can be delayed. Although some children exhibit symptoms early in childhood, others remain asymptomatic until adolescence or adulthood. Eventually, as the disease progresses, symptoms will manifest. In adults, fatigue, dyspnea on exertion, syncope, and chest discomfort may occur. As the obstruction to flow continues, signs of right and left ventricular heart failure develop.

The obstruction to forward blood flow causes an increase in chamber pressure, which effectively forces the stenotic valve open and leads to right ventricular hypertrophy. In addition to hypertrophy, there is dilatation of the right atrium and right ventricle.[44] Eventually, the lack of forward flow leads to clinical symptoms. Unavailability of the oxygenated blood needed to complete activities leads to fatigue and dyspnea. A low CO develops due to the backup of blood in the periphery. Chest discomfort or pain may occur because of right ventricular ischemia.

The hemodynamic signs of pulmonic stenosis include an elevated right atrial and right ventricular pressure with a decrease in PAP, pulmonary capillary wedge pressure, and CO. A pressure gradient will exist between the right ventricle and pulmonary artery. The severity of the disease can be assessed by measuring the gradient. A gradient of < 40 mmHg is considered mild pulmonic stenosis, a gradient of 40–80 mmHg is considered moderate, and a gradient > 80 mmHg is considered to be severe.[45]

In adults, physical examination reveals a hyperdynamic right ventricle with a palpable thrill. Auscultatory findings include a wide splitting of S2 due to delayed valve closure. There is a systolic ejection murmur heard best at the left sternal border. The intensity of the murmur increases with inspiration. Initially, the murmur is heard late and loud in systole. As the severity of the stenosis increases, the murmur moves closer to S1 and softens.[46] Eventually, when there is little valvular opening, the murmur and the second heart sound may be absent. The obstruction to forward blood flow also results in peripheral venous engorgement (i.e., jugular venous distention, liver and abdominal enlargement, and severe peripheral edema).

The tests used to confirm the diagnosis of pulmonic stenosis include an M-mode echocardiogram with a Doppler study and a chest radiograph. An ECG may reveal right ventricle hypertrophy. The echocardiogram will delineate the degree of valvular stenosis, any congenital abnormalities, and any subvalvular involvement. The echo Doppler study will reveal the presence and severity of valvular regurgitation; the transvalvular pressure gradient can be calculated, and the valve area can be measured. The echocardiogram will also reveal signs of rheumatic heart disease. The diameter of the valve annulus is measured to aid selection of the proper balloon size if valvuloplasty is planned. The chest X-ray will reveal dilatation of the pulmonary artery and right ventricular enlargement. An ECG may show signs of right axis deviation because of right ventricular hypertrophy and P wave abnormalities because of right atrial enlargement.

Once the clinical information is obtained, a decision is made regarding treatment. The time for treatment depends on symptom progression.

Often, treatment occurs in childhood. In a small number of patients, symptom progression does not warrant treatment until adulthood. Among children and adults, percutaneous balloon dilatation is the treatment of choice if the valve is not dysplastic or there is no subvalvular stenosis.

Pulmonic Valvuloplasty

The first percutaneous pulmonic valvuloplasty procedures were performed in 1982.[47] The procedure is similar to that of aortic valvuloplasty, but is somewhat easier to perform because it is within the lower pressured right side of the heart. The success of the procedure in both children and adults is well documented.[48] Pulmonic valvuloplasty is the treatment of choice in patients diagnosed with pulmonic stenosis. The procedure can be performed safely without risk of severe complications, and long-term clinical data look promising.

Procedure

The pulmonic valvuloplasty procedure begins with a diagnostic left and right heart catheterization. In adults over the age of 40, the existence of coronary artery disease is assessed and treated, if necessary, prior to the valvuloplasty procedure. Supportive right heart catheterization data is collected (i.e., right atrial pressure, right ventricular pressure, PAP, pulmonary capillary wedge pressure, and CO). A right ventriculography is performed to evaluate the level of the obstruction and the size of the pulmonic valve annulus, and the transvalvular pressure gradient is measured.

Once the diagnostic information has been collected, the valvuloplasty procedure can safely begin. IV heparin is administered, and a 12.5F venous sheath is inserted into the right femoral vein. The pulmonic annulus measurement is used as a guide in selecting the appropriate balloon; a balloon-to-artery ratio of 1.0:1.2 is considered ideal.[49]

Antegrade access to the pulmonic valve is achieved with a 0.035–0.038 inch extra-stiff guide wire. The wire is introduced into the sheath and positioned forward across the pulmonic valve. The distal end of the wire is left safely out in a branch of the pulmonary artery. Once the wire is in place, the balloon is passed over the wire, across the pulmonic valve. The Inoue balloon can be used for this procedure as well as the single- or double-balloon technique.[45] The Trefoil balloon, which maintains blood flow during the procedure, can also be used for pulmonic valvuloplasty.

Diluted contrast medium, connected via a high-pressure stopcock, is used to inflate the balloon. If a Trefoil balloon is not used, the inflation time is kept to less than 10 seconds, which helps prevent complications from occlusion of the right ventricular outflow tract. After each inflation, the balloon is withdrawn from the valve to allow the patient to recover and the hemodynamic effects to be evaluated. Additional inflations are performed until the desired result is obtained (usually a drop in the right ventricular pressure to less than half of the initial value).

Evaluation of the transvalvular pressure gradient postinflation is used to judge the success of the procedure. A procedure in which the gradient is decreased to < 35 mmHg is considered a success.[45] Once the procedure is complete, the balloon is removed and repeat hemodynamic measurements are taken.

Complications

The risks of the procedure are similar to those for the other valve procedures. The potential risks include perforation, damage to the valve, damage to the pulmonic valve, embolic events, and vascular compromise. The risk of major complications (i.e., death, stroke, or perforation) amount to less than 1%.[50] The occurrence of vascular compromise is 8%–10%.[45] Pulmonary valve regurgitation is clinically of little importance because of the minimal diastolic pressure gradient difference between the pulmonary artery and the right ventricle.

TRICUSPID VALVE

The tricuspid valve is a trileaflet valve located between the right atrium and right ventricle. In adults, the tricuspid valve measures 7 cm2. The tricuspid valve apparatus is composed of the three leaflets (referred to as the anterior, posterior, and septal leaflets), the chordae tendineae, and the papillary muscles. The chordae tendineae and papillary muscles provide the pulling mechanism necessary to keep the tricuspid valve in place. The tricuspid valve allows the oxygen-depleted blood returning from the peripheral circulatory system to pass from the right atrium into the right ventricle, and on to the lungs for reoxygenation.

Tricuspid Stenosis

Tricuspid stenosis is an uncommon valvular lesion, most often the result of rheumatic heart disease. The mitral and aortic valves are the principal valves affected by the rheumatic process, with tricuspid stenosis occurring in addition to the other valvular disease rather than by itself. The disease primarily occurs in adults, with women 30 to 60 years old most commonly affected.[44]

The rheumatic changes to the tricuspid valve resemble those seen with the mitral valve, but with less severity. With rheumatic tricuspid stenosis, there may be fusion of the valve commissures, fusion, and thickening of the leaflets and thickening and shortening of the chordae tendineae. Calcification is rarely present.[44] Other causes of tricuspid stenosis are rare and have congenital or carcinoid origins.

The symptoms of tricuspid stenosis occur as the result of the increase in pressure needed to force blood forward from the right atrium into the right ventricle through the stenotic valve. The impedance to forward flow results in right-sided

atrial hypertrophy and dilatation. Symptoms are noted when the valve area falls to 2 cm2 or less.[44]

Symptoms include fatigue, dyspnea on exertion, and peripheral edema.[30] There may be added symptoms due to the effects of the rheumatic disease on the other valves. Despite a concomitant presence of tricuspid and mitral stenosis, the symptoms of pulmonary congestion typical for mitral stenosis patients (i.e., hemoptysis, orthopnea, and pulmonary edema) are often not found. The limited forward flow available to the left side of the heart masks the mitral stenosis, and these symptoms are minimized.

Physical examination of these patients reveals an elevated jugular venous pressure, and signs of venous engorgement due to fluid retention.[51] There may be visible pulse waves in the neck due to the large "A" wave seen in the jugular vein. Auscultation reveals a diastolic murmur heard best at the left sternal border, at the fourth or fifth intercostal space. The murmur has a crescendo-decrescendo pattern ending before S1, increasing in intensity with inspiration. There may also be an OS due to leaflet tension. The auscultatory findings must be identified and separated from the findings resulting from the mitral and aortic valves.

The diagnostic testing used to evaluate the presence and severity of tricuspid stenosis includes an M-mode and 2-D echocardiogram with a Doppler study, a TEE, a chest X-ray, and an ECG. The echocardiogram will show evidence of right-sided chamber enlargement and reduced excursion of the tricuspid valve leaflets. The valve area can also be measured during the echocardiogram. The M-mode and 2-D echocardiogram is technically limited when evaluating the tricuspid valve, but a Doppler study can evaluate and document a transvalvular pressure gradient. In contrast to the mitral valve gradient, the tricuspid valve gradient is usually quite minimal. However, the presence of a transvalvular gradient as small as 2 mmHg can confirm the diagnosis and a gradient greater than 5 mmHg can elevate the right atrial pressure, resulting in noticeable symptoms.[44] A TEE is performed to view the tricuspid valve in detail. To better quantify the size of the tricuspid valve orifice, the transvalvular pressure gradient and the presence of valvular regurgitation, a TEE is necessary.

The chest X-ray may reveal right-sided chamber enlargement and prominence of the superior vena cava. The ECG may show right atrial enlargement, evidenced by tall peaked P waves in leads II, III, and AVF.[30] There are usually no ECG signs of right ventricular hypertrophy.

Once the history, physical and supportive diagnostic testing are complete, a decision is made regarding treatment. Presently, in the presence of tricuspid regurgitation or additional valve disease, surgery is the treatment of choice, while balloon valvuloplasty remains the best treatment option for isolated tricuspid stenosis.[52] There has been limited usage, however, because of the rarity of the disease. The double balloon technique has been performed most frequently, with good success. The technique is similar to the other valvuloplasty procedures.

REFERENCES

1. Nkomo V, Scott C, Sarano M. Prevalence of valvular heart disease in Olmsted County. *J Am Soc Echocardiog* 2005;18:500.
2. Wilkins GT, Weyman AE, Abascal VM, et al. Percutaneous balloon dilatation of the mitral valve: an analysis of echo-cardiographic variables related to outcome and the mechanism of dilatation. *Br Heart J* 1988;60:299–308.
3. Brunton L. Preliminary note on the possibility of treating mitral stenosis by surgical methods. *Lancet* 1902;1:352.
4. Cutler EC, Beck CS. The present status of the surgical procedures in chronic valvular disease of the heart. *Arch Surg* 1929;18:403–416.
5. Souttar HS. The surgical treatment of mitral stenosis. *BMJ* 1925;2:603–606.
6. Harken DE, Ellis LB, Ware PF, Norman LR. The surgical treatment of mitral stenosis, I: valvuloplasty. *N Engl J Med* 1946;239:801–809.
7. Ben Farhat M, Ayari M, Betbout F, et al. Percutaneous balloon versus surgical closed and open mitral commissurotomy: short and long term results. *J Am Coll Cardiol* 1993;21:428A.
8. Iung B, Cormier PD, Porte JP, et al. Immediate results of percutaneous mitral commissurotomy. A predictive model on a series of 1514 patients. *Circulation* 1996;94:2124–2130.
9. Bueno R, Andrade P, Nercolini D, et al. Percutaneous balloon mitral valvuloplasty vs open mitral valve commissurotomy: results of a randomized clinical trial. *J Am Coll Cardiol* 1993;21:429A.
10. Cardoso LF, Grinberg M, Rati MA, et al. A randomized study of open mitral commissurotomy versus balloon valvuloplasty for selected patients: immediate and one year follow-up results. *J Am Coll Cardiol* 1996;27:259A.
11. Reyes VP, Raju BS, Wynne J, et al. Percutaneous balloon valvuloplasty compared with open surgical commissurotomy for mitral stenosis. *N Engl J Med* 1994;331:961–967.
12. Patel JJ, Shama D, Mitha AS, et al. Balloon valvuloplasty versus closed mitral commissurotomy for pliable mitral stenosis: a prospective hemodynamic study. *J Am Coll Cardiol* 1991;18:1318–1322.
13. Ben Farhat M, Ayari M, Maatouk F. Percutaneous balloon verses surgical closed and open mitral commissurotomy. *Circulation* 1998;97:245–250.
14. Feldman T, Herrmann HC, Rothbaum DA, et al. Late outcome after percutaneous mitral commissurotomy: six year results of the N. American Inoue balloon registry. *J Am Coll Cardiol* 1997;29:226A.
15. Holloway S, Feldman T. An alternative to valvular surgery in the treatment of mitral stenosis: balloon mitral valvotomy. *Crit Care Nurse* 1997;17:27–36.
16. Feldman T. Hemodynamic results, clinical outcome, and complications of Inoue balloon mitral

valvotomy. *Cathet Cardiovasc Diagn* 1994;Suppl 2:2–7.

17. Pan M, Medina A, Suarez de Lezo J, et al. Cardiac tamponade complicating mitral balloon valvuloplasty. *Am J Cardiol* 1991;68:802–805.

18. Manga P, Singh S, Brandis S. Left ventricular perforation during percutaneous balloon mitral valvuloplasty. *Cathet Cardiovasc Diagn* 1992;25:317–319.

19. Complications and mortality of percutaneous balloon mitral commissurotomy: a report from the National Heart, Lung, and Blood Institute balloon valvuloplasty registry. *Circulation* 1992;85:2014–2024.

20. Vahanian A, Palacios I. Percutaneous approach to valvular disease. *Circulation* 2004;109:1572–1579.

21. Bassand JP, Schiele F, Bernard Y, et al. The double-balloon and Inoue techniques in percutaneous mitral valvuloplasty: comparative results in a series of 232 cases. *J Am Coll Cardiol* 1991;18:982–989.

22. Sharma S, Loya YS, Desai DM, Pinto RJ. Percutaneous mitral valvotomy using Inoue and double balloon technique: comparison of clinical and hemodynamic short term results in 350 cases. *Cathet Cardiovasc Diagn* 1995;29:18–23.

23. Park SJ, Kim JJ, Park SW, et al. Immediate and one year result of percutaneous mitral balloon valvuloplasty using Inoue and double balloon techniques. *Am J Cardiol* 1993;71:938–943.

24. Galloway AC, Colvin SB, Baumann FG, Grossi EA, Ribakove GH, Harty S, Spencer FC. A comarison of mitral valve reconstruction with mitral valve replacement: intermediate-term results. *Annals of Thoracic Surgery* 1989;47:655–662.

25. Alfieri O, Maisano F, DeBonis, et al. The edge to edge technique in mitral valve repair: a simple solution for complex problems. *J Thoracic Cardiovascular Surgery* 2001;122:674–681.

26. Feldman T, Wasserman HS, Herman H, et al. Percutaneous mitral valve repair using the edge-to-edge technique: six month results of the EVEREST phase 1 clinical trial. *J Am Coll Cardiol* 2005;46:2134–2140.

27. Braunwald E. Valvular heart disease. In: Braunwald E, ed. *Heart Disease: A Textbook of Cardiovascular Medicine*, Vol. 2, 5th ed. Philadelphia: WB Saunders; 1997:1007–1076.

28. Khan G. Valvular heart disease and rheumatic fever. In: Khan G, ed. *Heart Disease Diagnosis and Therapy: A Practical Approach*. Baltimore: William & Wilkins; 1996:415–460.

29. Abramaczyk E, Brown M. Valvular heart disease. In: Kinney M, Packa D, Andreoli K, Zipes D, eds. *Comprehensive Cardiac Care*, 7th ed. St. Louis, MO: Mosby Year Book; 1991:327–342.

30. Rackley C. Valvular heart disease. In: Bennett JC, Plum F, eds. *Cecil Textbook of Medicine*, 20th ed. Philadelphia: WB Saunders; 1996:319–327.

31. Lind O, Magnussen K, Knudsen M, et al. The potential for normal long term survival and morbidity rate after valve replacement for aortic stenosis. *J Heart Valve Dis* 1996;5:258–267.

32. Lababidi Z. Aortic valvuloplasty. *Am HeartJ* 1983;106:751–752.

33. Feldman T, Glagov S, Carroll JD. Restenosis following successful balloon valvuloplasty: bone formation in aortic valve leaflets. *Cathet Cardiovasc Diag* 1993;29:1–7.

34. Percutaneous balloon aortic valvuloplasty: acute and 30-day follow-up results in 674 patients from the NHLBI Balloon Valvuloplasty Registry. *Circulation* 1991;84:2383–2397.

35. Lewin RF, Dorros G, King JF, Mathiak L. Percutaneous transluminal aortic valvuloplasty: acute outcome and follow-up of 125 patients. *J Am Coll Cardiol* 1989;14:1210–1217.

36. Isner JM. Acute catastrophic complications of balloon aortic valvuloplasty: the Mansfield Scientific Aortic Valvuloplasty Registry Investigators. *J Am Coll Cardiol* 1991;17:1436–1444.

37. Carlson MD, Palacios I, Thomas JD, et al. Cardiac conduction abnormalities during percutaneous balloon mitral or aortic valvuloplasty. *Circulation* 1989;79:1197–1203.

38. Feldman T, Carroll J. Cardiac catheterization, balloon angioplasty, and percutaneous valvuloplasty. In: Wood L, Hall J, Schmidt G, eds. *Principles of Critical Care Medicine*. New York: McGraw-Hill;1992:343–360.

39. Bernard Y, Etievent J, Mourand J, et al. Long term results of percutaneous valvuloplasty compared with acute valve replacement in patients more than 75 years old. *J Am Coll Cardiol* 1992;20:796–801.

40. Peterson ED, Cowper P, Jollis J, et al. Outcomes of coronary artery bypass graft surgery in 24,461 patients aged 80 years or older. *Circulation* 1995;92:85–91.

41. Bonhoeffer P, Boudjemline Y, Saliba Z, et al. Percutaneous replacement of pulmonary valve in a right ventricle to pulmonary artery prosthetic conduit with valve dysfunction. *Lancet* 2000;356(9239):1403–1405.

42. Cribier A, Eltchaninoff H, Bash A, et al. Percutaneous transcatheter implantation of an aortic valve prosthesis for calcific aortic stenosis: first human case description. *Circulation* 2002;106:3006.

43. Friedman W. Congenital heart disease in infancy and childhood. In: Braunwald E, ed. *Heart Disease: A Textbook of Cardiovascular Medicine*, 4th ed. Philadelphia: WB Saunders; 1992:887–965.

44. Braunwald E. Tricuspid, pulmonic, and multivalvular disease. In: Braunwald E, ed. *Heart Disease: A Textbook of Cardiovascular Medicine*, Vol. 2, 5th ed. Philadelphia: WB Saunders; 1997:1054–1076.

45. Plauth W. Pulmonary valve stenosis. In: Hurst JW, ed. *Current Therapy in Cardiovascular Disease*, 3rd ed. Philadelphia: BC Decker; 1991:115–120.

46. Stapelton J. Clinical aspects of non-rheumatic valvular disease. In: Chizner M, ed. *Classic Teachings in Clinical Cardiology*. Cedar Grove, NJ: Laennec; 1996:1017–1048.

47. Kan JS, White RI, Mitchell SE, Gardner TI. Percutaneous balloon valvuloplasty: a new method for treating congenital pulmonary valve stenosis. *N Engl J Med* 1982;307:540–542.

48. Fawzy ME, Galal O, Dunn B, Shaikh A, Sri-ram R, Duran CM. Regression of infundibular pulmonary stenosis after successful balloon pulmonary valvuloplasty in adults. *Cathet Cardiovasc Diagn* 1990;21:77–81.

49. Narang R, Das G, Dev V, Goswami K, Saxena A, Shrivastava S. Effect of the balloon-anulus ratio on the intermediate and follow-up results of pulmonary balloon valvuloplasty. *Cardiology* 1997;88:271–276.

50. McCrandle BW, Kan JS. Long-term results after balloon pulmonary valvuloplasty. *Circulation* 1991;83:1915–1922.

51. Segal B. Clinical recognition of rheumatic heart disease. In: Chizner M, ed. *Classic Teachings in Clinical Cardiology*. Cedar Grove, NJ: Laennec; 1996:991–1015.

52. Sharma S, Loya YS, Desai DM, Pinto RJ. Percutaneous double-valve balloon valvotomy for multivalve stenosis: immediate results and intermediate-term follow-up. *Am Heart J* 1997;133:64–70.

SUGGESTED READING

Bonow O, Carabello K, DeLeon AC, et al. ACC/AHA 2006 guidelines for the management of patients with valvular heart disease. Executive summary. *Circulation* 2006;114:450–527.

Sorrentino MJ. Valvular heart disease. In: Wood L, Hall J, Schmidt G, eds. *Principles of Critical Care Medicine*, 2nd ed. New York: McGraw-Hill; 1998:467–482.

Hermann HC. Balloon valvuloplasty: indications, techniques, and results. In: Pepine C, Hill J, Lampert CR, eds. *Diagnostic and Therapeutic Cardiac Catheterization*, 3rd ed. Baltimore: William & Wilkins; 1998:764–786.

Chapter 22

ENDOMYOCARDIAL BIOPSY

Arlene Ewan, RN

HISTORICAL PERSPECTIVE

In 1958, Weinberg, Fell and Lynfield documented the myocardial and pericardial biopsy of five patients whose lack of specific symptoms hindered a definite diagnosis.[1] An incision in the fourth left intercostal space allowed cartilage resection while pleura reflection revealed the pericardium, enabling biopsy of the epicardium and myocardium. Two of these patients were found to have myocardial disease; one patient had lupus myocarditis, and amyloidosis could be excluded in another patient. However, the type of incision and surgical extraction necessary to the procedure prevented its widespread use.

In 1960, Sutton and Sutton documented 150 biopsies from 54 patients who were suffering from cardiomegaly or idiopathic myocardial disease. Sutton commented that diagnostic information (such as specific etiology or pathological diagnosis) was fundamental to the management of myocardial disease, and this information

formed the foundation of treatment.[2] However, inadequate tissue recovery often hindered a specific diagnosis. Timmis and colleagues undertook biopsy collection in 20 canine models. Adequate diagnostic tissue specimens were produced in 43 of 71 (60.5%) attempts.[3]

In 1965, Bulloch, Murphy, and Pearce introduced a heart biopsy needle designed for the biopsy of the right ventricle, inserting the needle into the right external or internal jugular vein. They highlighted the need for a routine biopsy technique that was reliable, easy to undertake and associated with low morbidity and low mortality. Several procedural principles of endomyocardial biopsy described in this paper are still in use today. These include percutaneous access, using the right external or internal jugular vein, definition of right heart boundaries prior to biopsy and advancement of the tip toward the interventricular septum.[4]

The era of modern transvenous endomyocardial biopsy began in Japan. In 1962, Konno and

Sakakibara developed a new technique for performing endomyocardial biopsy using a bioptome catheter. Endomyocardial sampling was performed by a "pinch" rather than the previous needle or incision biopsy methods. They successfully obtained 10 biopsy specimens from five patients, and a specific diagnosis was established for three patients. The Konno bioptome was large and very rigid, and required brachial artery cutdown for insertion. This bioptome enabled adequate multiple tissue sampling and gained acceptance due to safety and convenience.[5]

In 1972, Shirey and associates reported a series of left ventricular biopsies, obtaining 254 specimens from 198 people. Tissue sample size was adequate, and the biopsy of the unselected population revealed a non-specific diagnosis in nearly 50% of the cases. The authors concluded that the role of biopsy in patients suffering from cardiac disorders of diffuse etiology was minor.[6]

Following kidney transplantation, serial needle biopsy of the transplanted kidney allowed the histological diagnosis of graft allograft rejection.[7] Techniques for the biopsy of the human heart had been described previously, but the use of these methods following cardiac transplantation had not been established. Caves and associates successfully performed percutaneous endomyocardial biopsy in 20 dogs following orthotopic cardiac transplantation.[8]

In 1973, Caves and his colleagues documented the further use of serial endomyocardial biopsy in patients following orthotopic cardiac transplantation. Sixty-seven endomyocardial biopsies were performed in 17 heart transplant recipients. Complications were minimal; supraventricular arrhythmias occurred in two patients. The modified bioptome and new technique were simple and safe, ensured the ease of specimen sampling, allowed repeated periodic biopsies, and were associated with minimal patient discomfort. Biopsy results were accurate, and it was now possible to identify histological changes of allograft rejection prior to the associated functional changes of the transplanted heart.[9]

Within four decades endomyocardial biopsy has evolved from a primitive surgical technique to a routine percutaneous procedure that is safe and relatively free of pain.

BIOPTOMES

Bioptomes in use today are radiopaque, have stainless steel cutting jaws, are flexible, and promote ease of use by the operator (see Figure 22-1). Bioptomes are available in a variety of diameters, including a 9F, for right internal jugular vein or right subclavian vein access, and a 7F, for femoral vein cannulation. The length of bioptomes also differs and is determined by the venous approach undertaken. A bioptome approximately 50 cm long is used for neck access, and a bioptome approximately 100 cm long is used for femoral cannulation. The size of the endomyocardial biopsy specimen taken can also vary. The standard biopsy device in use in the United States and the United Kingdom is the Caves-Shultz bioptome. The basic structure and function of the bioptome has not changed radically, although modifications have occurred; for example, Kawai in 1980 designed a bioptome that enabled intracardiac monitoring.[10]

Bioptomes are either disposable or reusable. Disposable bioptomes are sterilized by ethylene oxide gas and designed for single use only. They are also preformed or preshaped to facilitate right ventricle entry. Manufacturers warn that they cannot guarantee the structural and functional integrity of the bioptome if used more than once. Likewise, due to difficulties with cleaning, adverse patient reactions may occur if the bioptome has been exposed to biological material through previous usage.

Prior to sterilization, reusable bioptomes must be cleaned thoroughly. Particular attention should be given to cleaning the biopsy jaws. Manufacturers recommend regular maintenance programs to prevent bioptome failure.

Figure 22-1. Biopsy forceps (bioptome). *Source:* Diagram courtesy of Cordis, a Johson and Johnson Company.

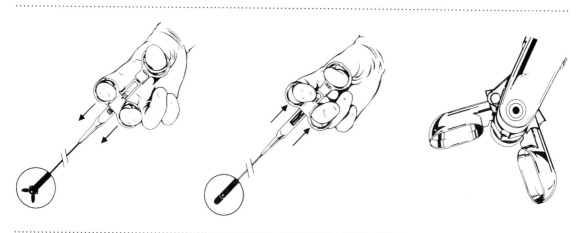

INDICATIONS FOR ENDOMYOCARDIAL BIOPSY

Endomyocardial biopsy is performed when a sample of cardiac tissue is needed to confirm or aid a diagnosis. Indications for endomyocardial biopsy include:

- Evaluation and management of allograft rejection
- Evaluation and management of idiopathic or drug-induced cardiomyopathy
- Evaluation and management of idiopathic ventricular arrhythmias
- Evaluation and management of restrictive or constrictive heart disease research

Cardiac disorders that can be diagnosed by endomyocardial biopsy are:

- Immune or inflammatory disease
- Degenerative cardiac disease

Initially, endomyocardial biopsy was considered a potentially valuable asset in providing essential diagnostic information regarding cardiac disease. The number of potential specific diagnoses that can be made from endomyocardial bi-opsy is large. However, the frequency of finding a causative agent is relatively small.[11]

Today the most common indication for endomyocardial biopsy is the detection and surveillance of allograft rejection following orthotopic or heterotopic cardiac transplantation. Endomyocardial biopsy also enables the mapping of the severity of histological changes within the transplanted heart and the monitoring of the effectiveness of rejection therapy. Non-invasive investigations are also available to assist in the diagnosis of rejection, but they are not as specific or as sensitive in accurately detecting rejection.

An initial stumbling block during the early days of heart-lung transplantation was the mistaken belief that the rejection of the transplanted heart and lungs would occur simultaneously. Findings highlighted that specimens from the endomyocardial biopsy of the heart showed no signs of rejection, while at the same time the function of the transplanted lungs deteriorated. Several theories have been put forward, including speculation that myocardial tissue is protected from rejection episodes or that pulmonary changes are detected earlier than those of the heart. Studies have also documented that episodes of rejection following combined heart-lung transplant occur less frequently. The role of endomyocardial biopsy following heart-lung transplantation is now limited in most centers.[11]

The frequency of routine surveillance endomyocardial biopsy is determined by each institution, and this may vary between patients. Since rejection is most common in the first few weeks following transplantation, endomyocardial biopsy is performed the most frequently then, usually weekly. Thereafter, the frequency is gradually reduced to biweekly, monthly, every 3 months, every 6 months and eventually annually.

PROCEDURE

Endomyocardial biopsy of the right or left ventricle can be performed using any one of the standard bioptomes currently available. Right ventricular endomyocardial biopsy can be performed via the right internal jugular vein, right subclavian vein, right femoral vein, or left femoral vein. Left ventricular biopsy can be performed using retrograde entry through the right femoral artery or left femoral artery.

Endomyocardial biopsy of the right ventricle via the internal jugular vein is the standard approach following cardiac transplantation. Cannulation of the right internal jugular vein is relatively simple, allows the serial introduction of the bioptome and carries minimal complications.

Hearts transplanted heterotopically are a challenge. The appropriate venous approach is partly determined by the angle of the anastomosis (donor right atrium and the recipient right atrium or superior vena cava). Left subclavian or left femoral veins are the preferred approaches.

Endomyocardial biopsy is undertaken in the cardiac catheterization laboratory with electrocardiographic monitoring and fluoroscopy control.

Patient Preparation

Informed consent is obtained. Preparation of the patient prior to endomyocardial biopsy may differ from center to center. Investigations (e.g., chest radiograph, electrocardiograph, echocardiogram) and premedication prior to the procedure are not routine unless clinically indicated. It is not always necessary for the patient to be NPO, in fact, some centers encourage fluids prior to biopsy to increase venous pressure.

Once the patient is in the laboratory, his ECG and blood pressure is monitored. The patient's head is turned to the left 30°–45°. The right side of the neck is prepped, a sterile field established, the right internal jugular vein identified, and the area anaesthetized. Once the anesthetic has taken effect, a small incision is made in the skin, and a needle is inserted. A guide wire is inserted through the needle into the superior vena cava, and a sheath is inserted over the guide wire. The guide wire should not be advanced into the right ventricle because this may initiate ventricular premature beats.

The bioptome is introduced into the sheath with the jaws closed and advanced to the right atrium. It is then rotated counterclockwise, whereupon it crosses the tricuspid valve. It should not be forced. Once inside the right ventricle, the rotation continues counterclockwise, and the tip is positioned near the interventricular septum. This is confirmed by the appearance of premature ventricular contractions on the ECG. The right ventricular free wall is only 1–2 mm thick, and biopsy of this wall could result in perforation. The position of the bioptome should also be verified by fluoroscopy.

Once the position has been confirmed, the bioptome is withdrawn 1–2 cm and the jaws opened. It is slowly advanced to engage the septum or the apex (avoiding the free wall), and the jaws are closed gently and slowly to obtain the myocardial specimen.

The bioptome should be carefully removed to prevent tension or inadvertent advancement. The specimen is removed gently from the bioptome forceps using a small needle or wet filter paper. The bioptome should be cleaned and wiped free of blood and tissue residue prior to another biopsy attempt (check the manufacturer's recommendations). The sheath should also be flushed often.

Pathologists report that previous biopsy sites are hard to identify and consist of small areas of mural thrombus. However, repetitive biopsies may lead to endomyocardial fibrosis and histological interpretation of specimens may be hindered as a result.[12] Visual examination of the specimen obtained by an experienced operator may help to reduce the incidence of fibrotic tissue taken.

If the biopsy is undertaken for diagnosis of infiltrative disease, biopsies should be taken from different endomyocardial sites as the pathological changes associated with infiltrative disease often occur in small localized areas. Histological changes associated with rejection occur globally.

To reduce the incidence of sampling error, a minimum of three biopsy specimens should be obtained from the right ventricle. A 9F bioptome gathers tissue samples of 2–3 mm in diameter. It has been documented that three biopsy specimens from a 9F bioptome result in a 5% false-negative biopsy error, while a 2% false-negative biopsy error is predicted from four specimens. The smaller the bioptome used, the smaller the tissue sample taken. Five to six specimens are required from a 7F bioptome to reduce sampling error. The International Society of Heart and Lung Transplantation has strict criteria and recommends that four to six biopsy specimens be taken depending on the investigations required and the size of the bioptome used.

Tissue specimens are placed in a formalin (10%) solution as soon as possible following the biopsy procedure to reduce the amount of contraction artifact. Formalin is kept at room temperature.

After fixation and processing, the biopsy tissue is embedded into paraffin wax (which allows for easier slicing). The sample is cut into thin slices (4–5 microns) and mounted onto slides for further evaluation. If an urgent diagnosis is needed, the biopsy tissue is frozen and then mounted onto slides (frozen section).

If allograft rejection is suspected, the following additional information should be included:

- Date and type of cardiac transplant
- Routine surveillance biopsy or urgent (if the patient is unwell)
- Presence of any clinical signs or symptoms suggestive of rejection
- Level of the patient's immunosuppression

If the patient is in for her yearly outpatient control, the following will also be performed:

- Coronary angiogram
- Right heart pressure measurements
- Complete blood and platelet count (because the patients are immunosuppressed)
- Cyclosporine level
- Renal/metabolic panels (cyclosporine is renal toxic and contrast media adds additional insult to kidney function)
- Prothrombin time/international normalized ratio (if these are prolonged, vitamin K is usually given, or the case rescheduled)

During the more frequent, earlier controls, the blood tests will normally be performed prior to the biopsy.

Complications

Virtually all complications relating to transvenous endomyocardial biopsy occur during the procedure itself. Complications include right ventricular perforation and pericardial tamponade, ventricular arrhythmias, supraventricular arrhythmias, transient heart block, pneumothorax, arterial puncture, nerve paresis, and venous hematoma formation. The appropriate emergency equipment should always be at hand and in working order in case these complications occur.

Right Ventricular Perforation and Pericardial Tamponade

The greatest risk associated with endomyocardial biopsy is right ventricular perforation that may lead to pericardial tamponade. Perforation results from the biopsy of the right ventricular free wall rather than the interventricular septum. Pericardial tamponade following ventricular perforation is rare, but its true incidence is not known.

Patients complaining of pain during the biopsy should be closely monitored, and biopsy attempts should be halted until the origin of the pain has been identified. An echocardiogram may be of benefit in determining pericardial accumulation. Cardiovascular collapse or electromechanical dissociation occurring during a biopsy procedure should be considered pericardial tamponade until the possibility has been excluded.

A pericardiocentesis tray should be immediately available. Reaccumulation of blood within the pericardial space may require insertion of a drain.

The risk of right ventricular perforation is reduced by carefully confirming the position of the bioptome prior to the biopsy. The bioptome is directed perpendicular to the interventricular septum (the bioptome handle is directed posteriorly or from the left shoulder to the right scapula). A septal contraction may be palpable on the bioptome shaft once the septum is engaged. Fluoroscopy should be used.

Ventricular Arrhythmias

Premature ventricular contractions are anticipated and considered to be normal during positioning of the bioptome. Short bursts of ventricular couplets or triplets occur routinely. These arrhythmias are usually self-terminating or resolve once the bioptome has been withdrawn. Sustained ventricular arrhythmias require pharmacological or electrical cardioversion. Antiarrhythmic drugs and a defibrillator should be within easy access whenever a biopsy procedure is underway.

Supraventricular Arrhythmias

During endomyocardial biopsy, the bioptome passes through the right atrium. Contact with the atrial wall is frequent, and this irritation of the atrial wall may cause atrial premature contractions or, rarely, sustained supraventricular arrhythmia. An atrial arrhythmia can be terminated by the removal of the bioptome (or sheath) from the right atrium. If the atrial arrhythmia is sustained, medical therapy (such as adenosine) should be initiated.

Heart Block

As with any procedure involving right heart manipulation, pressure against the interventricular septum may result in right bundle branch block and intraventricular conduction delay. Inappropriate biopsies (such as tissue taken high from the intraventricular septum) can result in intraventricular conduction delay. Care should also be taken in patients who have preexisting left bundle branch block and who then sustain right bundle branch conduction delay, as they may develop complete heart block. Complete heart block is transient, however, and usually resolves once the antegrade conduction pathways have returned.

Removal of the bioptome from the right ventricle may resolve the conduction delay. If the conduction delay persists, temporary pacing is indicated. Because of the risk of conduction delay or damage, continuous ECG monitoring should be undertaken throughout every biopsy. Access to temporary pacing (transvenous pacemaker and generator) is recommended.

Pneumothorax

The right lung is at risk of pneumothorax during endomyocardial biopsy when the venous access site is the internal jugular vein or the right subclavian vein. The risk of pneumothorax can be reduced by avoiding the apical pleura, by performing the jugular puncture in the mid-neck area and by the careful exchange of needles, sheaths, and guide wires into the venous port.

Arterial Puncture

The internal jugular vein and the subclavian vein lie adjacent to the carotid artery and the subclavian artery. An anomaly in anatomy or an incorrect technique can result in arterial puncture rather than venous access. If arterial puncture occurs with the probing needle, the needle should be removed and gentle but firm pressure applied to achieve hemostasis. Arterial puncture from a large instrument (e.g., a sheath) may require a vascular surgical referral or surgical opinion prior to sheath removal. The development of carotid insufficiency symptoms demands the immediate removal of the sheath. Usually the arterial puncture heals spontaneously. Gentle but firm pressure is applied for 15 to 20 minutes. The patient is observed for 24 hours.

Nerve Paresis

Infiltration of local anesthetic into the area surrounding the internal jugular vein may result in Horner's Syndrome, vocal cord paresis or, rarely, temporary diaphragmatic weakness. These complications can last for 1–2 hours provided that they are due to the local anesthetic and not to nerve damage caused by a needle. The risk can be lessened by avoiding the carotid sheath, limiting the deep infiltration technique and limiting the quantity of anesthetic given to reduce the chance of it dissemination into the surrounding tissue.

Venous Hematoma

This can result from excessive movement of the venous sheath by the operator resulting in excessive venous oozing, inadequate compression of the puncture site following sheath removal or venous bleeding as a result of high venous pressure. This complication is not life threatening, but it can significantly hinder future attempts at internal jugular vein cannulation.

POST-BIOPSY PROCEDURE

Following completion of the biopsy procedure, the sheath is removed. Firm pressure is applied to the venous cannulation site for 2–3 minutes or until hemostasis is achieved. Patients with arterial cannulation require pressure to the arterial site for 20–30 minutes or until hemostasis. A sterile dressing is placed over the puncture site, and this dressing is removed 24 hours later. A chest radiograph or other investigations post biopsy are not routine unless clinically indicated.

Patients returning to a hospital room following right internal jugular or subclavian venous biopsy can return to normal activities. Maintaining an upright position (such as sitting up) will help to reduce the risk of bleeding or oozing from the biopsy site. The patient's pulse and blood pressure are monitored and recorded every 15 minutes for 1 hour. Patients may eat after 1 hour.

Patients who have undergone femoral venous biopsies should remain supine 2–4 hours before ambulating. If arterial cannulation is undertaken, patients must remain supine for 4–6 hours (depending on the gauge of sheath used), and frequent observation of vital signs is necessary to detect bleeding or hemodynamic change.

Outpatient venous biopsy is common, particularly for transplant patients. These patients require observation for 1 hour, and then they may return home.

Nursing Care

The staff involved in endomyocardial biopsy include the physician, nurse, cardiology technician, and radiology technician. Not every laboratory may use such an extensive staff roster, and in some laboratories, staff working within the laboratory may serve multiple functions.

The nurse should be familiar with the equipment (guide wires, sheaths, bioptomes) and the individual procedural complexities of endomyocardial biopsy. In addition, the nurse must be familiar with the laboratory design and layout, exhibit an understanding of the principles of aseptic technique and radiation safety and have developed a working knowledge of cardiovascular medications.[13] All staff involved in endomyocardial biopsy should wear lead aprons during the procedure.

Prior to the biopsy, specific nursing responsibilities include:

- Ensuring that the defibrillator is in working order
- Checking the supply and expiration dates of emergency and stock medications
- Checking the resuscitation cart and equipment (oxygen therapy, suction equipment, intubation equipment)
- Checking the location of the pericardiocentesis tray and the temporary pacing box

The nurse prepares the patient by:

- Greeting the patient on arrival
- Ensuring that documented informed consent is in the patient's medical notes
- Checking the results of any prebiopsy investigations ordered and reporting any abnormalities
- Answering the patient's questions as needed
- Positioning the patient supine on the X-ray table

During the biopsy, the nurse will:

- Assist the physician with the initial preparation (gown and gloving)

- Assist with the draping of the patient; the drape on the patient's left side is usually placed over a frame so that the patient's head is not completely covered
- Prepare any medications or flush solutions as needed or requested
- Record the dosage and time of any medication given to the patient

After completion of the biopsy, the nurse should:

- Organize the patient's return to the nursing unit
- Assist the patient from the table
- Ensure the correct labelling of the endomyocardial specimens and arrange for their transfer to the pathology laboratory
- Ensure that the post-biopsy investigations are ordered where necessary
- Discard all non-reusable material (sharps disposal), wearing rubber gloves. Reusable material should be collected for cleaning and sterilization
- Complete the log book or hospital documentation as necessary

Standard local practices should be followed in addition to, or in place of, the preceding general guidelines.

REFERENCES

1. Weinberg M, Fell EH, Lynfield J. Diagnostic biopsy of the pericardium and myocardium. *AMA Arch Surg* 1958;76:825–829.
2. Sutton DC, Sutton GC. Needle biopsy of the human ventricular myocardium: review of 54 consecutive cases. *Am Heart J* 1960;60:364–370.
3. Timmis GC, Gordon S, Baron RH, Brough AJ. Percutaneous myocardial biopsy. *Am Heart J* 1965;70(4):499–504.

4 Bulloch RT, Murphy ML, Pearce MB. Intracardiac needle biopsy of the ventricular septum. *Am J Cardiol* 1965;16:227–233.

5. Sakakibara S, Konno S. Endomyocardial biopsy. *Jpn Heart J* 1962;3:537–543.

6. Shirey EK, Hawk WA, Mukerji D, Effler DB. Percutaneous myocardial biopsy of the left ventricle. Experience in 198 patients. *Circulation* 1972;46:112–122.

7. Kincaid-Smith P. Histological diagnosis of rejection of renal allografts in man. *Lancet* 1967;2:849–852.

8. Billingham ME, Caves PK, Dong E Jr, Shumway NE. The diagnosis of canine orthotopic cardiac allograft rejection by transvenous endomyocardial biopsy. *Transplant Proc* 1973;5:741–743.

9. Caves PK, Stinson EB, Billingham M, Shumway NE. Percutaneous transvenous endomyocardial biopsy in human heart recipients. *Ann Thorac Surg* 1973;16:325–336.

10. Baumgartner WA, Reitz BA, Achuff SC, eds. *Heart & Heart-Lung Transplantation*. Philadelphia: WB Saunders, 1990.

11. Cernaianu AC, DelRossi AJ, eds. *Cardiac Surgery: Current Issues* 4. New York: Plenum; 1995.

12. Shumway SJ, Shumway NE. *Thoracic Transplantation*. Cambridge, MA: Blackwell Science; 1995.

13. Lubell D. *The Cath Lab: An Introduction*, 2nd ed. Philadelphia: Lea & Febiger; 1993.

SUGGESTED READING

Williams BAH, Grady KL., Sandiford-Guttenbeil DM, eds. *Organ Transplantation: A Manual for Nurses*. New York: Springer, 1991.

Williams BAH, Sandiford-Guttenbeil DM, eds. *Trends in Organ Transplantation*. New York: Springer; 1996.

Chapter 23

ELECTROPHYSIOLOGY

Elizabeth A Ching, RN, CCDS, FHRS
Stephanie Lavin, RN, BSN
Henry L. Blair, C-CPT

Intracardiac electrophysiology is the study of the heart's conduction system, examined by placing electrode catheters inside the heart's chambers. These catheters may also be used to stimulate the heart in order to reproduce the arrhythmia causing the patient's clinical symptoms and to ablate the focus of the arrhythmia.

An invasive cardiac electrophysiology study (EP or EPS) is undertaken to evaluate the cardiac conduction system in order to relate associated findings with the patient's clinical symptomatology. It is performed using a systematic approach and can be diagnostic or therapeutic. Diagnostic purposes include locating and defining patterns of arrhythmogenic substrates, assessing antiarrhythmic drug efficacy or proarrhythmia, and evaluating current rhythm control therapy. The most common therapeutic purpose of an EP study is to identify the location of arrhythmogenic substrates in order to alleviate them with radiofrequency catheter ablation.

Patients undergoing EPS range in age from neonates with supraventricular tachycardia (SVT) to patients with ventricular arrhythmias following a myocardial infarction. The indications for an electrophysiology study include syncope/presyncope, ventricular tachycardia (VT), SVT, Wolff-Parkinson-White syndrome, and the evaluation of antiarrhythmic medication effectiveness or ability to cause proarrhythmia.

There are many terms that are specific to the EP. These are listed in the glossary at the back of this book.

HISTORY

Cardiac electrophysiology was introduced by the French in 1945 when Lenegre and Maurice first reported recording electrical activity from inside the heart of humans.[1] In 1967, the concept of intracardiac mapping during open-heart surgery was introduced,[2] quickly followed by successful surgical ablation of an accessory pathway in 1968.[3]

In 1969, Scherlag and colleagues described today's technique for recording His bundle activity utilizing an electrode catheter.[4] Many more advances were made during the early 1970s, with clinical applications that led to the first series of patients undergoing intracardiac radiofrequency catheter ablation (RFCA) in 1991.[5] This was an important advancement, because it allowed a cure for selected arrhythmias without the need for open-heart surgery or chronic antiarrhythmic drug therapy.

Catheter ablation was introduced in the early 1980s as a treatment for poorly controlled, drug refractory atrial fibrillation. The procedure was performed in conjunction with implantation of a permanent pacemaker. It was carried out using direct current shocks to the His bundle area causing complete heart block. These initial ablations were very crude when compared to today's, very high-tech procedures that use activation mapping and electro-anatomical mapping systems that can perform single-beat localization of the offending area within the heart. These exacting measurements and today's improved quality of ablation catheters enable the medical staff to destroy small pathways within the heart, rather than the whole His bundle.

ELECTROPHYSIOLOGY

The overall goal of ablation is to destroy the function of the conductive tissue within the heart that is causing an arrhythmia. Radiofrequency (RF) catheter ablation is the most common type of ablation performed. It is a low-voltage, high-frequency current, which is transmitted through an electrode catheter to a specific area of the heart to destroy arrhythmogenic tissue. The tissue must be heated to at least 50° Centigrade to render it devitalized. Because the indifferent electrode has a much larger surface area than the catheter electrode tip, there is only minimal heat production at the puncture site. Targeted cardiac tissue is destroyed by thermal injury using the principle of resistive heating. The tip itself does not heat, but passes on energy in the form of heat to the tissue. This localized heating is the same mechanism used in a variety of household appliances, such as toasters.

The amount of RF energy applied varies according to the location of the arrhythmogenic tissue within the heart. The duration of energy application is dependent on lesion size and site, and can range from 10–120 seconds. RF energy forms scar tissue around the catheter's electrode tip. The heat dries out the tissue and causes tissue death resulting from lack of blood. The lesions created with RF energy are well defined and homogeneous, and they are unlikely to be arrhythmogenic. The depth of the lesion will be determined by catheter contact and orientation of the tissue.

The source of energy is provided by an RF generator. RF energy levels of 1 to 60 watts may be achieved with most RF generators. The same energy is used for localized cautery in surgical procedures.

Equipment

The catheterization laboratory and its staff members must be prepared prior to the performance of electrophysiologic testing. In many institutions, there is no stand-alone electrophysiology laboratory, so the catheterization laboratory is used to perform EPS. The equipment necessary for performing an EPS includes:

- Multipurpose recorder
- Programmable stimulator
- Electrode catheters
- Junction box

The multipurpose recorder must be capable of instant replay and long-term storage and should have the ability to record at least six electrical channels (18 are preferred) with a paper speed of 100 to 500 mm/sec. A minimum of three channels (13 is preferred) must be free of current leakage and must allow filtering of waveforms of greater than or equal to 250 to 500 Hz and less than 30 to 50 Hz. Additionally, two to four channels to record surface electrocardiograms are needed. The filter settings should have a lower limit of DC and an upper limit of 200 Hz. To ensure optimal recordings, the electrophysiology/catheterization laboratory should be free of 50- and 60-Hz interference. Once positioned, two to five electrode catheters are connected to the recorder via a junction box, which can have up to 12 channels. The junction box also allows pacing and recording from a variety of sites within the heart.

Either a battery or a wall socket can power the programmable stimulator. If it is powered from the wall socket, an optical isolation device should be used to ensure that there is no current leakage from the stimulator to the patient. A pulse width of 1 to 2 ms and an output of 0.5 to 20 mA along with a variety of pacing modes should also be available. A pacing rate of 600 ppm should be attainable.[6] Although there are a multitude of vendors who can provide this equipment, it is also possible to customize a computer to perform stimulation protocols, automatically measure intervals, and generate a final report.

A multitude of introducers and electrode catheters should be available. In general, a 5F to 7F catheter is used in adults, while smaller sizes may be needed in the pediatric population.

In addition to the equipment just listed, the ability to document a 12-lead ECG is a must. A blood pressure monitoring system is also critical, whether it is manual, automatic, or via an arterial line. Some catheterization laboratories may use invasive arterial lines to constantly monitor blood pressure in select patients. Transcutaneous pulse oximetry is also vital.

The following emergency equipment should be readily available:[7]

- Oxygen
- Suction

- Biphasic defibrillator (and a backup device in case the first one fails), preferably one that can externally pace
- External pacemaker (if not part of the defibrillator)
- Resuscitation cart stocked with the necessary IV equipment, fluids, supplies, emergency drugs, surgical back-up in case of perforation, and airway management equipment. Airway management equipment should include a bag and mask, endotracheal tubes in a variety of sizes, laryngoscope handle, laryngoscope blades, batteries, suction, oral airways, and various oxygen delivery systems. A full range of medications should be available, including, but not limited to, cardiac medications, sedation and sedation reversal agents, local anesthetics, and a variety of emergency medications (e.g., epinephrine and sodium bicarbonate).

Personnel

Individuals working in the catheterization and/or electrophysiology laboratory should possess a basic understanding of sterile technique, infection control measures, and radiation safety, both for themselves and for the patient. All personnel should be proficient in basic life support measures. Airway management proficiency is a must in the event of respiratory complications related to hemodynamic compromise or secondary to the administration of sedative agents. It is optimal for all personnel to be educated in advanced life support maneuvers, which may include courses for neonates (NALS), children (PALS), and adults (ACLS).

The personnel caring for patients undergoing electrophysiology testing should have an understanding of basic electrocardiography and common arrhythmias. The effects of these arrhythmias (i.e., their potential hemodynamic sequelae) must be understood so they can be prepared for. Knowledge of all medications likely to be used, both cardiac and noncardiac, is vital for all personnel.

It is essential for individuals working in the electrophysiology laboratory to have a basic understanding of each procedure and its potential complications. Certain induction protocols may result in arrhythmias, causing hemodynamic compromise. Nursing and technical staff must be conversant regarding these protocols and be prepared for emergency situations before they arise.

PROCEDURE

A multitude of catheters (from two to five) can be placed in the heart to record electrical activity. These catheters are generally made of woven Dacron. They come in a variety of shapes and sizes and are steerable. The number of electrodes on the catheter tip varies from 3 to 14, with variable electrode spacing. Quadripolar catheters are most common, with multipolar catheters being used for coronary sinus placement or mapping.

In most cases, catheter access is obtained through the femoral vein(s). Alternate sites may include the subclavian, internal jugular, and median antecubital veins. The veins of the upper body allow for superior catheter placement into the coronary sinus. If there is a need to evaluate the left side of the heart, a transseptal or a retrograde (arterial) approach may be utilized. The choice of which approach to use is generally based on the experience of the physician performing the procedure.

The catheters are generally placed in four sites:

- The atrial catheter is placed in the high right atrium (HRA) and records electrical activity in and around the sinus node (see Figure 23-1).

Figure 23-1. ECG with 12 leads recorded during electrophysiologic testing with high right atrial (HRA) electrogram. The HRA electrogram correlates with the P wave on the surface ECG.

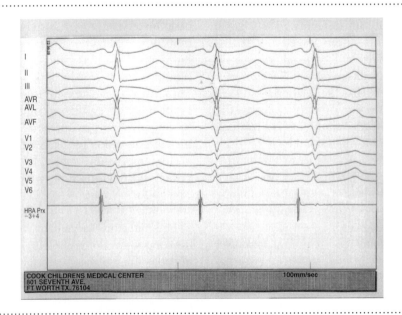

- The His bundle catheter is placed across the tricuspid valve and records the His bundle electrogram (HBE) (see Figure 23-2). It also allows recording of low atrial and ventricular activity, which allows for evaluation of AV conduction.
- The ventricular catheter is placed in the right ventricular apex (RVA) and allows electrical activity to be recorded from the base of the right ventricle (see Figure 23-3).
- The coronary sinus (CS) catheter, whether placed from above or below, records both atrial and ventricular activity from the base of the left atrium close to the AV groove (see Figure 23-4). The CS catheter also allows for retrograde atrial activation sequence determination in patients with SVT.

Occasionally catheters will be placed in the right ventricular outflow tract (RVOT), left ventricle, or left atrium, and ventricular activity is commonly recorded from two separate sites during electrophysiologic testing. The catheters are placed in their anatomic locations using single or bipolar fluoroscopy (see Figure 23-5), and a typical electrophysiologic tracing depicts surface ECG leads I, AVF, V1, and V6 along with the intracardiac electrograms (see Figure 23-6).

Resting Interval Measurements

Three intervals are commonly used in the EP lab: PA, AH, and HV.

The PA interval is an indirect measurement of atrial conduction. This is performed by measuring from the beginning of the earliest P wave activation to the rapid deflection of the atrial EGM on the HBE (see Figure 23-7). The normal PA interval ranges from 20 to 30 milliseconds.

Figure 23-2. ECG with 12 leads recorded during the electrophysiologic testing with the His bundle electrogram (HBE). There are three components to the HBE: the first deflection is low septal right atrium (LSRA) and correlates to the end of the P wave on the surface ECG; the second is the His bundle deflection (H) or "His spike" and occurs just prior to the beginnings of the QRS complex on the surface ECG; and the third is ventricular activity (V) and correlates with the QRS complex on the surface ECG.

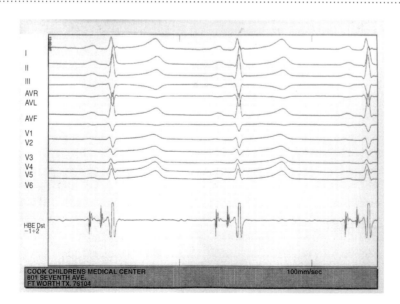

Figure 23-3. Surface ECH leads I, AVF, V1, and V6, and the right ventricular apex (RVA) electrogram. The RVA electrogram records electrical activity at the base of the RV and correlates to the QRS complex on the surface ECG.

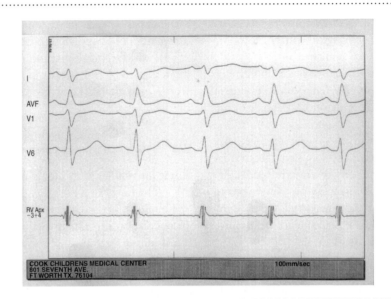

Figure 23-4. Surface ECG leads I, AVF, V1, and V6, and electrograms recorded from the coronary sinus (CS). As evidenced on the CS electrogram, electrical activity is recorded from the base of the left atrium close to the AV groove and includes both atrial and ventricular activity.

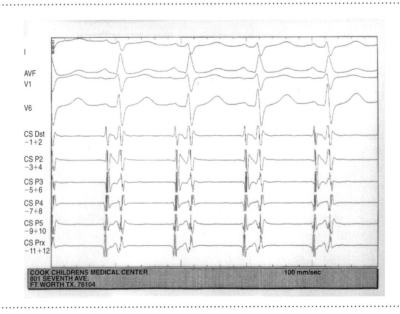

Figure 23-5. Fluoroscopic radiograph of electrophysiology catheter placement with annotation. The tip of the high right atrial (HRA) catheter is barely visible in the left side of the figure, but is placed high in the right atrium near the sinus node. This His catheter has three electrodes and is lying across the tricuspid valve. The right ventricular apex (RVA) catheter has four electrodes and is placed in the apex of the RV. All three of these catheters were placed via the right femoral vein. The fourth catheter, the coronary sinus (CS) catheter (arrow), has 10 electrodes (five pairs) and was placed from above via the left antecubital vein.

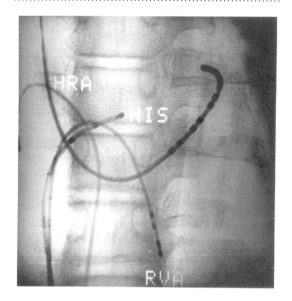

The AH interval is indicative of conduction through the AV node to the bundle of His. Measurement of the AH interval is performed by measuring from the earliest rapid deflection of the atrial EGM to the beginning of the His bundle deflection on the HBE (see Figure 23-8). Autonomic tone can cause the AH interval to vary. The normal range for the AH interval is 60 to120 milliseconds. Conduction from the bundle of His to the ventricular myocardium (or distal conduction system assessment) is manifested by the HV interval.

The HV interval is measured from the beginning of the His bundle deflection to the earli-est onset of ventricular activation on the surface ECG or the ventricular EGM (see Figure 23-9). The normal HV interval ranges from 30 to 55 milliseconds.

The LSRA-H interval is measured during intrinsic electrical activity, and is used to assess the AV node. The interval varies according to age in the pediatric population.[8,9] Additionally, these intervals vary with differing cycle length and autonomic tone. The function of the AV node can also be evaluated by determining various refractory periods (see the following section on refractory period determination).

Programmed Electrical Stimulation Protocols

Programmed electrical stimulation protocols are performed for a variety of reasons. They are used to determine sinoatrial conduction times, sinus and atrioventricular nodal conduction, and refractory periods of specific cardiac tissue. The primary goal of these protocols is to evaluate the patient's normal cardiac electrophysiology while attempting to induce any abnormal rhythms. Once the arrhythmia has been induced, the information collected can be used to determine an appropriate treatment modality. In many of the electrophysiology studies performed today, arrhythmia induction is used for "mapping," followed by the potentially curative procedure of catheter ablation.

Sinus Node Recovery Time

Sinus node function is evaluated by performing what is known as a sinus node recovery time or SNRT. The SNRT is performed by overdrive pacing the atrium at progressively faster rates than the sinus rate (cycle length) for a period of 30 seconds. The paced cycle length is decreased by 50 milliseconds each time until one of the following occurs: Wenckebach or 2:1 AV block, hypotension, or a cycle length of 300 milliseconds is reached.

Figure 23-6. Surface ECG leads I, AVF, V1, and V6, with typical introcardiac catheter placement revealing the proximal high right atrial (HRA Prx), coronary sinus (CS), His bundle electrogram (HBE), and right ventricular (RV) apex electrogram. The HRA recording, from electrodes 3 and 4, has atrial activity, but also some ventricular activity. The CS catheter, with six pairs of electrodes, starts with the distal (Dst) electrodes (1 and 2) and ends with the proximal (Prx) electrodes (11 and 12) and displays both atrial and ventricular activity, typical of CS recordings. The next three recordings are from the HBE catheter with recordings from electrodes 1 and 2, 2 and 3, and 3 and 4. The His bundle potential is most visable on the proximal (3 and 4) electrode recording. The RVA electrogram, recorded from electrodes 3 and 4, is seen last.

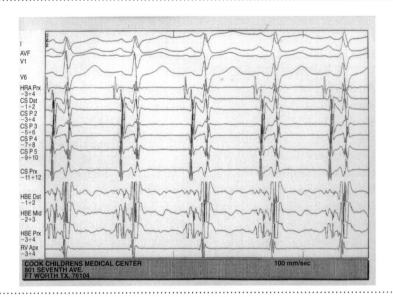

Figure 23-7. ECG with 12 leads obtained during electrophysiology testing with the His bundle electrogram (HBE) being recorded from electrodes 1 and 2. The PA interval is calculated by placing the caliper to the left at the beginning of the surface P wave, and placing the right caliper at the earliest deflection of the lower septal right atrium (LSRA) on the HBE catheter.

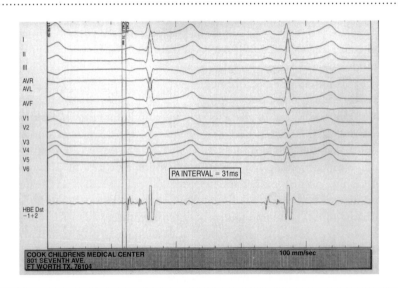

Figure 23-8. Surface ECG with 12 leads with the His bundle electrogram (HBE). The electrogram is recorded from electrodes 1 and 2 (distal) on the catheter tip. The initial deflection seen on the HBE is from the low septal right atrium (LSRA). The second deflection is the His spike and the third is ventricular activity. The AH interval (as noted with the calipers) is measured from the earliest atrial activation to the beginning of the His bundle deflection. The measurement of 89 msec is within the normal range.

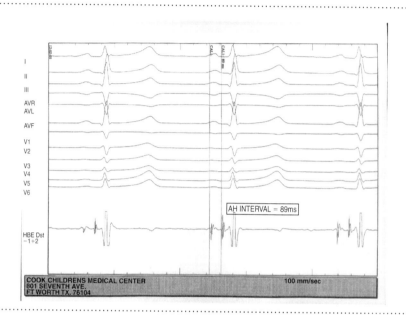

Figure 23-9. Surface ECH with 12 leads with His bundle electrogram (HBE) recorded in the same manner as in Figure 23-7. The HV interval is measured by placing the calipers at the beginning of the His bundle deflection to the earliest onset of ventricular activation. The measurement of 47 msec is within the normal range.

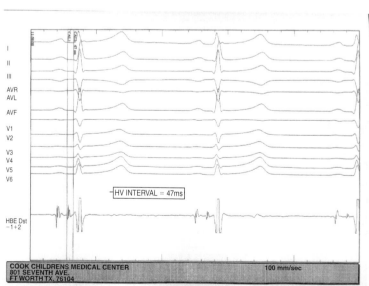

The corrected sinus node recovery time (CSNRT) is the standardized value used to measure sinus node automaticity. The CSNRT is obtained by subtracting the patient's basic sinus cycle length from the number obtained from the interval from the last paced beat to the first intrinsic sinus beat once overdrive pacing has been terminated (see Figures 23-10 and 23-11). A normal CSNRT ranges from 100 to 250 milliseconds. A CSNRT value of 600 milliseconds indicates mild dysfunction, while a CSNRT of 3 seconds or greater is indicative of severe sinus node dysfunction.

Refractory Period Determination

Refractory periods of the cardiac conduction system are determined using extrastimuli or simply, premature beats. These extrastimuli are delivered at various pacing cycle lengths and can be introduced during the patient's intrinsic rhythm or into a paced rhythm known as a drive train. Both the pacing cycle length and the pacing amplitude can affect refractoriness. The first extrastimulus is delivered at a cycle length 20 milliseconds shorter than the intrinsic or paced cycle length. Subsequent extrastimuli are decreased by 10 to 20 milliseconds until refractoriness is reached.

There are several types of refractory periods: absolute, functional, and effective. These refractory periods are used to evaluate atrial tissue, ventricular tissue, the AV node, and the His-Purkinje system as well as accessory pathways.

The absolute refractory period is the length of time from the onset of an action potential until repolarization is only one-third complete. The tissue being stimulated will be unresponsive.

The functional refractory period is a measure of how rapidly a structure can conduct from itself to another and is the minimum interval between two consecutively conducted impulses.

Figure 23-10. Surface ECG leads I, AVF, and with electrograms from the high right atrium (HRA), the His bundle electrogram (HBE), and the right ventricular apex (RVA). The PP interval is measured by placing the calipers at the beginning of the surface P wave on the atrial electrogram on two consecutive beats in the patient's resting state. The PP interval is 1128 msec.

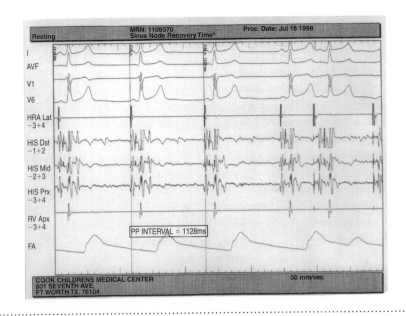

Figure 23-11. Surface ECG leads I, AVF, and V6 with electrograms from the high right atrium (HRA), the His bundle electrogram (HBE), and right ventricular apex (RVA) in the same patient as Figure 16-8. A sinus node recovery time (SNRT) is the interval from the last paced beat to the first intrinsic atrial beat (recovery beat). In order to calculate the CSNRT, the resting PP interval of 1128 msec is subtracted from the SNRT of 1232 msec, giving a corrected value of 104 msec, which is within the normal range. The pressure waveform is from the femoral artery (FA).

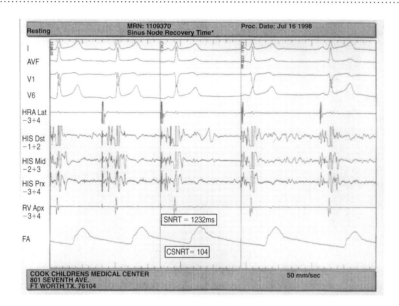

The most commonly calculated refractory period is the effective refractory period and is indicative of how fast select tissue can conduct. It is especially important in evaluating the properties of accessory pathways. It reveals the general health of the tissue being evaluated. The longer the effective refractory period, the more dilated and fibrotic the tissue might be.

The atrial muscle refractory period is determined by introducing an atrial extrastimuli into either an intrinsic or paced rhythm. Once the atrial stimulation fails to produce a response (or does not capture), the atrial tissue is considered refractory (see Figure 23-12). The effective atrial refractory period ranges from 159 to 360 milliseconds.

The AV node refractory period, used to assess AV node function, is accomplished in the same manner. Once AV node refractoriness is reached, the stimulus will capture the atrium, but will not conduct to the ventricles (Figure 23-13). The normal range for AV nodal refractory period is 230 to 425 milliseconds. In most cases, the AV node becomes refractory prior to the atrial tissue.

The ventricular muscle refractory period is determined by introducing a ventricular extra-stimuli into either an intrinsic or paced ventricular rhythm. Once this stimulus fails to capture the ventricle, the cycle length at which the extra-stimulus was delivered becomes the ventricular refractory period. The normal range is from 170 to 290 milliseconds (see Figure 23-14).

Decremental and Burst Pacing

Antegrade and retrograde conduction is assessed utilizing decremental pacing. Antegrade

Figure 23-12. Surface ECG leads I, AVF, V1, and V6, and electrograms from the high right atrium (HRA), the coronary sinus (CS), the radiofrequency catheter (RF), and the His bundle electrogram (HBE). The atrium is being paced, as evidenced on the HRA catheter. The fifth deflection on the HRA catheter does not capture the atrium. Due to prolonged AV conduction, there is delay from the atrial stimulus to the ensuring ventricular activity. By looking at the HBE, one can see by correlating the atrial pacing stimulus on the HRA to the stimulus on the HBE that no atrial activity is seen. The next deflection is that of ventricular activity that resulted from the previous paced atrial beat with prolonged conduction.

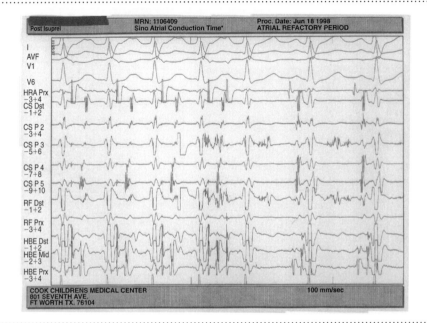

Figure 23-13. Surface leads II and III with electrograms from high right atrium (HRA) and the His bundle electrogram (HBE). The pacing artifact can be seen as S1 and S2. The two S1s stimulate and capture the atrium and conduct to the ventricles, as evidenced on the HBE. The premature beat or S2 captures the atrium, but does not conduct to the ventricles, thus the AV node refractory period has been reached. The lower curve is the femoral artery pressure (FAP).

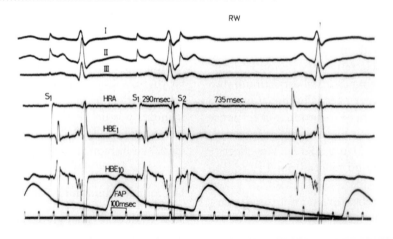

Figure 23-14. Surface ECH leads I, AVF, V1, and V6, and electrograms from the high right atrium (HRA Prx), the coronary sinus (CS), the radiofrequency catheter (RF), and the His bundle electrogram (HBE). During ventricular stimulation, one can see the ventricular pacing artifact best on the HBE catheter. The stimulus captures the heart until the fifth beat, where there is no ventricular activity on the HBE. This is known as the ventricular refractory period. The patient then has two spontaneous junctional beats, as evidenced by the atrial electrogram that is within the QRS complex.

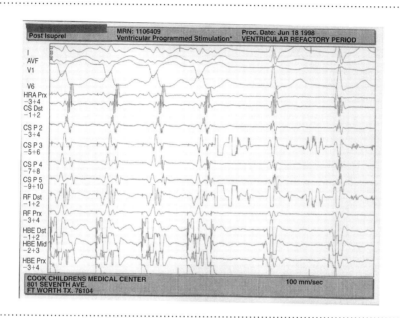

conduction is evaluated by pacing the atria from the HRA catheter at a rate slightly faster than the patient's intrinsic heart rate (see Figure 23-15). The pacing cycle length, measured in milliseconds rather than beats or pulses per minute, is gradually decreased (hence, the term decremental) until Wenckebach and/or 2:1 AV block occurs. The AH interval prolongs with faster and faster pacing rates until the atrial electrogram is no longer followed by a His bundle or ventricular electrogram. The normal Wenckebach rate ranges from 350 to 500 milliseconds.

Retrograde conduction is assessed by pacing the ventricle from the RVA (or RVOT) at a rate slightly lower than that of the patient. If retrograde conduction is present, there will be a one-to-one relationship between the ventricular and atrial electrograms (see Figure 23-16).

Burst pacing can be performed in either the atrium or ventricle. Atrial burst pacing can be used in an attempt to induce/reproduce supraventricular arrhythmias, whereas ventricular burst pacing is used to induce/reproduce ventricular arrhythmias. Generally, 8 to 10 beats are utilized for burst pacing. The initial burst cycle length is decremented by 20 milliseconds until Wenckebach or 2:1 AV block is reached.

Arrhythmia Induction

Any of the aforementioned stimulation protocols may result in an arrhythmia. There are additional protocols that may be used. Typically, arrhythmia induction begins with the least aggressive and progresses to the most aggressive protocol. As more aggressive techniques are used, the specificity of

Figure 23-15. Surface ECH leads I, AVF, V1, and V6, and the following intracardiac electrograms: high right atrium (HRA), coronary sinus (CS), a radiofrequency (RF) catheter, and a His bundle electrogram (HBE). Antegrade (from top to bottom) conduction is depicted in this tracing. The activation sequence goes from high (HRA) to low (ventricular activity on the HBE and CS catheters). The conduction progresses in a normal fashion from the sinus node, through the AV node followed by the His bundle to the ventricles.

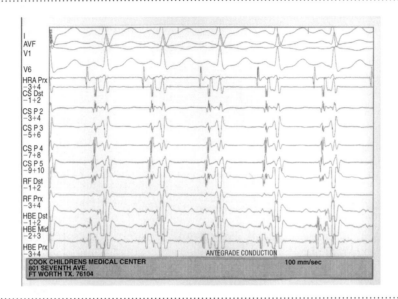

Figure 23-16. Surface ECG leads, 1 AVF, V1, and V6, and electrograms recorded from the high right atrium (HRA), coronary sinus (CS) (both distal and proximal), His bundle (HBE), and right ventricular apex (RVA). The ventricle is being paced to assess for retrograde (bottom to top) conduction. The arrows on the RVA recording are positioned to the ventricular pacing artifact. If there is 1:1 retrograde conduction, each ventricular pacing stimulus should be followed by atrial activity that can be seen on the HRA or CS electrograms. This recording depicts 1:1 retrograde conduction.

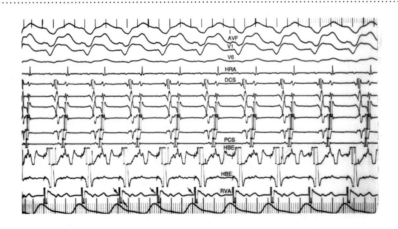

the arrhythmia induced may be decreased (i.e., it may be of little clinical significance).

In most cases, single or multiple extrastimuli are utilized first to attempt arrhythmia induction. Atrial and ventricular extrastimuli can be used; first with singles, then with doubles, and occasionally with triples. Once again, with triple extrastimuli, the specificity of the arrhythmia induced may be decreased due to the aggressive nature of the protocol.

Burst pacing is another method used for arrhythmia induction. As previously mentioned, it can be performed in the atria and ventricles. Once again, a nonclinical arrhythmia may be induced, requiring a determination of its significance, particularly if the burst cycle length is less than 200 milliseconds.

If the previous protocols do not produce an arrhythmia, isoproterenol can be utilized to simulate exercise. Isoproterenol is infused at 0.05 µg/kg/min to 0.1µg/kg/min to yield a 20%–30% increase in the patient's baseline heart rate. Once this increase has been achieved, the stimulation protocols are repeated. An additional technique, specifically for ventricular arrhythmia induction in coronary artery disease, is to move the catheter to an alternate site. For example, the RVA catheter may be repositioned to the RVOT or LV. The ventricular stimulation protocols are then repeated at the alternate site.

ARRHYTHMIAS

The electrophysiologic mechanisms demonstrated with the particular arrhythmia allow its classification. Arrhythmias can be classified as reentry, automatic, or triggered. Reentry mechanisms are the most commonly found arrhythmias. Examples of reentry arrhythmias include atrial tachycardia, Wolff-Parkinson-White, concealed bypass tract, and bundle branch reentry ventricular tachycardia. Automatic arrhythmias are usually occurring in the presence of an acute illness. Triggered arrhythmias are usually caused

by the leakage of positive ions into the cardiac cells, leading to a bump in the action potential in late Phase 3 or early Phase 4 of the action potential (PACs or PVCs). Both triggered and reentry arrhythmias are easily induced with PES (programmed electrical stimulation) in the EP lab.

Some arrhythmias are referred to as "focal." Atrial tachycardias can exist throughout the atrium and can either be focal or nonfocal in origin. The focal origins tend to be due to triggered automaticity, automaticity, and reentry. Nonfocal origins are anatomically or functionally mediated circuits or scar mediated due to congenital heart disease or surgery. The location can be left or right atrium. Nonfocal origins are anatomically or functionally mediated circuits or scar mediated due to congenital heart disease or previous cardiac surgery. Ablation therapy of ectopic atrial tachycardia (EAT) involves extensive mapping of both the right and left atrial in an effort to localize the site of earliest activation.

RADIOFREQUENCY ABLATION THERAPY

Steps taken within an ablation procedure usually include induction of the arrhythmia, mapping of the arrhythmia, ablation, and postablation attempts at arrhythmia induction.

One of the most common sites of ablation therapy is the AV Junction. RF catheter ablation of the AV junction is used to produce complete AV block for atrial tachyarrhythmias with uncontrolled ventricular rates (e.g., atrial fibrillation). Either the right- or left-sided approach can be used when ablating the AVJ. The right-sided approach is the most common. The catheter is positioned across the tricuspid valve and withdrawn until a large His bundle is recorded and energy is delivered into this area. Permanent pacing is required following the procedure.

While RF energy induces thermal lesion formation through resistive heating of myocardial tissue, other options including cold or cryoablation have been developed. Cryoablation destroys targeted cells only. This tool allows the electrophysiologist to slightly freeze the tissue, which tests whether it is responsible for conducting an arrhythmia. RF or other heat-inducing methods do not allow this. Catheters themselves have changed, reflecting the needs of the electrophysiologist diagnose and treat the particular arrhythmia. Large-tip catheters have become the standard of care for the ablation of Type 1 flutters. Issues regarding patient fluid overload with the irrigated tip catheters can be an issue for the patient undergoing a long ablative procedure.

The following are common arrhythmias that can be cured with catheter ablation.

Atrioventricular Nodal Reentrant Tachycardia (AVNRT)

This is one of the most common arrhythmias that are referred to electrophysiologist. In a reentrant tachycardia, there must be two parallel conducting pathways that are connected at both ends, one with slower conducting properties than the other. In classic AVNRT, the slow pathway is used for antegrade conduction and the fast pathway is used for retrograde conduction. Both pathways are needed for the tachycardia to be sustained. The objective of the EPS is to ablate the slower pathway, eliminating the AVNRT. The success rate for this ablation is extremely high. This concept of reentry can be applied to many arrhythmias from VT to SVT.

Atrial Fibrillation

AF ablation that involves the pulmonary vein isolation is currently evolving as an ablation target. The latest studies are showing that ablating around, rather than within, the pulmonary veins is more successful and causes fewer complications. The evolution of contact and noncontact mapping of atrial fibrillation has continued to expand rapidly. Advanced technology such as magnetic navigation, robotic catheter placement, and 3-D

mapping are becoming commonplace in many laboratories. New catheters and ablation energy sources are constantly being developed.

Atrial Flutter and Ventricular Tachycardia

These are clinically accepted indications for ablation therapy as well as atrial tachycardia. Continued investigation will broaden the use of RF ablation in the treatment of cardiac arrhythmias.

The Future of Ablation

The future of ablation as a cure for all types of atrial fibrillation is in rapid cycle development. Medical professionals are learning more and more about the electrical substrate or triggers that cause atrial fibrillation. As they make advancements in that area, the industry is continuing to improve catheters and ablation tools. As the tools improve, the length of the procedure decreases. As the ablation of AV nodal reentrant tachycardia has become a "cure" and a preferred method of care, so too will the ablation of the focus of atrial fibrillation. Currently, the professionals are focusing on the pulmonary veins as the trigger for atrial fibrillation but the ablation of this focus has been difficult. Again, the advancement of mapping tools is exploding and keeping up with these advances requires diligence on the part of the EP lab personnel. Constant training is needed as these tools become available. With the ablation tools becoming easier to use, a cure for atrial fibrillation may be on the near horizon.

NURSING CARE

Prior to the Procedure

Having an invasive procedure, especially one involving the heart, is very anxiety-provoking for the patient and family. All efforts should be made to alleviate the patient's fears and concerns. Patient education is pivotal and begins as soon as it becomes known that the patient will undergo the procedure. Any written information that can be provided to the patient and family beforehand is helpful. A preprocedure tour of the laboratory is optimal, so that the patient becomes familiar with the equipment and the personnel. The patient and family should be allowed time to ask questions about the procedure, as well as what to expect afterward.

In addition to explaining what to expect before, during, and after the procedure, the nurse must ensure that other tasks are completed. The patient must be instructed when, where, and at what time they are to report prior to the procedure. Many patients will undergo a preprocedure work-up the day before the procedure. In addition to obtaining preprocedure tests, this is an excellent opportunity for patient education. The preprocedure tests may include blood tests, ECG, echocardiogram, and exercise stress testing. A female of childbearing age must have a negative pregnancy test prior to the procedure. A history and physical should be performed and an informed consent obtained by the physician performing the procedure. The patient's antiarrhythmic medications may or may not need to be stopped prior to the procedure, for catheter ablation or antiarrhythmic drug efficacy, respectively.

The type of sedation to be used prior to and during the procedure should be reviewed with the patient. Many patients will receive a sedative prior to the procedure and will remain awake for its duration, while others will receive conscious sedation.[10,11] Regardless of the type of sedation used, the patient should be informed prior to the procedure. Lastly, when to withhold food and fluids must be reviewed with the patient.

Once the patient has arrived in the EPS laboratory, the nurse is responsible for bringing him or her to the table. Because the procedure can run for several hours, it is important that the patient is lying comfortably. Patient comfort can be increased with the use of a gel mattress and well-positioned arm supports. A support cushion under the knees will also take pressure off the patient's lower back.

During the course of the procedure, the patient will be continuously monitored, so placement of a fingertip oxygen saturation measurement device on one side (preferably the side with the infusion) and the cuff of a blood pressure monitor on the other arm is essential. The patient also needs an infusion with an extension and a three-way stopcock for drug administration. The stopcock should be positioned so that it is easily accessible and the sterile field does not have to be compromised to use it.

Surface ECG lead placement is very important for EPS. The skin should be clean and dry prior to electrode placement. Lead placement should be verified prior to the start of the EPS, especially since limb lead reversal can result in an abnormal ECG. Carbon leads should be used for the chest wall electrodes because they are radiotransparent and will not interfere with the radiograph. Baseline vital signs as well as an assessment of peripheral pulses should be obtained prior to starting the procedure.

It is important that the nurse uses this time of preparation to talk with the patient, describing what is being done and why, and answering any lingering questions. The patient should feel free to communicate when he or she experiences pain or discomfort during the procedure, and the patient should be told to ask for the bedpan when he or she feels the bladder is getting full.

When the patient has been positioned comfortably and the nurse is confident that the patient is ready to begin the procedure, the assistant can be notified and the patient can be draped. The preparations can be quite baffling for the patient, so the nurse should describe what is going on.

During the Procedure

The nurse's responsibility during an EPS may vary, depending on the number of additional personnel present and whether sedation is used. If conscious sedation is used and no anesthesia personnel are present, a nurse must be assigned to monitor the patient's airway. This nurse would have no other responsibilities during the procedure. Additionally, when using conscious sedation agents, one nurse should be assigned to administer the agents (if the physician does not prefer to do so) and be responsible for fluid administration or other pharmacological agents. One person must be assigned to monitor and record the patient's vital signs at predetermined intervals.

Although the procedure often seems tedious and boring, the nurse must be alert to the possibility of arrhythmia induction, vagal responses, and/or hemodynamic compromise. Any significant changes in the patient's vital signs should be reported to the physician immediately. The nurse should be proficient in the use of the external defibrillator and remain close to it throughout the procedure.

Because the patient is awake, the nurse may need to constantly reassure him or her in order to decrease anxiety. Certain protocols may be painful to the patient and arrhythmia induction may result in chest pain, hypotension, and/or syncope. Sensations that the patient might experience (i.e., rapid heart rates, skipped beats, and light-headedness) should be explained to the patient prior to protocol initiation.

After the Procedure

Once the procedure has been completed, the patient will be moved to a designated area of the hospital to recover. Although most complications occur in the catheterization laboratory, some can occur later, usually within the first 6 hours following the procedure. The nurse caring for the patient after EPS must be cognizant of these potential complications. They include bleeding, infection, cardiac tamponade, hematoma formation, and stroke.

During this recovery phase, the patient's vital signs must be closely monitored. This includes assessing the ECG for any rhythm disturbances such as arrhythmias, interval changes, or ST-segment changes. Typically, patients are placed on bed rest with little movement for 4 to 6 hours after the procedure. A sandbag or pressure dressing may be placed over the catheter site(s) to decrease the incidence of bleeding. A leg immobilizer may be used if the patient has difficulty with the movement restrictions.[12] The catheter site(s) and affected extremity(ies) must be assessed with each vital sign check. The site should be assessed for bleeding and/or hematoma formation, and the extremity should be checked for color, temperature, and pulse. Arterial site punctures are becoming increasingly common in the electrophysiology laboratory setting. If the patient has had an arterial puncture, the postprocedural assessment must include evaluation of pulses and quick intervention is vital if a decrease in pulses or change in temperature of the extremity is encountered.

Discharge Planning

Discharge planning should be initiated at the time of admission. Due to the fact that many of these procedures are now performed on an outpatient basis, the nurse must be preparing for the patient's discharge prior to their admission. Once again, any written information that can be given to the patient and family is helpful.

The findings of the EPS will affect any discharge planning, especially if treatments are to be initiated prior to discharge. Patients should be instructed on what signs to look for at home that requires physician contact. The signs and symptoms may include fever, infection of the catheter entry site(s), swelling, redness, purulent drainage, hematoma formation at the puncture site, and/or changes in the color and temperature of the affected extremity. Activity restrictions, if any, should be reviewed, such as when the patient may return to work or school. After an ablation for any type of tachycardia, it is very common for the patient to be aware of occasional palpitations. These should subside over time. Anything that is prolonged or causing symptoms must be evaluated in the physician's office or the emergency room.

Differences Between Children and Adults

Children are not small adults. They are physiologically, psychologically, emotionally, and developmentally different than their adult counterparts. Because of a child's cognitive and emotional immaturity, his or her response to, and understanding of, medical procedures will vary. A child's family should be involved in the procedure as much as they feel comfortable with. Written information is an effective adjunct. Explanations should be honest and factual in order to promote trust between the nurse and the patient and family. Explanations regarding the procedure should be brief, simple, and repeated often. Additionally, a child's communication skills are underdeveloped, so nonverbal communication between a nurse and a child is extremely important.

Children differ anatomically and physiologically from their adult counterparts. In a child, every component of the respiratory system is immature and smaller than that of an adult. Caring for children in the electrophysiology laboratory requires equipment that is suitable for smaller patients, such as smaller sizes of airways and endotracheal tubes. Pediatric diagnostic and ablation catheters are generally sized to suit the child, with catheters in the 3–4 French range available.

Children typically have faster heart rates than adults and, in contrast, their cardiac output is directly proportional to heart rate due to their smaller stroke volume. In children, hypotension is a LATE sign of decreased perfusion.

When compared to adults, the child has a larger surface area to volume ratio leading to greater heat loss to the environment. Maintaining a neutral thermal environment and monitoring the child's temperature during the procedure can minimize this heat loss.

The arrhythmias seen in the pediatric population are different, primarily due to the faster baseline heart rates in children.[13] For example, SVT in an infant can be as fast as 300 beats per minute and be tolerated for several hours, whereas an adult with a heart rate this fast would probably experience syncope. The most common arrhythmogenic substrate in the pediatric population is that of an accessory conduction.[14] Enhanced automaticity is a more common mechanism in a child as well.

Many children have arrhythmias as a result of surgery for congenital, structural heart disease.[15] When caring for these patients, the nurse must be cognizant of the child's anatomy and physiology as well as the potential effect of the arrhythmia on the child's overall hemodynamic status.

Finally, children undergoing invasive electrophysiology testing require more sedation than their adult counterparts. Also of note is the EP effects of sedation that can occur in the pediatric patient. This difference can cause changes in the refractory periods of accessory pathway. Various levels of sedation can be used in children, depending on their age, developmental status, and the anticipated duration of the procedure. These sedation levels range from conscious sedation to deep sedation to general anesthesia. Because children are different, the sedation agents and their routes of administration are variable.[16]

CONCLUSION

The field of invasive electrophysiology continues to grow, with the emphasis currently on the focus and cure of atrial fibrillation. The rapid growth of invasive electrophysiology almost parallels the growth of angioplasty in the early 1980s. Along with atrial fibrillation, the electrophysiologist is also increasingly focusing on the patient with heart failure and the implantation of biventricular devices. This is one field that is always trying to improve the mouse trap and find better ways to treat the patient with complex arrhythmias.

REFERENCES

1. Lenegre J, Maurice P. De quelques resultats obtenus par la derivation directe intracavi-taire des courants electriques de l'oreillette et du ventricule droit. *Arch Mal Coeur Vaiss* 38;1945:298–302.

2. Burchell HB, Frye RL, Anderson MW, et al. Atrioventricular and ventriculoatrial excitation in Wolff-Parkinson-White syndrome (type B): temporary ablation at surgery. *Circulation* 1967;36:663–672.

3. Cobb RF, Blumenschein SD. Successful surgical interruption of the bundle of Kent in a patient with Wolff-Parkinson-White syndrome. *Circulation* 1968;38:1018–1029.

4. Scherlag BJ, Lau SH, Helfant RH, et al. Catheter techniques for recording His bundle activity in man. *Circulation* 1969;39:13–18.

5. Jackman WM, Wang X, Friday KJ, et al. Catheter ablation of accessory pathways (Wolff-Parkinson-White syndrome) by radiofrequency current. *N Engl J Med* 1991;324;1605–1611.

6. Zipes DP, MiMarco JP, Gillette PC, et al. Guidelines for clinical intracardiac electro-physiological and catheter ablation procedures: a report of the ACC/AHA task force on practice guidelines. *Circulation* 1995;92:673–691.

7. Shewchik J, Tobin MG. Instrumentation. In: Schurig L, Gura M, Taibi B, eds. *Educational Guidelines Pacing and Electrophysiology*, 2nd ed. Armonk, NY: Futura; 1997:425–431.

8. Gillette PC, Buckles D, Harold M, et al. Intracardiac electrophysiology studies. In: Gillette PC, Garson A Jr, eds. *Pediatric Arrhythmias: Electrophysiology and Pacing*. Philadelphia: WB Saunders; 1990:216–247.

9. Kugler JD. Sinus node dysfunction. In: Gillette PC, Garson A Jr, eds. *Pediatric Arrhythmias: Electrophysiology and Pacing*. Philadelphia: WB Saunders;1990:250–300.

10. Bubien RS, Ching E. IV sedation/analgesia. In: Schurig L, Gura M, Taibi B, eds. *Educational Guidelines Pacing and Electrophysiology*, 2nd ed. Armonk, NY: Futura; 1997:585–596.

11. Rodeman BJ. Conscious sedation during electrophysiology testing and radiofrequency catheter ablation. *Crit Care Nurs Clin North Am* 1997;9:313–324.

12. Rosenberg BL. Laboratory procedures. In: Schurig L, Gura M, Taibi B, eds. *Educational Guidelines Pacing and Electrophysiology*, 2nd ed. Armonk, NY: Futura; 1997:415–431.

13. Gilette PC, Zeigler VL, Case CL. Pediatric arrhythmias: are they different? In: Zipes DP, Jalife J, eds. *Cardiac Electrophysiology: From Cell to Bedside*. Philadelphia, W.B. Saunders, 1995

14. Ludomirsky A, Garson A Jr. In: Gillette PC, Garson A Jr, eds. *Pediatric Arrhythmias: Electrophysiology and Pacing*. Philadelphia: WB Saunders; 1990:380–426.

15. Zeigler VL. Postoperative rhythm disturbances. *Crit Care Nurs Clin North Am* 1994;6:227–235.

16. Zeigler VL, Brown LE. Conscious sedation in the pediatric population: special considerations. *Crit Care Nurs Clin North Am* 1997;9:381–394

Chapter 24

CARDIAC PACING

Laura Nyren, RN, MS, ACNP
Lezlie Bridge, BSc, DMS, NASPE Testamur

INTRODUCTION

In general, cardiac pacing is used to treat symptomatic bradycardia, a term that describes a heart rate that is too slow to allow cardiac output to satisfy physiological demand. This can cause symptoms ranging from intermittent lightheadedness, fatigue, and shortness of breath on exertion, to near syncope and syncope. Syncope is caused by standstill of the ventricles lasting more than 5 to 7 seconds. Less commonly, pacing may also be used to overdrive both atrial and ventricular tachyarrhythmias and as a treatment for heart failure.

The first pacemaker was implanted in 1958.[1] Early pacemakers paced in a single chamber at a fixed rate and output. Since that time, cardiac pacing has become both more complex and more frequent. Today's pacemakers offer multichamber pacing, multisite pacing, two-way telemetry, multiprogrammable features, rate response, extensive diagnostics, and remote monitoring. Inpatient data for 2005 indicates there were 180,000 pacemaker implants in the United States alone.[2]

NORMAL CARDIAC CONDUCTION

The heart's normal rhythm is called sinus rhythm, and it is initiated in the sinoatrial (SA) node located in the posterior and superior wall of the right atrium. Automaticity of the SA node is largely due to slow calcium channels. The inward current results in depolarization and action potential propagation. The shape of the action potential determines conduction velocity (see Figure 24-1).[3] Phase 0 represents depolarization of a cardiac cell due to the opening of rapid sodium (Na^+) channels. Phase 1 represents the onset of cellular repolarization. The Na^+ channels are closed and a transient outward current of potassium (K^+) begins. Phase 2 is known as the plateau phase as the calcium (Ca^{++}) begins to slowly flow into the cell, prolonging the action

Figure 24-1. The cardiac action potential.

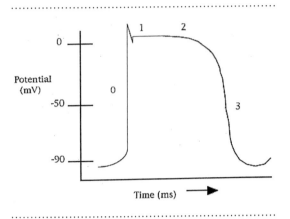

potential. Phase 3 is characteristic of an outward K^+ current. Normal ionic distribution is eventually restored by the sodium-potassium pump. Phase 4 represents the resting phase. Some movement of ions occurs at this phase. If threshold is reached, spontaneous depolarization occurs and is known as automaticity.

The impulse travels in concentric waves throughout the atria, generating a P wave on the surface ECG. It then spreads to the AV node, where there is an important conduction delay correlating with the P-R interval. This delay allows blood to passively fill the ventricles, prior to atrial contraction, or atrial kick. Electrical impulses are then conducted down the His bundle, which bifurcates into the left and right bundle branches. The left bifurcates again into the anterior and posterior fascicles. The left and right bundle branches ultimately culminate in the Purkinje fibres of the left and right ventricles. Depolarization of the ventricular cells produces the QRS complex. Repolarization of the large ventricular mass is depicted by the T wave on the surface ECG (atrial repolarization is not depicted on the surface ECG).

When defects or deficits develop in part of the conduction system, symptomatic bradycardia may arise. Etiologies of such faults may include myocardial ischemia or infarction, cardiac surgery and ablative therapy, drug therapy, the aging process, cardiomyopathies, congenital cardiac structural abnormalities, and congenital heart block. Commonly, it is only when a patient experiences symptoms as a result of these conduction defects or deficits that it is necessary to undertake pacemaker implantation on a temporary or permanent basis. In some cases, ECG patterns (e.g., incomplete trifascicular block or second-degree AV block of the Mobitz type) may lead to prophylactic pacemaker implantation in hitherto asymptomatic patients.

NBG CODES

There are many different modes of pacing. The one used is dependent on the arrhythmia for which the patient is being paced. An international coding system for describing these modes was designed in 1974. Originally, the code consisted of three letters; the first indicated the chambers paced, the second was for the chambers sensed, and the third indicated the response to what was sensed.[4] In 1987, the joint working party of the British Pacing and Electrophysiology Group (BPEG) and the North American Society of Pacing and Electrophysiology (NASPE) modified the pacemaker coding to a five-letter code. The code includes a fourth column for programmability and rate-modulation, and a fifth for antitachycardia functions.[5] The most recent revision was done in 2000, where the fourth letter reflects rate modulation only, and the fifth letter now reflects multisite pacing. This is referred to as the NASPE/BPEG generic (NBG) code, and is depicted in Table 24-1.[6]

For example, a pacemaker in the VVI mode paces and senses in the ventricle. If it senses intrinsic (the patient's own) ventricular activity, the output of the pacemaker will be inhibited. When the intrinsic activity falls below the programmed lower rate limit (LRL), the pacemaker will resume ventricular pacing. In DDD mode, the

Table 24-1. NASPE/BPEG (NBG) Generic Pacemaker Code

Category/ Position	I Chamber Paced	II Chamber Sensed	III Response to Sensing	IV Rate Modulation	V Multisite Pacing
Letter Codes	O=None	O=None	O=None	O=None	O=None
	A=Atrium	A=Atrium	T=Triggered	R=Rate Modulation	A=Atrium
	V=Ventricle	V=Ventricle	I=Inhibited		V=Ventricle
	D=Dual (A&V)	D=Dual (A&V)	D=Dual (T&I)		D=Dual (A&V)
Manufacturer Designation	S=Single (A or V)	S=Single (A or V)			

pacemaker paces and senses in both the atrium and the ventricle. If the pacemaker senses an intrinsic P wave before timing has elapsed for the ventricular to atrial (V-A) interval (DDD LRL timing is divided into V-A interval and the AV interval), it will inhibit atrial pacing. If no intrinsic atrial event is sensed by the pacemaker, an atrial paced event will occur at the timed V-A interval. A sensed or paced atrial event triggers ventricular pacing after a preset AV interval if no intrinsic ventricular depolarization occurs first.

INDICATIONS

Temporary Pacing

Temporary pacing is undertaken when there is insufficient time or inadequate facilities to proceed with permanent implantation or when there is the possibility that normal cardiac rhythm will be restored. These conditions may exist for the patient suffering acute MI. He or she may not be stable enough to undergo permanent implantation, or many times the bradyarrhythmia may be

only transient in nature. MI patients may experience varying degrees of heart block, sinus node dysfunction, or disorders of the intraventricular conduction system that require pacing.[7]

The pacing electrode is placed transvenously via the external (or internal) jugular vein, the subclavian vein, or the femoral vein to the heart, typically, the RV apex. Some centers prefer the fast method of transesophageal atrial pacing because the esophagus lies in close proximity to the posterior wall of the atrium. However, this requires high output and may result in esophageal burning. Temporary pacing is also used perioperatively for cardiac surgery. Temporary pacing wires are usually placed on the epicardial surface of the heart (ventricle and/or atrium) for optimizing cardiac output and treatment or suppression of arrhythmias. Within a few days, as the edema around the conduction system reduces and fluid balance returns to a preoperative state, rhythm disturbances often resolve. At this time, the physician may remove the pacing wires.

In some patients undergoing cardiac catheterization, profound bradycardia may also occur. Catheter manipulation in the right ventricle may produce transient right bundle branch (RBB) block. For patients with preexisting left bundle branch (LBB) block, this would result in complete heart block (CHB). In patients with preexisting RBB undergoing a left heart catheterization, CHB rarely occurs as the left bundle extends only a limited distance before its bifurcation. Contrast injection into the right coronary artery (RCA) may also produce severe bradycardia. However, this usually only results in several seconds of bradycardia or asystole and does not typically require temporary pacer placement.[7] When a procedure is expected to be prolonged, a temporary pacer may be maintained for the duration of the procedure. If no transvenous temporary pacing lead has been placed, it is possible to pace using a guide wire as the cathode (−), either in a coronary artery or in the left ventricle, and a skin patch electrode as the anode (+) pole.

Temporary pacing may also be used to serve as a bridge during pacemaker generator replacement. In patients who are pacer dependent (they have no discernible underlying intrinsic rhythm) and are undergoing revision of a permanent pacemaker system, it is often useful to insert a temporary pacemaker prior to starting the procedure. With this method, the temporary pacer is used to pace the patient while the existing pulse generator is disconnected from the lead system until the new generator is secured.

Please see Chapter 37 for more details on temporary pacemakers.

Permanent Pacing

The indications for the implantation of a permanent pacing system have broadened as technology has advanced. They now include the treatment of ablation-induced AV block, congestive heart failure, hypertrophic obstructive cardiomyopathy (HOCM) and dilated cardiomyopathy, paroxysmal atrial fibrillation, vasovagal syncope, long QT syndrome, and carotid hypersensitivity.[8–11] In addition, refinements have been made in the use of pacing in cardiac transplant recipients, and it has also been utilized in treatment of cardiomyoplasty patients.[12]

Pacemaker therapy is commonly used to treat SA and AV conduction defects or a combination of the two. SA disease, or sick sinus syndrome (SSS), encompasses abnormalities of the impulse arising from the sinus node and includes sinus bradycardia, sinus arrest, sinus exit block, and specific atrial tachyarrhythmias.[7] The term SSS indicates symptomatic sinus bradycardia.[13] AV conduction defects are those that affect the impulse travelling through the AV node, or distal to the AV node, and range from first-degree heart block (prolonged AV conduction) to CHB. Pacing is only necessary in prolonged AV conduction if it is associated with symptomatic bradycardia. Intraventricular conduction defects may also be indications for permanent pacing.[7] Examples may include bifascicular block (RBB block with a left anterior or posterior hemiblock, or complete LBB block), incomplete trifascicular block (bifascicular block with associated first-degree AV block), or second-degree AV block of Mobitz type.

Pacing indications are not always straightforward. For this reason, guidelines were developed and updated in 2008 by the American College of Cardiology (ACC), American Heart Association (AHA) and Heart Rhythm Society (HRS) (see Table 24-2). These guidelines provide a classification for specific diagnoses that indicates whether there is a consensus that pacing is indicated.[14] Class I refers to those diagnoses that are accepted indications for pacing, Class IIa are reasonable, IIb may be considered, and Class III are not indications and may be harmful.

The BPEG guidelines for selection of pacing mode states that the ventricle should be paced if there is actual or threatened AV block, and that the atrium should be paced and/or sensed unless

Table 24-2. Indications for Cardiac Pacemakers (Adults)[14]

	Sinus Node Dysfunction (SND)
Class I	With documented symptomatic bradycardia, including frequent symptomatic pauses (may be the result of drug therapy for medical condition)
	Symptomatic chronotropic incompetence
Class IIa	Sinus node dysfunction with heart rates < 40 bpm when a clear association has not been made between symptoms and bradycardia
	Syncope unknown etiology when abnormalities of SN function is discovered or provoked in electrophysiological studies (EPS)
Class IIb	Minimally symptomatic with HR < 40 bpm while awake
Class III	Asymptomatic SND
	Symptoms suggestive of bradycardia clearly documented in its absence
	SND with symptomatic bradycardia due to nonessential drug therapy
	Acquired AV Block
Class I	Third-degree and advanced second-degree at any level associated with: symptomatic bradycardia or ventricular arrhythmias presumed due to AV block arrhythmia or other medical conditions that require drug therapy that results in symptomatic bradycardia > 3 seconds asystole or escape rate < 40 bpm or escape below the AV node in awake, asymptomatic patients in SR 1 or more pauses > 5 seconds in awake, asymptomatic patients with atrial fibrillation (AF) and bradycardia catheter ablation of the AV junction postoperative AV block not expected to resolve after cardiac surgery neuromuscular diseases with AV block, with or without symptoms
	Third-degree AV block, persistent asymptomatic, with ventricular rates > 40 bpm if cardiomegally or LV dysfunction is present or the site of block is below the AN node
	Second-degree AV block associated with symptomatic bradycardia regardless of site of block
	Second- or third-degree AV block during exercise in the absence of myocardial ischemia
Class IIa	Asymptomatic complete heart block, persistent, without cardiomegally, with ventricular rates of > 40 bpm
	Asymptomatic second-degree AV block at intra- or infra-His levels at EPS
	First- or second-degree AV block with symptoms similar to those of pacemaker syndrome or hemodynamic compromise.
	Asymptomatic type II second-degree AV block with a narrow QRS
Class IIb	Neuromuscular disease with any degree of AV block (including first degree) with or without symptoms because of unpredictable progression of conduction disease
	AV block in the setting of drug use/or drug toxicity when block is expected to recur after drug is withdrawn

continues

Table 24-2. Indications for Cardiac Pacemakers (Adults)[14]   *continued*

Class III	Asymptomatic first-degree AV block
	Asymptomatic Mobitz I at the AV node level
	AV block that is likely to resolve and not recur

Chronic Bifasicular Block	
Class I	Advanced second-degree or intermittent third-degree AV block
	Type II second-degree AV block
	Alternating bundle branch block (BBB)
Class IIa	Syncope not demonstrated to be due to AV block when other likely causes have been excluded, e.g. VT
	Markedly long HV interval ($>$ 100 msec) in asymptomatic patient
	Pacing induced infra-His block that is not physiological found at EPS
Class IIb	Or any fasicular block in patients with neuromuscular diseases with or without symptoms
Class III	Fascicular block without AV block or symptoms
	Fascicular block with first-degree AV block, asymptomatic

After Acute Phase of Myocardial Infarct (MI)	
Class I	Post ST elevation MI with persistent second-degree AV block in the His-Purkinje system with alternating BBB or third-degree AV block within or below the His-Purkinje system
	Transient second- or third-degree AV block and associated BBB
	Persistent, symptomatic second- or third-degree AV block
Class IIb	Persistent second- or third-degree AV block at the AV nodal level, even in the absence of symptoms
Class III	Transient AV conduction disturbances in the absence of intraventricular conduction defects
	Transient AV block in the presence of isolated left anterior fascicular block
	New BBB or fascicular block in the absence of AV block
	Persistent asymptomatic first-degree AV block in the presence of BBB or fascicular block

Hypersensitive Carotid Sinus Syndrome and Neurocardiogenic Syncope	
Class I	Syncope caused by spontaneously occurring carotid sinus stimulation or $>$ 3 second ventricular asystole with carotid sinus pressure
Class IIa	Recurrent syncope without clear, provocative events and with hypersensitive cardioinhibitory response of $>$ 3 seconds
Class IIb	Significantly symptomatic neurocardiogenic syncope associated with bradycardia documented spontaneously or at the time of tilt-table-testing
Class III	Hyperactive cardioinhibitory response to carotid sinus stimulation in the absence of symptoms or with vague symptoms
	Situational vasovagal syncope in which avoidance behavior is effective or preferred

Following Cardiac Transplant	
Class I	Persistent inappropriate or symptomatic bradycardia not expected to resolve and for other Class I indications

Table 24-2. Indications for Cardiac Pacemakers (Adults)[14]

Class IIb	When relative bradycardia is prolonged or recurrent, which limits rehabilitation or discharge
	Syncope after transplant even when bradyarrhythmia not documented
Cardiac Resynchronization Therapy (CRT) in Patients with Severe Systolic Heart Failure	
Class I	Left ventricular ejection fraction (LVEF) < 35%, QRS duration > 0.12 seconds, and sinus rhythm, CRT with or without ICD is indicated for NYHA functional Class III or ambulatory Class IV heart failure symptoms on optimal medical therapy
Class IIa	LVEF < 35%, QRS duration > 0.12 seconds, AF, CRT with or without ICD is reasonable for NYHA functional Class III or ambulatory Class IV heart failure symptoms on optimal medical therapy
	LVEF < 35%, NYHA functional Class III or ambulatory Class IV heart failure symptoms on optimal medical therapy and who have frequent dependence on ventricular pacing
Class IIb	LVEF < 35% with NYHA Class I or II symptoms, receiving optimal medical therapy undergoing implantation of a permanent pacemaker and/or ICD with anticipated frequent ventricular pacing
Class III	Asymptomatic patients with reduced LVEF in the absence of other pacing indications
	Functional status and life expectancy are limited predominantly by chronic noncardiac conditions
Hypertrophic Cardiomyopathy	
Class I	SND or AV block as previously outlined
Class IIb	Medically refractory symptomatic patients and significant resting or provoked LV outflow obstruction (when risk factors of Sudden Cardiac Death present consider DDD ICD)
Class III	Asymptomatic or symptoms medically controlled
	Symptomatic patients without evidence of LV outflow tract obstruction
Detection and Treatment of Tachyarrhythmias	
Class IIa	Symptomatic, recurrent supraventricular tachycardia that is reproducibly terminated by pacing when catheter ablation and/or drugs fail to control the arrhythmia or produce intolerable side effects
Class III	Presence of an accessory pathway that has the capacity for rapid antegrade conduction
Prevention of Atrial Fibrillation	
Class III	In patients without any other indication for permanent pacing

contraindicated.[15] AAI/R pacing is contraindicated if a patient has any evidence of AV conduction block. This may be diagnosed either during electrophysiology (EP) testing, atrial pacing at the anticipated upper rate limit (URL), or during carotid sinus massage.

Chronic AF is also a contraindication. In this case, atrial pacing would be of no benefit because in this condition the electrical impulse is not able to stimulate the atrium. In a dual-chamber system, sensing of the rapid atrial rate would trigger ventricular tracking up to the pacer's programmed URL. If the atrial fibrillation occurs only intermittently (paroxysmal atrial fibrillation) tracking at the upper rate can be overcome by programming mode switching on. This will cause the pacemaker to revert to pacing the ventricle alone until the restoration of orderly atrial rhythm. AAI/R pacing had been used infrequently, due to concern for AV block developing at a later time but is frequently used now in devices that will automatically revert from AAI/R to DDD/R should AV block occur. This is beneficial as ventricular pacing > 40% of the time has been associated with heart failure.[16]

PACEMAKER COMPONENTS

The basic components of any pacemaker circuit, whether temporary or permanent, include a pulse generator, lead system, and myocardium. Pulse generators contain a power source (or battery), output circuitry, sensing circuitry, and possibly other specialized features. Pulse generators connect to the heart muscle by one, two, or more leads that are composed of insulated conducting coil(s) and uninsulated electrode(s).

Temporary External Pulse Generators

Batteries that are used to power pacemakers must be reliable and long lasting. Temporary pacers are typically powered by 9-volt batteries. In temporary generators, batteries are usually changed before instituting pacing and at regularly scheduled intervals. Generators may have a light indicator or some other means of alerting the user to a low battery. Many temporary pacemakers on the market today will operate for several seconds after the battery is removed, enabling quick battery replacement while the device is connected to a patient. It should not be assumed, however, that every generator has this capability. Always refer to the manufacturer's instruction manual. If this function is not present, a second temporary pacing device with a new battery, set to identical parameters, can provide a means of rapid battery replacement. The existing temporary generator is disconnected from the patient's pacing leads and the new generator connected immediately.

The patient should experience minimal delay in pacing output but should be warned that they may experience an episode of dizziness if they are pacer-dependent.

Permanent Pulse Generators

The outer casing of the implantable pulse generator is made from titanium or stainless steel.[1] The casing is hermetically sealed to avoid seepage of body fluids. Pulse generators are designed as single, dual, or multichamber. They are used in conjunction with bipolar and/or unipolar lead systems, or strictly unipolar lead systems. Headers (see Figure 24-2) mounted on the pulse generator provide connector ports for insertion and connection of the lead system.

Permanent pulse generators are typically powered by a 2.8-volt lithium iodine battery. These batteries are designed for long life, are small in size, and are highly reliable. They do not produce any gas and are capable of functioning in a sealed environment. The battery consists of an inner layer of lithium and an outer iodine layer. A middle layer of lithium iodide forms as the battery is used, and this gives rise to the characteristic battery voltage drop. By increasing the pulse

Figure 24-2. Header. This header is for a dual-chamber bipolar lead system.

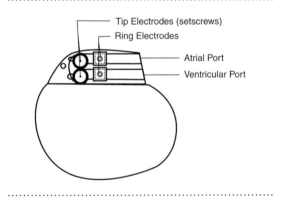

duration (the length of time over which a pacing stimulus is delivered), the delivered voltage remains the same despite the fact that the battery voltage has dropped. An early indication of battery depletion given by the manufacturer provides sufficient time to allow elective replacement of the pacemaker. This is known as the elective replacement (ERI) or "end-of-life" (EOL) indicator. Typically, this takes the form of an altered pacing rate known as the magnet mode. Booklets are available from manufacturers of permanent pacemakers that list ERI or EOL behaviours of all pulse generators. Battery replacement requires the entire generator to be changed. It is not possible to replace just the battery.

Other integral components of a permanent pacer include its output, timing, and sensing circuitry guided by a read-only memory (ROM) microprocessor. The output voltage of a pacemaker is powered by the battery and conducted via the pacing electrode to the myocardium. The programmed output in volts is drawn to the capacitor from the battery and delivered via the lead system. When more than 2.8 volts are required for pacing, small capacitors, or multipliers, increase the output capability of the generator. Energy is drawn to multipliers and delivered to the output capacitor in sequence, resulting in a greater delivered energy.

Pacemaker output is regulated by the timing circuit. When a spontaneous beat is sensed, the output of the pacemaker is inhibited, and the lower rate timing is reset. Dual-chamber pacing also involves upper rate timing, V-A interval, and an AV interval. In order to sense intrinsic beats, an intracardiac electrogram (IEGM) must be received from the pacing lead. The IEGM is then amplified, filtered, and compared to the set sensitivity. Signals of too low an amplitude or too high or low a frequency are disregarded. T waves and muscle signals are typically examples of low- and high-frequency signals.

A noise reversion circuit is often used and serves as a safety mechanism when electrical signals exceed sensing threshold, but occur at a faster rate than the noise reversion rate. In this event, the pacemaker will pace in an asynchronous mode. Another time a pacer will revert to an asynchronous mode is when a magnet is placed directly over the pulse generator. The internal reed switch is closed, disabling the sensing circuitry and, again, the pacer will function in an asynchronous mode.

The pulse generator is protected from large external voltages such as defibrillation by a zener diode.[7] However, after a defibrillation, each patient's pacemaker should be evaluated, because the high-voltage shock may harm the pacemaker system (e.g., alter the program or increase the pacing threshold).

Pacemakers today will also have telemetry coils for sending programming commands and receiving diagnostic information. Programmable features may include, but are not limited to: pacing mode, LRL, URL, AV interval (paced and sensed), hysteresis rate, sleep rate, pulse amplitude, pulse duration, blanking periods, refractory periods, and pacing and sensing polarities. Diagnostic data are stored in random-access memory (RAM) and can be valuable in evaluating performance and troubleshooting. Diagnostic information typically includes battery status information, lead impedances, atrial and ventricular high rate diagnostics, IEGMs, a summary of paced and sensed events, and rate distributions, heart failure diagnostics, and semiautomatic pacing and sensing threshold tests.

Many additional specialized features may also be available and vary with different models and manufacturers. One such feature, safety pacing, is depicted in Figure 24-3. The pacemaker senses an intrinsic ventricular beat closely following an atrial-paced beat. The programmed AV interval is shortened from the programmed interval of 280 milliseconds to 120 milliseconds. The purpose is to prevent R on T phenomenon and arrhythmia induction, or the inhibition of ventricular pacing due to far-field sensing of atrial activity, known as crosstalk.

Figure 24-3. Safety pacing.

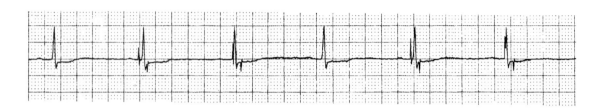

Another feature is mode switching. This is used in DDD/R pacemakers to prevent tracking of paroxysmal atrial tachyarrhythmias. Mode switching occurs when an atrial rate is detected above the set atrial tachycardia rate. The pacemaker switches from DDD/R mode to DDI, DDIR, or VVIR depending on how the device has been programmed. The pacer will then revert back to the originally programmed mode when the atrial rate falls below the tachycardia detection rate. Rate-adapter sensor circuits also become quite popular and accounted for approximately 48% of implants in 1993[8] and are seen more frequently today.

RATE ADAPTATION

During exercise, body tissues require more oxygen and produce more metabolic byproducts requiring removal. The body has mechanisms to deal with these demands, such as distributing more blood to the working muscles, increasing their ability to absorb oxygen, increasing respiratory rate and, most importantly, increasing cardiac output (CO). CO is a function of heart rate (HR) multiplied by stroke volume. HR is generally determined by the sinus node in response primarily to hormones and autonomic tone. In demand states, increasing HR is the most effective way to increase CO. In normal subjects, CO at peak exercise may be about four times higher than it is at rest. Typically, appropriate heart rates are reached within seconds or minutes of the onset of activity and level off at that rate. If HR does not

appropriately increase with exercise, it may not necessarily mean that the patient will be symptomatic of low CO, because slow rates may be compensated for by the increased stroke volume. For those individuals who do not compensate, extreme fatigue, dyspnea on exertion, dizziness, chest pain, or CHF may be experienced.

Rate-responsive pacing provides a means of increasing the heart rate in the absence of an appropriate spontaneous increase. This may be beneficial to patients with no appreciable atrial activity, atrial fibrillation, or chronotropically incompetent patients (inability to reach 100 beats per minute in response to an exercise test).[11] This includes those patients in whom incompetence stems from necessary medication or medical therapy. In order to increase rates, a sensor is added within the pacing system. The sensor identifies a physical or physiological change indicative of exercise and increases the heart rate in a linear fashion. The response rate can be limited by a separately programmable URL.

Sensors can be divided into two categories: closed loops and open loops (see Figure 24-4).[17] In a closed-loop system, a physiological change (for example, oxygen saturation or desaturation) is detected by the sensor, and, by the use of an algorithm, the pacing rate is increased accordingly. The increased rate then causes a change in the physiological parameter (oxygen saturation) in the opposite direction. Thus, as oxygen saturation rises, the pacing rate falls unless the increased oxygen demand persists. In the closed loop system, the change in rate has a negative

Figure 24-4. Types of rate-response systems.[17,18]

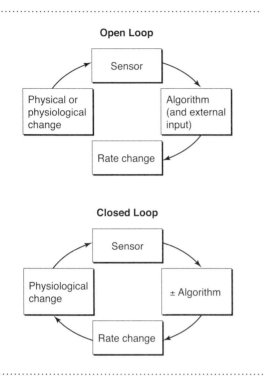

amount of rate increase for the level of exercise being undertaken. It is possible to program the threshold to tailor the sensor to the individual patient's needs. If a low level is programmed, very little activity is needed before the sensor will respond. Conversely, if a high level is selected, the patient will need to be more active before any rate response is seen. The degree of responsiveness, called the slope, is also programmable. Programming a lower slope value will provide a lesser degree of heart rate response to a particular level of exercise, and a higher slope value will create more response.

There are two types of motion sensors: activity and accelerometer. In an activity-sensing device, the piezoelectric crystal is bonded to the inside of the pacemaker can (see Figure 24-5). The accelerometer's crystal is bonded to the circuit board (see Figure 24-6). The activity sensor responds to vibration while the accelerometer is more sensitive to forward motion.

The advantages of motion sensors are that they rapidly respond to the onset of exercise and can

feedback effect on the physiological parameter to which the sensor responds.[18]

In an open-loop system, there is no negative feedback. A physical or a physiological change is detected by the sensor and, through an algorithm, the pacing rate is changed. There is no effect on the physical or physiological parameter in response to the change in rate.

Motion (Activity) Sensor

Motion sensors detect mechanical vibrations that increase with body movements, and therefore, exercise. A piezoelectric ceramic crystal inside the pacemaker flexes and deforms in response to mechanical vibrations. This generates an electric current that the sensor circuitry processes for both frequency and amplitude and then determines rate response via an algorithm. This enables the pulse generator to give an appropriate

Figure 24-5. Activity sensor. *Source:* Courtesy of Medtronic, Inc., Minneapolis, MN.

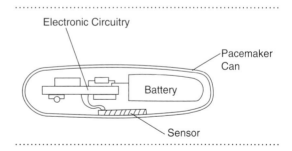

Figure 24-6. Accelerometer. *Source:* Courtesy of Medtronic, Inc., Minneapolis, MN.

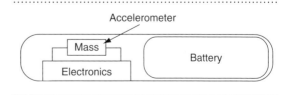

distinguish between varying levels of work. Because the piezoelectric crystal is within the pacemaker can, they are extremely easy to implant and are the most commonly used sensor implanted to date. They can be used in atrial, ventricular, and dual-chamber devices. However, they are not directly related to metabolic function and will not respond to psychological demands. Forms of work that involve relatively little vibration—for example, bicycle riding—may not be responded to adequately. Walking downstairs usually produces more vibration through the body than going upstairs does, so the heart rate may be inadequate when ascending. The sensors may, in fact, respond inappropriately to the motion of excessive arm movements or rocking. Motion sensors may also detect extracorporeal vibrations such as that from driving along a particularly bumpy road or from pressure on the pulse generator. If the generator is situated near the heart, a patient who has an enlarged hyperdynamic heart could also have inappropriate rate increase.

Respiration Sensor

Transthoracic impedance increases with inspiration and decreases with expiration. Impedance can be defined as electrical resistance, and this resistance is greater across an air-filled space than across one that contains only body fluids and tissue. With respiratory sensors, subthreshold, low-energy pulses of known current are emitted from the ring electrode of a standard bipolar pacing lead. Thoracic impedance can be calculated by measuring the resultant voltage between the tip electrode and the pacemaker can. The amplitude of the impedance change is proportional to the tidal volume or the depth of respiration. Minute ventilation is calculated from the frequency of respiration (breaths per minute) and tidal volume. Resting shallow breaths (that is those with a low tidal volume) will not be detected as they will be below the programmable detection level. With exertion, the rate and depth of breathing

increase, in turn, the pacing rate is increased by the pulse generator's sensor.

Because the continuously emitted pulses are of extremely low energy, they have very little effect on pacemaker battery longevity. They are also of too little amplitude to stimulate the myocardium or to induce arrhythmias. The early respiratory sensing pacemakers required an additional lead to be implanted subcutaneously across the chest wall to measure the transthoracic impedance. This made implantation of this system complicated. Today, a standard bipolar pacing lead can be used. A tripolar system that allows transthoracic impedance measurement is created between the two poles of the bipolar lead and the single pole, or electrode, of the pulse generator. Frequencies greater than 60 Hz are filtered out in order to minimize sensing of activities such as cardiac motion and arm movement that can also cause a change in transthoracic impedance.

Minute volume sensing is effective for a variety of different exercises, but it can often be slow to respond to the onset of activity. If rapid deep breathing continues after termination of exercise, the sensor driven rate may continue to increase in the initial postexercise phase. Additionally, patients receiving artificial mechanic ventilation may have inappropriate activation and require the sensor to be programmed to an inactive mode. This sensor is used for atrial, ventricular, and dual-chamber pacemakers.

QT Interval Sensor

This sensor technology has been used to a lesser extent. The QT interval is measured from the beginning of the QRS complex to the end of the T wave. Its duration is dependent on circulating catecholamines. At rest, the QT interval is greater than that measured during exercise. In normal subjects, the QT interval shortens as the heart rate increases with exercise or emotional stress. In individuals with a fixed heart rate, such as those with a fixed-rate pacemaker or chronotropic incompetence, it is also seen to shorten on exercise despite the lack of rate increase. Pacemakers that utilize QT interval sensing measure the QT interval from the ventricular pacing stimulus to the end of the T wave. As the sensor detects the shortening of the QT interval it, in turn, accelerates the pacing rate. A blanking period prevents the pacemaker from sensing the paced R wave and interpreting it as a T wave. This period begins with the pacing stimulus and renders the pacemaker blind to any activity, but terminates before the anticipated onset of the T wave.

With this type of sensor, there is no need for any special implant technique; a standard low-polarization pacing lead is all that is required. However, the QT interval is measured on paced beats because it is calculated from the pacing stimulus to the end of T wave. Therefore, if an intrinsic rhythm is present no rate modification will occur. Additionally, this type of sensor is not suitable for atrial implants due to the insufficient repolarization waves (T waves) in the atrium. It can be used for single-chamber ventricular pacing or dual-chamber rate-responsive systems. With a dual-chamber system, an increased rate of atrial pacing results from the QT interval shortening measured on the ventricular lead.

Right Ventricular Pressure

The rate of change of right ventricular pressure (dP/dT) increases with exercise and can be measured by a piezoelectric crystal mounted on the lead tip. Measurements can occur on both spontaneous and paced beats. Pressure on the crystal creates a voltage that is monitored by the pacemaker and is used to increase the pacing rate. A specialized lead is required. A similar method to looking at peak endocardial acceleration has been used which requires a microaccelerometer housed inside the tip of a standard unipolar pacing lead.[19]

An ideal rate-responsive sensor should mimic normal SA node activity in response to physical or emotional stressors. It should respond quickly and be accurate. Ideally, the sensor should be easy to implant and not consume much battery energy. Generally, sensors that respond to body motion have a fast response, while physiologic sensors tend to be more accurate.

LEAD DESIGN

The pacing lead is the conduit that carries electrical stimuli from the pulse generator to the heart muscle and electrical signals from heart muscle back to the pulse generator. The lead body is composed of insulation material, conductor(s), and electrode(s). The insulation layers are made from either polyurethane, silicone, or a combination. Both materials are inert and will not react with body fluids. Polyurethane is slippery, making it easier to implant than silicone. However, it has been shown that certain polyurethanes have been prone to environmental stress, cracking, and insulation failure.[20,21] Silicone offers more flexibility, but previously required thicker walls, resulting in a larger lead diameter.[7] However recent advances in lead manufacturing have overcome this. The connector (see Figure 24-7) is used as a means of securing the lead to the pulse generator. In the past, variations in connector pins between manufacturers led to confusion over lead generator compatibility. This confusion preempted industry standardization (IS-1)[22] for compatibility.

Pacing leads are either bipolar or unipolar in configuration. Bipolar leads have two conductors: an inner negative conductor and an outer positive conductor. The conductors are separated by insulating material. There is a second layer of insulation covering the entire lead (see Figure 24-8).[23] For this reason, most bipolar leads have larger diameters than unipolar ones. The conductor forms the electrode at the tip of the lead and is not covered with insulation. A bipolar lead also has an additional electrode located about 1–2 cm proximal of the tip electrode. This

Figure 24-7. Lead connectors. Lead connectors vary in diameter, pin length, and the presence or absence of sealing rings. A: various connectors (top to bottom): the 5-mm unipolar, 5-mm bifurcated bipolar, two differing 3.2-mm low profile connectors, and the 3.2-mm IS-1 (industry standard) bipolar or unipolar connector. B: a detailed view of the IS-1 connector. *Source:* Courtesy of Medtronic, Inc., Minneapolis, MN.

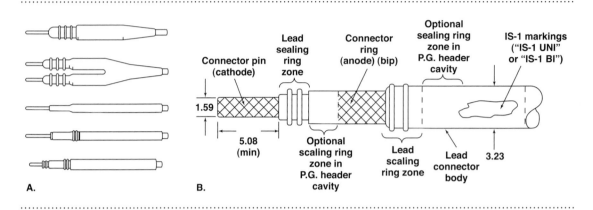

appears as an uninsulated ring around the body of the electrode (see Figure 24-9).[23] In all pacing systems, regardless of the polarity of the lead, the distal electrode is the negative (cathode) or active pole. On bipolar leads, the positive (anode) or indifferent pole is formed by the proximal ring electrode.

Original lead designs were unipolar. Unipolar leads have only one conductor within the lead body. The conductor forms the cathode as it does in the bipolar lead. The anode is formed by the pulse generator casing, or area on the casing that is not covered with insulating material. Thus, the current of energy travels to the active pole (cathode), then to the myocardium, and completes its circuit by returning via the indifferent

Figure 24-8. Bipolar lead construction.

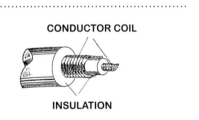

Figure 24-9. Bipolar lead. The bipolar lead has both a distal tip electrode and a proximal ring electrode. This differs from the unipolar lead, which consists only of a tip electrode.

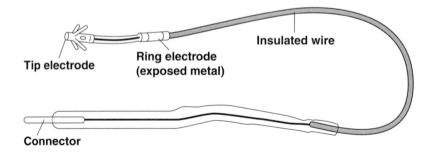

pole (anode) (Figure 24-10). One advantage to pacing in a unipolar mode is the resultant large deflection of the pacer output seen on tracings. However, this mode of pacing and sensing also has disadvantages. Pectoral muscle, or other muscle masses, may be stimulated at high output. Programming the voltage amplitude down may solve the problem, but an adequate safety margin for capture of the heart still needs to be maintained (see the section on pacing threshold). The distance between unipolar electrodes may also pose a problem with sensing. The pulse generator might see muscle potentials generated by nearby muscles (typically, pectoral) and interpret them as being intrinsic heartbeats. This would result in inappropriate inhibition of pacing output, a phenomenon known as myopotential inhibition (see Figure 24-11).

When connecting the lead(s) at implant, capture will not occur until the energy circuit is complete. The proximal pole (anode) located on the generator must have contact with the patient's tissue.

Permanent pacing leads are inserted either transvenously or epicardially. Epicardial leads are attached to the external surface of the heart. This is usually done at the time of cardiac surgery, using a midsternotomy approach. If the patient

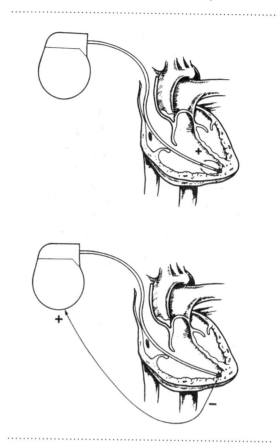

Figure 24-10. Bipolar and unipolar systems.
Source: Courtesy of Medtronic, Inc., Minneapolis, MN.

Figure 24-11. Myocardial inhibition. Skeletal myopotentials are sensed by the pacemaker and interpreted as intrinsic beats. As a result of this oversensing, the patient's rate decreases from the programmed rate of 62 bpm to a rate of about 30 bpm.

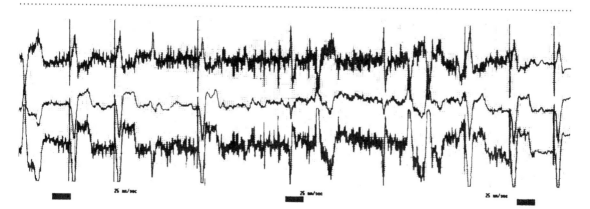

has difficult venous access, has a prosthetic tricuspid valve, or difficulty placing/positioning an LV lead, epicardial pacing may be undertaken as a stand-alone procedure through either a subxiphoid or thoracotomy approach. Epicardial leads may be unipolar or bipolar.

Methods of securing a pacing lead within the heart are categorized into either passive or active fixation. Classically, passive fixation leads have several appendages at the end of the lead that are designed to be encapsulated or wedged by the trabeculae (see Figure 24-12A). These appendages are made from the insulation material and are in the shape of tines, fins, cones, or helices. With time, the endocardium grows over the tip of the lead, making future explantation of a redundant passively fixed lead an extremely difficult and often hazardous procedure. LV leads may be designed to wedge into a branch of the coronary sinus (CS).

Active fixation leads are designed for transvenous and epicardial lead placement (see Figure 24-12B). Transvenous leads have a sharpened helical screw at the end that is inserted into the myocardium. Damage to the vein is avoided by retracting the screw into the lead body or by covering it with a soluble substance that dissolves after several minutes of contact with fluid. If the screw is permanently extended, the implant physician rotates the lead counterclockwise in order to prevent damage to the venous system. Epicardial lead placement also requires leads that are actively fixed either by sewing them in place or by using leads that have hooks, barbs, or helical screws.

Actively fixed leads often prove easier to remove than those that have been passively attached. By rotating the sharpened helix, it may be possible to unscrew it from the endocardium. However, endothelialization will also occur with these leads, so removal is not always ensured.

Active fixation leads are particularly beneficial when it is not possible, or viable, to implant a

Figure 24-12. Lead Fixation (23) *A.* Passive fixation. *B.* Active fixation.

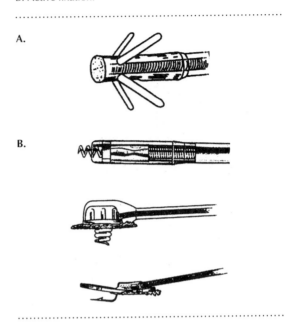

passive fixation lead. This is typically the case when implanting an atrial lead in a patient who has had previous cardiac surgery. Cannulation of the right atrium during bypass surgery removes the atrial appendage, making it difficult to entrap a passive lead in the remaining smooth muscular wall. Pacing from the right ventricular outflow tract (RVOT) may also require an active fixation lead. In other cases, such as in young patients, active fixation devices may be preferred in anticipation of multiple lead replacements.

Permanent pacing leads typically have steroid elution to minimize the rise in pacing thresholds historically seen directly following implant.

IMPLANT PROCEDURE

Preparation

If possible, preparation should begin in the preadmission period. This includes psychological preparation on the part of the patient and family, as well as the physical preparation of the patient. Written instruction may be essential, because there are many internal and external barriers to both patient and family learning at this point. Written booklets can be obtained commercially or developed specifically for a facility. They may describe the indication and function of a pacemaker as well as the peri-implant period, discharge care, routine follow-up, and restrictions. The NASPE Council of Associated Professionals has prepared guidelines[24] that may be used in development of educational materials. Generally, written material should be at the sixth-grade level. Visual representation, such as a model, of a pacemaker system assists in providing concreteness. Additionally, video and oral instruction will provide more variability and assist in gaining the learner's attention. Reinforcement is essential.[25] Sometimes, other patients who have previously had a pacemaker implanted (or the families of such patients) may offer additional support. Patients should display a basic understanding of the preparation, implant procedures, and follow-up of a permanently implanted pacemaker system. However, lengths of stay are short, pacers may even be done on an outpatient basis, and goals may need to be simplified.

Physical preparation may begin one or more days prior to the anticipated implant. Routine preadmission laboratory studies, including complete blood count $+/-$ differential, basic metabolic panel, coagulation studies, urinalysis, ECG and chest radiographs, and possibly liver function studies may be ordered. If the patient is on anticoagulants, they are usually discontinued in order to ensure an international normalized ratio (INR) of less than 2 at implant. Some physicians will perform pacemaker implant under anticoagulation provided the INR is at or below 2. The patient, or nurses, may be asked to scrub the proposed implant site with an antimicrobial solution beginning one or more days prior to the implant

procedure. No electrodes or adhesive should remain at the site.

The patient is kept NPO after midnight or for at least 4 hours prior to the procedure. The patient should preferably have at least one 20-gauge (or larger bore) patent intravenous (IV) catheter ipsilateral to the anticipated implant site. IV hydration may be ordered to ensure that the patient does not become dehydrated. Diabetic patients should be scheduled for their procedure earlier in the day, as schedules permit. Oral antidiabetic agents are held, and insulins held or adjusted, accordingly. Antibiotic coverage is generally ordered on call to the procedure room or within 1 hour of the surgical incision. An ECG of the patient's intrinsic rhythm should be obtained upon arrival in the procedure area.

Strict adherence to sterile technique is required for the implantation procedure itself. Ideally, an operating room or a dedicated pacemaker laboratory should be used for the implantation of all permanent systems and, if possible, for temporary pacing systems. Nurses, technicians, and physicians directly involved perform a full surgical scrub. The instrument tray (see Table 24-3) should be set up immediately prior to the procedure. Pacing leads and pulse generators are only opened as needed, because the anticipated needs of the patient may change.

The site of implantation is shaved and prepped as close to the procedure time as possible. The site is typically cleansed with either iodine or chlorhexadine wash. Sterile towels and drapes are used to cover the patient leaving only the operative area and patient's face exposed. A sterile transparent surgical dressing may be used over the operative site. A barrier, typically formed by the sterile drape, separates the patient's face from the operative site. The conscious patient should be discouraged from moving his or her hands to the incision site and should keep the face averted. If it should become necessary to change operative sites, the staff rescrubs and the patient is prepped and draped again.

Table 24-3. Common Sterile Implant Supplies

1 large and 1 small self-retaining retractor	1 pair wire cutters
2 Catspaw retractors	4 towel clips
1 each long and short arterial hooks	2 gallipots
1 each No. 3 and No. 4 blade handles	1 6-inch bowl
1 straight Iris forceps	1 receiver
1 curved Iris forceps	10 radiopaque sponges
2 Largenbecks retractors	1 Roberts clamp
1 each toothed and non-toothed forceps	5 curved mosquito clips
1 each 2, 10 and 20 mL syringe	2 straight mosquito clips
1 each No. 11 and No. 22 blade	1 utility drape
1 pair Mayo/Metzenbaum scissors	1 laparotomy drape
1 each 19, 21, and 25 G needle	1 table cover
1 pair fine curved McIndor scissors	1 X-Ray tube cover
1 pair Iris scissors	1 stitch holder
1 Hohn dilator	3 sponge holders
suture, ties	1 connector cable
sheaths	gowns, gloves

Staffing

Staffing typically consists of the scrub person, a room nurse, and the implanting physician(s). The implanting physician may be a surgeon, cardiologist, electrophysiologist, or a surgeon and cardiologist together. An anesthesiologist is present for procedures requiring general anesthesia. A radiographer and a cardiac technician should also be available if needed. It is recommended that the patient be monitored on more than one cardiac monitor.[24] Typically, one monitor would also have external pacing and defibrillation capabilities. Throughout the implant procedure, the nurse monitors and records the patient's heart rhythm, heart rate, blood pressure, respiratory rate, oxygen saturation, and level of comfort and/or sedation. Pacemakers are usually implanted under local anesthetic. When conscious sedation is administered, the patient is monitored at intervals of 1 to 5 minutes.[26] One nurse should be dedicated to conscious sedation administration and patient monitoring. Emergency medications, suction equipment, oxygen, and oxygen delivery devices should be immediately available.

Surgical Procedure

The physician may choose the patient's left or right side for pacemaker implantation, depending on the patient's routine activities. Generally, the implant site is chosen on the less-dominant side (e.g., if the patient is right-handed, the left side will be used). Other considerations such as sporting activities may also be taken into account. Individuals who shoot firearms should have the unit implanted on the side opposite to that on which they hold their weapon. Recoil may damage the skin over the generator, the generator, or lead system. Others who engage in contact sports such as football or basketball may prefer to have their pacemaker implanted in the axilla or behind the great pectoral muscle to avoid damage. In other instances, pacemaker generators may be implanted submammary or abdominally.

Transvenous lead placement is preferred by most physicians implanting pacemakers. When a permanent pacemaker system is being implanted, the subclavian or cephalic veins are commonly selected for access. An approximately 4 cm to 6 cm incision is made in the subclavian region, below and parallel to the clavicle (may be made after access is confirmed). A subcutaneous pocket in which the pulse generator will lie is formed inferior to the incision.

The subclavian vein will then be punctured using the Seldinger technique. With this technique, a large-bore (18-gauge) needle is inserted into the vein, then a guide wire is passed through the bore of the needle. This is done under fluoroscopic guidance. Over the guide wire, dilators may be passed as needed to allow entrance of the peel-away (or split) sheath into the vein.[7] The pacing lead is introduced into the vein through the sheath. The sheath is then removed by peeling it apart. If the guide wire is to be retained for placement of a second lead, the sheath may be two sizes larger than the lead in diameter.

The cephalic vein can also be used. It is isolated via a direct cut-down method, and a venotomy is then performed to gain access into the vein. Both of these veins may be of sufficient size to facilitate the passage of two pacing leads, although the cephalic may prove more difficult.[7] However, the cephalic vein may be preferred over the subclavian vein by some implanters. With the subclavian approach, the lead may form a rather sharp angulation as it extends up from the generator site and enters into the vein. It then travels between the clavicle and first rib. Movement of the arm and shoulder may cause crushing of the lead or leads implanted, leading to possible insulation and/or conductor fractures, especially if introduced too medially. The cephalic or a lateral subclavian approach may avoid this. On rare occasions, other veins such as the external or internal jugular may be used. This is typically only done when the subclavian and cephalic veins do not supply sufficient access. Additionally, if pacing leads made with differing insulations are used, separate veins prevent adherence to one another.

Temporary pacing leads should be inserted at a site other than the one anticipated for permanent implant. This minimizes the risk of infection occurring at the permanent site. The internal jugular and subclavian veins are preferred entry sites for temporary leads, although the external jugular, brachial, and femoral veins are also used. However, using the femoral vein means that the patient is rendered relatively immobile throughout the period of time the temporary pacer is maintained.

If a temporary pacing system is in place at the time of permanent implantation, it is typically removed under fluoroscopic guidance once the permanent system is functioning appropriately, because the tip of the permanent electrode may be displaced during removal of the temporary electrode. In rare instances, it may be left in place for 24 hours to be used in the event of permanent pacemaker lead dislodgment.

Measurements

Sensing

Intrinsic P (atrial) and R (ventricular) waves are measured in their respective chambers to ensure sensing of intrinsic activity by the pulse generator. The IEGM is the signal used by the pacemaker to sense the patient's own heart rhythm. The amplitudes of these signals are measured in peak-to-peak voltage.[7] Although they can be measured from an ECG machine, the filters within the ECG machine may clip the signal. Typically, a pacing system analyzer (PSA) is used. (Note: Filtering of signals differs slightly among manufacturers; signals measured by one company's PSA may not correlate exactly with others or possibly with the implanted generator.) This is done by connecting a sterile cable from the pacing lead to the PSA and will soon have remote capability as do some ICDs. Acceptable values are depicted in Table 24-4.

If suboptimal peak-to-peak values of the intrinsic signal are recorded, they may be accepted if it is unlikely that the patient's own heart rhythm is going to be sensed. For example, a patient whose underlying ventricular rhythm is less than the anticipated LRL may not necessarily need

Table 24-4. Acceptable Implant Measurements

	Atrium	Ventricle
Acute stimulation	≤ 1.0V	*≤ 1.0V
Chronic stimulation threshold	2–2.5V	2–2.5V
Sensed P wave/R wave	≥ 1.5 mV	≥ 4.0 mV
Lead impedance	300–1500 Ohm	300–1500 Ohm
Slew rate	0.3 V/sec	0.5 V/sec

Acceptable measurements for acute and chronic lead placement. Stimulation thresholds are based on pulse duration of 0.5 millisecond.

*LV lead may be slightly higher.

ventricular sensing. In this instance, proper lead positioning is based on other implant criteria. If there is any likelihood that the patient's own rhythm will increase, it is vital that the intrinsic amplitude be large enough to allow for adequate sensing. If the intrinsic deflection is not of sufficient amplitude, the pacemaker will not sense or see the intrinsic activity. This may lead to inappropriate pacing. Delivery of a pacing stimulus during the relative refractory period may induce ventricular arrhythmias (paced R on T), as well as atrial arrhythmias. However, factors other than amplitude will affect sensing by the pulse generator.

The slew rate is the measure of voltage over time of the peak slope of the intracardiac signal (see Figure 24-13). It is also used by pacemakers to assist sensing of intrinsic activity. It is measured in volts per second (V/sec). Normal values are also depicted in Table 24-4. Slew rates tend to correlate with the frequency content of the signal. Pulse generators accept certain frequency signals as intrinsic and filter out signals of higher or lower frequency.[7] T waves tend to be of low frequency and have lower slew rates. They are generally of a lower peak-to-peak amplitude than R waves, and thus are not typically sensed. An atrial IEGM that also records a ventricular signal (see Figure 24-14) may not be an issue as the far-field R wave amplitude is typically smaller and of lower frequency. Even if the peak-to-peak signal

is large and the slew rate is low, a beat may not be sensed. This may be true of ventricular ectopic beats or normal intrinsic beats. Therefore, it is important to measure the slew rate at implant in addition to the intrinsic amplitude.[8]

The sensing threshold is the minimal intrinsic signal to be consistently sensed. When programming sensing, it is important to remember that the higher the value programmed (in millivolts), the less sensitive the system is. In other words,

Figure 24-13. The slew rate is equal to the change in amplitude (volts) per change in time (seconds) and is measured at the steepest portion of the IEGM signal.

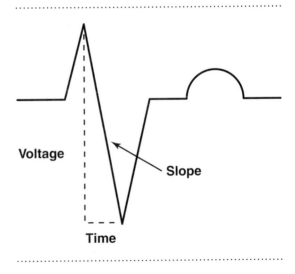

Figure 24-14. Atrial IEGM recording with farfield ventricular IEGM.

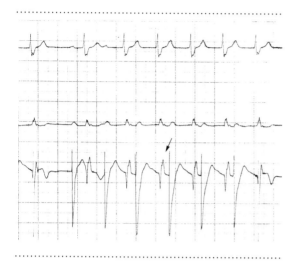

a high value is less sensitive and a low value is highly sensitive or less = more! An analogy may also be made with a brick wall. The higher the wall is raised (value in millivolts), the less one will be able to see. If the wall is lowered, more will be seen (sensed).

Intracardiac Electrogram

The intracardiac electrogram (IEGM) is a filtered, localized recording of intrinsic electrical activity between the distal electrode (cathode) tissue interface and a second electrode or pole (anode). It is used as a means of ensuring that the pacing lead has sufficient contact with viable myocardium. Additionally, recording at least one simultaneous surface ECG lead ensures that the lead is positioned in the appropriate chamber of the heart. The IEGM may only be recorded in patients who have an underlying rhythm. If the patient is in a paced rhythm, pacing should be weaned slowly, at increments of 10 paces per minute (ppm), until intrinsic activity is obtained. Typically, if no intrinsic rhythm greater than 30 ppm in noted, no further attempt is made at obtaining an electrogram.

The IEGM may be recorded via the PSA, ECG machine, or EP recording system. To record an IEGM via the ECG machine, a sterile connector cable is attached to the connector pin (see Figure 24-15) of the pacing lead (negative pole) and the other end connected to a V lead on an ECG recorder. The limb leads are connected to the patient in the usual way. The V-lead tracing will reflect the unipolar IEGM. A bipolar signal may also be obtained by connecting the connector pin to the right arm lead and the connector ring (positive pole) to the left arm lead. The lower ECG limb leads are connected to the patient as usual. In a laboratory with an electrophysiology recording system, a unipolar recording can be obtained by setting the distal pole (connector pin) as negative and the proximal pole (connector ring or tissue ground) as Wilson's central terminal (WCT). In a bipolar recording, the proximal pole is set as positive.

The unipolar IEGM allows evaluation of lead position by the current of injury. Its presence shows that the lead is in contact with healthy myocardium that has become transiently injured by the pacing lead. With proper positioning, the unipolar electrogram should have a large, positive current of injury. This is depicted as PT-elevation on an atrial lead, and ST-elevation on a ventricular lead (see Figure 24-16). The amplitude of the injury current will vary according to the type of pacing lead being implanted. It is most pronounced with active fixation leads and often less marked with soft, or passive, fixation leads. No injury current may mean that either there is no contact or that the tissue is necrosed, ischemic, or scarred. Damaged tissue requires high energy to stimulate, or may not be stimulated at all, and is not suitable for pacing. The lead must be repositioned in the absence of a current of injury. It is important to note that injury current resolves with time, so it will not be present on chronically implanted leads.

The IEGM of a chronic lead will show an ST- or PT-segment that has returned to the isoelectric

Figure 24-15. Recording of the IEGM (27). *A:* The set-up used to obtain a unipolar IEGM recording. *B:* The set-up for a bipolar recording.

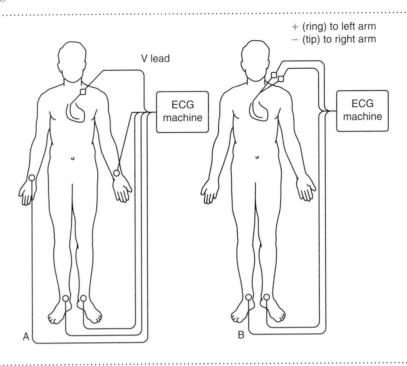

Figure 24-16. Acute IEGMs. Tracing A shows acute PTa elevation (arrow) recorded at the time of implantation on an atrial IEGM. Tracing B shows acute ST elevation (arrow) on a ventricular IEGM, also recorded at implantation.

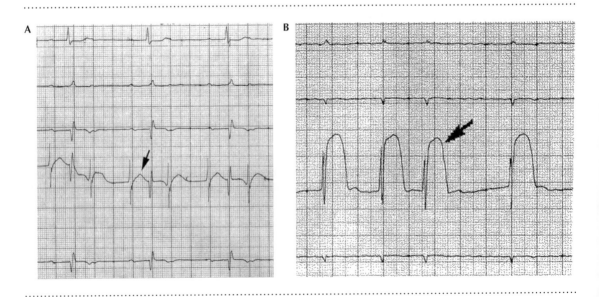

line or below and an inverted T wave (see Figure 24-17). If a unipolar IEGM acutely displays a negative injury current and T wave inversion, it suggests that the myocardium has been perforated by the lead. On a bipolar IEGM, the polarity of the injury current is dependent upon the lead from which it is being recorded.

Pacing Threshold

After ascertaining that the lead is positioned in healthy myocardium and sensing appropriately, a pacing threshold is measured. The pacing or stimulation threshold is the minimal electrical stimulus required to consistently cause cardiac muscle contraction. It is measured in volts/pulse duration or current (mA). Permanent pacing thresholds are expressed as x volts at y pulse duration. To measure this, a sterile connector is used to connect the lead to the PSA. If a PSA is not available, a temporary pacing box may be used. However, this is less desirable because all measurements for implantation may not be obtained. Care should be taken to ensure that the connections are made correctly. On a bipolar lead, the distal electrode is active (negative) and the proximal (ring electrode) is indifferent (positive). In a unipolar system, the generator, or skin, acts as the positive electrode. The international convention is that negative connectors are colored black and

that positive ones are colored red. A mnemonic for remembering this is:

R.I.P. (Red Indifferent Positive)
B.A.N. (Black Active Negative)

If the connections are reversed, the stimulation threshold may be significantly higher. In addition, anodal (positive) stimulation can induce ventricular fibrillation even at subthreshold outputs.[27]

In order to measure the stimulation threshold, one must pace at a rate about 10 to 15 bpm faster than the patient's intrinsic rhythm. For an acutely implanted lead, one typically begins pacing with a pulse duration of 0.5 millisecond and a voltage of 5.0 V. If capture is noted, voltage may quickly be lowered to 2.0 V. Continue decrementing the voltage slowly until loss of capture is noted. Then, the voltage is increased until capture is reestablished. It is often seen that loss of capture while reducing voltage is at a lower value than that which is needed to regain capture when the voltage is subsequently increased. This is known as the Wedensky effect (see Figure 24-18). Threshold is the value at which capture was reestablished, or that which consistently captured the heart.[28]

If no capture is achieved at 2.0 V and 0.5 milliseconds with an acutely implanted pacing lead, it is usually repositioned. At this point, previously

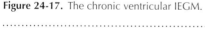

Figure 24-17. The chronic ventricular IEGM.

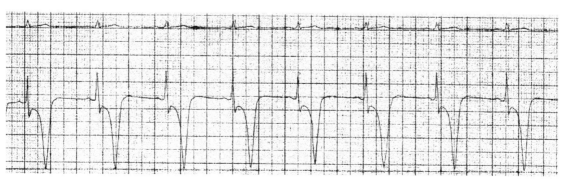

Figure 24-18. As the atrial output is gradually decremented to 1.5 V, atrial capture is lost. The atrial output is then gradually increased. Note that capture is not regained until the output reaches 1.8 V.

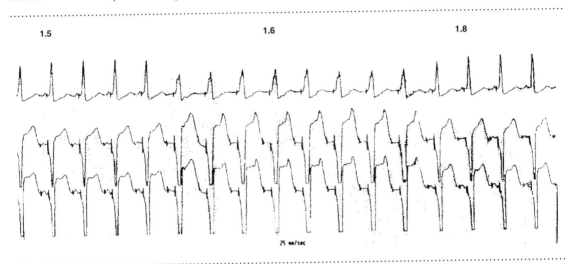

1.5   1.6   1.8

25 mm/sec

obtained measurements are repeated. If the initial threshold measurement is too high but a good injury current was obtained, one should wait for about 5 minutes and then retest. The threshold may have dropped because initial high values may be seen due to localized myocardial damage by the pacing lead and subsequent release of potassium ions, particularly with active fixation leads. The age and health of the patient, difficulty of venous access, and the length of the procedure should be taken into account before rejecting high thresholds. The risks of a prolonged and/or difficult procedure may potentially be more dangerous for the patient and high thresholds may ultimately be accepted despite faster battery depletion. When pacing thresholds have been obtained, the rate may again be slowly decreased until the patient's intrinsic rhythm is noted or temporary pacing support is resumed.

The voltage strength-duration curve (SDC) may also be plotted. This is done by measuring voltage threshold at different pulse durations, typically 0.1 milliseconds, 0.5 milliseconds, and 1.0 milliseconds. Some pacemakers have semiautomated software for plotting a SDC. The SDC plots threshold amplitude on the vertical axis and threshold pulse duration on the horizontal axis (see Figure 24-19). In general, the curve shows that at short pulse durations, a small change can dramatically affect threshold voltage, but has little effect at longer pulse durations.

There are two important points on the curve: rheobase and chronaxie. Increasing the pulse duration will lower the voltage required for capture until the rheobase value is achieved. Rheobase is the point at which voltage threshold has reached its lowest value and no matter how much farther the pulse duration is stretched, the voltage threshold cannot be reduced. It is the lowest stimulation threshold achievable at any pulse duration.[7] This is represented by the flattened region of the SDC. Typically, it is at around 1.0 milliseconds that the rheobase is seen and it never occurs at greater than 2.0 milliseconds. Chronaxie is the pulse duration threshold at twice rheobase voltage.[7]

Thresholds are obtained in the clinical setting either by decrementing voltage at a constant pulse width (0.5 milliseconds) or by decrementing pulse width at a constant voltage (2.5 V).

Figure 24-19. Strength duration curve.

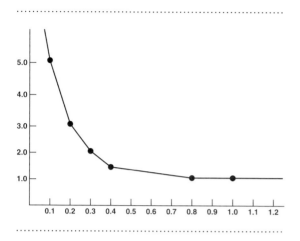

Table 24-5. Basic Electrical Relationships in Pacing

$$E = VIT$$

$$E = \frac{V^2}{R} \times T$$

Ohm's Law

$$I = \frac{V}{R} \qquad or \qquad R = \frac{V}{R} \qquad or \qquad V = IR$$

In the equations, E represents energy (microjoules), V represents voltage, I current (mA), T pulse duration (ms) and R resistance, or impedance.

In general, the same chronic 2:1 safety margin can be achieved by doubling the threshold voltage or by tripling the threshold pulse duration. However, in looking at the SDC, one can see that this is only possible at very short pulse durations. In fact, this may not necessarily be true for pulse width threshold values greater than 0.2 milliseconds.[7] At pulse durations greater than chronaxie, there is little effect on threshold voltage, but there is wastage of pacemaker battery energy. With newly implanted leads, a greater safety margin is programmed due to potential threshold rise.

Current and Lead Impedance

Current is measured while pacing at a fixed output (5.0 V and 0.5 millisecond). It is the rate the electrical charge passes through any point within the circuit.[24] Its unit of measurement is milliamperes (mA) and can be obtained using the PSA. PSAs also have the ability to measure lead impedance. However, if this is not available it can be calculated using Ohm's law (see Table 24-5) when the voltage and current are known, and were obtained at the same pulse duration. In general, impedance is analogous to the resistance

within the circuit.[24] Acceptable values for lead impedance are, generally, between 300 and 1500 ohms. Bipolar systems tend to have higher lead impedances than unipolar systems. Some leads are designed as *high-impedance* leads in order to minimize current drain and pacing threshold. It is useful to measure the impedance in the polarity to which it will be programmed for permanent pacing. A beat-to-beat variation in lead impedance of up to 50 ohms may be seen with an error range as much as 30%.[24]

Retrograde AV Conduction

When a ventricular pacing lead is implanted, a retrograde atrioventricular conduction (RAVC) test should be done. In the presence of ventricular pacing, the surface ECG is observed for P waves falling within ST-segment or T waves on the surface ECG leads (see Figure 24-20). If an atrial lead is also being implanted, the intracardiac signal can be used to assist in determining if there is atrial activity following each paced ventricular beat. The significance of retrograde conduction is the loss of AV synchrony. The atria contract against closed AV valves resulting in increased chamber pressure and loss of atrial kick. If a single chamber ventricular system is implanted and RAVC is present, the patient has a greater risk of pacemaker syndrome.[13]

Figure 24-20. While ventricular pacing is at 86 bpm, 1:1 retrograde conduction is noted as indicated by the negative deflected P waves following each QRS complex.

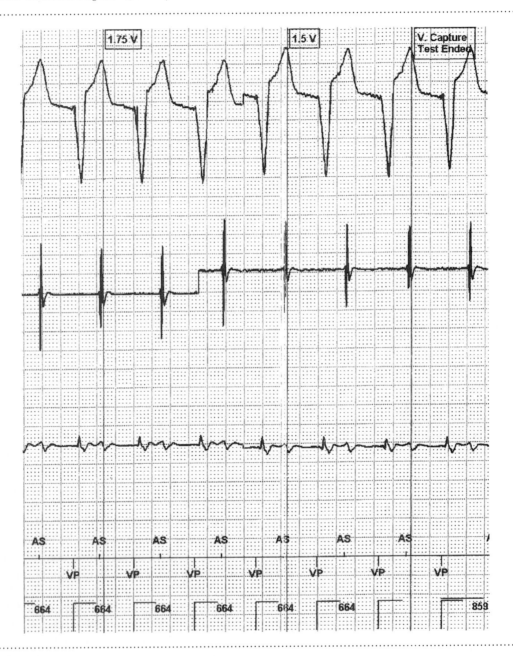

Pacemaker syndrome encompasses a variety of signs and symptoms attributed to ventricular pacing. It results from the hemodynamic com- promise attributed to RAVC. Signs of pacemaker syndrome include increased atrial and jugular ve- nous pressures, cannon A waves, decreased cardiac output, and a decrease in blood pressure. Symptoms are variable but may include malaise, fatigue, weakness, dizziness, dyspnea, paroxysmal nocturnal dyspnea, palpitations, neck throbbing, and possibly syncope.[7] If RAVC is noted at the implantation of a ventricular single-chamber pacemaker, the implanter will typically consider changing to a dual-chamber system, because pacemaker syndrome can prove intolerable to the patient.

Dual-chamber pacemakers maintain AV synchrony and thus prevent pacemaker syndrome. However, the presence of retrograde conduction may subject the patient to pacemaker-mediated tachycardia (PMT). This form of reentry is initiated if a retrograde P wave is sensed, triggering ventricular pacing output, and the scenario is perpetuated. It may be initiated by a premature ventricular contraction (PVC) or with the loss of atrial capture. This may occur in DDD, VDD, or DDDR modes. Therefore, when a dual-chamber system is implanted and RAVC is present, it is important to measure the RAVC time. This is measured from the pacing stimulus to the beginning of the retrograde conducted P wave, or to the A deflection of the IEGM. It will be necessary to program the pacemaker's postventricular atrial refractory period (PVARP) to a value beyond this (generally, 30 ms) thus avoiding sensing and tracking retrograde P waves. Pacemakers may have a safety feature in which the PVARP is automatically extended when a PVC is sensed. Others may have PMT termination algorithms. PMTs may occur as the result of rapid atrial rhythms, however, all are limited by the programmed URL and may be alleviated by appropriate mode switching.

Stability

Once all other measurements have been obtained, lead position stability is evaluated. This may be done by asking the patient to perform a variety of maneuvers such as sniffing, panting, deep breath-

ing, and coughing while continuously pacing at a rate faster than the patient's intrinsic rate. The ECG is observed throughout the stability test to be sure that there is no loss of capture. The physician monitors the lead tip under fluoroscopy during these maneuvers to observe lead position radiographically and evaluate for excess lead tension that may occur with deep inspiration.[7]

Diaphragmatic Stimulation

Finally, diaphragmatic stimulation is assessed. While pacing faster than the patient's intrinsic rhythm, at an output of 10 V and 0.5 milliseconds, the implanting physician places his or her hand over the region of the patient's diaphragm to feel for contraction. This should be done for both atrial and ventricular leads, because laterally positioned right atrial leads may stimulate the phrenic nerve. If diaphragmatic stimulation, or twitching, is felt at 10 V the voltage should be reduced gradually until the twitching ceases. The lead position may be accepted only if diaphragmatic stimulation occurs at output values greater than those that are expected to be programmed. RV leads should be assessed for possible perforation of the ventricle. LV leads may require repositioning if not able to program to avoid diaphragmatic or chest wall stimulation.

Pulse Generator Implantation

After the leads are appropriately positioned, nonabsorbable suture is used to secure them to the underlying fascia. The pocket is irrigated with an antibiotic solution and evaluated for bleeding. If the procedure has been prolonged for 4 or more hours, additional IV antibiotics are given. The pulse generator, still in its sterile package, is programmed to the appropriate settings, then opened. The physician inserts the lead pin(s) into the connector block (see Figure 24-21) of the pulse generator and set screws secured as directed by the manufacturer. Care is taken to ensure the

Figure 24-21. Insertion of lead to connector block. *Source:* From Thera DR: Product Information Manual. Minneapolis, MN: Medtronic; 1995:UC9403918EN.

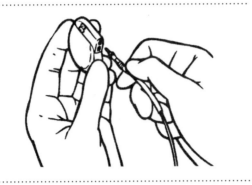

atrial lead is inserted in the atrial port, and then the ventricular lead is inserted (see Figure 24-22). With bifurcated bipolar leads, the connecting pin of the distal electrode is inserted into the cathode port in the block and the proximal in the anode (+).

Once the set screws have been tightened in the connector block, or header, the lead(s) are gently tugged to ensure that they are secure. Failure of the pin to extend fully into the header can result in no contact with the proximal pole and lack of bipolar pacing (and an extremely high measured bipolar lead impedance). The excess length of the lead(s) is then coiled behind the pulse generator and implanted in the pocket (coiling the lead under the generator prevents damage to the leads if, or when, the pocket is reopened). The incision is then sutured closed, then steristrips and a sterile dressing are applied. Alternatively, the outer layer may be closed with a cyanoacrylate skin glue that permits showering.

OTHER METHODS OF PACING

Temporary pacing can be achieved by methods other than the transvenous or epicardial approach. Short-term, transcutaneous electrodes may be used. These are large self-adhesive patches that are attached to the chest wall and connected to a transcutaneous pacing generator. Modern generators and the large size electrodes allow low thresholds when using long (40 millisecond) pulse durations. This diminishes stimulation of skeletal muscle and cutaneous nerves that in the past caused excruciating pain to the patient.[24] However, their use is still associated with considerable pain. This method of pacing is more commonly used as a standby procedure should emergency pacing be required. Transcutaneous pacers provide simple and efficient noninvasive VVI support.[7,24]

Esophageal electrodes are also available. These require high-output generators and may result in esophageal burning. They are not frequently used because they also tend to cause the patient discomfort. In addition, this method of pacing may not always be reliable for ventricular support.[24] The electrodes may be more useful in obtaining IEGMs, but even so, they are somewhat cumbersome to have to swallow. They have been effective in atrial overdrive pacing and in infants and children with difficult venous access.

Transthoracic pacing may also be achieved by inserting a cannula and pacing lead through the chest wall and into the right ventricle. This is only considered in an extreme emergency and is rarely used. The transthoracic lead can be attached to a normal temporary pacing box. However, thresholds tend to progressively rise and insertion of a transvenous system is recommended only when the patient is in a stable condition.[7]

Biventricular Pacing

As pacemaker technology has evolved, so have the indications for which pacing therapy can be used. Biventricular devices are increasingly used to treat heart failure because they can provide cardiac resynchronization therapy (CRT). In the normal heart, both ventricles contract synchronously following atrial contraction. When a person suffers heart failure and reduced LVEF, ventricular synchrony can be lost. This can be

Figure 24-22. *A.* Reversed atrial and ventricular leads. The ECG (A) shows ventricular capture following each atrial pacing artifact. *B.* The marker channels retrieved (B and C) reveal atrial sensed (AS) occurring with each QRS and ventricular sensed events occurring with each P wave. *C.* The marker channels retrieved (B and C) reveal atrial sensed (AS) occurring with each QRS and ventricular sensed events occurring with each P wave.

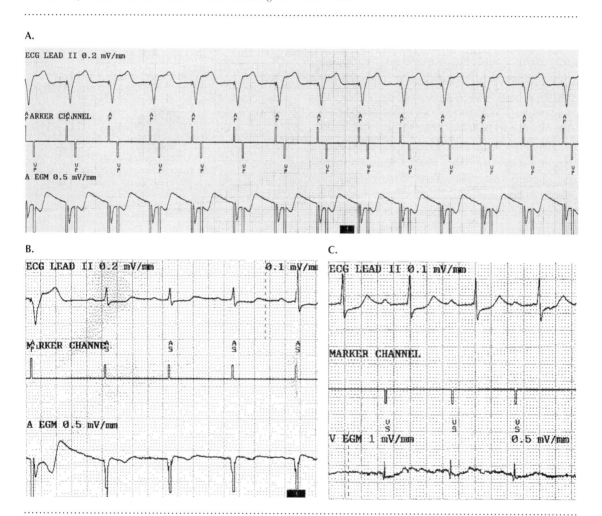

seen as a widening of the QRS complex on the surface ECG. Heart failure signs and symptoms may include shortness of breath, dyspnea on exertion, orthopnea, paroxysmal nocturnal dyspnea, lower extremity edema, fatigue, activity intolerance, and often rapid, irregular heart rhythms. By resynchronizing ventricular activity, symptoms may be reduced and LVEF improved. Implant is indicated for patients with an LVEF less than or equal to 35 percent, QRS duration greater than or equal to 120 ms and NYHA Class III or IV heart failure (see Table 24-2). Class III patients are at high risk of life-threatening arrhythmias, and in some instances Class IV, in which case, a biventricular ICD rather than a pacemaker may be considered.[14]

Initially, a standard dual-chamber device was implanted with two ventricular leads connected into the ventricular port using a bifurcated connector. The atrial lead was connected to the atrial channel as normal, unless there was chronic atrial fibrillation. In this case, one ventricular lead could occupy the atrial port. Now, dedicated biventricular devices are available with two separate ventricular ports and an atrial port, making a triple-chamber device. One ventricular lead is inserted into the RVA; the other paces the LV. This lead is inserted transvenously into the CS with a guide catheter and possibly injection of contrast material. LV venous tributaries are identified and the lead is advanced to a lateral branch midway between the AV groove and apex. The IEGM should fall in the later aspect of the surface QRS tracing.[29] Higher pacing thresholds are generally accepted if no diaphragmatic stimulation is noted. LV pacing should produce a RBBB pattern in lead V1 and be positive in lead III on a surface ECG verses RV apical pacing which produces a LBBB pattern in V1 and is positive in lead I. Additional consideration is given to programming of CRT devices. If possible, the lowest pacing threshold should be used in order to maintain device longevity.

Biventricular pacemakers now have independently programmable outputs for each ventricle. If these are not available, it is necessary to program the sole ventricular output with an adequate safety margin to ensure capture of the chamber with the highest threshold (normally the LV), but possibly forgoing a 2:1 safely margin for this lead. Capture is still ensured due to the redundancy of ventricular leads. Echo guidance with programming may ensure optimal diastolic filling, and mechanical synchrony both inter- and intraventricular.[29] The goal is to provide 100% biventricular pacing and hopefully improve LVEF and reduction of heart failure symptoms and hospitalizations.

Complications

Complications may arise acutely in association with the implantation procedure or chronically as a result of the presence of the pacemaker system within the body. Common complications of pacemaker therapy can be found in Table 24-6. Additional risks with LV lead implant may include dissection, coronary vein or artery occlusion, and possibly contrast-induced nephropathy.[29] It is imperative that the nursing staff be familiar with possible complications so that they can be anticipated, quickly identified, and treated. Of particular concern are signs of impending erosion or infection that may necessitate removal of the pacing system hardware. However,

Table 24-6. Complications of Pacemaker Therapy[7]

1. Venous access
   A. Secondary to Seldinger technique
      i. Pneumothorax
      ii. Hemothorax
      iii. Other (e.g., injury to thoracic duct, nerves)
   B. Secondary to sheath insertion
      i. Air embolism
      ii. Perforation of central vein or heart
2. Lead placement
   A. Arrhythmia
   B. Perforation of heart or vein
   C. Damage to heart valve
   D. Damage to lead
   E. Displacement/Twiddler's syndrome
3. Intravascular thrombosis/fibrosis
4. Generator
   A. Misconnection
   B. Pain
   C. Migration
   D. Erosion
   E. Infection

complication rates are relatively low, estimated at 2.9% for dual-chamber systems and 1.5% for single chamber,[8] although data suggests infection rates rose to more than 5% for pacer patients in 2003.[30]

POSTOPERATIVE CARE

Patient Evaluation

Patients typically return from the implant procedure awake and alert. However, both swallow and gag reflexes should be checked. Cardiopulmonary status should also be evaluated. Vital signs and incision site inspection may be ordered at frequent intervals over the initial 2 to 3 hours. If the patient has a transparent dressing, the incision may be easily inspected for approximation of the incision line, hematoma, seroma, or signs of infection. If the patient has a bulky opaque dressing, one can gently palpate the surrounding tissue and evaluate for other signs and symptoms of possible complications such as crepitus indicating possible pneumothorax, or hematoma and seroma.

The mode of pacing and other parameters should be noted in the patient's chart. The patient should be attached to a telemetry monitor, and his or her rhythm noted at routine intervals. This should include whether the pacer is sensing and pacing appropriately as well as if capture occurs with each pacing output.

An ECG with and without a magnet should be obtained. The magnet application reverts the pacer to an asynchronous pacing mode to assist in evaluating capture and confirms an adequate battery status of the pulse generator. Pacing from the RVA should have an LBB block pattern, although RBB has been infrequently reported with RV lead positions.[31] If an RBB block pattern is noted, further investigation of lead position is warranted.

Some physicians may choose to obtain a portable chest radiograph upon the patient's arrival on the ward to rule out pneumothorax. PA and lateral chest radiograph is typically done the following morning for inpatients. This may assist in detection of acute lead dislodgment or confirm a stable lead position. A formal chest radiograph following the implant procedure also serves as a means of comparison should lead placement be questionable in the future.

Patient Care

Bed rest is maintained for the first 3 hours or up to 24 hours. The head of the bed should be maintained at 30° (pectoral implants) to avoid edema in the head and neck region. A sling may be used to immobilize the ipsilateral arm overnight. Chest physical therapy or other activities that may provoke lead dislodgment are avoided. Typically, preprocedure diet and medications are resumed. Analgesics may be required over the first 24 hours.

If an inpatient, the initial dressing is removed by the implanting physician the following morning. Anticoagulation therapy may be resumed if it had been held. At the discretion of the physician, anticoagulants may be withheld for a prolonged period to prevent bleeding into the pacemaker pocket. A predischarge evaluation of pacing and sensing thresholds, IEGM, and programmed parameters may be done to confirm appropriate pacer function.

Individual institutions generally develop their own guidelines for the care of a temporary pacing system. These guidelines should encompass site care, battery changes, sensing and pacing thresholds, and electrical safety precautions. Site care may vary, but a sterile technique should be maintained. As previously discussed (in the section on temporary pulse generators), batteries should be changed prior to use. It is recommended that a log be kept of each pulse generator. If a temporary generator should have a faceplate covering controls, it should be maintained, because it serves as a means of protection from inadvertent reprogramming. Daily pacing and sensing thresholds are generally done to protect the patient from loss of capture or sensing due to inflammation at the electrode-tissue interface resulting in acute threshold rise. Threshold evaluation may be the responsibility of the physician or nursing staff and is done in the same manner as for a permanent pacemaker.

Electrical safety is a major concern for this patient population, because the pacing lead provides a direct route for current flow to the heart tissue. Pacing leads must always be protected from any potential source of electrical current whether environmental or equipment related. Nurses caring for patients should ensure proper maintenance and grounding of equipment. In addition, they should discharge any potential static electricity on a metal surface prior to contact with patients. Rubber gloves should be worn when handling pacing leads (wires) and exposed pacing wires should also be protected with insulating material (i.e., a rubber glove). Contact between two pacing wires should be avoided. Nurses should not simultaneously touch electrical equipment and pacing wires. There has been past concern that policies for electrical safety may not be adequate in many facilities.[32]

Postprocedure Education

Written discharge instructions should be reviewed, emphasizing care of the incision, activity restrictions, and a name and phone number of a healthcare provider who can answer any questions that may arise. For example, many patients believe that at the moment of death, the pacemaker will keep them alive for a longer time. This problem, which does not exist in reality, must be discussed with every patient.

The patient and/or caretakers should observe the site as a reference for comparison when at home. Any redness, swelling, discharge, increased bruising or pain, or a persistent temperature greater than 100°F should be reported to the implanting or follow-up physician. For pectoral implants, it should be emphasized that the ipsilateral arm should not be raised above shoulder height for at least the first few days, postoperatively. Activity such as sweeping or lifting heavy (more than 5 to 10 lb or 2 to 5 kg) objects should be avoided for 3 to 4 weeks. This is to protect the surgical site and to allow endothelialization of the lead tip within the heart chamber.

Precautions regarding lifestyle choices that may impact pacemaker function should be reviewed with the patient and family. These may include activities that may damage the pacer or impact appropriate function. There are many sources of potential device interactions as depicted in Table 24-7.[24] Generally, household appliances and electric tools are not a concern provided they are properly maintained and grounded. If the patient works with current-carrying conductors or near high-powered electromagnetic fields, arrangements should be made to evaluate the safety of that environment. Cellular telephones should be held on the contralateral side and kept at a distance of at least 6 inches (15 cm) from the pulse generator. In addition, the antenna of portable and mobile cellular phones transmitting more than 3 watts should be maintained a distance of 12 inches (30 cm). Cellular phones may temporarily inhibit pacing or trigger asynchronous pacing.[33] If patients become symptomatic, they should distance themselves or be removed by another person from the potential source of interference. Rate-response sensors may also need to be evaluated in the patient's environment.

Laws regarding the operating of a motor vehicle or airplane vary between states and countries. The AHA and the NASPE have issued a formal statement addressing the safety of operating motor vehicles or airplanes when arrhythmia poses the risk of loss of consciousness.[34] In the United Kingdom, pacemaker recipients who wish to continue to hold a valid driver's license

Table 24-7. Device Interactions[24]

Sources	Possible Effects	Precautions*
Surgical electrocautery	Reprogramming, noise reversion, component damage, transient or permanent malfunction, myocardial damage	Bipolar cautery, distance from site, ground pad placement (minimize current path), low energy setting, monitoring, asynchronous pacing, evaluate pacer postprocedure
Cardioversion/defibrillation	As above, also may cause transient loss of capture	Distance, paddle placement, energy settings, pacing system evaluation
Magnetic resonance imaging	Transient or permanent malfunction, runaway pacing, noise reversion	Avoid procedure, emergency equipment, contraindicated
Lithotripsy	Transient malfunction, activity sensor malfunction/damage	Distance beam 8 to 10 cm, asynchronous pacing, pacing system evaluation
Therapeutic radiation	Reprogramming, component damage, transient or permanent malfunction, cumulative damage	Distance, shielding, relocation of device
Arc welders	Transient or permanent malfunction, noise reversion	Avoid, distance, equipment maintenance, pacing system evaluation
Diathermy	Transient or permanent malfunction, component damage	Distance, monitoring, pacer system evaluation
Transcutaneous electrical nerve stimulation (TENS) units	Transient malfunction, inhibition, triggering	Distance, pacing system evaluation
Electroconvulsive therapy		Monitoring, emergency equipment
Internal combustion engines	Transient malfunction	Distance, do not lean directly over running engine
Airport metal detectors	Transient malfunction	Caution with walk-through detectors, distance with hand-held detectors
Ham radio	Transient malfunction, noise reversion, reprogramming	Distance, power settings

*Detailed precautionary guidelines are available from individual manufacturers.

must attend a pacemaker check annually. Failure to do so may mean the loss of their license.

All patients should receive a temporary ID card for their pacemaker. In the United States, this card provides the date of implant, pacemaker and lead model numbers, and following physician. In Europe, a European standard is used to code pacing indication, symptoms, and the prepacing rhythm. The manufacturer issues a permanent ID card once the Device Registration Form has been received. The information on the card facilitates prompt evaluation of the patient's pacemaker status should the patient present to a physician, or facility, other than the one that typically follows them. Before discharge, a follow-up appointment should be provided.

Follow-Up

Records

A record pertaining to the follow-up and management of each individual patient should be initiated at the time of implant. Records ideally should be computerized. Each patient's record should contain his or her demographic information, referring physician information, past medical history, allergies, implant diagnosis, symptoms, and operative notes. In addition, specific device information such as model and serial numbers of all leads, generators, adapters, or other hardware should be documented. Device specifications and/ or warranties, as well as technical information and advisories, should be posted in the patient record. Patient notification of any device recall or advisory should be clearly documented.

With each evaluation, current device settings should be posted with notation of any changes and the rationale for those changes. Patients' rhythm, battery and data, and magnet rate can be documented with any remote visit. Other additional data such as pacing and sensing thresholds, stored arrhythmias, percent pacing, alerts, and hemodynamic data such as heart rate variability and activity level may be documented at patient office visits.[35] Well-kept records, which include trends over time, enable the follower to quickly identify potential or actual complications. Records should be accessible 24 hours a day.

A cross-reference system, such as a computer database, facilitates identification of patients with specific leads or generators should a product alert or advisories arise. Specific model and serial numbers as well as patient name and address, implant date, and explant date should be included. Although medical device manufacturers strive to maintain quality and reliability in their products, device alert, advisories, and recalls have historically occurred. When this does occur, the manufacturer notifies the implanting center (manufacturers maintain their own databases). However, patients frequently change follow-up centers, and properly maintained databases will allow each follow-up center to notify their patients who have had a specific device implanted.

Frequency

Frequency of follow-up may vary between individual patients, physicians, and clinics. Follow-up schedules should be based on HRS and European Heart Rhythm Association consensus statement (see Table 24-8).[35] These are the minimum recommended follow-up examinations and may be conducted more often at physician discretion. In general, patients may return to the follow-up center for wound evaluation and pacer evaluation 7 to 10 days after implantation. After 6–12 weeks, stimulation thresholds have generally stabilized at values slightly higher than the initial implant values and the pacemaker output, or voltage, can be safely decreased. Patients with dual-chamber or rate-responsive pacers are generally evaluated at a minimum of 6-month intervals. Patients with single-chamber devices that are not rate respon-

Table 24-8. HRS/EHRA: Minimum Frequency of Pacemaker Follow-up

Pacemakers/CRT	
Within 72 hours of implant	In person
2–12 weeks post implant	In person
Every 3–12 months	In person or remote
Annually until battery depletion	In person
Every 1–3 months at signs of battery depletion	In person or remote

sive may be followed on a yearly basis, although frequency will depend on the patient, rhythm, battery status, or any other device-related issues.

Transtelephonic and Remote Monitoring

Transtelephonic monitoring requires that patients have a specialized transmitter and the clinic a receiver. Typically, the patient calls the clinic, turns on the machine, and attaches wrist bracelets designated for the left and right wrists. The metal tabs on the bracelets are positioned on the inner aspect of the wrist. Moisture under the metal tabs enhances conduction, so many patients use a small amount of water or lotion. The patient then places his or her phone on the transmitter cradle as directed. While the phone is on the transmitter, the ECG signal is converted to an audible tone, transmitted over the telephone line, and converted back to an ECG tracing by the receiving device. The patient is then asked to transmit a second tracing. A few seconds after the second tracing begins, the patient places a magnet, supplied with the transmitter, directly over the pulse generator. The patient is encouraged to sit still while transmitting.

Transtelephonic monitoring provides the clinician with some basic information regarding pacemaker function. Without magnet application, the transmission may indicate whether the device is sensing and possibly pacing appropriately. If pacing occurs on the ECG strip, it is evaluated for capture. When the magnet is applied, the pacer begins to pace asynchronously. If capture was not evaluated previously, it may be at this time. Battery status is also evaluated. The magnet rate is compared with normal and EOL magnet rates for the specific pulse generator. In addition, some devices will display stretching of the pulse width as the battery ages. A threshold margin test may be available with some model pulse generators. This provides a quick evaluation of the programmed safety margin. Typically, the pulse width decrements by 25%–50%

on a specific pacing cycle after magnet application.[36] Examples of ECG transmissions with and without magnet are ultimately evaluated by the physician and documented in the patient record.

Remote monitoring may be patient initiated or device initiated. The patient-initiated monitoring may be done at scheduled intervals or as needed should symptoms arise. The monitoring initiated by the device is due to a significant finding such as low battery voltage. The device links with the home monitoring device, the interrogated information is sent to a server, and ultimately the responsible physician. Battery, lead (including automated threshold data), stored arrhythmias, alerts, and additional hemodynamic monitoring data are all transmitted.

Clinic Evaluations

When a patient comes to the pacemaker clinic for pacemaker evaluation, a more thorough assessment of pacemaker function can be made. This provides the clinician with an opportunity to evaluate any potential pacemaker-related symptoms or potential sources of pacemaker malfunction. A brief history and physical examination should also be obtained. The focus is toward the pacemaker, including its relation to patient symptomatology, and the site of implant. Questioning the patient about relevant symptoms can disclose a problem with the pacing system. Symptoms of interest are those such as lightheadedness, dizziness, presyncope, syncope, palpitations, activity intolerance, or any other symptom that may have preceded implantation. If the patient has a single-chamber VVI pacer, pacemaker syndrome should also be ruled out.

Classically, the patient is then attached to the ECG cable of the pacemaker programmer. An ECG tracing with and without the magnet is obtained. The pacemaker is interrogated via a programming wand held over the pulse generator, and the initial parameters and measured data are printed. Diagnostic counters are also retrieved, printed/saved, and cleared at this time. The data should be evaluated for inadvertent device reprogramming, battery and lead status (see Figure 24-23), and percentage of time pacing.

Assessment of the percentage of time the patient has paced or sensed events may allow reprogramming that is beneficial to the patient. For example, hysteresis may be considered for a patient with a good underlying rhythm and with counters showing a high percentage of time pacing. Rate hysteresis allows for longer interval timing after sensed events. Thus, the patient may have an intrinsic rhythm in the 60s, and a hysteresis rate of 50 bpm. Once the rate falls below 50, the pacer begins to pace at a programmed LRL, such as 70 ppm. For dual-chamber pacers, ventricular pacing can be minimized by extending the AV delay or changing to an AAI/R mode that automatically reverts to DDD/R should heart block occur.

Heart-rate histograms allow the assessment of chronotropic competence while the patient is at home and is useful in deciding if activation of a rate-response feature is indicated. This can either be turned on to the manufacturer's nominal settings or, preferably, tailored to the patient's needs by the use of an exercise test. Formal exercise test protocols are often of little benefit in assessing rate response settings. They, typically, do not reflect the level of work done by many of these patients at home. Many pacemakers now have the ability to perform a semiautomated exercise test that assists in tailoring the rate-response parameters specifically to individual patient needs. Careful assessment should then be carried out to ensure that they are achieving the desired maximal heart rate during activity and that at rest the rate is returning to baseline. In patients with a history of angina, the upper rate may be limited to avoid increased angina symptoms. Any other special diagnostics available, such as mode-switching

Figure 24-23. Measured data regarding battery and lead status retrieved at clinic follow-up.

Battery/Lead Values: **Collected: 10/29/97 15:27**

Battery Status: OK
  Estimated Time to
    Replacement (Average)   64 months (past history)
  Battery Voltage   2.76 V
  Battery Current   11.4 uA
  Battery Impedance   122 Ohms

Lead Status:	**Atrial**	**Ventricular**
Pulse Duration	0.34	0.55 ms
Pulse Amplitude	2.22	2.22 V
Output Energy	2.2	3.0 uJ
Lead Current	3.0	2.6 mA
Lead Impedance	695	799 Ohms
Pacing Configuration	Bipolar	Bipolar

events, or heart failure diagnostics should also be assessed.

Sensing Measurements

The pacemaker's ability to sense any intrinsic cardiac activity should be assessed. Chronic sensing thresholds may be somewhat smaller than those obtained at the initial implant as depicted in Table 24-4. If not automated, the sensitivity threshold is obtained using the same technique as during the implant procedure, the difference being the pacemaker programmer is used instead of the PSA. If the intrinsic rhythm (P wave or R wave) is not initially present, the rate is gradually lowered to a lower value than the patient's intrinsic rate, if possible. It is often necessary to leave the rate at the lowest programmable setting for some time before an underlying rhythm presents itself. Asking the patient to cough may also help to reestablish intrinsic cardiac activity. Assessing the sensing threshold first lets the clinician know what the patient's intrinsic rhythm is before attempting a pacing threshold. The underlying rhythm should be documented in the patient record. T wave inversion is frequently noted when intrinsic activity resumes. This is a normal phenomenon following prolonged periods of ventricular pacing and is referred to as cardiac memory.[37]

Once the intrinsic rhythm is present, a semi-automatic sensing test can be performed (if available), or a manual test can be carried out. The automated test generally involves pressing a button to obtain a value. The manual test requires programming progressively less-sensitive values (increasing the programmed millivolts) until the intrinsic signal is no longer sensed. The least-sensitive setting where the signal was still sensed consistently is said to be the threshold. Sensitivity settings are typically left set at the manufacturer's nominal setting or half of the threshold amplitude, whichever is the most sensitive. This allows for fluctuations in the size of the intrinsic signal caused by changes in posture and metabolic function. Care must be taken to ensure that no oversensing occurs at the programmed setting, particularly for unipolar devices.

In unipolar pacing systems, testing for myopotential inhibition should be performed. This is especially important if the patient complains of lightheadedness when doing certain activities that involve the arm and the great pectoralis muscle on the same side as the pacemaker, such as reaching, pulling, lifting, or even shaving. To assess, the patient should be asked to perform a variety of maneuvers using the upper extremities (pectoral implants) while recording a paced ECG. This may include pushing, pulling, reaching, and swinging motions. If the unit has been implanted abdominally, the patient may perform sit-ups, or tense abdominal muscles to elicit myopotential inhibition. During the maneuvers, the ECG should be observed for inappropriate inhibition of pacing output. The marker channel would depict oversensing of multiple myopotential artifacts.

If oversensing is demonstrated, the sensitivity should be reprogrammed to a less-sensitive value until myopotential inhibition can no longer be reproduced. Note, however, that undersensing is usually less dangerous than oversensing. A pacing output occurring during the vulnerable period of the T wave only rarely induces ventricular fibrillation, while oversensing may produce ventricular asystole in some patients. Care should be taken to ensure that the native rhythm can still be sensed, and a 2:1 safety margin is maintained. In pacemakers programmed to the DDD mode, sensing of skeletal myopotentials by the atrial lead may lead to triggered ventricular pacing up to the URL.

Pacing Threshold

Stimulation thresholds are done while pacing at approximately 10 ppm faster than the patient's underlying rhythm. They may also be measured via automated, semiautomated tests, or manually. Auto thresholds would be stored with the diagnostic data retrieved. Semiautomated tests are done in the office, generally by either decrement voltage at a constant pulse width or vice versa. In some instances, both methods may be done and a SDC plotted, as previously discussed. The test is terminated when loss of capture is noted on the ECG. Manual testing can be performed by gradually decrementing either the pulse width or voltage until capture is lost. The value where consistent capture was last seen is noted as the capture threshold. It is imperative that the operator knows how to quickly regain pacing. A temporary screen may be used that quickly returns to permanently programmed parameters once loss of capture is noted. In addition, a button on the programmer should provide high-output emergency pacing, typically in the VVI mode. Emergency equipment should always be readily available.

Typically, patients are discharged with more than a 2:1 safety margin. The rationale is that the lead causes edema and inflammation in the surrounding myocardial tissue and ultimately, fibrotic capsule formation surrounding the tip electrode. This process distances the lead from excitable myocardial tissue and is known as the lead maturation process. Generally, this process begins on the first day. The thresholds may rise dramatically in nonsteroid electrodes and much less dramatically in steroid electrodes, and return near implant values at about 6 weeks (see Figure 24-24).[7] Thresholds usually stabilize at this point to chronic values depicted in Table 24-4. When the patient returns for his or her initial clinic evaluation (at 6 to 12 weeks), programmed outputs are reduced to a 2:1 safety margin. This increases longevity while still maintaining patient safety. Some devices with automated thresholds may safely operate at much lower pacing outputs.

Factors Influencing Thresholds

If thresholds remain high during the first 2 months, or exceed pacemaker output (exit block),

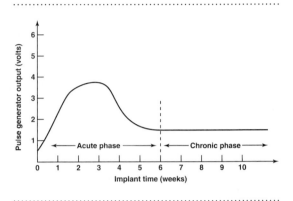

Figure 24-24. Thresholds typically begin to rise postimplantation (nonsteroidal leads) and peak at about 2 weeks.

a course of oral steroids may be prescribed to help reduce inflammation where the lead tip electrode meets the tissue. This results in thinner fibrotic capsule formation. After 1 week of oral steroid treatment, pacing thresholds have been shown to continually decline over a period of 1 month.[38] Corticosteroids have more recently been incorporated into pacemaker-lead technology. Steroid-eluting leads may consist of a porous steroid-eluting electrode or collar. The steroid is slowly released over time and has been associated with virtually no acute threshold rise. Other lead technologies focusing on reduced pacing thresholds have also emerged. They include, but are not limited to, smaller electrodes, larger surface areas (microporous electrode), low polarization, activated carbon, and platinum-iridium electrodes.[39]

Other factors may also affect both pacing and sensing thresholds. Glucocorticoids, exercise, ephedrine, and epinephrine have a positive effect on thresholds;[23] however, these do not seem to serve a practical purpose in pacemaker technology. Conversely, thresholds may be adversely affected by hyperkalemia, acidosis,[7] alkalosis, hypercapnia, hypoxia, hyperglycemia, ischemia, and many medications.[23] Antiarrhythmics such as 1C agents are of particular concern, and 1A agents, propranolol, verapamil, amiodarone, glucose and insulin, hypertonic saline, and mineralocorticoids may also adversely effect thresholds. Clinicians should carefully evaluate for possible reversible causes should pacing and sensing thresholds adversely change with a chronic pacing lead. However, changes with a chronic lead may not always be reversible.

Thresholds may also permanently rise due to progressive myocardial fibrosis. This may be related to myocardial infarction or a primary myopathic process. Other lead complications such as conductor fracture or insulation failure should be carefully ruled out. Lead impedances would typically reflect either of these problems. If a conductor fracture is intermittent, it may be elicited by those maneuvers used in evaluating for myopotentials. For each of these complications, it is likely that the lead will need to be replaced. In myocardial fibrosis, repositioning of the lead is a theoretical option, but chronic leads are not easily repositioned. A chest radiograph may be useful to assess for lead dislodgment or for tension on the lead as may be caused by growth of a pediatric patient.

At the end of every pacemaker check, the device should be reinterrogated, and the final program compared to the initial one. Careful cross-checking will ensure that only those parameters intended to be changed were changed, and that appropriate safety margins were maintained. All findings should be compared to the previous follow-up for abrupt changes. In addition, they should be compared to all previous findings for trends over time. The final parameters should then be posted in the patient record and significant findings documented. Time should be taken to reassess patient and family learning needs. When evaluation and education are complete, a follow-up appointment should be provided.

ICD PATIENTS

Recent advances in technology have enabled the incorporation of DDD pacing into the implantable cardioverter defibrillator (ICD). Patients no longer need to have both a separate pacemaker and an ICD implanted. Historically, separate pacemaker therapy may be a source of interference in the appropriate function of ICDs due to double or triple counting of the paced rhythm by the sensing circuitry of the ICD, especially with asynchronous pacing following magnet application. There was also a failure to detect VF if pacer artifact was sensed at the time of the arrhythmia.[40,41] During implantation, if the patient had an existing ICD, the ventricular lead of the pacemaker was positioned at the RV septum or RVOT. The leads were positioned at perpendicular vectors and separated by at least 2 to 3 cm. Dedicated bipolar (will not revert to unipolar) pacing leads were used. These precautions helped avoid sensing of the pacemaker artifact.

Testing was done at the time of implant to be sure VF was detected appropriately while the pacemaker was programmed to its maximal output and AV delay. The pacer was evaluated postdefibrillation for loss of sensing, loss of capture, power on reset, or reversion to ERI. Generators were positioned a distance of 20 cm apart to avoid misprogramming.[40] Consideration was given to the URL of the pacer and the detection rate of the ICD for tachyarrhythmias. ICD oversensing of pacer artifact was also evaluated at follow-up by means of asynchronous pacing at the programmed output. Inhibition of the ICD during pacemaker interrogation and programming helped to prevent potential inappropriate therapy during telemetry.

SUMMARY

Pacemaker technology has become very complicated in recent years and will continue to advance in the years to come. New technology that increases device longevity will continue to develop, as will new specialized features and pacemaker indications. All nurses need to have a basic understanding of pacemaker function and potential complications, because pacemakers are quite common in the general population. However, nurses working in this specialty area need to keep abreast of new technology in this area in order to provide optimal care to their patients.

Despite these advances, an implanted device may be very traumatic for the patient. This very often has an impact on their body image, self-esteem, and independence and these factors need to be taken into consideration when dealing with pacemaker patients.

REFERENCES

1. Rozkovec A. Basic principles of permanent cardiac pacing. *Br J Hosp Med* 1996;55:31–37.
2. Rosamond W, Flegal K, Fluie K, et al. Heart disease and stroke statistics 2008 update: a report from the American Heart Association statistics committee and stroke statistics subcommittee. *Circulation* 2008:117:e25–e146.
3. Olson J. *Clinical Pharmacology Made Ridiculously Simple*. Miami, FL: MedMaster, Inc.; 1992.
4. Parsonnet V, Furman S, Smyth NPD. Implantable cardiac pacemakers: status report and resource guideline: a report of the Inter-Society Commission for Heart Disease Resources. *Am J Cardiol* 1974;34:487–500.
5. Bernstein AD, Camm AJ, Fletcher RD, et al. The NASPE/BPEG Generic Pacemaker Code for antibradyarrhythmia and adaptive-rate pacing and antitachyarrhythmia devices. *PACE* 1987;10:794–799.
6. Bernstein AD, Daubert JC, Fletcher RD, et al. The revised Naspe/BPEG generic code for antibradycardia, adaptive rate and multisite pacing. *PACE* 2000;25:260–264.
7. Ellenbogen KA, ed. *Cardiac Pacing*. Boston: Blackwell Scientific; 1992.
8. Bernstein AD, Parsonnet V. Survey of cardiac pacing and defibrillation in the United States in 1993. *Am J Cardiol* 1996;78:187–196.
9. Nishimura RA, Symanski JD, Hurrell DG, et al. Dual-chamber pacing for cardiomyopathies: a 1996 perspective. *Mayo Clin Proc* 1996;71:1077–1087.
10. Glikson M, Espinosa RE, Hayes DL. Expanding indications for permanent pacemakers. *Ann Intern Med* 1995;123:443–451.
11. Dreifus LS, Fisch C, Griffin JC, et al. Guidelines for implantation of cardiac pacemakers and antiarrythmia devices: a report of the American College of Cardiology/American Heart Association Task Force on Assessment of Diagnostic and Therapeutic Cardiovascular Procedures (Committee on Pacemaker Implantation). *Circulation* 1991;84:455–467.
12. Magovern GJ Sr, Simpson KA. Clinical cardiomyoplasty: review of the ten-year United States experience. *Ann Thorac Surg* 1996;61:413–419.
13. Fogoros RN. *Electrophysiology Testing*, 2nd ed. Cambridge, MA: Blackwell Science; 1995.
14. Epstein AE, DiMarco JP, Ellenbogen KA, et al. ACC/AHA/HRS 2008 Guidelines for device-based therapy of cardiac rhythm abnormalities: Executive summary: A report of the American College of Cardiology/American Heart Association Task Force on Practice Guideliines writing committee to revise the ACC/AHA/NASPE 2002 guideline update for implantation of cardiac pacemakers and antiarrhythmia devices) developed in collaboration with the American Association for Thoracic Surgery and Society of Thoracic Surgeons. *J Am Coll Cardiol* 2008;51:2085–2105.
15. Clarke M, Sutton R, Ward D, et al. Recommendations for pacemaker prescription for symptomatic bradycardia: report of a working party of the British Pacing and Electrophysiology Group. *Br Heart J* 1991;66:185–191.
16. Sharma AD, Rizo-Patron C, Hallstron AP, et al. (DAVID Investigators). Percent of right ventricular pacing predicts outcomes in the David trial. *Heart Rhythm* 2005;2:830–834.
17. Lau CP. *Rate Adaptive Cardiac Pacing*. Mount Kisco, NY: Futura;1993.
18. Griesbach L, Grestrich B, Wojciechowski D, et al. Clinical performance of automatic closed-loop stimulation systems. *PACE* 2003; 26:1432–1437.

19. Greco EA, Ferrario M, Romano S. Clinical evaluation of peak endocardial acceleration as a sensor for rate responsive pacing. *PACE* 2003;26:812–818.

20. Raymond RD, Nanian KB. Insulation failure with bipolar polyurethane pacing leads. *PACE* 1984;7:378–380.

21. Hanson JS. Sixteen failures in a single model of bipolar polyurethane-insulated ventricular pacing lead: a 44 month experience. *PACE* 1984;7:389–394.

22. Calfee RV, Saulson SH. A voluntary standard for 3.2 mm unipolar and bipolar pace-maker leads and connectors. *PACE* 1986;9:1181–1185.

23. Moses HW, Moulton KP, Miller BD, Schneider JA. *Practical Guide to Cardiac Pacing*, 4th ed. Boston: Little Brown; 1995.

24. Schurig L, ed. *Educational Guidelines: Pacing and Electrophysiology*. Armonk, NY: Futura; 1994.

25. Redman BK. *The Process of Patient Education*, 7th ed. St. Louis, MO: Mosby Year Book; 1993.

26. Association of Operating Room Nurses. Proposed recommended practices: monitoring the patient receiving IV conscious sedation. *AORN J* 1992;56:316–324.

27. Furman S, Hayes DL, Holmes DR. *A Practice of Cardiac Pacing*, 3rd ed. Mount Kisco, NY: Futura; 1993.

28. Medtronic. *Temporary Stimulation and Sensing Threshold Procedure*. Minneapolis, MN: Medtronic;1992:UC9202138aEN.

29. Ellenbogen KA, Kay GN, Wilkoff G. *Device Therapy for Congestive Heart Failure*. Philadelphia, PA: Saunders:2004.

30. Stiles S. ICD, pacemaker infection rates seen to grow faster than number of implants. May 26, 2006. Available at: www.theheart.org/article/704841.do. Accessed September 1, 2009.

31. Coman JA, Trohman RG. Incidence and electrocardiographic localization of safe right bundle branch block configuration during permanent ventricular pacing. *Am J Cardiol* 1995;76:781–784.

32. Baas LS, Beery TA, Hickey CS. Care and safety of pacemaker electrodes in intensive care and telemetry nursing units. *Am J Crit Care* 1997;6:302–311.

33. Medtronic. *Thera DR: Product Information Manual*. Minneapolis, MN: Medtronic; 1995:UC9403918EN.

34. Epstein AE, Miles WM, Benditt DG, et al. Personal and public safety issues related to arrhythmias that may affect consciousness: implications for regulation and physician recommendations. A medical/scientific statement from the American Heart Association and the North American Society of Pacing and Electrophysiology. *Circulation* 1996;94(5):1147–1166.

35. Wilcoff BL, Auricchio A, Brugada J, et al. HRS/EHRA expert consensus on the monitoring of cardiovascular implantable electronic devices (CIEDs): description of techniques, indications, personnel, frequency and ethical considerations. *Heart Rhythm* 2008.5:1–19.

36. Medtronic Technical Services. *Pacemaker and ICD Encyclopedia*. Minneapolis, MN: Medtronic; 1997:UC89032031EN.

37. Tsutsumi T, Izumo K, Sekiya S, Harumi K. Post-pacing T loop abnormalities. *Jpn Heart J* 1985;26(6):897–908.

38. Yesil M, Bayata S, Postaci N, et al. The effect of oral corticosteroid on acute pacing thresholds in patients with nonsteroid ventricular pacing leads. In: Adornato E, Galassi A, eds. *How to Approach Cardiac Arrhythmias: Proceedings of the IVth Southern Symposium on Cardiac Pacing*, Vol. 2. Rome, Italy: Edizioni Luigi Pozzi; 1994:63–66.

39. Yesil M, Bayata S, Postaci N, et al. The effect of oral corticosteroid on acute pacing thresholds in patients with steroid-eluting leads. In: Adornato E, Galassi A, eds. *How to Approach Cardiac Arrhythmias: Proceedings of the IVth Southern Symposium on Cardiac Pacing,* Vol. 2. Rome, Italy: Edizioni Luigi Pozzi; 1994:67–70.

40. Medtronic Technical Services. *Tech Note: Implantation of Pacemakers with Defibrillators*. Minneapolis, MN: Medtronic; 1994.

41. Geiger MJ, O'Neill P, Sharma A, et al. Inter-actions between transvenous nonthoracotomy cardioverter defibrillator systems and permanent transvenous endocardial pacemakers. *Pacing Clin Electrophysiol* 1997;20(3 Pt1):624–630.

SUGGESTED READING

Ellenbogen KA, Kay GN, Wilkoff G. *Clinical Cardiac Pacing and Defibrillation*, 2nd ed. Philadelphia: W.B. Saunders; 2000.

Barold SS, Stoobandt RX, Sinnaeve AF. *Cardiac Pacemakers Step by Step: An Illustrated Guide*. Mount Kisco, NY: Futura; 2004.

Chapter 25

IMPLANTABLE CARDIOVERTER DEFIBRILLATORS

Laura Nyren, RN, MS, ACNP
Joan M. Craney, RN, PhD
Phyllis J. Gustafson, RN, BSN

HISTORY

The concept of the implantable cardioverter defibrillator (ICD) occurred to Dr. Michel Mirowski in the late 1960s as the result of the unfortunate death of a friend, colleague, and mentor, Dr. Harry Heller, from recurrent ventricular arrhythmias. Following Dr. Heller's passing, Dr. Mirowski moved to Baltimore, Maryland, to serve as director of a new coronary care unit at Sinai Hospital. There, he and others began work on the development of the automatic defibrillator and within a few months, began device testing in dogs.[1]

Early models used pressure sensors mounted in a right ventricular catheter for ventricular arrhythmia detection. Defibrillation energy was delivered between a subcutaneous electrode and the right ventricular catheter electrode or a single lead with dual electrodes. However, concern arose over lead stability within the right ventricular apex (RVA) and epicardial patch electrodes were

developed (see Figure 25-1).[2] Investigational device exemption (IDE) was approved by the U.S. Food and Drug Administration (FDA) in 1979, and the first human implant of the implantable defibrillator took place at Johns Hopkins Hospital on February 4, 1980.

The first-generation implantable defibrillators were implanted in 37 patients, and it was found that that many patients experienced ventricular tachycardia (VT) before the onset of ventricular fibrillation (VF). Cardioversion capabilities were then added to the second-generation devices, but retrievable diagnostic information was limited to the number of device discharges at what output.[1,3]

Probability density function (PDF) technology had been used to differentiate ventricular tachyarrhythmias based on the time the intracardiac electrogram (EGM) spent at the isoelectric line, or baseline. In 1982, separate rate sensing leads were added, because PDF was noted to be impaired by electrode polarization postshock.

Figure 25-1. Early ICD system using epicardial patches and rate sensing leads. *Source*: Courtesy of Medtronic, Inc., Minneapolis, MN.

....

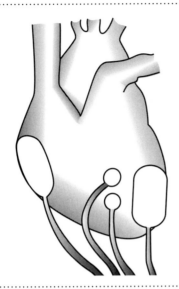

Figure 25-2. Early ICD system utilizing a transvenous lead system and SQ patch. Defibrillation occurs between the RV coil, SVC coil, and SQ patch. *Source*: Courtesy of Medtronic, Inc., Minneapolis, MN.

....

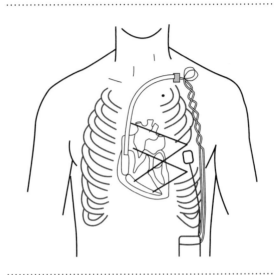

The automatic implantable cardioverter defibrillator (AICD) received FDA approval in 1985, and Medicare reimbursements were approved in 1986. By the end of the same year, the first nonthoracotomy lead system was implanted. Additional manufacturers began introducing ICDs for clinical trials in 1989. The nonthoracotomy lead system (see Figure 25-2) and these additional ICDs were market released in 1993.[1]

These third-generation devices represented significant advances in technology. The weight of the ICDs implanted in humans had gone from as much as 250 grams[4] to 197 grams.[5] Devices were multiprogrammable with bradycardia and antitachycardia pacing (ATP), in addition to cardioversion and defibrillation for tiered patient therapy. Many had programmable detection zones for "slow" and "fast" tachycardia rates. Less-aggressive therapy was now permitted with the slowing of a tachycardia rate. Biphasic and sequential shock waveform delivery methods were also introduced.[5] These alternative shock waveform methods were associated with lower patient defibrillation thresholds (DFT).[6] Arrhythmia detection criteria were added to increase detection specificity. Noncommitted shocks evolved to prevent inappropriate shocks in the event of nonsustained tachyarrhythmias, as did the ability to do noninvasive electrophysiology studies (NIPS) via the device. This generation also introduced more complex memory in devices, including R-R interval data and stored electrograms.[5] In 1996, more than 65,000 ICD systems were implanted worldwide.[7] Device diagnostic, therapy capabilities, and indications have continued to evolve. In 2005, implants in the United States alone reached an estimated 91,000 for the year.[8]

SUDDEN CARDIAC DEATH

In the United States alone, more than 400,000 deaths are caused each year from sudden cardiac death (SCD).[9] This represents 1 to 2 deaths per

1000 annually and is consistent with the incidence reported in Europe.[10] It is estimated that 60% of these deaths are from ventricular arrhythmias.[6] Survival for patients who experience cardiac arrest outside a hospital is poor, but it is difficult to identify those who will experience SCD. Specific high-risk subgroups of the population, such as those convalescing after an MI, actually represent a small number of the absolute deaths. The higher the known risk of SCD in a specific subgroup, the lower the absolute number of deaths reported. This is due to the fact that high-risk groups are, in comparison, small, but identifying characteristics are useful to assess risk in the general population.[11]

Mechanisms of VT

Ventricular tachycardia has been classified into three basic mechanisms: enhanced automaticity, triggered activity, and reentry.

Enhanced Automaticity

Automaticity is the result of acceleration of Phase 4 depolarization. It characteristically exhibits a gradual warm up and cool down. This mechanism probably accounts for less than 10% of VT, though.

Triggered Activity

This is the result of oscillations in membrane potential, resulting in afterdepolarizations occurring during Phase 3 (early afterdepolarization), early Phase 4 (delayed afterdepolarization), or of the action potential. If there is sufficient influx of positive ions, the threshold is reached and a new action potential is generated. This, in turn, may perpetuate a repetitive cycle of VT. Triggered activity may also display a gradual acceleration and deceleration of rate versus the abrupt onset and termination seen in most VT. It has been associated with digitalis-toxic arrhythmias, torsade de pointes, and calcium sensitive VT.[12] This mechanism appears to be rare.

Reentry

This mechanism is thought to be the most common mechanism for VT. It is dependent on a functional circuit in which one of the connecting limbs has slowed conduction and another limb has a prolonged refractory period. Thus, if a premature event (e.g., premature ventricular contraction) arrives at such a circuit, one limb is blocked due to the prolonged refractory period. The wave of depolarization will travel down the slow conduction limb only, and by this time, the other limb has recovered. The wave of depolarization now circles back to the slow conducting limb, which has a more rapid recovery, and is ready to receive the impulse. The depolarizing wavefront can then perpetuate in this circular motion. In addition, each time the electrical wavefront circles around, it is also exiting the circuit and causing depolarization of the ventricle. Most of these malignant ventricular reentry tachycardias are associated with scar tissue interspersed within the myocardium, the result of infarction or cardiomyopathy.

INDICATIONS

Patients were initially required to have survived two previous cardiac arrests in order to be eligible for implantation of an ICD, and one of the two cardiac arrests had to be on what was presumed to be effective medication therapy.[2] Over time, accepted device indications have gradually broadened. The most recent ACC/AHA guidelines were issued in 2008 (see Table 25-1). Each ACC/AHA indication is ranked as to its level of supporting evidence. Level A has the support of multiple, randomized clinical trials with large numbers of individuals. Level B supported trials consist of comparably smaller numbers of participants or are from nonrandomized studies

Table 25-1. Indications for ICD Therapy

Class I	Evidence level
Cardiac arrest due to VF or hemodynamically unstable sustained VT (not due to a transient or reversible cause)	A
Spontaneous sustained VT in association with structural heart disease (whether hemodynamically stable or unstable)	B
Syncope of undetermined origin and inducible at EPS (for clinically relevant, hemodynamically significant sustained VT or VF)	B
LVEF ≤ 35%, prior MI (at least 40 days post), **and NYHA Class II or III**	A
Nonischemic DCM LVEF ≤ NYHA Class II or III	B
LV dysfunction due to prior MI (at least 40 days post) **with LVEF ≤ 30% and NYHA class I**	A
NSVT due to prior MI, LVEF ≤ 40%, and inducible for VF or sustained VT at EPS	B
Class IIa	Evidence level
Unexplained syncope, significant LV dysfunction, and nonischemic DCM	C
Sustained VT and normal or near-normal ventricular function	C
Hypertrophic CM and one or more major risk factors of sudden death	C
Arrhythmogenic RV dysplasia/CM who have one or more risk factors for sudden death	C
Long-QT syndrome who are experiencing syncope and/or VT (while receiving beta blockers)	B
Non-hospitalized patients awaiting transplantation	C
Brugada syndrome with syncope	C
Brugada syndrome with documented VT (that has not resulted in cardiac arrest)	C
Cholaminergic polymorphic VT and syncope and/or documented sustained VT while receiving beta blockers	C
Sarcoidosis, giant cell myocarditis, or Chagas disease	C
Class IIb	Evidence level
Nonischemic heart disease with LVEF ≤ 35% and NYHA Class I	C
Long-QT syndrome and risk factors for SCD	B
Syncope with advanced structural heart disease (invasive and noninvasive studies have failed to identify cause)	C
Familial CM associated with sudden death	C
LV noncompaction	C
Class III	Evidence level
Patients who do not have reasonable expectation of survival with an acceptable functional status for at least one year (Even if they meet Class I, IIa, and IIb indications)	C
Incessant VT or VF	C

Class III	Evidence level
VT or VF resulting from arrhythmias amenable to ablation (i.e., Wolff-Parkinson-White syndrome, right ventricular outflow tract VT, idiopathic left ventricular VT, or fascicular VT in the absence of structural heart disease)	C
Ventricular tachycardias due to reversible causes in the absence of structural heart disease (e.g., electrolyte imbalances, drugs, or trauma)	B
Significant psychiatric illness (presumed to preclude follow-up or when illness may be aggravated by ICD implant)	C
Syncope of undetermined cause without ventricular tachyarrhythmias or without structural heart disease	C
NYHA Class IV drug-refractory CHF in patients not transplant candidates or CRT-D	C

Table 25-1. ICD Indications. Class I indications are generally agreed upon. Class IIa have the weight of evidence in their favor, while for Class IIb the evidence or opinion is less well established. For Class III conditions, ICD is generally agreed not to be useful or effective and may be harmful.

Data adapted from Epsein et al. ACC/AHA/HRS 2008 guidelines for device based therapy of cardiac rhythm abnormalities: A report of the American College of Cardiology/American Heart Association Task Force on Practice Guidelines. Writing committee to revise the ACC/AHA/NASPE 2002 guideline update for implantation of cardiac pacemakers and antiarrhythmic devices. *Circulation* 2008;e350–e408.

with well-designed data analysis or observational data registries. Level C indicates that supporting evidence is based primarily on the recommendation of expert opinion.[13] The guidelines reflect the surge of clinical evaluations that looked at the effectiveness of ICD therapy and helped to identify groups at risk for SCD.

Since the 2002 guidelines were published, indications have continued to expand. The Sudden Cardiac Death-Heart Failure Trial (SCD-HeFT) and The Defibrillators in Nonischemic Cardiomyopathy Treatment Evaluation (DEFINITE) have expanded implant indications to patients with nonischemic cardiomyopathy (NICM).[14,15] While the cost effectiveness of ICDs has been of question,[16] recent data suggests ICDs are cost effective in primary prevention.[17,18] Exclusion criteria has been established for patients who have had MI within 40 days.[19] New guidelines for the management of patients with ventricular arrhythmias were established in 2006 by the ACC/AHA.[20]

DEFIBRILLATOR CODES

The North American Society of Pacing and Electrophysiology (now known as the Heart Rhythm Society) and the British Pacing and Electrophysiology Group have developed a separate defibrillator code, which is depicted in Table 25-2. This four-letter code provides a detailed description of the tachycardia therapies provided. For example, a VVED device would denote the capability to shock in the ventricle, provide ATP therapy in the ventricle, use electrogram (rate/morphology) for detection, and provide dual-chamber pacing in the setting of bradyarrhythmias. In addition, they have also established a short-form code. This code uses ICD as the first three letters. The letter S, B, or T may then be added preceded by a dash. It is hierarchical in nature; S indicating shock-only capability, B indicating bradycardia pacing as well as shock, and T indicating tachycardia pacing in addition to the bradycardia pacing and shock capabilities.[21] For the most part, ICDs implanted today will have all these capabilities.

Table 25-2. NASPE/BPEG Defibrillator Codes

Position I	Position II	Position III	Position IV
Shock Chamber	Antitachycardia Pacing Chamber	Tachycardia Detection	Antibradycardia Pacing chamber
O = None	O = None	E = Electrogram	O = None
A = Atrium	A = Atrium	*H = Hemodynamic	A = Atrium
V = Ventricle	V = Ventricle		V = Ventricle
D = Dual (A + V)	D = Dual (A + V)		D = Dual (A + V)

*Devices that denote H for hemodynamic are assumed to incorporate electrograms in addition.

Adapted from Bernstein AD, Camm AJ, Fletcher RD, et al. The NASPE/BPEG defibrillator code. *Pace* 1993;16: 1776–1780.

ICD SYSTEM COMPONENTS

Pulse Generator

The ICD system consists of a pulse generator and lead(s) that interact with the patient's myocardium. Today, ICDs typically weigh 68–90 g. The outer casing of the generator is generally made of titanium. Within the casing are one or two lithium/silver vanadium-oxide (3.2V) batteries, which provide device longevity greater than 5 years in most models. There are one or two aluminum electrolytic capacitors capable of storing high voltage (HV) for cardioversion or defibrillation therapy. When needed, voltage is drawn from the batteries, amplified by a transformer, rectified, and then stored on the capacitor(s) for delivery. Additional electronic circuitry is housed within the casing for sensing, output, and information storage. Information storage may be in the form of read-only memory and random access memory. Current devices offer extensive programmability and diagnostic reporting capabilities, as well as a multitude of therapy options. They may incorporate sophisticated biventricular resynchronization therapy, ATP, and therapies for atrial arrhythmias. The generator itself typically serves as the cathode or anode in shock therapies. Mounted on the generator casing is a connector block, or header. There are various headers available to allow for various pacing and defibrillation leads to be connected.

Lead System

In general, ICD leads serve two purposes: They send energy to the myocardium for the delivery of therapy, and they transmit cardiac signals to the generator for rate sensing. Transvenous leads for pectoral implants are typically 65 cm in length. The materials used in their construction are similar to those used for pacemaker leads. The lead design may be coaxial, as with pacing leads, or multilumen. RV leads are available with active or passive fixation mechanisms and steroid-eluting tips to maintain low pacing thresholds. However, ICD lead defibrillation electrodes are of a significantly larger surface area. RV leads are commonly tripolar or quadrapolar, having one or two defibrillation electrodes, or coils, and two electrodes, for pacing and sensing. Single-coil leads positioned in the RVA are used with generators capable of serving as the second defibrillation electrode (anode or cathode). With this type of system, defibrillation occurs between the coil located on the lead and the ICD generator (see Figure 25-3). The generator may also serve as a third defibrillation electrode when the lead is a dual coil.

Other, less commonly used lead systems are also available. Epicardial lead systems, including rate-sensing leads and defibrillation patches, may be used for a patient undergoing concomitant cardiovascular surgery. Separate unipolar defi-

Figure 25-3. Pectorally implanted generator and transvenous lead system. Defibrillation occurs between RV coil and generator. *Source*: Courtesy of Medtronic, Inc., Minneapolis, MN.

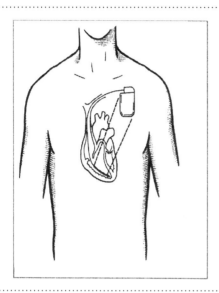

brillation leads may be used for additional, or varied, lead placement such as the superior vena cava (SVC), coronary sinus (CS), or innominate vein. If the DFT is high, subcutaneous leads or patches may be added to encompass the critical mass of myocardium necessary for successful defibrillation.

The pace/sense portion of the tripolar and quadrapolar leads may consist of a tip and ring electrode like a standard pacemaker lead or the proximal ring may be integrated into the right ventricular defibrillation coil. These configurations are commonly referred to as *true bipolar* and *integrated bipolar* sensing. When dual-chamber devices are implanted, an atrial pacing lead is also required. Although no special design characteristics are required, they are typically bipolar and may employ reduced tip to ring spacing designed to reduce far-field oversensing.

An International Standard-1, or IS-1, connector pin is used for pacing and sensing, and a standardized DF-1 connector pin is used for

high-voltage leads. However, when patients have existing lead systems, it is important to be aware of connector pin size.

Biventricular pacing provides cardiac resynchronization therapy for New York Heart Association (NYHA) class III or IV patients with idiopathic dilated or ischemic cardiomyopathy. They must also have a QRS interval $\geq$ 130 ms, left ventricular (LV) end diastolic diameter $\geq$ 55 mm, and EF $\leq$ 35%.[13] LV leads are available designed specifically for placement in a cardiac vein. These leads are 4 to 6 French in diameter and are passively fixated, or wedged. They are delivered to the CS via a guiding catheter, and typically positioned in the posterior or lateral tributary (see Figure 25-4) using a stylet, or an over–the-wire system. If lead placement via the CS is unsuccessful, an epicardial pacing lead may be placed on the left ventricle in the operating room. LV leads may be unipolar or bipolar.

Figure 25-4. RAO view of biventricular lead system. A dual coil defibrillation lead is seen positioned with the distal coil in the RV apex. A unipolar LV pacing lead is seen coarsing posteriorly via coronary sinus with the tip wedged in a tributary. *Source*: Rhode Island Hospital.

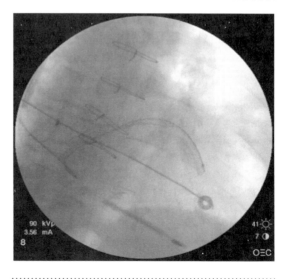

With unipolar LV leads, pacing occurs from the LV lead tip to the distal coil or proximal ring electrode in the RV.

Programmer

A programmer is a brand-specific external computer used to communicate with the ICD. It operates using two-way telemetry or radiofrequency signals. Clinicians use the programmer to set device detection, therapy parameters, and diagnostics based on the needs of the patient. The programmer is used to facilitate arrhythmia induction and therapy delivery during the DFT testing at implant and for NIPS. At follow-up visits, the programmer permits evaluation of device function and lead integrity, and retrieval of stored data.

BASIC DEVICE OPERATION

The two functions of the ICD device are detection of the cardiac rhythm, and emitting therapeutic impulses when necessary.

Detection

Heart Rate (HR)

Traditionally, ICD systems have continuously monitored a patient's HR to determine the need for intervention. The device looks at the cycle length of each intrinsic interval and classifies it as *slow*, *normal*, or *fast*. Slow heart rates are defined by the programmed lower rate, or bradycardia pacing rate, of the device. If the HR drops to the programmed lower rate, the ICD will pace at that programmed lower rate. ICD pacing capabilities are similar to bradycardia pacemakers and may include single-chamber, dual-chamber, or multisite pacing.

Normal rates fall between what is classified as slow and what is classified as fast. When rates are in this range, the device simply monitors the rhythm. However, with certain dual-chamber or rate-responsive modes, atrial and/or ventricular pacing may be noted.

Tachycardia

Tachycardia is defined by rate and duration of rate, as programmed by the practitioner. Most devices allow for the definition of two or three different tachycardia zones, based on rate. A maximal duration, or number of intervals, for the HR to be in each zone may also be programmed. If rate and duration criteria are met, therapy is initiated. For example, a VT may be defined as a HR of 150–180 bpm for 16 consecutive beats. VF may be defined as a HR above 180 bpm. The criteria for the duration of VF are typically less stringent. Instead of requiring 16 beats in a row, any 12 of 16 beats may need to be classified as VF to meet detection. This is to allow for the occasional *drop out* or *undersensing* that may occur during VF.[22] In some devices, the practitioner may simply program a shorter duration or number of intervals to meet detection.

Atrial Tachyarrhythmias

Detection is programmed based on rate and may be divided into two zones: atrial fibrillation (AF), and atrial tachycardia and/or flutter (AT). Duration is separately programmable for ATP and cardioversion therapies. Depending on the device, additional algorithms may be used to differentiate AF from more organized atrial tachyarrhythmias. These devices are also fully functional ventricular defibrillators.[23]

Sensitivity

This must be programmed to ensure appropriate detection of atrial and/or ventricular tachyarrhythmias. ICDs must be capable of sensing the very small potentials that often accompany AF or VF, yet avoid oversensing. In addition to a programmed sensitivity setting, the ICD sensitivity automatically adjusts, based on the patient's rhythm or signal size, in order to accommodate sensing of small electrogram amplitudes, but avoid signals such as T waves in sinus rhythm.

Arrhythmia Detection

Programmable criteria can assist in increasing the specificity of arrhythmia detection. The various algorithms help the device distinguish between sinus tachycardia (ST), supraventricular tachycardia (SVT), and true VT, thus avoiding inappropriate therapy.

Onset Criterion

Onset criterion monitors cycle length to detect the sudden onset of a tachycardia that is consistent with VT. Onset criterion is helpful in appropriately rejecting ST, which typically exhibits a slow, gradual rate increase, not an abrupt onset.[24] Thus, the patient avoids inappropriate shocks if his or her rate were to exceed detection rate during exercise.

Stability Criteria

These programmable criteria enable the device to look at the regularity of the rhythm. Based on the variability in cycle length of a tachycardia, it may meet detection or be rejected. The purpose of this algorithm is to avoid treating irregular rhythms such as rapid AF or atrial flutter.

QRS Width

The width of the QRS waveform can also be evaluated, and the rhythm rejected based on narrow QRS that often represents an SVT.[25] More recently, algorithms have been developed that as-

sess the tachycardia QRS morphology and compare it with the baseline, sinus QRS morphology. Similar EGM morphologies are classified as SVT, whereas dissimilar morphologies are classified as VT/VF. In some instances, baseline rhythm templates may be continually updated.[26]

Electrogram

Dual-chamber devices may also use EGM from the atrial lead to assist in rhythm interpretation. Based on the rates and relationships of atrial and ventricular activity, dual-chamber algorithms increase the accuracy of arrhythmia detection.[27]

Although these arrhythmia detection criteria are designed to increase specificity, it is important to keep in mind that programming of these criteria reduces sensitivity of the ICD to detect potentially life-threatening ventricular tachyarrhythmias. Therefore, increasing specificity reduces sensitivity.

Therapy

ICD therapy is tailored to the individual patient needs. It is based on the clinical rhythms displayed, the tolerance to those rhythms, and the effectiveness of therapeutic modalities. It can include ATP, cardioversion, defibrillation, or bradycardia pacing support (see Table 25-3).

Tachyarrhythmias

The device delivers the first therapy assigned to the classification of rhythm detected. After therapy delivery, the rhythm is reassessed for continuation of the tachycardia, acceleration of rhythm, or termination of the arrhythmia. Should the tachycardia still be present, the next programmed therapy or therapy sequence is delivered. Manufacturers typically have separate redetection parameters to expedite subsequent

Table 25-3. Common Arrhythmia Detection Zones and Corresponding Therapies of Ventricular ICDs

Arrhythmia Detection	Therapy
Ventricular and atrial fibrillation	
Rate	Defibrillation
Stability	50 Hz burst (atrial only)
Ventricular and atrial tachycardia	
Rate	ATP
Duration	Ramp
Onset	Burst
Stability	50 Hz burst (atrial only)
Morphology	Cardioversion
Other	
Bradycardia	
Rate	VVI/R +/− biventricular
	DDD/R +/− biventricular
	AAI/R→DDD/R +/− Biventricular

therapy if more than one therapy is required to terminate an episode.

Antitachycardia Pacing

This may be effective in terminating organized atrial or ventricular tachyarrhythmias. To do so, the paced impulse must penetrate the excitable gap of the reentry circuit. The tachycardia wavefront terminates when it collides with the paced wavefront or encounters recently depolarized, refractory tissue. If successful, ATP eliminates the need for painful cardioversion or defibrillation shocks. It may also be programmed to be delivered while the device is charging to deliver a shock therapy. ATP is included into a patient's therapy regime when proven effective or may be programmed empirically. Various types of antitachycardia-pacing therapies are available through different manufacturers.

Overdrive Burst Pacing

Overdrive burst pacing delivers a selected number of paced beats (typically 1 to 25) at a fixed pacing rate that automatically exceeds the rate of the tachycardia (see Figure 25-5).[28] The number of pacing sequences, or attempts at burst pacing, is also programmable. The number of sequences prescribed is based on the patient's history and his or her hemodynamic response to the arrhythmia. Scanning is a feature that employs progressively faster pacing rates with each burst sequence.[29]

Adaptive Burst or Ramp Pacing

This is another form of ATP in which the pacing sequence is delivered at a rate faster than the detected tachycardia. It differs from burst pacing in that each successive paced beat is delivered at

Figure 25-5. Monomorphic VT is initially below detection rate. Rate accelerates and detection is met. Clear AV dissociation is seen. A single sequence of burst pacing is delivered and four additional beats of VT are seen (Type II termination).

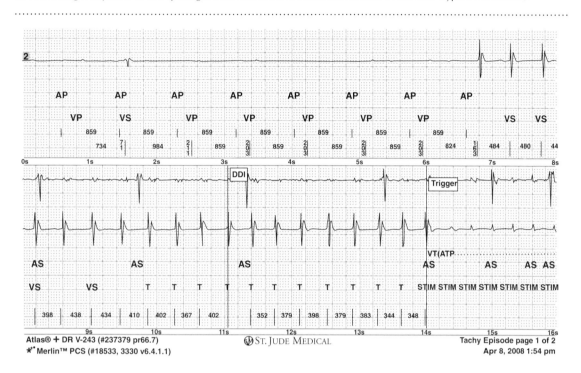

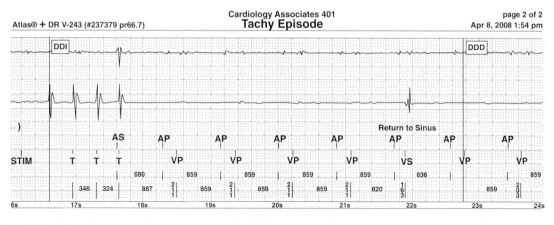

progressively faster intervals. It may also be referred to as incremental ramp. Decremental ramp pacing is also available in some devices. With decremental ramp pacing, each successive paced beat is delivered at progressively slower intervals.

50 Hz Burst Pacing

Yet another type of ATP available in atrial defibrillators for the treatment of AF is 50 Hz burst pacing. With this type of pacing, AOO burst pulses are delivered at 20 ms intervals for a specific duration, typically 2 seconds.

Shock Therapy

Both cardioversion and defibrillation are referred to as shock therapies. Today, ICDs are capable of aborting shocks should the tachycardia be nonsustained. When charging of the capacitor is complete, a reconfirmation process occurs. If the tachycardia persists, therapy is delivered; if not, therapy is withheld.[30] This is termed *noncommitted shock*. Generally, up to six or eight shocks may be programmed in one zone. The shock energy levels programmable range is from 0.1 to 41 joules (J).

Cardioversion

This is a synchronized shock to terminate AT, AF, or VT. Delivery is synchronized to an R wave. It is usually programmed to follow ATP, should pacing therapies fail (see Figure 25-6). It may also be used as an initial therapy in patients with poorly tolerated VT or in patients in whom ATP has been ineffective. Energy levels can be programmed based on the strength of shock that successfully terminated the patient's tachyarrhythmia during testing.[28,31] Cardioversion may also be programmed empirically at energies much less than that required for defibrillation.

High-Energy Defibrillation

Defibrillation is an asynchronous shock to terminate VF, and it is the only therapy for this arrhythmia (see Figure 25-7). Depending on the device, the energy is programmable from 0.1 J to 41 J. The number of shocks available for delivery varies among devices but may be up to eight, should initial attempts fail to terminate the arrhythmia. The first shock may be programmed to reconfirm the arrhythmia prior to delivery. Subsequent shocks are generally committed.

Shock Waveforms

Biphasic (or bidirectional) waveforms have proven to be more efficient than unidirectional or monophasic waveforms, providing lower DFTs.[29] Waveform tilt, or the percentage of decay in the defibrillation pulse, is allowed before truncation, and generally ranges from 40%–65%.[32] Depending on the device, waveform type and tilt may be programmable options. Pathway polarity, which determines the direction of energy flow, may also be programmable.

Atrial Cardioversion

When this therapy is available, it requires additional programming. Programmable parameters allow control of the time of day shocks are given (generally during sleep), maximal number of shocks available per day, and time at which cardioversion therapy is suspended should an episode persist for days. Patient-activated atrial cardioversion is also available in selected devices.

Antibradycardia Pacing

Antibradycardia pacing is available for individuals with pacing indications, or for transient bradycardia pacing support, such as following cardioversion or defibrillation. Often, output (voltage) is programmed higher postshock and for ATP, because thresholds may be elevated. Depending on the specific ICD model, single-chamber (VVI/R/D) or dual-chamber modes (DDD/R/D) of pacing may be available with or without rate-responsive sensors or multisite pacing.

Hysteresis

This function allows a longer escape interval following a sensed event. The hysteresis rate is generally set 10 pulses per minute below the lower rate limit to allow intrinsic rhythm over pacing in this range.

Figure 25-6. Strip illustrating surface ECG, EGM, and device marker annotations of an episode of VT. Initial ATP therapy is unsuccessful. Second therapy, cardioversion, converts VT to sinus rhythm. *Source:* Courtesy of Medtronic, Inc., Minneapolis, MN.

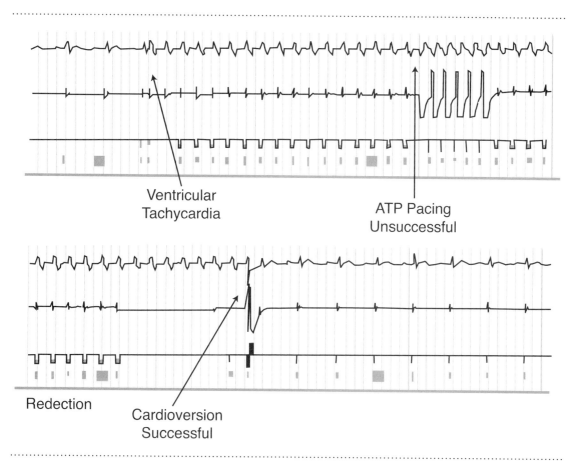

Rate Smoothing

This is an algorithm that only allows the intrinsic cycle length to vary by a determined percentage. If a beat is not sensed within this interval, a pacing pulse is delivered. The purpose is to decrease the incidence of atrial or ventricular arrhythmias induced by long-short sequences.

Data Storage

Devices have greatly expanded their ability to store and report diagnostic information. Current devices may incorporate a considerable amount of memory, 512 Kb, for EGM storage and event counters. Date and time stamps are recorded with each arrhythmic event. Analysis of these stored events and associated information, including the clinical scenario, can assist the clinician in evaluating the appropriateness or effectiveness of therapy.[33] ICDs may also incorporate information on nonsustained tachycardia episodes, SVTs, mode switch episodes, HR trends, HR variability, fluid volume status, pacing percent, and patient activity. Impedance trends may be available for pace/sense leads and HV leads. Some ICDs may also incorporate trending information

Figure 25-7. Strip illustrating surface ECG, electrogram (EGM), and device marker annotations of an episode of VF successfully terminated with a defibrillation shock and subsequent temporary pacing support. *Source:* Courtesy of Medtronic, Inc., Minneapolis, MN.

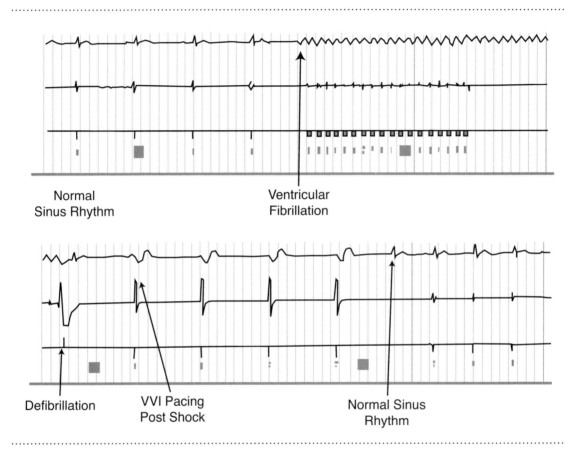

on P wave amplitude, R wave amplitude, impedance, and measured-pacing thresholds.

IMPLANT PROCEDURE

Patient Preparation

Preoperative patient preparation focuses on both emotional and physical care. The patient and his or her family may already be experiencing anxiety or fear concerning the implant procedure, the device, or the patient's underlying disease. A comprehensive educational plan should ad-dress basic device operation, anticipated medication regime, and disease process. A discussion of how the device may affect the patient's lifestyle after the implantation is also important. A review of the implant routine and anticipated postoperative course may allay fears. Educational brochures and films are readily available through device manufacturers or may be individualized to each facility.

Once all of the patient's questions have been answered, informed consent is obtained, and the routine presurgery work-up is performed. This includes laboratory work, a chest X-ray, and a

12-lead ECG. Patients should fast the night before the procedure.

Medication

The nurse should be alert to special instructions regarding anticoagulation, because in most cases, anticoagulation medication may be changed or discontinued prior to device implantation. Similarly, antiarrhythmic medications may be held or adjusted prior to implant and testing. A large-bore IV line is typically started in the arm ipsilateral to the anticipated implant site, and IV fluids are initiated. Preprocedure medications may include a mild sedative and antibiotic prophylaxis. Special care is given to the skin near the location of the anticipated pocket, and ECG patches are not placed in this area (see Table 22-4). While most devices are implanted using the transvenous approach today, additional teaching and physical preparation is required should the patient be scheduled for a thoracotomy.

Physical

Hands-free external defibrillation/pacing electrodes connected to a defibrillator are placed on the patient. The patient is connected to a pulse oximetry monitor, ECG monitor/recorder, and a noninvasive BP monitor. More invasive monitoring may be used at the discretion of the physician. Skin preparation may be limited to the anticipated implant site in some centers, but others may prefer a more extensive scrub should a procedural change be encountered. Prophylactic antibiotics should be given with the infusion timed to end 30 minutes before incision.

Room Preparation

Preparation for a pectorally implanted ICD is similar to that of pacemaker insertion with strict adherence to sterile technique. Although some institutions use operating rooms, others may use

Table 25-4. An ICD Preoperative Pathway/ Checklist

DIET
    Low cholesterol, low fat, sodium restriction as
        indicated
    Fasting after midnight
ACTIVITY
    Unrestricted
ASSESSMENT
    Vital signs
    Cardiopulmonary status
    Height
    Weight
EDUCATION
    Review ICD booklet
    Provide ICD video
    Review postoperative and discharge restrictions
    Overview of ICD
    Instruct to report:
        lightheadedness
        dizziness
        palpitations
    Patient/family verbalize:
        readiness for surgery/procedure
        understanding of ICD function
        postprocedure restrictions
        reduced anxiety
MEDICATIONS
    Routine medications as ordered
    Anesthesia preprocedure medications, PRN
    Anticoagulation: discontinue heparin at midnight
CONSULTS
    Anesthesia, PRN
    Nutrition, PRN
    Psychiatry, PRN
    Social service, PRN
DISCHARGE PLAN
    Identify potential date for discharge
    Identify preliminary plans for discharge
    Identify potential resources needed
TREATMENTS
    Remove electrodes from left chest
    Initial antimicrobial scrub left chest
    20-gauge angiocatheter left forearm
TESTS
    12-lead ECG
    Chest radiograph
    Coagulation studies, metabolic panel, and complete
        blood count
    Type and screen, PRN

rooms such as the catheterization or electrophysiology laboratory with proper negative air flow, after they have been rigorously cleaned.

Instrument Tray

Introducers appropriate for the selected lead system should be available; sizes may range from 7–11F. An instrument for tunneling leads, such as a trocar or chest tube, ought to be available if leads need to be tunneled.

Equipment

The procedure room must contain a full array of emergency equipment for resuscitation; oxygen, suction, and equipment for intubation and mechanical ventilation must be on hand. Medications for advanced cardiac life support and temporary or external pacing must also be readily available. Two external defibrillators, one used in conjunction with the hands-free defibrillation/pacer electrodes, and a backup defibrillator are recommended. Other standard equipment includes a multichannel recorder, electrocautery equipment, fluoroscopic equipment, and a radiolucent patient table. Should an LV lead be placed, contrast material and the ability to store images may be helpful.

Pacing System Analyzer

A pacing system analyzer (PSA) is used for testing the ICD. The equipment includes the PSA itself, PSA patient cable(s), programmer, and sterile wand or sterile sleeve for the programming wand (unless the system is able to communicate wirelessly). With any implant, it is advisable to have on hand not only the specific ICD generator and leads anticipated, but also backup and alternate systems.

Generator Replacements

Replacement procedures present special challenges and require additional planning and sup-plies. Manufacturer encyclopedias are available to look up what connectors are on existing headers and leads and what size wrench is required to disconnect the leads. It is essential to obtain information on the implanted system prior to change out so that a generator with a proper connector block can be on hand. Lead adapters are available if the proper connector block is not available, but are generally avoided. Appropriate lead end-caps should also be readily available during a generator replacement.

Staffing

A safe and successful ICD implantation requires the coordinated effort of different members of the healthcare team. Personnel involved with the procedure of device and lead insertion may include a surgeon, cardiologist, and electrophysiologist. A nonscrubbed physician may also be available to perform inductions, and assess device function. Support staff may include a scrub person, circulating nurse, X-ray technician, and a cardiac technician to assist with electrophysiology recording equipment. Depending on the type of anesthesia to be administered (deep versus conscious sedation), a member of the anesthesia team may also be present. With the advent of pectoral implantation, several sources have documented the use of conscious sedation as a safe and effective alternative to general anesthesia.[33–35]

Implant Technique

Transvenous, subcutaneous ICD systems are associated with decreased complication rates[36] and faster postoperative recovery times[31] and are the preferred method of implantation. The operative technique for pectoral implantation of the lead and device is similar to that discussed with pacemaker implantation. Either the cephalic, axillary, or the subclavian vein is accessed, and the lead is advanced under fluoroscopic guidance. With dual coils, the distal coil is typically positioned in the RVA and the proximal in the SVC. Although a subcutaneous pocket is most often made, a submuscular approach may also be used.

With active or hot-can technology, the device is typically implanted on the left side, thus encompassing more myocardial mass in the shocking vector.[6] Right-sided implants, however, have been used successfully when anatomical situations preclude a left-sided implant.[37] Depending on the system selected, additional defibrillation coils or patches and pacing leads may be added.

Care should be taken throughout the procedure to avoid inadvertent device discharges that may result from the device sensing noise. The device is turned off, or detection suspended, during the use of electrocautery or connection of leads to the generator. If not, noise may be detected by the ICD and shock therapy delivered.

Threshold Testing

Critical to the overall function of the ICD is the ability to effectively pace and sense. Pacing, sensing, and lead impedance measurements are evaluated using a PSA, and acceptable values are similar to those for pacemakers. The presence of diaphragmatic stimulation is also assessed at implant.

Prior to defibrillation threshold testing, the testing device is checked for proper battery voltage and charge time. The device is preprogrammed to the desired detection rates and shock outputs. Sensitivity is set to a less-sensitive setting than will be ultimately programmed. HV lead impedance (approximately 20 to 200 ohms) may be determined to assess lead/device connections and HV lead integrity. Many ICDs now utilize an HV impedance test that is not felt by the patient, otherwise, sedation is required.

VF is then induced one or more times to evaluate the sensing and defibrillation function of the system. VF can be induced by several methods, including rapid ventricular burst pacing, 50 Hz burst pacing, or a low-energy shock on the T wave.[38] With each induction, an external defi-

brillator is charged and ready to deliver a full energy shock should the device fail to convert the rhythm.

Sensing is evaluated during VF by observing the device's sense indicators and EGM amplitude on the programmer screen. It is critical that adequate sensing of ventricular fibrillation be present to avoid underdetection of VF. The manufacturers' recommendations should be followed to test for an adequate sensing safety margin during VF. If sensing is inadequate, the lead is repositioned. Sufficient time ranging from 2 to 5 minutes is allowed between inductions for hemodynamic stabilization.

The DFT can be defined as the lowest energy at which successful defibrillation occurs, provided that a failure occurred at a lower output. Various DFT protocols exist that attempt to estimate energy requirements needed to consistently terminate VF. Some employ a simple protocol of two successive attempts at 10 J less than the maximum output of the device or on three of four attempts. Other protocols employ a step-down procedure, decreasing the delivered energy on successive inductions until failure occurs.[38] The binary search DFT protocol begins testing at lower initial defibrillation energy, and steps output up or down, depending on success or failure of each induction.[22] Upper limit of vulnerability testing may also be used and is based on the relationship between the lowest shock energy that does not induce VF and the DFT.[39]

It is recommended that at least a 10 J safety margin be available regardless of the DFT protocol used. If the given lead system does not demonstrate an adequate defibrillation safety margin, the lead can be repositioned, polarity reversed, or defibrillation waveform adjusted. If needed, an additional transvenous or subcutaneous defibrillation patch or coil may be added.

Testing for therapy efficacy of ATP or cardioversion for ventricular tachycardia may also take place at the time of the initial implant. This testing may be done via the programmer using programmed electrical stimulation for induction of VT.

After testing has been completed, the lead(s) and device are secured to prevent lead dislodgment or generator migration. The incision is closed, and a sterile dressing is applied. Final parameter settings including sensitivity, detection criteria, and programmed therapies should be carefully reevaluated. The data collection of the device may be cleared, and any desired diagnostic parameters selected. Device status and programmed parameters are then documented in the medical record.

Following implantation, the patient is transferred to a recovery area, telemetry unit, or intensive care unit depending on level of consciousness postsedation and acuity.

Complications

The type and number of complications related to ICD therapy has decreased significantly with the advent of pectoral implantation techniques. However, staff members should still be aware and anticipate possible complications that may occur (see Table 25-5).[40]

POSTOPERATIVE EVALUATION AND CARE

Ward Care

Table 25-6 lists tasks that are undertaken between the operation and discharge. Special orders may be written regarding antiarrhythmic medication, antibiotic coverage, and anticoagulation.

It is essential that staff members are familiar with the basic programmed parameters, such as cutoff rates for VT and VF, and the therapies programmed for each rhythm. Institutions should post programmed information so that it is readily accessible to all members of the healthcare team. Personnel should also be aware of whether the device is on or off.

Emergency Care

Should an arrhythmia occur, the device detects and starts therapy in typically less than 10 or 20 seconds. During an emergency, however, care of the patient must be based on basic and advanced cardiac life support protocols, and standard emergency treatment is not delayed. If one is touching the patient during ICD discharge, a slight tingling sensation may be felt, but the person will not be harmed. Rubber gloves will minimize any sensations felt. If external defibrillation is required, avoid placing the paddles directly over the implanted device. Should the standard anterior-lateral paddle placement fail to convert the rhythm, consider changing to anterior-posterior paddle placement.

Device Monitoring

If device therapy occurs while the patient is still in the hospital, the ECG recording, patient

Table 25-5. Potential Complications During or After ICD Implantation

Air embolism	Seroma
Blood loss	Spurious shocks
Cardiac tamponade	Stroke
Diaphragmatic stimulation	Pericarditis
Hematoma	Pneumothorax
Inability to terminate arrhythmia	Vein thrombosis
Infection	Perforation of atrium or ventricle
Myocardial infarction	

Table 25-6. Pathway/Checklist for Day of ICD Implantation

DIET

Preoperative fasting

Postoperative advance diet as tolerated; low fat, low cholesterol, sodium restriction PRN

ACTIVITY

Bedrest overnight

Head of bed > 30°

Limited range of movement/splinting of left arm

ASSESSMENT

Preoperative INR < 1.8

Continuous telemetry:

call MD if HR > 110, < 40

Pulse oximetry: maintain SAO2 > 92%

Postoperative vital signs

every 15 minutes × 4

every 1 hour × 4

every 4 hours, and PRN

Temperature upon arrival, every 4 hours, and PRN

call MD if temperature > 100° F (38° C)

Breath sounds Q 4 hours

Input and output every 4 hours

urine output > 30 cc/hr

Effective cough/airway clearance

Moving all extremities

Dressing dry, intact

No hematoma/seroma

ICD "ON"

Parameters posted

EDUCATION

Explain postprocedure routine

Instruct to call for bleeding/pain

Provide family with contact numbers

Verify phone numbers of family contact

Ask family if they have received adequate information regarding patient condition

MEDICATIONS

Antibiotic within 1 hour of implant

Resume preprocedure medications

Resume anticoagulation per MD/NP

Analgesics for pain control per MD/NP

Patient expresses adequate pain control

CONSULTS

Reassess needs (i.e., PT, Social Service)

DISCHARGE PLAN

Discuss with patient/family readiness for discharge

Complete referral forms as needed

TESTS

12-lead ECG

Postprocedure portable chest radiograph

symptoms, and hemodynamic status should be documented before, during, and after events. Any signs of inappropriate device operation, such as the device treating sinus rhythm, ST, or other SVTs should be monitored, recorded, and reported. Any ineffective therapy should be noted. Occasionally, device therapy may accelerate VT or convert it to VF. Device undersensing may be present if a tachycardia is observed and no device therapy is given. Evidence of inappropriate pacing or loss of capture on telemetry may also signal sensing issues, lead dislodgment, or a loose set screw.

Operation Site

A final assessment of the implant site, pacing thresholds, EGM amplitude and programmed parameters may be done by a physician or other allied health professional prior to patient discharge. A PA and lateral chest X-ray is obtained to document lead and generator position (see Table 25-7). Selected patients may require additional postoperative testing in the catheterization or electrophysiology laboratory under sedation.

Noninvasive Electrophysiology Study

A NIPS is performed using the device and programmer to initiate and terminate arrhythmias. The purpose is to set up VT detection and evaluate therapies. Testing may also be performed predischarge if a marginal defibrillation energy safety margin is found at the time of the initial implant.

Magnet Application

Nursing staff on the postoperative unit need to be familiar with magnet operations specific to the implanted device. Magnet application does not cause asynchronous pacing as in a standalone pacemaker, and the effect may be manufacturer, device, or patient specific. In many instances, a

Table 25-7. An ICD Implantation Patient Discharge Pathway/Checklist

DIET
　Tolerating diet
ACTIVITY
　Independent in ADLs (or baseline)
　Ambulating independently
　Able to climb stairs
　Tolerating activity: no dyspnea on exertion
　BP within 20 mm Hg of baseline, no decrease in
　　BP, pulse within 20 bpm of baseline
ASSESSMENT
　Discharge order
　Laboratory work stable
　HR > 40, < 100 × 12 hours
　Normal sinus rhythm, or baseline, on telemetry
　Systolic BP > 90, < 160 mm Hg
　Temperature < 100° F (38° C) for 12 hours
　Respiratory rate > 12, < 20 at rest
　Lungs clear to auscultation
　Free from symptoms or signs of infection
　No hematoma/seroma
EDUCATION
　Review medications and discharge instructions
　Patient/family should be able to describe:
　　care of incision
　　restrictions (e.g., driving)
　　activity progression
　　medication instructions
　　diet
　　"warning" signs
　　action to take if receives shock
　　phone numbers of physicians/clinicians
　　follow-up appointments/plan
　　how to take radial pulse
DISCHARGE PLAN
　Patient/family received:
　　prescriptions
　　written discharge instructions
　　temporary ID card
　　Medic Alert pamphlet
　　ICD support group information
　　Instructions to carry medication list in wallet
　　Awareness of CPR courses (optional)
TREATMENTS
　Final ICD evaluation/programming
　Remove intravenous line at discharge
TESTS
　Formal PA/lateral chest radiographs
　Additional laboratory examinations as needed

magnet may be placed over the device to suspend detection and therapy. This interaction can be useful in the event of inappropriate device operation. With other devices, the magnet may be capable of permanently deactivating or reactivating the device. In other instances, the magnet may have no effect on ICD function. One should be familiar with institutional guidelines regarding magnet placement. It is important to remember that some ICDs are turned off with magnet application.

Patient Education

Readiness for learning should be assessed in the ICD recipient prior to educational sessions beginning. Particularly in patients with secondary prevention implant indications, the time from the decision to implant to time of implant is so short that patients do not have a chance to process the consequences of ICD implant. In other instances, patients may have lingering neurologic deficits secondary to cardiac arrest, such as short-term memory loss. Additionally, patients who are in denial regarding the seriousness of their diagnosis may not be ready to accept ICD placement as necessary for survival. Attempts to educate may go unheard in all of these situations if the patient is not ready to hear preoperative teaching or discharge instructions.

　In general, education for the ICD recipient should address the topics of physical activity, wound care, pain management, and what to do should an ICD shock occur. The patient's significant other(s) are encouraged to be present during educational sessions, especially if the patient has neurologic deficits. Time should be allotted for the patient and the significant other(s) to ask question of the healthcare provider. Patients should be given the name and telephone number of a contact person should questions develop after discharge. All instructions should also be provided in writing and given to the patient to take home (see Table 25-8).

Table 25-8. An ICD Discharge Instruction Sheet

Date _____

Device manufacturer _____, Model _____

Incision care:
   Maintain steri-strips
   You may shower on _____.

Call your doctor/device clinic for:
   redness, swelling, or drainage from incision site
   increased bruising, discoloration, or tenderness
   fever of 100° F (38° C) or higher
   if you plan to take a vacation or relocate

Please carry:
   defibrillator ID card
   a list of current medications
   your Medic Alert bracelet

Please avoid the following activities until your 1 month visit:
   lifting more than 10 pounds (5 kg) with your left arm (same side as defibrillator implant)
   reaching, swinging, pulling, or pushing with your left arm

If you receive a shock:
   Call your doctor/nurse.
   Call immediately if you receive more than one shock.
   Call emergency personnel for symptoms as you did before your defibrillator implant.

Long term:
   Remind your dentist and doctors treating you that you have an ICD.
   Avoid rough contact in the area of your defibrillator.
   Avoid strong magnetic fields.
   Avoid tight or restrictive clothing over the defibrillator.
   Use your cellular telephone on the opposite ear to your ICD implant side.
   Do not carry your cellular telephone in your breast pocket.
   You may resume sexual activity as tolerated.

You have a follow-up appointment with _____
Address: _____
                                                  Telephone: _____
Date: _____

EMERGENCY NUMBERS:

_____

Movement Restrictions

After pectoral ICD placement, patients are cautioned to limit range of motion of the ipsilateral arm. This activity restriction is used to minimize potential for lead dislodgment. Generally, for the first 4 weeks after ICD implant, specific arm movements such as carrying heavy objects, reaching overhead, or using swinging motions, such as those in golfing or swimming, are discouraged. Combing one's hair or feeding oneself is, of course, allowed. Routine use should be encouraged, because patients who do not allow some shoulder movement may get a frozen shoulder. Once the lead has endothelized and lead stability is ensured, more rigorous physical activities are permitted. Conversely, no restriction is placed on arm activity with an epicardial implant. Regardless of implant approach, general physical activity may be limited until the first follow-up visit to promote healing at the incision site.

Concerned that an increased HR might exceed the ICD's cut-off rate and trigger a shock, many ICD recipients avoid exercise. In fact, decreased overall activity is often due to a combination of factors: fear of being shocked, poor LV function, and postsurgical recovery. The ICD, however, does not prohibit physical activity any more than other cardiac conditions do in patients without ICDs. These findings, in a population with an ICD for an average of 4.5 years, are important to share with new ICD recipients who fear a decrease in quality of life after ICD insertion.

ICD Discharge

If an ICD discharge occurs or the patient thinks a discharge has occurred, he or she should be instructed whether to notify the healthcare provider or go to the emergency room. Patients with a recent implant may need to be reassured by the healthcare provider when a shock occurs for the first time. Other patients may feel comfortable waiting until the next follow-up visit to notify the physician.

Monitoring

Some manufacturers may employ programmable audible patient alerts to monitor certain device conditions, such as low battery voltage, abnormal lead impedance, prolonged charge time, and excessive therapy utilization. Demonstration, explanation, or both of the tone emitted and action to take should be reviewed with the patient. Other devices may now provide data to caregivers via remote home monitoring systems.

Driving

Driving a motor vehicle or using mechanical equipment is generally restricted for 6 months in patients with loss of consciousness (LOC) and may be restricted without LOC. If a recurrence occurs after the patient has resumed driving, an additional restriction may be recommended until the patient is free of arrhythmia. Patients who drive a vehicle as an occupation, such as bus or truck drivers, are evaluated separately, because their percentage of driving time is much greater and therefore their risk of injury greater. For patients who have not experienced loss of consciousness, driving is typically restricted until their first follow-up. Practitioners should be aware of any laws governing driving restrictions in their area.

Identification

Patients are encouraged to wear a medic alert bracelet or necklace and carry the ICD identification card in their wallet. They are instructed to inform all medical personnel including their dentist that they have an ICD. This is important because some medical equipment used may be contraindicated and require programming off detection or temporary suspension of the device during the procedure. MRI is contraindicated.

Device Interactions

Patients should be instructed regarding possible device interactions with equipment in their home or work environment that may possess electromagnetic fields or use strong electricity. The risk is temporary or permanent deactivation with a magnetic field and spurious shocks with electrical noise. Some ICDs may warn the patient by emitting beeping tones when a magnet is placed near the device. In this instance, patients are instructed to move away from the source. Examples of items to avoid include arc welding units, bingo wands, radiofrequency transmitters, alternators of running motors, transformers, and

12 V starters. Most items are safe if kept at least an arm's length away. Microwave ovens, hair dryers, and other low-level power sources have no effect on the ICD unless there is a lead fracture or insulation break already present.[41] Cellular telephones, when used on the ear opposite the pectorally implanted ICD, pose no problem as long as they are held greater than 6 inches from the ICD. In telephones transmitting more than 3 watts, separation of 12 inches is generally recommended.[42]

Precautions should also be reviewed for other equipment commonly encountered. Patients should be instructed not to linger in entryways with electronic article surveillance.[43] In airport terminals or other facilities with metal detectors, patients should show their ID and ask to be checked by hand. Patients may walk directly through the detector and not linger, but the alarm is often triggered and serves no purpose. Use of a hand-held screening wand is not recommended near the device.

Support Groups

Participation in ICD support groups is encouraged but emphasized as optional because a patient's readiness for sharing his or her concerns and experiences may not be present. Significant others' attendance at a cardiopulmonary resuscitation (CPR) course should also be encouraged, though some may either not be able to perform the skills or not be emotionally ready to contemplate performing CPR on a loved one. If unable to participate in a CPR course, the significant others must, at a minimum, know how to activate the emergency medical system, should it become necessary.

Follow-Up

Patients are scheduled to return to the clinic or physician's office for follow-up 1 to 4 weeks after ICD implantation. At the first visit, the wound is

assessed for healing. Any signs of infection, such as redness, swelling, or persistent low-grade fever are noted. Some puffiness and tenderness may still exist at the pocket site. This is not uncommon and may persist for up to 2 months after generator insertion. Tenderness or swelling, lasting longer than 2 months or any persistent redness is abnormal, and a more intense follow-up and treatment should be pursued. Blood cultures, CBC with differential, and antibiotic therapy should be considered for suspected infections. Pocket infections can have potentially lethal consequences, resulting in septicemia and even death if left untreated.

Evaluations thereafter are generally quarterly.[44] These may be in the form of office visits, or office visits supplemented with remote monitoring data evaluation. More frequent follow-ups may be necessary if multiple shocks are delivered, unstable lead impedance or pacing thresholds are obtained, or pocket infection is suspected. The site should be evaluated at each visit. The ICD is interrogated to determine parameter settings for brady- and tachyarrythmias, battery and lead status, charge time at last capacitor formation, and evaluation of stored diagnostic data. Tachycardia episodes are evaluated for appropriate sensing, detection, and treatment of the arrhythmia. The stored EGM is useful in determining the rhythm that precipitated therapy. The scenario in which the episode occurred and any patient symptoms are evaluated. Pacing thresholds, sensing thresholds, and lead impedances are obtained. All data collected must be reviewed and needed changes made.

Reprogramming

Reprogramming of sensitivities or defibrillation therapies is not recommended unless testing has been done at these settings, and appropriate safety margins maintained.

Frequently in patients with only RVA pacing, AV delays are lengthened, nontracking modes are used, or pacing is programmed to VVI at 40 bpm to avoid ventricular pacing. This programming arose from data showing that patients with intrinsic conduction do better those with RVA pacing, which results in dyssynchrony.[45] Many devices now offer modes that effectively AAI/R pace unless persistent AV block occurs, then they revert to DDD/R pacing.

If the patient has had spurious or inappropriate shocks, further investigation is indicated. This may merely include an assessment of what equipment the patient may have been in contact with at the time. Oversensing may also be evaluated in the office. Patients are asked to perform isometric arm exercises and reach across their chests while EGM and annotation channels are observed for the sensing of noise. This "noise" may be reflective of lead fracture or insulation break. Rarely, diaphragmatic oversensing has been noted with deep breathing. Further assessment of system integrity may include overpenetrated radiographs or testing of the HV system under sedation, if needed.

Data Transmission

Technology has been developed that allows patients with certain ICDs to transmit device data to their follow-up clinics over the telephone via a remote monitoring system. The information sent may be similar to that obtained during an in-office follow-up. Depending on the manufacturer, clinicians may be able to assess programmed parameters, lead impedances, EGM amplitudes, battery voltage, most recent charge time, arrhythmia episodes, stored electrograms, and other diagnostics. This type of follow-up may be helpful in reducing the frequency of in-office visits and in triaging patients receiving shocks. Devices may be set up to automatically query the device and transmit data at regular intervals or may automatically transmit should a preprogrammed device condition (e.g., impedance out-of-range) be met. Other testing and programming are not available with this form of follow-up.

Psychosocial Functioning

The patient or significant others may voice questions regarding the ICD's functioning and its ability to terminate lethal arrhythmias. Reassurance by the healthcare provider about the functioning of the device helps to alleviate fear and anxiety. Depending on the patient's diagnosis, and on whether the ICD was placed after cardiac arrest, symptomatic VT or implanted prophylactically, levels of anxiety, fear, and depression may differ. As time in recovery continues, persons who experience no or few shocks will have diminished anxieties, fears, and concerns as compared with those who receive multiple shocks.[46]

Recovery from ICD insertion requires more than usual attention to physical needs, such as wound healing and restricting physical activity. Physical and psychosocial concerns of both the patient and significant others may overwhelm the recovery process and inhibit the return to activities of daily living.[47–49] Anxieties develop around uncertainty or fear about the ICD's failure to function, or functioning but inflicting pain with shock delivery.[50,51] Changes in body image and concerns about what bystanders would think if the ICD fires in public are also a source of anxiety. Other concerns reported in the literature include insomnia,[52,53] depression,[54] and overprotectivenesss of family members. Long-term outcomes on patients with an ICD suggest that those who are emotional are likely to be psychologically distressed and adapt poorly to social and domestic life, while those who can problem-solve have less distress.[55]

How or whether a patient can resolve these anxieties, fears, and concerns affects their recovery. The causes of anxiety can differ depending on one's stage of recovery. Soon after ICD placement, the patient is usually anxious about when the ICD will fire, if ever, and what it will feel like.[47] As the wound heals and activity restrictions lift, new anxieties develop about what could trigger the ICD to fire. Could arguments or stressful situations cause a tachycardia? What would happen if the ICD fired while driving a car? Resumption of each activity including social activities such as attending church, family gatherings, resuming hobbies, or physical activities such as driving were difficult to resume in those with low self-efficacy.[49]

As recovery continues, patients who receive shocks from their ICD have very different anxieties than those who receive no or few shocks.[46,49] Higher levels of anxiety were experienced not only by the ICD recipient of multiple shocks, but also by the significant other. Anxiety levels continue to remain high as long as the shocks recur but diminished over time in those who received few or no shocks.[54] Significant others are often anxious about the uncertainty of knowing what to do should a shock occur.

Education Programs

Comprehensive education programs are designed to educate and inform ICD patients and family members about ICD functioning, physical activity restrictions, risks and benefits of ICD placement, and what to anticipate during hospitalization and after discharge. In addition to education, emotional support is also provided. A contact person is identified to answer questions and impart information in a timely manner to the patient and significant other(s). Explanations are consistent since the contact person is reinforcing earlier instruction and understands what information has been shared with patient and family previously. Patients, especially those who experienced short-term memory loss as a result of cardiac arrest, benefit from a comprehensive program because it seeks to reinforce educational topics pre-ICD implant to 1 year postimplantation. The need for additional education during follow-up varies with the patient's recovery. Those who receive ICD discharges might require further explanation as to the necessity of medication changes, tachycardia induction, and repro-

gramming of the ICD. Emotional comfort and support would also be provided to both patient and family while the education takes place.

SUMMARY

Mortality related to sudden death has been estimated at approximately 1%–2% annually in the ICD patient population. This is a significant improvement over a 15%–25% annual sudden death rate for such patients without an ICD. As the focus has turned toward preventing SCD by identifying those at high risk and directing new and future technology at arrhythmia prevention, indications are growing. It is imperative that healthcare providers understand ICD technology and the impact it has on both patients and their families. This is essential to provide quality patient care.

REFERENCES

1. Mower MM. Clinical and historical perspective. In: Singer I, ed. *Implantable Cardioverter-Defibrillator*. Armonk, NY: Futura; 1994:12.
2. Mower MM, Hauser RG. Historical development of the AICD. In: Estes NAM, Manolis AS, Wang PJ, eds. *Implantable Cardioverter-Defibrillators: A Comprehensive Textbook*. New York: Marcel Dekker; 1994:173–186.
3. Mower MM, Hauser RG. Developmental history, early use, and implementation of the automatic implantable cardioverter defibrillator. *Prog Cardiovasc Dis* 1993;36:89–96.
4. Schuder JC. The ICD: progress, prospects, and problems. *PACE* 1997;20:2367–2370.
5. Marchlinski FE, Kleiman RB, Hook BG, et al. Advances in implantable cardioverter defibrillator therapy. In: Josephson ME, Wellens HJJ, eds. *Tachycardias: Mechanisms and Management*. Mount Kisco, NY: Futura; 1993:405–420.
6. Kuck KH, Cappato R, Siebels J. ICD therapy. In: Camm AJ, ed. *Clinical Approaches to Tachyarrhythmias*, Vol. 5. Armonk, NY: Futura; 1996.

7. Kamalvand K, Gill JS. The implantable cardiac defibrillator. *Br J Hosp Med* 1996;55:37–41.

8. Rosamond, W, Flegal, K, Furie, K, et al. Heart disease and stroke statistics—2008 update: A report from the American Heart Association Statistics Committee and Stoke Statistics Committee. *Circulation* 2008; 117: e1–e122.

9. CDC. State-specific mortality from sudden cardiac death—United States 1999. *MMWR Weekly* 2002;51(06):123–126.

10. Priori SG, Blomstrom-Lundqvist C, Bossaert L, et al. Task force on sudden cardiac death, European society of cardiology: Summary of recommendations. *Europace* 2002;4:3–18.

11. Myerburg RJ, Kessler KM, Castellanos A. Sudden cardiac death: structure, function, and time-dependence of risk. *Circulation* 1992;85(suppl I):I2–I10.

12. Fogoros RN. *Electrophysiologic Testing.* Cambridge, MA: Blackwell Scientific; 1991.

13. Epstein AE, DiMarco JP, Ellenbogen KA, et al. ACC/AHA/HRS 2008 Guidelines for Device-Based Therapy of Cardiac Rhythm Abnormalities *Circulation* 2008;117;e350–e408.

14. Bardy GH, Lee KL, Mark DB, et al. Amiodarone or an implantable cardioverter-defibrillator for congestive heart failure. *N Engl J Med* 2005; 352(3):225–237.

15. Schaechter A, Kadish AH. Defibrillation in non-ischemic cardiomyopathy treatment evaluation (DEFINITE). *Cardiac Electrophysiology Review* 2003;7(4):457–462.

16. O'Brien BJ, Connolly SJ, Goeree R, et al. Cost-effectiveness of the implantable cardioverter-defibrillator: Results from the Canadian implantable defibrillator study (CIDS). *Circulation* 2001;103(10):1416–1421.

17. Al Khatib SM, Anstrom KJ, Eisenstein EL, et al. Clinical and economic implications of the multicenter automatic defibrillator implantation trial-II. *Ann Intern Med* 2005;142:593–600.

18. Mark DB, Nelson CL, Anstrom KJ, et al. Cost-effectiveness of defibrillator therapy or amiodarone in chronic stable heart failure: results from the Sudden Cardiac Death in Heart Failure Trial (SCD-HeFT). *Circulation* 2006;114:135–142.

19. Hohnloser SH, Kuck KH, Dorian P, et al. Prophylactic use of an implantable cardioverter-defibrillator after acute myocardial infarction. *N Engl J Med* 2004;351(24):2481–2488.

20. Zipes DP, Camm AJ, Boggrafe M, et al. ACC/AHA/ESC 2006 guidelines for management of patients with ventricular arrhythmias and the prevention of sudden death: a report of the American College of Cardiology/American Heart Association Task Force and the European Society of Cardiology Committee for Practice Guidelines *J Am Coll Cardiol* 2006;48:247–346.

21. Bernstein AD, Camm AJ, Fletcher RD, et al. The NASPE/BPEG defibrillator code. *PACE* 1993;16:1776–1780.

22. Ellenbogen KA. *Cardiac Pacing,* 2nd ed. Cambridge, MA: Blackwell Scientific; 1996.

23. Medtronic. *Medtronic Gem III AT 7276 Dual Chamber Implantable Cardioverter Defibrillator System Reference Guide.* Minneapolis, MN: Medtronic, Inc.; 2001:UCX198834001.

24. Furman SF, Hayes DL, Holmes DR. *A Practice of Cardiac Pacing,* 3rd ed. Mount Kisco, NY: Futura; 1993.

25. Echt DS, Lee JT, Hammon JW. Implantation and intraoperative assessment of antitachycardia devices. In: Saksena S, Goldschlager N, eds. *Electrical Therapy for Cardiac Arrhythmias.* Philadelphia, PA: WB Saunders; 1990.

26. Medtronic. *Wavelet Dynamic Discrimination Criterion in the Marquis VR ICD Model 7230.* Minneapolis, MN: Medtronic, Inc.; 2002:UC200201513aEN.

27. Olsen, WH. Dual chamber sensing and detection for implantable cardioverter-defibrillators. In: Singer I, Barold SI, Camm AJ, eds. *Nonpharmacological Therapy of Arrhythmias for the 21st Century: The State of the Art.* Armonk, NY: Futura; 1998.

28. Davidson T, VanRiper S, Harper P, et al. Implantable cardioverter defibrillators: a guide for clinicians. *Heart & Lung* 1994;23:205–216.

29. Moses HW, Moulton KP, Miller BD, et al. *A Practical Guide to Cardiac Pacing*, 4th ed. Boston: Little, Brown and Company; 1995.

30. Nichols K, Collins J. Update on implantable cardioverter defibrillators: knowing the differences in devices and their impact on patient care. *AACN Clinical Issues* 1995;6:31–43.

31. Knight L, Livinston NA, Gawlinski A, et al. Caring for patients with third-generation implantable cardioverter defibrillators: from decision to implant to patient's return home. *Crit Care Nurse* 1997;17:46–65.

32. Hayes DL, Lloyd MA, Friedman PA. *Cardiac Pacing and Defibrillation: A Clinical Approach.* Armonk, NY: Futura; 2000.

33. Sarter BH, Callans DJ, Gottlieb DS, et al. Implantable defibrillator diagnostic storage capabilities: evolution, current status, and future utilization. *PACE* 1998;21:1287–1302.

34. Stix G, Anvari A, Grabenwogert C. Implantation of a unipolar cardioverter/defibrillator system under local anesthesia. *Eur Heart J* 1996; 17:764–768.

35. Natale A, Kearney MM, Brandon MJ, et al. Safety of nurse-administered deep sedation for defibrillator implantation in the electrophysiology laboratory. *J Cardiovasc Electr* 1996;7:301–306.

36. Block M, Hammel D, Bansch D, et al. Prevention of ICD complications. In: Allessie MA, Fromer M, eds. *Atrial and Ventricular Fibrillation: Mechanisms and Device Therapy.* Armonk, NY: Futura; 1997.

37. Kirk M, Shorofsky S, Gold M. Comparison of the effects of active left and right pectoral pulse generators on defibrillation efficacy. *Am J of Cardiol* 2001,88:1308–1311.

38. Stanton MS, Hayes DL, Munger TM, et al. Consistent subcutaneous prepectoral implantation of a new implantable cardioverter defibrillator. *Mayo Clinic Proc* 1994;69:309–314.

39. Hui RC, Rosenthal L, Ramza B, et al. Relationship between the upper limit of vulnerability determined in normal sinus rhythm and the defibrillation threshold in patients with implantable cardioverter defibrillators. *PACE* 1998;21:687–694.

40. Bubien R. Therapeutic modalities: device therapy-antitachycardia pacing. In: Schurig L, ed. *Educational Guidelines Pacing and Electrophysiology.* Armonk, NY: Futura; 1994:393–400.

41. Fogel RI, Hemer ME, Sample R, et al. ICD implant does not preclude working around industrial equipment. *J Am Coll Cardiol* 1998;31:435A.

42. Medtronic. Questions About Electromagnetic Interference (EMI). Minneapolis, MN: Medtronic, Inc.; 2001:UC199300962e EN.

43. Levine PA. *Electronic Article Surveillance and Pacemakers.* Sylmar, CA: St. Jude Medical; 1999:No. P0061.

44. Winters SL, Packer DL, Marchlinski FE, et al. NASPE policy statement: consensus statement on indications, guidelines for use, and recommendations for the follow-up of implantable cardioverter defibrillators. *PACE* 2001;24(2):262–269.

45. Wilkoff BL, Cook JR, Epstein AE, et al. Dual-chamber pacing or ventricular backup pacing in patients with an implantable defibrillator. *JAMA* 2002:24:3115–3122.

46. Dougherty CM. Psychological reactions and family adjustment in shock vs no shock groups after implantation of internal cardioverter defibrillator. *Heart & Lung* 1995;24:281–291.

47. Burke LJ. Securing life through technology acceptance: the first six months after transvenous internal cardioverter defibrillator implantation. *Heart & Lung* 1996;25:352–366.

48. Dougherty CM. Family-focused interventions for survivors of cardiac arrest. *Journal of Cardiovascular Nursing* 1997;12:45–58.

49. Schuster PM, Phillips S, Dillon DL, Tomich PL. The psychosocial and physiological experiences of patients with an implantable cardioverter defibrillator. *Rehabilitation Nursing* 1998;23:30–37.

50. Cooper DK, Luceri RM, Thurer RJ, et al. The impact of the automatic implantable cardioverter defibrillator on quality of life. *Clin Prog Electrophys Pacing* 1986;4:306–309.

51. Dunbar SB, Warner CD, Purcell JA. Internal cardioverter defibrillator device discharge: experiences of patients and family members. *Heart & Lung* 1993;22:494–501.

52. Sneed NV, Finch N. Experiences of patients and significant others with automatic implantable cardioverter defibrillators after discharge from the hospital. *Prog Cardiovasc Nurs* 1992;7:20–24.

53. Vitale MB, Funk M. Quality of life in younger persons with an implantable cardioverter defibrillator. *Dim Crit Care Nur* 1995;14:100–111.

54. Dougherty CM. Longitudinal recovery following sudden cardiac arrest and internal carioverter defibrillator implantation: survivors and their families. *Am J Crit Care* 1994;3:145–154.

55. Craney JM, Mandle CL, Munro BH, Rankin S. Implantable cardioverter defibrillators: physical and psychosocial outcomes. *Am J Crit Care* 1997;6:445–451.

SUGGESTED READING

Bubien RS, Fisher JD, Gentzel JA, et al. NASPE expert consensus document: use of IV (conscious) sedation/analgesia by nonanesthesia personnel in patients undergoing arrhythmia specific diagnostic, therapeutic, and surgical procedures. *PACE* 1998;21:375–385.

Ellenbogen KA, Wood M. *Cardiac Pacing*. Hoboken, NJ: Wiley, John & Sons, Inc.; 2005.

Ellenbogen KA, Wilkoff BL, Kay GN. *Clinical Cardiac Pacing, Defibrillation and Resynchronization Therapy*. St Louis, MO: Elsevier Health Sciences; 2006.

Hayes DL, Lloyd MA, Friedman PA, eds. *Cardiac Pacing and Defibrillation: A Clinical Approach*. Armonk, NY: Futura; 2000.

Moss AJ, Hall WJ, Cannom DS, et al. Improved survival with an implanted defibrillator in patients with coronary disease at high risk for ventricular arrhythmia. *N Engl J Med* 1996;335:1933–1940.

Moss AJ, Zareba W, Hall WJ, et al. Prophylactic implantation of a defibrillator in patients with myocardial infarction and reduced ejection fraction. [comment]. *N Engl J Med* 2002;346(12):877–883.

Schurig L, ed. *NASPE Council of Associated Professionals Educational Guidelines: Pacing and Electrophysiology*, 2nd ed. Armonk, NY: Futura; 1997.

Chapter 26

HEMOSTASIS AND VASCULAR CLOSURE DEVICES

Kenneth A. Gorski, RN, RCIS, RCSA, FSICP
Thomas H. Maloney, MS, RCIS, RT(N), FSICP

Hemostasis is a term that means to control or stop bleeding, a process that can be vital to survival when blood vessels are damaged. This same process can also be catastrophic when a thrombus forms in a vital vessel, such as a coronary or cerebral artery. The first part of this chapter will briefly review the science behind how a thrombus forms; the second part will review the different means of safely achieving and maintaining hemostasis after a percutaneous vascular procedure.

BASIC PHYSIOLOGIC MECHANISMS OF HEMOSTASIS

When trauma, spontaneous hemorrhage, or a needle stick damage a blood vessel, the first physiological response is vessel spasm. Spasm occurs when the vessel's endothelium is denuded, and there is a loss of nitric oxide. This loss increases sensitivity to local vasoconstrictors (i.e., serotonin from aggregating platelets) and decreases sensitivity to local vasodilators. This process is most ef-

fective in small vessels and serves as the vessel's first line of defense against hemorrhage.[1] This reflex may only last for a few minutes; however, a platelet plug begins to form within seconds. While the platelet plug is forming, serotonin is released by the platelets causing further vascular constriction.[2]

The initiation of the coagulation cascade (see Figure 26-1) is now in motion. The clotting cascade is delineated by a series of Roman numerals.[3] Each numeral describes a specific factor based on the order of its discovery. Each factor has an exposed phospholipid on the platelet surface membrane, which is the site where coagulation factors congregate. The coagulation proteins form an enzymatic cascade that eventually forms a fibrin clot. The intrinsic pathway is stimulated by blood coming into contact with foreign substances in the absence of tissue damage. This pathway can be measured in the laboratory by the activated partial thromboplastin time. The extrinsic pathway is stimulated by broken blood

Figure 26-1. The coagulation cascade.

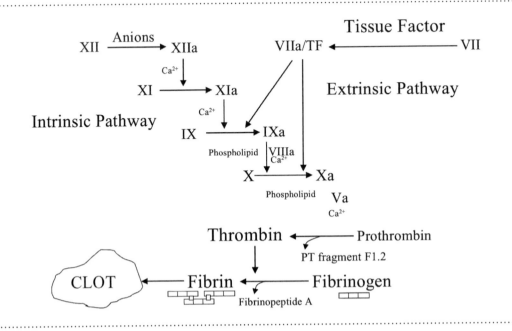

vessels or damaged tissues and can be measured by prothrombin time.[4]

The extrinsic pathway is triggered when blood comes into contact with damaged vessel walls or tissue outside blood vessels. Damaged tissues release a complex of substances from the cell membrane called *tissue thromboplastin*. Tissue thromboplastin initiates a series of reactions involving several clotting factors. These factors depend on calcium for the composition of each step leading to the production of prothrombin activator. The amount of prothrombin activator appearing in blood is directly proportional to the degree of tissue damage, and it is responsible for converting prothrombin into thrombin. Thrombin then acts as an enzyme and causes a reaction in the fibrinogen. Small portions of fibrinogen are split off and develop an attraction to similar molecules. The activated fibrinogen molecules join end to end, forming fibrin strands. Once the fibrin strands have formed, a meshwork is created

that serves as a means of entangling blood cells and platelets to form a blood clot.[3]

Once a clot begins to form, the promotion of further clots is initiated. This is due to the fact that thrombin begets more thrombin, promoting further clot propagation. This feedback creates an unstable environment that favors a prothrombotic state. Human life is dependant upon a relatively stable environment, and this feedback mechanism normally only lasts for a short time.

In contrast to the extrinsic pathway, the intrinsic clotting mechanism occurs within the blood. The intrinsic pathway in initiated with factor XII, when blood is exposed to a foreign substance (such as collagen from a mechanical closure device). In the presence of calcium ions, prothrombin is converted to thrombin by prothrombin activator, just as in the extrinsic pathway.

Balancing the effects in the blood is the fact that normally, rapidly moving blood keeps thrombin concentrations too low to enhance further clot formation. In addition, endothelial cells secrete antithrombin into the plasma, which limits the formation of thrombin. Thrombin generation is usually limited to slow-moving or stagnant blood and typically ceases in fast-moving, circulating blood.

Platelet plug, or white clot formation, is the process that ensues after initiation of the extrinsic or intrinsic pathways. Platelets in circulation are typically smooth and disc shaped. Platelets tend to stick to the exposed ends of injured blood vessels. Platelets are also attracted to the collagen found in the subendothelial layer of the blood vessel. In a very similar manner, platelets are attracted to the collagen found on many hemostasis devices commercially available. When platelets contact collagen, their shapes are altered, and many pseudopodia are expressed from the platelet surface membrane. This is known as platelet activation (see Figure 26-2). There are nearly 100 different pathways known for platelet activation.

Almost simultaneously, when platelets activate, they adhere to the endothelium. Once adhesion takes place, platelets also adhere to each other and form a monolayer of cells that may be able to control blood loss if the injury is small.[4] In addition, the stimulus of platelet activation from the subendothelium becomes covered by the monolayer of platelets, thus preventing further exposure to the prothrombotic environment of the vessel wall.

The pseudopodia that were expressed are now fully exposed from the platelet membrane. Platelets begin to aggregate and form the platelet plug. In order for platelets to aggregate together, they cross-link via the glycoprotein IIb-IIIa receptor sites. Once the platelets begin the process of aggregation, cytokines such as adenosine diphosphate are released to recruit additional platelets.[5] As additional platelets are recruited, a platelet plug forms, providing an effective barrier to further blood loss. The platelet plug traps additional

Figure 26-2. Platelet activation.

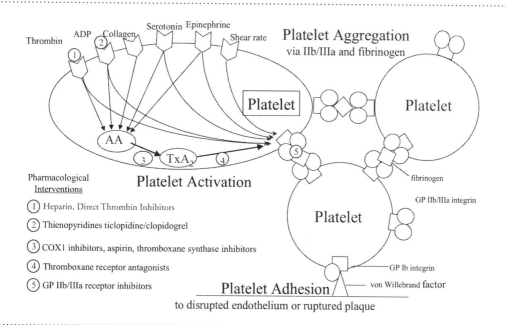

blood cells and begins fibrin strand formation to stabilize the clot.[6]

Many anticoagulants can alter the clotting cascade (see Figure 26-2). These medications inhibit factors that lead to hemostasis or prolong the process of hemostasis. In interventional cardiology, where mechanical trauma is induced to treat atherosclerotic disease, some form of anticoagulation must be administered to prevent acute vessel thrombosis. Altering various segments of the coagulation cascade with anticoagulants can achieve significant reductions in future major adverse cardiac events (MACE).[7]

The coagulation cascade is a delicate interplay of coagulation factors that can achieve lifesaving hemostasis without progressing to acute vascular thrombosis. Despite potent anticoagulation used in modern-day percutaneous coronary interventions, the coagulation cascade is still able to form a thrombus at sites of vessel trauma. This is because platelets and existing thrombin can generate a thrombus.

There are many ways to activate the coagulation cascade either intrinsically or extrinsically. The use of aspirin, heparin, direct thrombin inhibitors, glycoprotein IIb/IIIa inhibitors, and ADP inhibitors such as Clopidogrel and the currently under approval drug Prasugrel only effectively blocks a small number of pathways to thrombus formation. Platelets are still able to adhere to the site of injury for appropriate hemostasis. It is the delay in platelet plug formation that these agents have affected.

Many of the commercially available mechanical hemostasis devices promote thrombus formation by using collagen and other biologic prothrombotic materials. Complete vessel occlusion at the site is prevented (in most cases) because there is rapidly circulating blood in the vessel, and this allows for just a helpful amount of thrombus formation.

HEMOSTASIS METHODS

Proper technique, without shortcuts, is essential to achieving successful femoral artery hemosta-sis without complications. There are many ways to achieve hemostasis following a percutaneous catheterization. These include manual compression, mechanical compression, vascular plugs, percutaneous vascular suturing or staples, and topical hemostasis accelerators. Each of these methods will be briefly reviewed.

Manual Compression

Percutaneous vascular sheath insertion creates a subcutaneous tract to the vessel. Patient recovery is dependent upon the assessment skills and knowledge of proper hemostasis techniques of the cardiovascular invasive specialist. Correct technique is essential to stop bleeding and minimize potential complications such as hematomas and pseudoaneurysms. Prior to sheath removal, assess the distal pulses (dorsalis pedis and posterior tibial) and the access site for signs of an existing hematoma (discussed later in this chapter).

When venous and arterial sheaths are present in the same groin, it is recommended that the venous sheath should be removed prior to the arterial sheath to minimize the risk of atrioventricular fistula formation. When the sheath is removed, some patients will have a vasovagal response, exhibiting nausea, vomiting, diaphoresis, bradycardia, and hypotension. It is for this reason that some institutions prefer the removal of the arterial sheath first, allowing the venous sheath to stay in place if the need arises to rapidly administer intravenous fluids and medication.

For arterial sheath removal, place the fingers with folded, dry sterile gauze about 2 cm proximal and slightly medial to the skin incision, and palpate the artery. If a venous sheath is in place, finger position should be directly below the skin incision. Instruct the patient to take a deep breath in and then slowly exhale. As the patient exhales, gently remove the sheath. A small spurt of blood is normal and may help purge the artery of thrombi forming around the sheath. While removing the sheath, be careful not to compress or crush the sheath, because this may strip clots that may have formed within the sheath since the end of the procedure. Maintain occlusive pressure for 5 minutes. After 5 minutes of occlusive pressure, slowly decrease the pressure until distal pulses can be palpated. Maintain this amount of compression for an additional 5 minutes, then slowly let up pressure and assess the puncture site. If the site is oozing, apply gentle pressure for an additional 5 minutes. If an active bleed or pulsatile flow is present, quickly apply enough pressure to regain control and achieve hemostasis.

If the patient has not received any anticoagulation and proper technique is followed, hemostasis can be achieved for venous sheaths smaller than 9F in about 5 minutes. For arterial sheaths of 4F or 5F, hemostasis may be achieved in under 10 minutes; for 6F to 8F, 10–15 minutes of manual compression is generally sufficient. If arterial sheaths of 9F or greater are used, compression time will need to be adjusted accordingly.

Problems associated with manual pressure for hemostasis include poor technique, application of inconsistent pressure, staff fatigue, and predisposition to carpal tunnel syndrome related to hand and wrist strain. Adjunctive use of C-clamps or FemoStop can relieve the manual strain associated with holding the femoral site for extended lengths of time.[6]

Mechanical Compression

C-Clamp

A number of companies manufacture "C-clamp" devices to assist in achieving hemostasis. The original product, the Instromedex CompressAR system (from Advanced Vascular Dynamics of Vancouver, Washington), was introduced in the 1970s. The CompressAR 6000 C-Clamp consists of a flat, metal base; a pivoting metal shaft attached to the base; an adjustable arm lever with arm slide; and upper and lower arm lock mechanisms to hold the desired level of pressure (see Figure 26-3). Disposable plastic compression discs, attached to the arm, apply pressure over

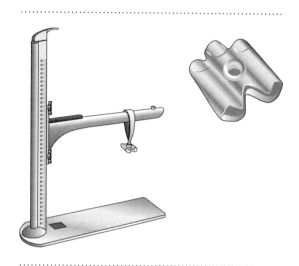

Figure 26-3. CompressAR StrongArm system.
Source: Adapted from Advanced Vascular Dynamics.

the desired area. The discs come in a variety of sizes and shapes, such as flat-round or oval discs, concave-round or oval discs, and Advanced Vascular Dynamic's "3-Finger Jack" disc. Each has a V-shaped notch for placement around the sheath prior to removal.

Prior to sheath removal, assess the patient's distal pulses. Loosen the arm locks, and position the base beneath the bed mattress directly below the patient's hip. Lift the lever at the top of the C-clamp arm; some brands allow you the pivot the arm for optimal placement. Adjust the arm slide into the desired position. Using aseptic technique, attach the desired disc to the tip of the slide arm. As with manual and other compression techniques, palpate the access site about 2 cm proximally and medially to the skin puncture, and gently lower the C-clamp arm into position. The sheath needs to be centered with the sheath hub within the notch of the disc. The shaft is then locked in position. With one hand on top of the arm and lever, remove the sheath with the other hand. Enough pressure should be applied to the arm to stop any bleeding once the sheath is completely removed. Lower the upper arm lock and relock to secure the arm lock. As with manual compression, be careful not to crush the sheath as it is removed from the vessel.[7]

Occlusive pressure should be maintained for 5 minutes. After the first 5 minutes, loosen the upper arm lock and slowly lift the arm lever no more than 45° to gradually release pressure. Palpate the distal pulse to ensure there is flow, and re-lock the arm in place. Maintain this pressure over the next 10 minutes. After a total of 15 minutes of C-clamp pressure, unlock the upper arm and slowly pump the arm lever to gradually release pressure. If at any time bleeding reoccurs, lower the lever to increase compression until hemostasis is achieved. Larger sheaths, use of anticoagulants, IIb/IIIa inhibitors, or thrombolytics may require longer compression times to achieve hemostasis.

Hand-Held Compression Assists

C-clamps provide one alternative for hemostasis, but many cardiovascular professionals favor the feel and control achieved with manual compression. A number of companies market products to reduce hand fatigue, strain, and the risk of carpal tunnel syndrome associated with repetitive manual holds. The EZ Hold (from TZ Medical of Portland, Oregon) and D-Stat Handle are weighted T-shaped devices designed to combine manual hold techniques with a compression disc (see Figure 26-4). Advanced Vascular Dynamics offers the Compass, which resembles a weighted air hockey paddle After applying the C-clamp disc to the device, which is positioned as described in the previously section, the sheath is removed, and manual pressure is applied on the handle sufficient to control the bleeding.

The weighted devices reduce the amount of strength required to achieve hemostasis, while the disc allows the cardiovascular professional to apply a more consistent pressure to the site and still palpate the patient's distal pulse with the free hand. Some of these products are available in varying weights of 1–2 lbs to accommodate personal preferences.

Figure 26-4. The EZ Hold. *Source:* TZ Medical.

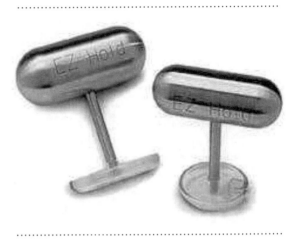

FemoStop

The FemoStop (from RADI Medical Systems of Reading, Massachusetts) is a pneumatic pressure device. It was first approved in 1992 by the FDA as an alternative to manual compression of vascular access sites. The FemoStop is composed of a plastic arch, inflatable transparent dome, connection tubing, a stopcock, an elastic belt, and a handheld FemoStop manometer (see Figure 26-5). The FemoStop's transparent dome offers clear visualization of the puncture site, allowing for very accurate placement.

Prior to sheath removal, note the patient's systolic blood pressure, and assess his or her distal pulses. The elastic belt is placed under the patient's hips and positioned in line with the puncture site. It is important that the belt be even and not twisted.

The FemoStop arch should be positioned so that the shorter arm of the arch is on the side of the sheath to be removed. The ends of the belt are threaded through the clips located on each arm of the arch. The center of the compression dome is placed about 2 cm superior and slightly medial to the skin puncture site (see Figure 26-6). This is extremely important. Although it varies with each

Figure 26-5. Femostop. *Source:* Reprinted with permission from St. Jude Medical™, © 2010 all rights reserved.

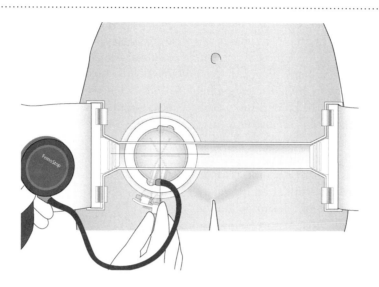

patient's anatomy, the sheath typically enters the artery through the skin at an angle of 30°–45°. Once the dome is positioned, retract the sheath far enough to allow the hub of the sheath to be free from underneath the dome. The arch should be as even and level as possible, and the dome should be flat prior to sheath removal. The belt

Figure 26-6. Femostop positioning. *Source:* Reprinted with permission from St. Jude Medical™, © 2010 all rights reserved.

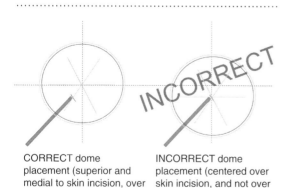

CORRECT dome placement (superior and medial to skin incision, over the puncture in the artery)

INCORRECT dome placement (centered over skin incision, and not over the arterial puncture)

should tightened so that the arch is snug on the patient without exerting significant pressure.

If a venous sheath has been used, the dome should be inflated to 30 mmHg and the sheath removed. Venous hemostasis should be obtained prior to removal of the arterial sheath. For arterial sheaths, the dome should be inflated to 60–80 mmHg. The arterial sheath is removed, and the dome is quickly inflated to 20 mmHg above the patient's systolic blood pressure. Observe the dome to assure that initial hemostasis is achieved. If the puncture site is still bleeding, slowly inflate the dome further until the bleeding ceases. After 3–5 minutes, the dome pressure should be slowly decreased until a palpable distal pulse is present. For diagnostic catheterizations without anticoagulation, the manometer pressure should be maintained at this pressure for the next 10–15 minutes; after that, the pressure may be decreased by 20 mmHg every 2 minutes until the manometer pressure has been completely released.[8] Some facilities will keep the manometer at 30 mmHg until bed rest is complete and the patient is ready to ambulate.

If at any time oozing or active bleeding appears beneath the dome, reinflate the manometer enough to regain hemostasis. Gradually decreasing the pressure is also important; a sudden return to full arterial flow at the puncture site can be enough to "pop the cork," and full manometer pressure may need to be reapplied. Depending on the size of the arterial sheath and the use of anticoagulants, thrombolytics, or IIb/IIIa agents, the amount of total compression time will vary.

The FemoStop permits hand-free operation and compression, less patient discomfort than manual or C-clamp compression, and increased freedom of movement for the patient. The manometer accurately controls pressure, allowing sustained blood flow to the lower extremity while maintaining hemostasis. Direct contact with blood is less than other compression methods for hemostasis. The soft, latex-free pneumatic dome is generally more comfortable for the patient than manual or C-clamp compression. Additionally, the FemoStop is indicated for nonsurgical, compression repair of pseudoaneurysms.[9]

The FemoStop HD addresses both deep and topical hemostasis simultaneously. The new sterile, occlusive dressing facilitates hemostasis at the skin incision site. The dressing is impregnated with a hemostatic agent to accelerate clotting time at the skin surface. When the m-doc particles are in contact with blood, the substance stimulates the initiation of the intrinsic pathway of the coagulation cascade.

Modified Pressure Dressings

Wedge Pressure Dressing

The Wedge pressure dressing (from Steri-Systems Corporation of Auburn, Georgia) is comprised of sterile, absorbent gauze surrounding a firm, high-density foam core (see Figure 26-7). The wedge is positioned on the femoral puncture site, and elastic tape is applied in a criss-cross fashion to provide firm pressure. The Wedge pressure dress-

Figure 26-7. The Wedge pressure dressing.
Source: Courtesy of Steri-Systems Corporation.

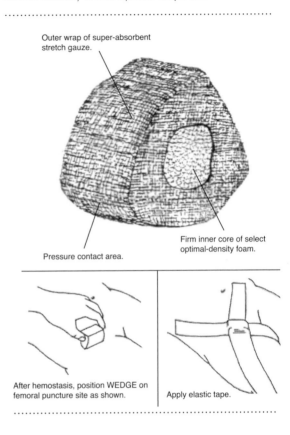

Outer wrap of super-absorbent stretch gauze.

Firm inner core of select optimal-density foam.

Pressure contact area.

After hemostasis, position WEDGE on femoral puncture site as shown.

Apply elastic tape.

ing should stay in place while the patient is on bed rest and may be left on overnight.

Minimal tape should be applied to the patient when utilizing pressure dressings. Too much tape or too bulky of a dressing may obscure site complications such as bleeding or growing hematomas.

Safeguard Pressure-Assisted Dressing

The Safeguard pressure-assisted dressing (from Datascope Maquet of Mahwah, New Jersey) may be used to assist manual hemostasis by reducing active compression time or as a posthemostasis site dressing. The Safeguard combines a latex-free sterile dressing, a transparent window, and a built-in inflatable pressure bulb to provide consistent pressure to the puncture site (see Figure 26-8). The window allows the invasive cardiovascular professional to directly visualize the access site without removing the dressing. The Safeguard should be applied with the access site visible in the dressing window. A luer-lock syringe is attached to the valve that controls the bulb inflation. The pressure bulb may be inflated to achieve a constant pressure, the sidearm of the sheath is aspirated to remove any residual clots, and the sheath is withdrawn.

Once hemostasis has been achieved, the Safeguard may be left in place or applied as a posthemostasis pressure dressing. If hemostasis is compromised, the pressure bulb may be reinflated or inflated higher, with a maximum of 50 ml of air.[13] The puncture site and distal pulses should be periodically assessed per hospital protocol.

Vascular Plugs and Sealers

Protein collagen is a major component of skin, bone, and vasculature. As described in the earlier portion of this chapter, collagen is considered to be the most thrombogenic component of vascular

walls, attracting and binding platelets. Collagen also plays an important role in healing wounds through carrying of growth factors and providing a matrix for cellular proliferation. For this reason and because it is highly biocompatible and easily manufactured in a number of different forms, collagen is an ideal component for hemostasis products. Some products use collagen alone to plug the vessel or tissue tract; some use collagen and thrombin combined. Thrombin converts fibrinogen to fibrin, accelerating and strengthening clot formation.

Prior to device deployment, it is good practice to assess the access site by injecting contrast through the sidearm of the existing sheath under fluoroscopy. If the sheath enters the vessel near or at a branch point, the side of the vessel, or is in a branch vessel, there is an increased risk (with certain products) of device failure or embolization, and an alternative method of hemostasis should be utilized. With any closure device, proper technique must be followed. Failure to follow any of the steps properly could result in bleeding complications, embolization, thrombosis or infection.

Vascular plugs and sealers may either be completely extravascular or have some absorbable intravascular component.

Figure 26-8. The Safeguard pressure-assisted dressing. *Source:* Courtesy of Datascope.

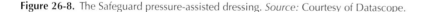
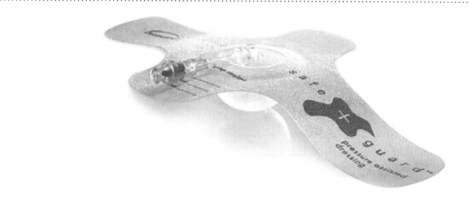

Earlier extravascular plugs and sealants had several drawbacks affecting success rates. VasoSeal and SubQ had high failure rates in fully anticoagulated patients; Duett's liquid thrombin had the potential to seep into the vessel, causing a thrombotic event within the associated limb. However, a successful extravascular passive closure device expands the ability to treat patients in several important ways. The sealant/plug is delivered to the surface of the artery, eliminating intraluminal and artery wall manipulation that may cause discomfort or pain. Additionally, patients with peripheral vascular disease or with arterial punctures at the bifurcation of the common femoral artery usually receive manual or mechanical compression techniques to achieve hemostasis of the access site. This is due to the concern that devices with intravascular components may compromise the lumen and blood flow in these patients.

Gel-foam is a passive, extravascular plug made from purified gelatin. It absorbs blood, and provides an area for expedited clot formation. There are also several other products that use a medical polyethylene glycol (PEG) or similar, which swell within the tissue tract and absorb blood within its matrix to rapidly produce hemostasis.

Angio-Seal

The Angio-Seal from St. Jude Medical (of Minnetonka, Minnesota), was approved by the FDA in 1996. The Angio-Seal mechanically closes the site by sandwiching the arteriotomy site between an intravascular bioabsorbable polymer anchor and an extravascular collagen sponge covering the arterial surface within the skin tract.

The Angio-Seal has gone through a number of modifications since its introduction and is available in 6F and 8F. Inserting the Angio-Seal consists of three steps: locating the artery, deploying and setting the polymer anchor, and deploying the collagen sponge.

The current Angio-Seal does not deploy through the existing sheath. The Angio-Seal components include an insertion sheath, an arteriotomy locator, a 0.032-inch (6F) or 0.038-inch (8F) × 70 cm J-tipped guide wire with wire straightener and the Angio-Seal device. Earlier versions of the device included a postplacement tension spring that would remain in place for a period of time postdeployment to secure the collagen.

Angio-Seal components are reabsorbed by the body in approximately 90 days. The FDA has approved the Angio-Seal for immediate repuncture of the same vessel, although many physicians still prefer to access the opposite groin if a procedure is necessary within 90 days.

Mynx

The Mynx, from Access Closure (of Mountain View, California), is an extravascular plug that can be delivered through the existing 6F or 7F arterial sheath. The plug is composed of 95% water and 5% PEG, which is freeze dried and integrated into the delivery catheter. The sealant is a hydrophilic, bioinert polymer with a well-established safety profile. It fully dissipates from the closure site within 30 days, leaving nothing behind in the artery.

The Mynx works by temporarily placing a small, semicompliant balloon within the artery to create temporary hemostasis. The dry PEG sealant is delivered above the arteriotomy, and the balloon is deflated and withdrawn. The PEG rapidly expands within the tissue tract by absorbing blood and subcutaneous fluids. As the sealant's porous structure fills with blood, it provides a platform for clot formation that facilitates natural hemostasis and subsequent healing of the tissue track. Both the arterial puncture and the tissue tract are sealed, minimizing oozing.

Percutaneous Vascular Sutures and Staples

Perclose

The Perclose product line from Abbott Vascular (of Redwood City, California) received initial

FDA approval in 1997. The Perclose products contain no collagen or thrombin and are based solely on nonabsorbable surgical sutures.

The early product line was originally launched with 9F and 11F devices with four needles and two suture lines. A major drawback to these early products was that to deploy the needles and sutures, the skin insertion site needed to be widened and the tissue tract dilated to 21F. This resulted in skin tract oozing, which could be decreased by using 2% xylocaine with epinephrine, and securing the tract incision with Steri-Strips or a stitch of absorbable suture. This also caused a greater amount of patient discomfort as the site healed and a potentially higher risk of infection due to the larger incision. The 9F and 11F products have since been discontinued, but 8F and 10F Perclose products are still available, most often used for cases requiring large sheath access, such as atrial or ventricular septal defect, patent foramen ovale closures, and aortic stent graft deployments. With the development of catheter-based structural heart procedures (such as percutaneous aortic valve replacement and mitral valve repair), sheaths of 18F and greater are being used. These puncture sites generally require surgical closure, but the "pre-close" technique is being utilized at some institutions.[10]

The latest generation products are lower profile 6F devices. They simplify the suture knot tying, and they do not require the skin tract to be further dilated for deployment. They are designed for 5–6F access sites. An off-label, modified "pre-close" technique, where the Perclose system is deployed at the beginning of the case without tying the knot followed by insertion of > 6F sheaths has been used successfully by many operators. The kits are composed of a specialized sheath and guide that houses the needles and the foot system that guides the needle placement around the puncture site. A marker lumen contained in the guide precisely locates the vessel lumen. A Knot-Pusher is included to assist in positioning the suture knot in the tissue tract to the arteriotomy (see Figure 26-9).

Suture is the gold standard for closure of open arteriotomies. The Perclose products offer an alternative to other percutaneous plugs and seals. Although absorbable suture would be preferred, the Perclose stitch quickly becomes covered with neointimal tissue. The site can be immediately repunctured, should the need arise.

StarClose

StarClose (from Abbott Vascular of Santa Clara, California) is an extravascular clip that mechanically closes the arteriotomy to ensure rapid hemostasis. StarClose is designed not to leave behind any intraluminal foreign body.

The StarClose is the clip applier and a 6F exchange system (which includes an exchange sheath, dilator, and J-tip guide wire). The clip itself is 4 mm in diameter, star shaped, and comprised of nitinol, which is mounted on the clip applier. The clip applier is attached to the introducer sheath hub and advanced. Vessel locator wings are positioned against the arteriotomy. The shaft of the sheath is split as the StarClose clip is advanced. The StarClose is deployed with a trigger mechanism onto the anterior surface of the femoral artery. The StarClose clip has inward facing tines designed to grasp the vascular tissue in a purse string fashion, cinching it against the outer ring cuff of the clip.

Skin tract oozing is not too uncommon with the StarClose device, especially with patients who have received anticoagulation. Like older generation Perclose products, the mechanism by which the clip is deployed dilates the skin tract to a larger degree than the original sheath. Skin tract dilation occurs when the clip applier splits the introducer sheath. While annoying, this oozing is rarely problematic and can generally be controlled by subcutaneous injection of lidocaine with epinephrine. Alternately, a topical hemostasis accelerator or Safeguard pressure-assisted

Figure 26-9. Perclose® ProGlide™. *Source:* Courtesy of Abbott Vascular.

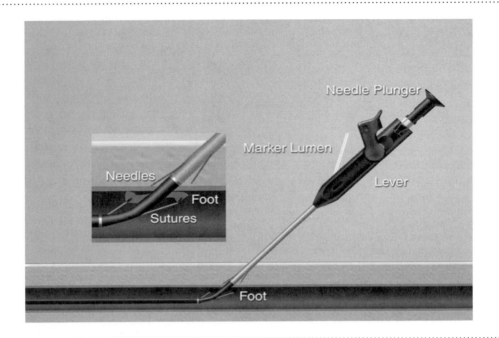

dressing (discussed elsewhere in this chapter) may also manage oozing.

It is important that the nurse or technician caring for a patient post procedure who has had any mechanical closure device be able to access the puncture site and distinguish between skin tract oozing and an active arterial bleed.

Topical Hemostasis Accelerators

A new approach to obtaining hemostasis combines the time-proven method of manual compression with topical agents that hasten localized clotting of the puncture site. Completely external, the tissue tract is sealed without an arteriotomy and leaves no subcutaneous foreign material behind.

Application of these topical products is relatively simple. Each of the patch products are packaged individually in a sterile pouch. The groin site is cleaned prior to sheath removal with sterile, nonheparinized saline, betadine, or both. The patch is opened into the sterile field and placed on a folded, dry sterile gauze. Palpate the artery—about 2 cm proximal and slightly medial to the skin incision—and apply firm occlusive pressure while placing the hemostasis patch over the puncture site. Instruct the patient to take a deep breath in, then slowly exhale. As the patient exhales, gently remove the sheath. A small spurt of blood is normal and may help to activate the hemostatic agent on the patch. After 3 minutes of occlusive proximal pressure, slowly release, maintaining firm pressure directly over the puncture site and the hemostasis pad.

After hemostasis has been achieved, these topical patches should be covered with a dry, sterile gauze and a transparent dressing, which remain in place for 24 hours. The patient may remove the dressing the next day, soak the patch with warm, soapy water, and gently peel it off. Disadvantages or problems associated with the use of these products are identical to manual pressure, as previously described. The following are descriptions of the topical hemostasis products commercially available in the United States.

Syvek Patch and Syvek NT

The Syvek Patch from Marine Polymer Technologies (of Danvers, Massachusetts) was introduced in the United States in 1998. The Syvek Patch is a 3 cm $\times$ 3 cm woven patch composed of a biopolymer, poly-N-acetyl-glucosamine, originally isolated from marine algae. A laboratory study has shown that poly-N-acetyl-glucosamine not only accelerates clot formation through red blood cell and platelet aggregates in contact with the patch, but it may also have a localized vasoconstrictive effect as well.[11]

The Syvek NT is a newer variation of the Syvek Patch. This version increases the amount of active poly-N-acetyl-glucosamine and gives the patch a foam backing. The increased active material decreases the time to hemostasis, while the foam backing gives the user greater tactile sensation of the product.

Clo-Sur P.A.D.

The Clo-Sur P.A.D. (pressure-applied dressing) developed by Scion Cardio-Vascular, Inc. (of Miami, Florida) has been available in the United States since 2001. It is a nonwoven, porous pad classified as a hydrophilic wound dressing. The active ingredient in the Clo-Sur P.A.D. is a naturally occurring biopolymer, polyprolate acetate, which is a proprietary form of chitosan.[11] Chitosan is derived from chitin, a natural hemostatic agent commercially extracted from crustacean shells. The polyprolate is cationically charged. This positive ionic charge, coupled with the porous pad, helps to attract and bind red blood cells, promoting hemostasis.

Chito-Seal

Chito-Seal from Abbott Vascular Devices (of Redwood City, California), is a sterile, nonwoven 4 cm $\times$ 4 cm wound dressing coated with chitosan. This chitosan is made by removing acetyl groups (deacetylation) from chitin molecules, forming a strong positive ionic charge. Similar to the Clo-Sur P.A.D., the Chito-Seal's strong positive ionic charge helps to attract and bind red blood cells. Theoretically, the higher the degree of deacetylation, the greater the number of positive receptors available to act on the negatively charged red blood cells, increasing the hemostatic properties.

One concern with chitin and chitosan-based products is a potential allergic reaction for patients with shellfish allergies. Chito-Seal chitosan is derived from shrimp and crab shells; the major allergen identified in shrimp and crab is a structural protein, tropomysin, found within their muscle tissue. The chitosan utilized in the Chito-Seal is deproteinated and denatured, making allergic reactions very unlikely, and no allergic reactions have been reported to date.

D-Stat/D-Stat Dry

D-Stat Dry (from Vascular Solutions of Minneapolis, Minnesota) are nonwoven gauze sponges impregnated with bovine thrombin, carboxylmethylcellulose (cellulose gum), and calcium chloride packaged sterilely in a foil pouch. The cellulose gum serves as the matrix for the sponge and provides a suspension media for the thrombin. Hemostasis is achieved through the combination of manual compression and the coagulation properties of the thrombin.[12] D-Stat Radial is a compression band with a D-Stat pad to control bleeding from radial artery puncture sites.

Unlike the other topical products, D-Stat Flowable uses procoagulant components, thrombin, and collagen mixed with a diluent to form a "flowable hemostat." Vascular Solutions states that this D-Stat product is not intended for primary hemostasis, but to control oozing after various procedures, such as after peripherally inserted central catheter line removal, atrioventricular fistula post dialysis, or postfemoral closure device (i.e., AngioSeal, Perclose).

The diluent is drawn into a syringe and is used to reconstitute 5000 units of thrombin. The syringe with the reconstituted thrombin is attached to another syringe that contains 200 mg of bovine-derived collagen, and the contents are mixed between the two syringes 10–20 times to achieve the desired consistency. Mixing increases the viscosity of the product. The D-Stat kit includes three different applicators to use in a variety of situations. The small-bore catheter is intended for application to large tissue areas. A 20-g, 3-inch echogenic right-angle needle is included for localized delivery, and a 20-g, 2.75-inch needle is provided for delivery directly into the skin tract if desired.

HemCon

The HemCon bandage was developed out of a partnership with the U.S. Army to save lives of the soldiers suffering from hemorrhage on the battlefield. The soldiers required a quick and easy-to-use solution to stop bleeding and allow for the time needed to transport to critical care units. HemCon products are fabricated from chitosan, a naturally occurring biocompatible polysaccharide derived from shrimp shells. HemCon's manufacturing process creates chitosan bandages which have a positive charge and attract red blood cells and platelets, which have a negative charge. This ionic interaction creates a strong seal at the wound site. This supportive, primary seal allows the body to effectively activate its coagulation pathway. The platelets and red blood cells continue to be drawn into the bandage and travel up the access tract to strengthen the initial seal.

In addition to its hemostasis properties, HemCon dressings also offer an antibacterial barrier by interacting with the bacteria's outer phospholipid membrane, causing the cell to rupture, collapse, and die.

Neptune Pad /Neptune Disc

The Neptune Pad (from TZ Medical of Portland, Oregon) is a topical dressing made from calcium alginate derived from seaweed. Calcium alginate has high absorptive properties and has been used in various surgical wound dressings. This property may decrease the time required to achieve manual hemostasis. The Neptune Disc applies the calcium alginate to the undersurface of a compression disc. The Neptune Disc is compatible with various mechanical C-clamps and the EZ-Hold manual compression device.

SafeSeal

The SafeSeal patch (Possis Medical) utilizes MPH (microporous polysaccharide hemospheres) to rapidly dehydrate blood cells, concentrating platelets and fibrin at the access site. MPH is nontoxic and completely bioabsorbable. The SafeSeal patch is placed over the access site upon removal of the sheath. The product is an adhesive bandage with a clear center window and a pull tab. While controlling the site with one hand, the nurse or tech pulls the tab, which releases the MPH over the puncture site and removes excess blood. The clear center window allows the nurse or tech to view the site and verify hemostasis. Its mechanism of action rapidly gelatinizes blood at the puncture site.

Boomerang

The Boomerang Wire (from Cardiva Medical of Mountain View, California) is a guide wire with a deployable low-profile nitinol disc that works through an existing 5–7F sheath. Once inserted through the sheath, the disc is opened, the sheath withdrawn, and the wire pulled back to the arteriotomy site within the vessel. A clip is placed on the wire at the skin to apply site-specific compression and provides temporary hemostasis. The smooth muscle of the artery relaxes naturally around the wire, recoiling back to its predilated, 18-gauge needle puncture state.

The newest generation Boomerang products are enhanced with a hemostatic coating on the wire to accelerate the coagulation within the skin tract. The Boomerang products are designed to retain the inherent benefits of manual compression and leave no foreign materials within the body.

FEMORAL SITE CARE AFTER HEMOSTASIS

After femoral artery sheath removal, the puncture site needs to be dressed appropriately. Infection can be a major concern with closure devices, particularly with obese, diabetic, and elderly patients. Collagen-based products, or products that increase the size of the skin tract incision, offer an open door for microorganisms to invade the body.

The femoral access site should be cleaned of any remaining blood, and the skin immediately around the skin tract should be cleaned with chlorhexadine (betadine or another topical antimicrobial solution of choice may also be used). Allow the solution to dry, swab the immediate area with a benzoin applicator, and allow it to dry. Betadine gel, bacitracin zinc, or some other antibiotic ointment is applied to the puncture, and a sterile 2-inch × 2-inch gauze pad is placed over the site and covered with a transparent dressing. In the case of the topical hemostasis products, clean the surrounding skin of any blood, and cover the hemostasis pad with a transparent dressing; no ointment should be applied.

Traditionally, patients were kept supine with a 2.5–10 lb sandbag over the groin. However, use of a sandbag only increases patient discomfort postprocedure without any documented clinical benefit. A large, occlusive dressing may mask bleeding and delay discovery of a hematoma. If the patient received an intervention, anticoagulation, or antiplatelet therapy or had a hematoma that was successfully controlled, a modified pressure dressing should be applied to the site.

Patient Recovery Postsheath Removal

Patient recovery is variable, depending on the access site, sheath size, anticoagulation use, and procedure performed. Recovery times, when mechanical hemostasis devices are used, are generally 30–120 minutes. Some facilities may practice immediate ambulation with some devices, if no sedation or anticoagulants are administered, and the patient has normal arteries (see Table 26-1).

When manual hemostasis techniques are used for removal of femoral artery sheaths, the patient should be kept supine post hemostasis. Some facilities may use the rule of 1 hour per sheath French size (i.e., 6 hours for 6F sheath). Other facilities may recover their patients for 2–4 hours with sheaths of 6F or smaller.

The patients must be instructed to:

- Keep their head down to avoid placing additional pressure on the site.
- Hold the groin site if they cough, sneeze, or laugh.
- Keep the leg used for the procedure straight and flat.
- Call for assistance, if they feel anything warm or wet near the groin site, and immediately press on the site.
- Stay in bed until ambulated with assistance/direct observation by the recovery nurse.

Some facilities will allow patients to have their head elevated 30°–45° after sheath removal if there are no signs of bleeding or a

Table 26-1. Factors Predisposing to Vascular Access Site Bleeding

Anatomic Factors
Calcified (inelastic) vessels
Elderly patient
Obese patient
Female patient
Patient movement

Procedural Factors
"Through-and-through" backwall puncture
High puncture (above inguinal ligament)
Low puncture (profunda or superficial femoral artery)
Multiple punctures
Large sheath size
Kinking of sheath due to acute angulation
Prolonged procedure time (higher heparin doses)
Prolonged indwelling sheath time (higher ACT levels)

Hemodynamic Factors
Increased pulse pressure (aortic insufficiency or
    non-compliant vessels)
Severe hypertension

Hematologic Factors
Multiple platelet antagonists (aspirin, clopidogrel, IIb/
    IIIa receptor antagonists)
Antithrombotic agents (heparinoids, warfarin)
Thrombolytic agents (tPA, SK)
Underlying coagulopathy or thrombocytopenia

Human Factors
Inexperience
Inability to gain "control" of site upon sheath removal
Short duration of pressure applied to obtain hemostasis

hematoma. If an intervention was performed, many facilities may have the patient on bed rest overnight.

On discharge, patients should be instructed to watch the access site for the following:

- Signs of infection
- Increasing swelling
- Increasing redness/warmth
- Pain
- Discharge
- Signs of vascular occlusion
- Numbness, tingling, dull aching
- Limb that is cool to touch
- Mottling or discoloration

If any of these should occur, the patient should seek immediate medical attention.

All patients should be instructed to avoid lifting more than 10 lbs for the next 3–5 days. In addition, patients who received a mechanical closure device should be instructed to avoid soaking in water (baths, hot tubs) for 1 week.

COMPLICATIONS RELATED TO SHEATH REMOVAL AND CLOSURE DEVICES

A number of complications are associated with the insertion and removal of vascular sheaths and closure devices. The two most commonly encountered are vasovagal reactions and hematoma formation; other complications include late bleeding, pseudoaneurysm, retroperitoneal bleeding, infection, vessel thrombosis, and death.

Vasovagal Reactions

Vasovagal reactions are not uncommon with sheath removal. Vasovagal reactions occur when the vagus nerve is stimulated, resulting in hypotension, bradycardia, nausea, and diaphoresis. Patients should be on an ECG and a noninvasive blood pressure monitor and have IV access with fluids running during sheath insertion and removal. Signs of a vasovagal reaction include a 15–20 mmHg drop in systolic blood pressure, a 20–30 beat per minute drop in heart rate, diaphoresis, and nausea or vomiting. Should a vasovagal reaction occur, the patient can be placed in Trendelenburg position, fluids opened, and atropine and an antiemetic agent given (if needed). If these measures do not resolve the problem, advanced cardiac life support protocols will need to be initiated, and the patient should be admitted to a step-down or intensive care bed for observation or further treatment once stabilized.

Hematomas

Hematomas occur when blood collects beneath the skin around the arteriotomy. They are most common when using larger sheaths (i.e., > 6F), anticoagulation, or in cases of preexisting vascular disease. The hematoma may form from the sheath insertion, poor manual compression sheath removal technique, incomplete or failed closure device deployment, or patient restlessness pre- or postsheath removal. Initially, the immediate area has a soft, spongy feeling. As more blood collects within the tissue, it becomes hard and painful for the patient. As the hematoma progresses, the thigh increases in firmness, and may continue to the knee or lower, and the peritoneal area. The patient may begin to complain of groin, leg, flank, or lower back pain. Distal pulses may become decreased, and the patient may become tachycardic. If the hematoma is caught early, additional manual compression may resolve the problem. The FemoStop is also an alternative. If the hematoma cannot be resolved by external compression techniques, distal pulses may be obliterated, and surgical intervention will be necessary.

Pseudoaneurysms

Pseudoaneurysms are another form of hematoma. A pseudoaneurysm is a communication between the arterial lumen and an area of separation within the arterial layers. Pseudoaneurysms associated with vascular sheaths are the result of inadequate compression after sheath removal or initial low sheath access (i.e., superficial femoral or profunda artery). The classic diagnosis of a pseudoaneurysm includes a pulsatile mass with a systolic bruit. Pseudoaneurysms may be avoided by careful, fluroscopic landmark-guided sheath

insertion and proper compression technique to achieve postsheath hemostasis. Pseudoaneurysms can be effectively treated by ultrasound-guided FemoStop compression.

Retroperitoneal Bleeds

Retroperitoneal bleeds are a potentially fatal complication and may occur if the femoral artery puncture is proximal to the inguinal crease, making effective compression very difficult. Retroperitoneal bleeds may also occur due to guide wire perforation or sheath dissection. They may also be spontaneous, related to anticoagulation or IIb/IIIa inhibitors. Bleeding above the inguinal ligament moves posteriorly into the retroperitoneum and is extremely difficult to detect until a problem occurs. The patient may begin to complain of acute abdominal or back pain and may have hypotension, tachycardia, and abdominal distention. Often, bleeds are first suspected with a drop in hemoglobin. CT scans offer the most reliable method of diagnosis. Retroperitoneal bleeds can be treated by discontinuing any anticoagulation or antiplatelet therapy, prolonged FemoStop compression, fluid replacement, and blood transfusion and pressure support agents. Surgical exploration and correction may be necessary.

Vessel Thrombosis

Vessel thrombosis may also occur. The vascular sheath should be removed carefully, without compressing the shaft and stripping clots that may have formed within. Aspirating the sheath sidearm immediately prior to removal may reduce this potential risk. If the patient has vascular disease, compression methods of hemostasis can restrict distal blood flow, resulting in thrombus formation. Prolonged occlusive pressure on the site should not be applied for more than 5 minutes to control initial bleeding; then use only enough manual or mechanical pressure for hemostasis while maintaining distal pulses. Vascular dissection related to the sheath insertion may also cause thrombus formation after the sheath is removed.

Groin Infection

Groin infection is also a potential complication, particularly with mechanical plug hemostasis devices. The material in the plug can theoretically act as a "wick," drawing external microorganisms down into the skin tract. Infections may also occur with manual techniques as well. It is important that the patient understand that the site dressing should be removed the following day. The site may be washed with soap and water, dried, and covered with a clean bandage. The patient should be instructed not soak in a tub, whirlpool, or swimming pool for the next 7–10 days.

If infection does occur, the patient may experience redness and warmth, swelling, pain, and discharge. Under most circumstances, the treatment will consist of oral antibiotics. In severe cases, the patient may need to be hospitalized for IV antibiotic treatment, surgical intervention, or both. As with most infections, those at highest risk include the elderly, diabetics, patients with poor hygiene, and immunosuppressed patients.

SUMMARY

As more and more endovascular therapies are developed and refined, procedural volume in catheterization laboratories will continue to grow. With the increased volume comes the additional problem of safely increasing patient throughput by decreasing postprocedure recovery time. A variety of compression devices, vascular plugs, sutures, staples, and topical hemostasis accelerators are becoming more popular because they allow quicker patient turnover.

Ultimately, patient recovery postcatheterization is dependent upon the assessment skills and knowledge of proper hemostasis techniques of the cardiovascular invasive specialist. Proper technique is essential to stop access site bleeding and minimize potential complications.

REFERENCES

1. Cohen RA, Shepherd JT, Vanhoutte PM. Inhibitory role of endothelium in the response of isolated coronary arteries to platelets. *Science* 1983;221:273–274.
2. Hole JW. *Human Anatomy & Physiology*, 6th ed. Dubuque, IA: William C. Brown Publishers; 1993.
3. Stein B, Fuster V. Antithrombotic therapy in acute myocardial infarction: prevention of venous, left ventricular and coronary artery thromboembolism. *Am J Cardiol* 1989;64:33B–40.
4. Fischbach DP, Fogdall RP. *Coagulation: The Essentials*. Baltimore, MD: Williams & Wilkins; 1981.
5. Phillips DR, Charo IF, Parise LV, Fitzgerald LA. The platelet membrane glycoprotein IIb-IIIa complex. *Blood* 1988;71(4):831–843.
6. Juran NB, Rouse CL, Smith DD, et al. Nursing interventions to decrease bleeding at the femoral access site after percuatneous coronary intervention. *Am J Crit Care* 1999;8(5):303–313.
7. Semler HJ. Transfemoral catheterization: mechanical versus manual control of bleeding. *Radiology* 1985;154(1);234–235.
8. Beaver K. Femoral artery hemostasis with the femostop compression system: the importance of proper dome placement. *Cath Lab Digest* 2002:10(9).
9. Chatterjee T, Do DD, Mahler F, Meier B. A prospective, randomized evaluation of nonsurgical closure of femoral pseudoaneurysm by compression device with or without ultrasound guidance. *Cathet Cardiovasc Interv* 1999;47:304–309.
10. Kahlert P, Eggebrech H, Erbel R, Sack S. A modified "Preclosure" technique after percutaneous aortic valve replacement. *Catheter Cardiovasc Interv* 2008;73(6):877–884.

11. Scion Cardio-Vascular website. Available at: http://www.scioncv.com. Accessed December 27, 2004.

12. Vascular Solutions, Inc. D-*Stat Dry hemostatic bandage: instructions for use*. Minneapolis, MN: Vascular Solutions, Inc.; 2003.

13. Datascope Corp. *Safeguard pressure assisted dressing; instructions for use*. Mahwah, NJ: Datascope Corp.; 2003.

SUGGESTED READING

Coleman RW, Hirsh J, Marder VJ, Salzman EW, eds. *Hemostasis and Thrombosis: Basic Principles and Clinical Practice*, 4th ed. Philadelphia: Lippincott; 2001.

Fischbach DP, Fogdall RP. *Coagulation: The Essentials*. Baltimore, MD: Williams & Wilkins; 1981.

Hole JW. *Human Anatomy & Physiology*, 6th ed. Dubuque, IA: William C. Brown Publishers; 1993.

Verstraete M, Fuster V, Topol EJ, eds. *Cardiovascular Thrombosis: Thrombocardiology and Thromboneurology*, 2nd ed. Philadelphia: Lippincott; 1998.

Chapter 27

PEDIATRIC INTERVENTIONAL CARDIOLOGY

Monica Arpagaus-Lee, RN, MN, MHA
Loren D. Brown RN, BSN, CCRN

INTRODUCTION

The safety, comfort, and well-being of the child are the primary responsibilities of the nurse during pediatric heart catheterization. Being able to assess the needs of the sedated child and provide a calm, quiet environment for him or her is essential. An understanding of congenital heart defects and the resultant changes in the anatomy and physiology of the heart is needed in order to anticipate which catheters will be used, where they will be placed, and what pressures and blood samples must be obtained and their expected values.

Since the 1960s, when the first angioplasty and balloon atrioseptostomy were performed, pediatric cardiology has seen enormous growth and development. Radiofrequency catheter ablation (RFCA), dilatations of vessels and valves, closures of patent ductus arteriosus (PDA) and atrial septal defects (ASD), embolizations, and stent implantations are techniques that are com-

monly seen today in most pediatric CCLs. With the change from diagnostic to interventional procedures, a broader knowledge base and a more flexible role for the nursing staff are required.

PATIENT PREPARATION

Ideally, children who are scheduled for a heart cath are seen shortly prior to their catheter procedure for their preprocedure history, physical assessment, and, if necessary, anesthetic consultation. Any other examinations, such as chest radiographs, lab work, 12-lead ECG, and echocardiography may also be done at this time. The lab work includes a complete blood count, pregnancy test for female patients 12 years or older, electrolytes, clotting times, and a type-and-cross match. Blood type and cross match are necessary in most interventional procedures and for infants under 5 kg. In most interventional labs, a unit of packed red blood cells is in the lab for the procedure.

In many cases, this precatheterization visit precludes the need for the traditional "evening before" admission and allows the child to spend what can be an anxious night at home in a familiar environment. This method necessitates a patient teaching program, with the goal of optimally preparing families, both psychologically and physically, for the pending procedure.

Teaching

Preprocedural preparation of both parents and child greatly reduces their anxiety. Practical information covering the catheterization procedure, its length, and what the child will experience should be discussed openly.

A visit to the nursing unit and the CCL will introduce the family to the surroundings in a calm and nonthreatening way. A videotape or age-appropriate book showing a child undergoing a heart cath is another tool being used in many institutions.

Nursing assessment of the developmental age of the child, followed by selection of age-appropriate precatheterization teaching tools can greatly aid the success of a teaching program. Adolescents are a good example of patients with special needs that must be met. Fear of disfigurement and disability and the potential loss of privacy and freedom are issues of particular concern to adolescents. A nurse's sensitivity to these issues and individualized nursing care can greatly ease the anxiety of an adolescent undergoing a cardiac catheterization procedure.

Written information reiterating what was discussed during the precatheterization teaching should be available for the family to reinforce what is discussed. A list of who and where to call if questions arise, with telephone numbers should be part of the information that the family takes with them.

GENERAL ANESTHESIA VERSUS SEDATION AND ANALGESIA

The selection of either general anesthesia or sedation and analgesia via intramuscular or IV routes differs between institutions. The goal of sedation is to provide some degree of analgesia and amnesia for the procedure.[1] Controlling pain and anxiety is important. These factors may change important clinical data such as blood pressure and heart rate.[2] In addition, the success and timely completion of the procedure depends on the cooperation of the child. Some institutions have an anesthesiologist who is assigned to the catheterization laboratory at all times and who accompanies every child. Others utilize procedural sedation, administer by trained nursing staff, with anesthesia available for failed sedation.

In making the decision about which method of sedation and analgesia to use, these factors should be considered:

- The safety and comfort of the child (this factor is of utmost importance)
- Nature of the procedure (because the cooperation of the child must be ensured during certain periods of the interventional procedure; some interventional procedures require an anesthesiologist to be present who can ensure the cooperation of the child at a given moment)
- Age or developmental level of the child
- Length of the procedure
- Ability of the child to cooperate (developmentally delayed children or those with special language needs can provide communication challenges, thus making cooperation difficult)
- Presence of cyanosis or proclivity to blue spells
- Elevated right ventricular or pulmonary artery pressures
- Prior experience with anesthesia or sedation including any adverse reactions

DIAGNOSTIC PROCEDURES

With the advent of more sophisticated echocardiographic equipment, better visualization of heart structures is possible, thus eliminating the need for invasive diagnostic heart catheterization in most cases. Currently, cardiac catheterization is indicated[3] when:

- Precise physiological measurements are needed.
- Anatomic features are poorly visualized by echocardiography.
- Electrophysiology studies are indicated.
- Interventional procedures are planned.

Safety

Patient safety in the catheterization laboratory depends on the proper monitoring of the patient's vital signs as soon as the patient enters the laboratory. This safety process also includes the ability of the catheterization staff to interpret and respond to the information derived from the various monitoring devices.

Indispensable patient monitoring devices in the pediatric catheterization laboratory are varied and include the following.

Transcutaneous Oxygen Saturation Monitor

Knowledge of the patient's baseline transcutaneous oxygen saturation and the monitoring of any changes during the procedure can alert the laboratory staff of the changing status of the child.

Blood Pressure Monitor

The noninvasive recycling blood pressure monitor is a direct reflection of cardiac output status. Cardiac output can change during the catheterization procedure due to factors such as changes in the fluid balance of the child, occlusion of vessels due to catheter placement, pain and anxiety that the child may be experiencing, or as a result of sedation.

ECG

Continuous auditory and visual monitoring of the child's ECG is imperative from the time the child enters the laboratory until he or she leaves. Knowl-

edge of the child's baseline ECG will ensure that the nurse quickly recognizes any ECG changes. Catheter-induced dysrhythmias (such as premature atrial or ventricular contractions) are not an uncommon occurrence in the catheterization laboratory, and quick recognition and early identification can help prevent a potential emergency situation. The nurse's ability to interpret the data from these monitors, and to react accordingly, is imperative. The cardiologist's main focus is on the catheterization procedure; the priority of the nursing staff is the safety, comfort, and well-being of the child.

Defibrillator

A synchronized cardioverter/defibrillator is standard emergency equipment in any CCL. It must be in correct working order, and within easy access to the patient at all times. The defibrillator remains ready for use and set to the appropriate level (2 J/kg) as long as the child is in the room. The correct paddle size must be chosen, attached, and ready to use. In procedures where the possibility of ventricular tachycardia is high (e.g., dilatation of a valvular aortic stenosis with left ventricular hypertrophy), multifunction defibrillator pads may be used. These are defibrillator/pacing patches that are attached to the patient before the procedure begins. The patches are transparent on X-ray, thus not disturbing the procedure, but are already in place in the event that cardiac defibrillation becomes necessary. A pacemaker mode is also available should immediate pacing be required.

Resuscitation Equipment

A well-stocked emergency cart that includes appropriately sized masks, endotracheal tubes, oral and nasal airways, suction catheters, and laryngoscope blades must be readily accessible.

Emergency Medication

The standard resuscitative medications (i.e., epinephrine, atropine, sodium bicarbonate, calcium) must be on hand as well as antiarrhythmic medications (i.e., lidocaine, adenosine, isoproterenol). Nurses should be familiar with the medications and know the appropriate dosages. In light of the procedures being performed, and the potentially dehydrated state of the child, it is a good idea to have a dopamine drip ready to infuse if necessary.

Catheters

The selection of the appropriate catheter is important for the success of the procedure. With the appropriate catheter, the cardiologist can achieve access to difficult-to-reach areas with minimal trauma to the heart. Angiography can be performed safely, and the quality of the pictures can be ensured.

Catheters differ not only in the size (length and inner diameter) and shape, but also in the different types of material used, which affects their rigidity.

End-hole catheters are used in the wedge position to measure pressures and obtain oxygen saturations, but they cannot be used safely for angiography because of the potential for myocardial injury caused by the concentrated jet of contrast dye from the end hole.

Closed-tip, multiple side-hole catheters are preferred for angiography.

Balloon flow-directed catheters are very useful in reaching difficult areas and in angiography. During angiography, the balloon can be inflated to distally occlude the vessel and give a more contrast-saturated angiogram. The balloon is inflated with carbon dioxide, which is soluble in blood, so that the risk of an air embolus occurring from balloon rupture is minimized.

Pigtail catheters are the catheter of choice for retrograde left ventricular angiography. Due to their special shape, the side holes, and the material used to make them, the cardiologist is able to use high-flow rates safely, with minimal risk of inducing myocardial injury or precipitating ventricular arrhythmias.

Specially shaped coronary catheters provide safe and easy access to the coronary arteries and allow for contrast injections.

The Procedure

The child is usually premedicated prior to entering the catheterization laboratory. The child is moved to the catheterization table, and the monitoring devices are appropriately placed. A warming device should be used to prevent hypothermia. The temperature is monitored either by temporal thermometer strip or, in anesthetized patients, a continuous transesophageal temperature probe during the procedure.

Immobilization of the child is achieved by soft restraints placed on the wrists and ankles, which are then tied to the table. If additional restraint of the lower extremities is necessary, tape or straps can be placed over the mid-thigh and the lower calf. By appropriately padding potential pressure areas, one can ensure the comfort of the child and prevent development of pressure sores. For long procedures or for patients who are at risk for decubitus ulcers, special foam, gel, or eggshell mattresses may be used.

The arms are positioned with elbows flexed at a 90° angle, hands near the ears, and elbows padded and internally rotated toward midline to prevent brachial plexus injury. Restraints should be released immediately at the end of the procedure.

After preparation with an antibacterial cleansing solution, followed by the appropriate sterile draping of the bilateral inguinal area, the procedure begins with percutaneous access via the femoral vessel. The femoral vein or artery is the preferable catheter insertion site because of their relatively large size and the direct access to the heart that they provide. The right femoral vein is preferred, but the left side is used if the right side is unavailable for use (i.e., because of stenosis or vein anomaly). If percutaneous puncture is unsuccessful on either side, a cutdown of the femoral vein may be attempted. When femoral access is not available, the subclavian may be used. In the newborn infant, the umbilical vessels provide easy access to both arterial and venous circulation and often can be used for the complete cardiac catheterization procedure.[1]

When the child is lying sedated, monitored, warmed, and in position, the cardiologist administers a local anesthetic to the catheter insertion site. This is usually lidocaine 1% for infants under 1 year and lidocaine 2% for over 1 year. Sodium bicarbonate with the lidocaine local anesthetic reduces the acidity of the lidocaine, making a painful process a little more comfortable.

A wire is inserted through the lumen of the introducing needle, the needle is removed, and the appropriate-size sheath is placed over the wire. The wire is then removed, and the sheath is ready for catheter insertion.

If an arterial catheter is needed, systemic heparinization of the child is performed to prevent thrombosis of the artery. Heparinization is achieved through a bolus of 100 IU/kg heparin IV. If the arterial catheter remains in place for more than an hour, activated clotting time (ACT) monitoring is recommended, and additional heparin may given unless the ACT is > 200 sec.

Hemodynamic measurements should be performed before angiography, because the contrast medium may alter the patient's immediate hemodynamic situation. Interventions typically follow angiography once precise demarcation of anatomy has been made.

Interventions such as placing a stent, device, or coil necessitate prophylactic antibiotic administration, typically 50 mg/kg (max. 2 grams) intravenous Cefazolin. Subsequent doses of 25 mg/Kg Cefazolin will follow in 8-hour intervals for two additional doses.

Which structures need to be visualized for complete diagnosis or surgical preparation will determine which parts of the anatomy need to be filmed. Careful planning of the structures to be filmed and understanding how best to visualize them is imperative as the cardiologist is limited to 7 ml/kg of contrast medium for the procedure.[1] Biplane equipment will help to reduce the fluoroscopy time and the amount of contrast medium needed.

After the catheter has been removed, the insertion site is manually compressed until hemostasis is achieved. This is usually about 5 minutes for a venous puncture or 10 minutes for arterial puncture. A dry sterile dressing covered with tegaderm is then applied and the patient is transferred to postanesthesia care unit.

Complications

Cardiac catheterization of children involves a very small chance that the patient will experience complications, or even death, on the table. Newborns tend to be at highest risk because of the precarious status of many of the newborns undergoing cardiac catheterization.

Serious complications such as cerebral emboli or perforation of heart structures due to catheter manipulation are rare, but must always be considered when catheterization is being performed. Modern balloon catheters and guide wires with soft or flexible tips have reduced the risk of perforation considerably over the last few decades.

The creation of air emboli is another risk during cardiac catheterization. Frequent flushing of the catheter and contrast medium injection pump during angiography are two tasks where careful attention will reduce the risk of air emboli. Frequent wiping of catheters and wires and frequent catheter flushes with heparinized saline also aid in decreasing the risk of thrombosis.

Thrombus in, or trauma to, the cannulated vein or artery is one of the most common complications. It can be minimized by frequent puncture site checks, and careful catheter manipulations. Regular pulse checks of the affected extremity as an integral part of the postcatheterization nursing care plan.

Catheter-induced arrhythmias are common during the procedure, and should disappear with movement of the catheter away from the sensitive area.

Pump injection of contrast media into the myocardium (due to catheter misplacement) can lead to transient ST changes that will usually resolve spontaneously. The recognition of ECG changes by trained heart catheterization personnel, and prompt assessment and initiation of treatment where necessary, will avoid what could otherwise develop into emergency situations.

Changes in fluid and electrolyte status caused by excessive flushing of the catheter and the use of contrast media for angiography should also be considered and watched for during and after the procedure.

Care should be taken to minimize blood loss during the catheterization. Especially with newborns and small infants, the blood samples should be carefully planned, and the minimal amount taken.

Hypothermia in the newborn or infant during a procedure may lead to bradycardia and can compromise the status of the child. This can be prevented by having a warming device on or under the child during the catheterization and keeping the temperature of the room controlled.

Postprocedure Care

In many pediatric facilities, the same-day admission patient is cared for both pre- and postcatheterization by the same nurse. This nurse has done an initial assessment of the patient the morning of the procedure and is familiar with both the child's baseline condition and the patient's medical history. This continuity of care ensures that the child receives the best care possible.

When the child is returned to the post anesthesia care or nursing unit, the cardiac catheterization laboratory nurse gives a complete report to the receiving nurse, including the type of procedure performed, venous and arterial catheter sites, significant hemodynamic values, interventions performed, medication amounts and time, the condition of the patient during the procedure, and any specific problem areas or complications that arose.

Heparin infusions may be started in patients with certain device placements, postperipheral pulmonary artery dilations, or if a narrow shunt was crossed with a catheter.

Although the postcatheterization care plan varies between institutions, the majority include strict bed rest with the affected extremity kept straight for 4 hours for venous access and 6 hours for arterial access.[4] Vital signs and postprocedural sedation scoring are checked every 15 minutes for at least 1 hour. The frequency decreases to every 30 minutes, and then to every hour as the child becomes more alert and his or her condition stabilizes.[5] When checking vital signs, the catheter insertion sites should be assessed for bleeding, edema, or discoloration. Pulses and peripheral perfusion are also checked on the catheterized extremity. Use of a Doppler device may be helpful in locating difficult-to palpate peripheral pulses and checking the tone quality of the pulse for possible stenosis. Dressings are typically removed the morning following the procedure whether in the hospital or at home. The use of a dry sterile dressing covered with a transparent dressing allows direct visualization of the catheterization site and is more comfortable to remove than an elastized tape pressure dressing.

INTERVENTIONAL PROCEDURES

Balloon Atrial Septostomy

Balloon atrial septostomy is a palliative treatment of transposition of the great arteries (TGA). In complete TGA, the aorta rises anteriorly from the right ventricle and the pulmonary artery posteriorly from the left ventricle. Functionally this means that systemic blood coming into the heart is misdirected back into the systemic circulation, and oxygenated pulmonary venous blood is returned to the pulmonary circulation. To sustain life, the creation of an atrial septal defect is necessary to enhance mixing of pulmonary and systemic venous blood, therefore improving oxygen saturation.

Indications for a balloon atrial septostomy (BAS) have since then increased to include:

- Total anomalous pulmonary venous return with a restrictive atrial septum
- Tricuspid atresia with restrictive atrial septum
- Pulmonary atresia with intact ventricular septum

Balloon atrial septostomy uses a catheter with a balloon tip to enlarge an already existing interatrial opening such as an open foramen ovale. The atrial septum must be amenable to tearing, so the procedure is best performed in infants less than 6 weeks of age. When the septum is too tough or thickened, the chance of success is reduced. Some institutions may not perform a BAS if the infant is adequately oxygenated with prostaglandin E1 (a medication used to keep the PDA open). Early surgical repair can be performed if the surgeon is satisfied with diagnostic echocardiographic data.

The Procedure

The newborn entering the cardiac catheterization laboratory is usually intubated and under general anesthesia for the procedure. Prostaglandin E1 is started as soon as the diagnosis of TGA is made.

The stability and oxygenation status of the newborn will determine the sequence of the procedure. In an unstable newborn, the Rashkind procedure will precede the diagnostic catheterization, whereas with a stabilized infant, it is up to the cardiologist's preference. The diagnostic catheterization will confirm the initial cardiac di-

agnosis and look for any other associated anomalies. This is especially important when deciding on the definitive surgical correction.

After prepping the groin, a 5F balloon angiographic catheter (the preferred diagnostic catheter) is introduced via the femoral vein. The right side of the heart is reached; oxygen saturations are performed, and pressures are recorded. A left-to-right atrial pull-back is performed, which will indicate how large the open foramen ovale is. The left ventricle can be reached either in a retrograde direction from the PDA or from the left atrium through the mitral valve. After pressures and saturations have been taken, right- and left-ventricle angiography is performed. An aortic root angiography is also performed to visualize and define the coronary artery orientation. This is important in patients with TGA anticipation of arterial switch surgery.

In preparation for the septostomy, the sheath must be exchanged for a 7F-sized one, to accommodate the balloon tip of the 5F atrioseptostomy catheter. The atrioseptostomy catheter is passed from the right atrium through the open foramen ovale to the left atrium. When the catheter's position in the left atrium is assured through fluoroscopy, the balloon is inflated with diluted contrast medium. The inflated balloon is drawn back against the atrial septal wall, then pulled with a short jerk into the right atrium, thus tearing the atrial septum. It is important to establish a defect of at least 10 mm to 12 mm.[1] With the successful creation of an adequately sized ASD, arterial oxygen saturations should improve rapidly.

After completion of the procedure, the infant is returned to the intensive care unit for postoperative care.

Postprocedure Care and Complications

Keeping in mind the already tenuous state of this critically ill newborn, the stress of the cardiac catheterization procedure may have serious consequences for the rest of the child's life, so careful monitoring during and after the procedure is vital.

Hypovolemia, due to both poor cardiac output and blood loss during the procedure, will require anticipation of fluid boluses to improve intra-atrial mixing. The patient may enter the catheterization lab in an extremely acidotic state and could possibly be in a state of constant resuscitation; fluid volume and electrolyte balance should be carefully monitored. Bradycardia during the Rashkind maneuver is not uncommon, but it should spontaneously resolve after the balloon has been deflated in the right atrium. Other rhythm disturbances such as supraventricular tachycardia and partial or complete heart block have been known to occur during or after the atrioseptostomy.

Depending on the size of the left atrium, risk of myocardial perforation with a wire or catheter exists. Accidental tearing or rupturing of valves or vessels can be avoided by proper positioning and the slow inflation of the balloon under fluoroscopy. Due to the large-size sheath, damage to the femoral vein (including tearing and thrombosis) may occur and should be considered in the post-catheterization care plan.

Radiofrequency Perforation for Pulmonary Atresia with an Intact Ventricle Septum

Pulmonary atresia with an intact ventricular septum is a life-threatening condition that is initially treated with the maintained patency of the PDA through prostaglandins. Relief of the right ventricular obstruction by the creation of a right-ventricle-to-pulmonary-artery connection is the next treatment consideration. Depending on the anatomy, surgical correction could require multiple procedures.

With the recent advances in interventional catheters, a method was sought to address the problem of pulmonary atresia with an adaptation of the successful technique of dilating stenotic pulmonary valves. The problem pulmonary atre-

sia poses is the need to first create an opening through the fused valvular leaflets that will allow a balloon dilatation catheter to be passed. Laser energy was used first in the attempt to perforate the valve. This method proved successful, but the prohibitive cost of lasers led to the search for another method. The use of radiofrequency energy to destroy aberrant conduction pathways in the heart is widely practiced in many pediatric institutions. The transfer of this technique to the use of radiofrequency catheters to perforate the fused pulmonary valve has now proven to be successful, with the added advantage that the equipment is already available in most catheterization laboratories.

To provide adequate forward blood flow to the pulmonary vasculature and to prevent avoidable complications, a few anatomical considerations must be determined before perforation and dilatation of the pulmonary valve is attempted.

These include the following:

- The child must be a candidate for a biventricular repair, where the right ventricle is not prohibitively small.
- The right ventricular outflow tract must be well developed.
- The infundibulum must be close to the pulmonary artery.
- The right ventricle is not the source of coronary blood flow.

Procedure

The newborn will be intubated and placed under general anesthetic. IV prostaglandin E1 is infusing to keep the PDA open. After routine monitoring and positioning, a grounding pad (to complete the radiofrequency circuit) is placed under the patient's buttocks.

After obtaining venous access, a balloon angiographic catheter is often used to reach the right side of the heart, and right heart hemodynamics and oxygen saturations are performed. The left side of the heart is reached from the right atrium through the open foramen ovale. Angiography may be performed in the left ventricle to confirm the patency of the septal wall. Angiography of the right ventricle is performed to confirm the diagnosis and visualize the pulmonary valve. The venous catheter may then be exchanged for a Judkins right coronary catheter, which is helpful in positioning the catheter in the right ventricular outflow tract, directly under the valve.

After femoral artery access is obtained, a catheter is passed from the descending aorta, through the PDA to the main pulmonary artery, where it will provide a reference point during the perforation. The radiofrequency perforation catheter is then passed through the Judkins catheter until its tip protrudes from the catheter's tip. When correct placement of the perforation catheter is confirmed through hand injections of contrast medium, the radiofrequency energy is applied. Hand injections showing a contrast medium jet passing through the valve will confirm perforation.

The cardiologist will then try to push the catheter through the perforated valve, but in some cases the catheter will be too wide. Thinner (0.012- to 0.035-inch) guide wires may be used to cross the valve. Once the wire or catheter is successfully across the valve, it is advanced further through the PDA and stabilized in the descending aorta. It is helpful to have a snare catheter on hand in the event the cardiologist has trouble advancing the guide wire. The snare catheter may be passed from the arterial side to grasp the wire once the wire has crossed the valve.

The Judkins catheter is then removed and replaced with the balloon dilatation catheter. The balloon catheter is then advanced over the guide wire and into position, with the balloon straddling the valve. The cardiologist may need to start with a smaller balloon to dilate the orifice sufficiently to allow a larger balloon to enter the valve. The valve is then dilated. After dilation, right ventricle pressure is checked, and a control

angiography is performed to visualize and measure the opening area of the valve and to check for forward flow into the pulmonary artery.

Postprocedure Care and Complications

Inadvertent guide wire perforation of the infundibulum, pericardium, or other cardiac structures may occur during the valvular perforation procedure. Thus, careful monitoring for signs and symptoms of cardiac tamponade is important during and after the procedure.

Antegrade flow across the pulmonary valve may not increase significantly in the neonate until the right ventricular compliance improves, therefore, a prostaglandin infusion may need to continue postcatheterization.

The chances of postprocedure complications increase following a prolonged procedure with multiple catheter changes. Catheter insertion sites should be monitored for postprocedure bleeding, and any bleeding should be prevented. The chance of thrombus formation is higher the longer the arterial catheter is in place.

Balloon Dilatations

Balloon dilatation to relieve stenotic vessels and valves has opened a new door to the treatment of pulmonary and aortic valvular stenosis, coarctation of the aorta, peripheral pulmonary stenosis, and stenosis of surgical conduits. Balloon dilatation for the relief of pulmonary valve stenosis and recoarctation of the aorta has become the primary treatment of choice for these diagnoses.[4,6,7]

With stenotic valves, the fused commissures are split, thus producing an open valve. In a recoarctation of the aorta or stenosis of the pulmonary vessels, the abnormal cardiac structures are dilated, producing deliberate tears to the intimal and medial layers, which will then heal in the open position.

Balloon dilatation has also been used to relieve stenosis or obstruction in Blalock-Taussig shunts. Classic Blalock-Taussig shunts (BTS) are subclavian-to-right pulmonary artery or subclavian-to-left pulmonary artery connections performed in children where blood flow to the pulmonary structures is reduced or nonexistent (i.e., pulmonary atresia or tetralogy of Fallot). It is also performed in children where left-sided heart structures are small (hypoplastic left heart syndrome) and the pulmonary artery is used to augment the aorta, and pulmonary blood flow is supplied via the BTS.

Current surgeries now use a conduit between the subclavian artery and the pulmonary artery (PA) rather than direct anastomosis of the subclavian to the PA. By avoiding the need for open-heart surgery for these children, not only is hospital time decreased to a day or two, thus offering substantial cost savings, but the child is also spared a potentially painful operation, a long postoperative recovery period, and the disfigurement of a sterna incision.

Pulmonary Valve Stenosis

The most frequent lesion-producing obstruction to right ventricular outflow is pulmonary valve stenosis.[8] Stenosis of the valve may be caused by either fusion or dysplasia of the valvular leaflets. Dysplasia produces thickened, immobile leaflets that often do not react to dilatation, whereas simple fusion of the pulmonary valve leaflets, in which the leaflets are relatively thin and mobile, will open beautifully with balloon dilatation. Balloon dilation of the pulmonary valve will decrease right ventricular pressure and transpulmonary gradients in most patients and is the treatment of choice for pulmonary stenosis. Patient selection is confirmed by a cardiac echo, and candidates generally include a transpulmonary gradient greater than 50 mmHg for a patient with normal cardiac output. Balloon dilation of the pulmonary valve is performed in patients with tetralogy of Fallot or other forms of cyanotic heart disease where pulmonary stenosis

is an important feature. Because there is minimal blood flow across the pulmonary valve to start with, the procedure is usually well tolerated.

Procedure

After sterile preparation and draping of the groin area, the right side of the heart is reached with the percutaneous catheterization of the femoral vein. Pulmonary and right ventricle pressures are measured. An antero-posterior and lateral right ventricular cineangiography is performed to confirm the diagnosis already obtained with echocardiography. The pulmonary annulus is measured to determine the balloon size, which should be 120%–140% of the annulus diameter.[9]

An end-hole catheter is then inserted, through which a stiff guide wire is passed, and anchored in a stable position in a branch of the pulmonary artery. The stiff guide wire will be used to stabilize the balloon catheter during dilatation. The end-hole catheter is then removed, leaving the guide wire in place. It may now be necessary to exchange the sheath for a larger one to accommodate the balloon catheter and, ideally, reach the right ventricle.

The balloon catheter is flushed with heparinized saline, checked for patency, and advanced over the guide wire into position with the balloon straddling the pulmonary valve. The balloon is filled with diluted contrast media so that it is visible on fluoroscopy, allowing the cardiologist to control the positioning. The cardiologist will inflate the balloon until the "waist" around the middle of the balloon disappears, signaling the relief of the stenosis. During the inflation, the cardiologist may use a pressure gauge placed between the balloon catheter and the inflation syringe to monitor the balloon inflation pressure so that the recommended balloon burst pressure is not exceeded.

When the balloon is inflated to its maximum capacity, blood flow to the patient's lungs is inhibited, thus producing a reduction in cardiac output with a resultant decrease in blood pressure. This resolves quickly as the balloon is deflated. When dilatation is completed, the balloon catheter is withdrawn. The end-hole catheter is replaced, and a pulmonary-artery-to-right-ventricle pull back is done to check for a residual gradient. Afterwards, the angiographic catheter is replaced, and a control angiography is performed to visualize and measure the opening area of the valve.

Postprocedure Care and Complications

Because dilatation catheters may require a larger size sheath, the recovery room nurse should be aware that special care must be observed in monitoring for bleeding at the insertion site or thrombosis of the affected vessel.

Aortic Valve Stenosis

Valvular aortic stenosis occurs in approximately 3%–6% of patients with congenital heart defects.[10] As with valvular pulmonary stenosis, the more dysplastic the valve, the less chance a successful result will be achieved. The indication for a balloon intervention is the same as for a surgical intervention, although supravalvar and subvalvar stenosis are not eligible for balloon dilation. The criteria for intervention in congenital aortic stenosis is a peak systolic ejection gradient across the aortic valve of 50 to 60 mmHg.[10,11]

Critical valvular aortic stenosis in the newborn is considered an emergency. Hemodynamically unstable due to their low cardiac output, these newborns have a high surgical mortality, thus the indications for an immediate catheter intervention are given.

The Procedure

This procedure can be performed with either general anesthesia or procedural sedation. Generally, the procedure can be tolerated by older children with sedation. The nurse will need to assure that the patient is adequately sedated prior to balloon dilation, so that the balloon position is not compromised during dilation. General anesthesia is preferred in patients with decreased LV function. As the chance of ventricular arrhythmia (especially ventricular tachycardia) is increased due to left ventricular wall hypertrophy, the use of the multifunction defibrillator pads or placement of a transvenous pacing wire is recommended. Some facilities will prophylactically atrial pace the patient at an increased heart rate (140 beats per minute) to increase cardiac output and minimize hemodynamic changes and risk of arrhythmia.

The left heart can be approached from the femoral artery in either a retrograde direction (femoral artery, aortic valve, left ventricle) or by an antegrade approach (right atrium, left atrium, mitral valve, left ventricle, aortic valve).

With the introduction of the appropriately sized sheath, a catheter with end and side holes, whose form is conducive to slipping through the stenotic aortic valve with minimal trauma, is placed in the left ventricle. It is important that the catheter is able to produce a high enough flow rate for a clear left ventricular angiogram. After pressures are measured in the left ventricle, an angiogram is performed to clearly visualize and measure the aortic valve. One of the complications of aortic valve dilatation is aortic regurgitation due to valvular insufficiency. Thus the size of the balloon becomes very important, and extreme care should be taken to choose the appropriate size. The optimal balloon-to-valve diameter ratio should be 90%–100%, with undersized balloons resulting in significant residual obstruction, and oversized balloons resulting in aortic regurgitation.[10,12]

A stiff guide wire is then passed through the catheter into the left ventricle. The guide wire must be stiff enough to support the balloon catheter during the dilatation, but it should have a soft tip to prevent irritation of the hypertrophic left ventricle. There are a number of stiff guide wires on the market with soft, flexible tips that are ideal for these cases.

The balloon is then passed over the guide wire, and filled with diluted contrast medium. It is inflated to check that it is in the correct position, with the balloon straddling the aortic valve. When the correct position is confirmed, rapid inflation and deflation of the balloon is performed, because cardiac output falls rapidly with the occlusion of the aortic valve. Enough recovery time must be given between dilatations to ensure that the vital signs have stabilized.

When the balloon waist disappears (signaling relief of the stenosis), the balloon catheter is removed and the original catheter replaced. Pressures are measured and a left ventricular control angiogram is performed. An aortic angiogram is also performed to check for any resultant aortic valvular insufficiency.

Postprocedure Care and Complications

After completion of the procedure, the catheter and sheath are withdrawn, and manual compression of the insertion site is initiated to achieve hemostasis. With successful hemostasis, a dry, sterile dressing is applied, and the child is released to the recovery room.

Postoperative bleeding or thrombosis of the catheterized artery are well-documented complications, and the patient must be monitored for them in the recovery period. Arrhythmias can occur, not only during the procedure, but also postoperatively. Rare but serious complications include inadvertent perforation of the left ventricular wall, resulting in cardiac tamponade, and damage to the valve that causes aortic insufficiency (regurgitation), leading to an acute low cardiac output state. The recovery room nurse must be aware of these possible complications to be able to appropriately monitor the patient.

Peripheral Pulmonary Artery Stenosis

Peripheral pulmonary artery stenosis is found as a primary or secondary lesion after surgery for right ventricular outflow tract reconstruction (see Figure 27-1). Balloon catheter dilation of primary and postoperative stenosis in the distal pulmonary vasculature offers a chance for improved survival and decreased morbidity in patients who were previously unable to be treated or had only minimal chances of surgical success.[11]

Precatheterization evaluation includes an echocardiogram to estimate the severity of right ventricular outflow tract obstruction and an estimate of flow distribution to the two lungs. The lung with the least amount of obstruction should be dilated first. Factors that determine anesthesia versus sedation include the extent of balloon dilation, duration of the procedure, anticipated complications, and right ventricular (RV) function. If RV pressure is anticipated to be greater than three-quarters systemic, then anesthesia should be employed.

The Procedure

The right side of the heart is catheterized and pressure measurements are performed. The cardiologist will be especially interested in the pressure gradients proximal from, and distal to, the stenotic area, and the pressure in the right ventricle. Angiography is performed in the right ventricle, and usually in the main pulmonary artery, with the cardiologist choosing a projection to best visualize the area of stenosis. If multiple stenoses are to be dilated, selective injections are performed in the vessels to be dilated.

Once the stenosis has been defined, an end-hole catheter is placed through the stenotic area, and a stiff guide wire is placed distal to the area to be dilated. With the guide wire securely anchored, the end-hole catheter is withdrawn and the balloon catheter is introduced. The most

Figure 27-1. Angiogram showing peripheral pulmonary artery stenosis.

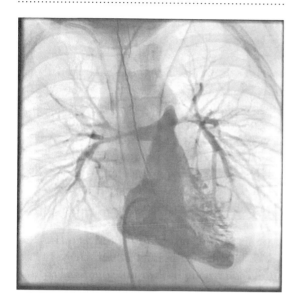

distal lesion is dilated first to avoid unnecessary passage through already dilated areas. Balloon inflation can weaken the dilated area, leaving the structures at risk for perforation; therefore, a catheter should never pass the dilated area without a guide wire.

The balloon chosen should be three to four times the diameter of the stenotic portion of the vessel,[9] but not more than two times the size of the adjacent normal pulmonary artery.[10,11] An initial inflation is done to check the position of the balloon. Ideally, the waist produced by the stenosis should be at the central portion of the balloon, because that is where the maximal inflation diameter is located. Inflation and deflation are performed until the waist of the balloon disappears or maximal inflation pressure (burst pressure) has been reached. High-pressure balloons are used because the lesions are difficult to disrupt and dilate. Due to the changed pulmonary vasculature (which may result in either cal-

cification or elastic recoil of the involved vessels), dilatation may require high inflation pressures to achieve a successful result or, in the case of elastic recoil, the dilation may not be successful. Cutting balloons (balloons with three or four longitudinal microsurgical blades), are now being used in vessels that are resistant to conventional balloon therapy.

Postdilation angiography is performed to visualize the result of the dilation and to check for aneurysm of the dilated vessel.

Postprocedure Care and Complications

Trauma to the catheterized vein in the form of tearing, dissection, or thrombosis may occur, so frequent checks of the catheterized extremity are necessary. Transient high-flow pulmonary edema due to increased flow and pressure in the dilated lung segment is a serious complication and must be carefully monitored postoperatively. It often results in an ICU admission postcatheterization for ventilator support and diuretic management. Other complications can include aneurysms and hemoptysis due to vessel trauma. Bleeding not confined to a lung segment can be catastrophic and life threatening. Urgent surgery may be required, although a balloon inflated in the branch pulmonary artery to occlude flow can stem the flow of blood.

Coarctation of the Aorta

While balloon dilatation of native coarctation of the aorta is still controversial due to the low success rate of the procedure as opposed to surgery, balloon dilation to relieve restenosis following surgical correction is now considered the therapy of choice.[7,9] Aortic arch restenosis following a surgical repair usually occurs within the first few months following the surgical anastomosis. It is most often related to residual duct tissue within the aortic wall. Balloon dilation is a useful procedure for the infant or child who is at high risk for standard surgical management.[10]

The Procedure

After percutaneous arterial access is achieved , a Judkins right coronary catheter is often used to reach the ascending aorta and passed through the stenotic area. The pressure gradient across the coarcted segment is measured by catheter pullback. Angiography is performed in the ascending aorta to visualize the narrowed aortal segment.

The balloon chosen should be 2.5 to 3 times the diameter of the stenosis.[11] To avoid injury, long balloons (greater than 3 cm) and balloons greater than 50% of the unaffected aorta are not used.

A guide wire is then inserted through the Judkins catheter and anchored in the ascending aorta. After careful flushing with heparinized saline, the balloon catheter is introduced and positioned with the recoarted segment in the middle of the balloon. Rapid inflation and deflation of the balloon is necessary because cardiac output drops during balloon inflation.

When the balloon waist disappears or dilation is considered adequate, the balloon catheter is withdrawn and pressure measurements are taken. Angiography is performed to confirm the success of the procedure and to check for aneurysm of the aortic wall.

Postprocedure Care and Complications

After completion of the catheterization, the usual procedure of insertion site hemostasis is initiated. After hemostasis has been achieved, a dry, sterile dressing is applied, and the child is released to the recovery room.

The most common complication is femoral artery damage. Therefore, pulse checks to the affected extremity are important. Aneurismal formation at the site of the dilation may be found either during the catheterization or at follow-up,

and should be monitored with an echocardiogram. Further complications and care are the same as with aortic valve balloon dilation.

Device Placement

Interventional device placements can be performed instead of a surgical procedure, such as in the case of the PDA closure device or to augment surgery, such as pre- or postsurgical coil closures of unwanted systemic-to-pulmonary-artery collateral vessels. Stent implantations have been useful in overcoming the elastic recoil of vessels, thus offering relief of stenoses in instances where balloon dilation has failed.

Patent Ductus Arteriosus Closure

A PDA is the persistence of an open connection between the descending aorta and the pulmonary artery. This vessel, open during fetal circulation, usually closes after birth. Its failure to do so can lead to arterial blood recirculating in the lungs with resultant pulmonary hypertension and left ventricular dilatation. This connection also provides a risk of bacterial endocarditis, requiring antibiotic treatment for any situation that may provoke a bacterial infection (such as routine dental work).

Before the golden age of pediatric interventional cardiology, PDA was treated with surgical ligation, a safe and straightforward procedure with a mortality of less than 1%.[13] Despite the low mortality rate and success of the surgical closure, the procedure entailed a hospital stay of at least 5 days at a substantial cost and necessitated a thoracotomy incision with the resulting scar. This motivated the development and resultant success of transcatheter closure of PDA.

The Procedure

Percutaneous access of both the femoral vein and the femoral artery is achieved, and a sheath is placed in each. The right side of the heart is catheterized, usually with an end-hole catheter, and right ventricle and pulmonary artery pressures and oxygen saturations are measured. Using a pigtail catheter through the arterial sheath, angiography is performed in the descending aorta to visualize and measure the PDA in a lateral projection (see Figure 27-2).

After careful measurement of the PDA, the correctly sized coil or ductal closure plug is selected by the cardiologist. There are several factors to consider when choosing one PDA closure method or another. A PDA with an internal diameter of < 2.5 mm responds well to closure with an occlusion coil (see Figure 27-3), whereas larger PDAs can be successfully closed with a ductal occlusion device.[13,14]

Occluding spring coils are made of surgical stainless steel covered with Dacron strands to promote thrombus formation (see Figure 27-4). Coils are usually delivered retrograde from the femoral artery, with the two-thirds of the coil loop placed into the pulmonary artery, and the remaining two-and-one-half to three-and-one-half loops delivered into the aortic ductal ampulla.[15]

Occlusion devices such as the Amplatzer ductal occluder can be used for PDAs as small as 5 mm using a 5F or 6F sheath, or as large as 12 mm through a 7F sheath (see Figure 27-5). The occlusion device is placed antegrade from the pulmonary artery side of the PDA. The device is opened slightly so that its cap is deployed just inside the aorta. The catheter is then pulled back against the aortic ampulla, and the remainder of the plug is deployed within the ductus, leaving a small portion protruding into the pulmonary side. An angiogram following deployment of either the coil or plug is obtained to evaluate position and residual leak.

Postprocedure Care and Complications

It is possible for a coil to be misplaced or detached in an undesirable position; thus, it is important

Figure 27-2. Lateral view of PDA.

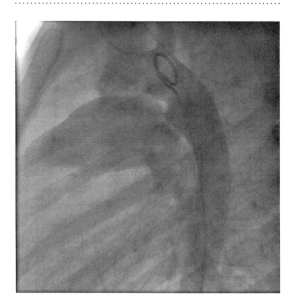

Figure 27-3. After device closure.

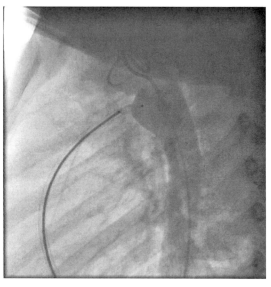

Figure 27-4. Coil occlusion devices.

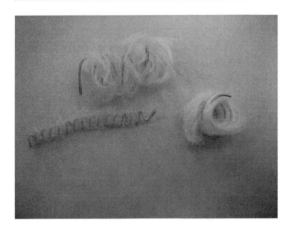

Figure 27-5. Amplatzer ductal occluder. *Source:* Courtesy of AGA Medical Corporation.

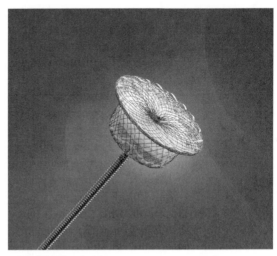

AMPLATZER® Duct Occluder
© AGA Medical Corporation

to have the necessary retrieval forceps or snare wire on hand. Migration of the coil into the heart can lead to cardiac arrhythmias, thrombus formation, pulmonary embolization, myocardial damage, and hemorrhage.

A large-sized sheath is often used, so the possibility of postprocedure bleeding or thrombosis of the affected vessel must be considered.

Whether MRI scanning can cause migration of a coil has yet to be determined. The manufacturer recommends that patients with coil placements refrain from MRI scans for the first week following implantation, and MRI compatible coils have recently appeared on the market.

Embolization Coil Closures

Transcatheter coil closures have been proven useful in instances in which collateral vessels, fistulas, and shunts need to be closed to improve the patient's hemodynamic situation. Systemic to pulmonary artery collateral vessels are those most commonly embolized. Coils vary in diameter, as well as in the number of loops they can form. Advances in the size, shape, and material of the coils allow for easier coil placement in vessels that are difficult to reach and whose shape is difficult to fit.

The Procedure

An angiogram in the aorta will show the position of the collateral vessel to be embolized. With further hand injections of contrast media, the size and shape of the vessel can be analyzed. The catheter chosen to deliver the coil is dictated by the location of the vessels to be embolized. The catheter must be nontapered, with an end hole. Side holes are not desirable, because the coil can catch on one of the side holes during deployment. Catheters that have proven useful in these situations are Judkins coronary catheters or multipurpose catheters.

The distal tip of the catheter is placed well into the vessel to be occluded. The coils come encased in a delivery pod, and this is placed against the hub of the catheter, and a wire is used to push the coil out of the pod and into the catheter. The coil is advanced to the end of the catheter, where it is carefully deployed in the vessel under fluoroscopic control. A control angiogram is then performed to check the patency of the occluded vessel.

Postprocedure Care and Complications

Complications and postoperative care are similar to PDA coil closures.

Stent Implantation

Collapsed stainless steel balloon expandable intravascular grafts (see Figure 27-6) (commonly known as stents) have been successfully used in treating stenoses when the elasticity of the vessel has caused balloon dilatation to fail. By mechanically supporting the vessel wall, the stent can provide relief in hemodynamically significant stenoses, such as those resulting from elastic recoil of the vessel or caused by resilient scar tissue as a result of previous surgery. By controlled expansion of the stent with the balloon catheter, the stent can be carefully fitted to the vessel wall. Self-expanding stents will also conform perfectly to the vessel contours if the size is selected correctly.

The most commonly used locations for stents in congenital heart patients are aortic coarctations and conduits after surgery as in tetralogy of Fallot. Stents may also be used to maintain atrial septal patency in patients with a single ventricle physiology and in management of systemic

Figure 27-6. Vessel stent.

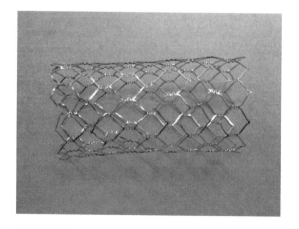

venous and pulmonary venous baffle obstructions.[15] Stent implantation is an acknowledged treatment option in the handling of peripheral pulmonary stenosis resistant to balloon dilation. In distal branch pulmonary stenosis in which the narrowing is found within the hilus or behind the aorta, surgical correction can prove to be challenging. In such difficult-to-reach areas, stent implantation has proven to be useful. Stent implantation has also been found to be effective in systemic venous obstructions such as found with superior and inferior vena cava obstructions following surgery. The treatment of pulmonary vein stenosis, however, has shown a very poor success rate. Because stent implantation may not halt the progression of pulmonary vein stenosis in children with diffuse involvement, the risk exists that the stent could become part of an inoperable stenotic area. Use of stents in the pediatric population presents the challenge of redilatation of the stent to accommodate vessel growth at a later date.

The Procedure

The child enters the cardiac catheter laboratory and is prepared as usual. After femoral access is achieved, hemodynamics are measured in the stenotic area. An angiogram is then performed to measure the stenosis and the vessel's anatomy immediately distal from and proximal to it. A guide wire is placed through the stenotic area, with the tip well distal to it.

If a balloon expanding stent is being placed, it will usually come premounted on a balloon catheter. The catheter is passed over the guide wire, and the stent is positioned within the stenosis. It is then inflated by hand with diluted contrast medium. As the balloon is inflated, the stent expands. The inflation is held until the waisting in the balloon disappears, signaling the relief of the stenosis. The balloon is then deflated, leaving the expanded stent in place, and the catheter is carefully removed.

Self-expanding stents are deployed by retracting the sheath once the distal end of the stent has been positioned correctly. During deployment, the stent shortens, which has to be taken into account when the size of the stent is being selected.

When the stent has been expanded within the lesion, a control angiogram is performed to check the success of the procedure and the position of the stent. If warranted, additional balloon dilatations can be performed to ensure effective expansion of the stent.

The catheter and sheath are removed and hemostasis is achieved by manual compression. After application of the dry, sterile dressing, the child is transported to the recovery room.

Postprocedure Care and Complications

Long-term aspirin therapy is started when there is pulsatile flow through the stent. With non-pulsatile flow, anticoagulation is required, with heparin administered in the acute phase followed by warfarin for 6 months.[10] Potential complications are similar to those of PDA coil closure.

Atrial Septal Defect

One of the most common congenital cardiac anomalies is the ASD. ASDs can be divided into three common types: ostium primum, ostium secundum, and sinus venosus defects. The most common of these, the ostium secundum defect, lies within the region of the fossa ovalis, and is surrounded by a rim of atrial tissue. This complete rim allows for ideal device placement; it is able to support the implanted device as well as provide a separation between the device and other surrounding heart structures.

Although surgical closure of ASD is considered one of the safest and most effective of the cardiac surgical procedures,[11] the inherent risks of open-heart surgery still remain. Coupled with the lasting thoracotomy scar, long postoperative recovery period, and the expense of a long hospital stay, devices that can close an ASD through a catheter have been developed. Modern device placement is a relatively simple procedure requiring small-gauge sheaths, resulting in a safe procedure for small children.

The precatheter echocardiogram assures that the size and position of the ASD are appropriate for a device closure. Several ASD devices on the market allow cardiologists to choose whichever device best suits their individual technique.

The Procedure

The sedated child enters the catheter lab and is placed comfortably on the table. The usual monitors are connected, and the patient's body is positioned and padded as appropriate. Because transesophageal echocardiography is often used to aid in accurate device placement, intubation of the child may be desirable.[7] Implant endocarditis prophylaxis with Kefzol is started as previously described. Systemic heparinization is also started when device placement is assured.[14]

The right side of the heart is reached via the femoral vein access and right-sided hemodynamics are measured. A technique called balloon sizing is performed to accurately measure the size of the defect and aid in visualizing its position. This technique involves pulling an inflated balloon from the left to the right atrium until it fits snugly within the ASD. A device that is about twice the size of the balloon-stretched diameter of the ASD is considered adequate.[13,14]

As with the PDA delivery system, a long sheath is placed through the ASD, across the atrial septum into the left atrium. The device delivery system is then loaded into the sheath and advanced through the right atrium. The device is pushed forward to the tip of the sheath, in the middle of the left atrium. The sheath is then retracted, allowing the distal portion of the device to unfold. The whole unit (sheath, guide wire, and device) is then pulled back until the distal device fits snugly against the defect in the left side of the interatrial septum. The sheath is further retracted, allowing for the proximal device to unfold in the mid-right atrium. With correct positioning of the device confirmed, the device is released and the delivery system is removed. A control angiogram is performed to confirm closure of the ASD.

After the completion of the procedure, the sheath is removed. Once hemostasis is achieved, a dry, sterile dressing is applied, and the child is released to the recovery room.

Postprocedure Care and Complications

Depending on the cardiologist's experience, this procedure may be lengthy with a resultant increase in postprocedure complications. Because a large sheath may be required, monitoring for bleeding in the insertion site or thrombosis of the femoral vessels is mandatory. The recovery room should be aware that embolization of the device may be manifested in a sudden decrease in oxygen saturations. Arrhythmias due to device placement too close to conduction tissue may occur. A long-term aspirin course is recommended to prevent excessive platelet aggregation on the device.[14] Residual leaks may occur from the device, so continued clinical follow-ups, including an echocardiogram, are prescribed.

Radiofrequency Catheter Ablation

RFCA uses radiofrequency energy to destroy aberrant pathways within the heart's conduction system. Before the advent of RFCA, intractable arrhythmias that were resistant to pharmacologic therapy caused ventricular dysfunction with resultant congestive heart failure. They were surgically mapped and treated and required open-heart surgery with all the inherent risks. Since its initiation in the pediatric population nearly two decades ago, RFCA has shown excellent treatment results with low complication rates. Due to the possible complications and long-term toxicity of the antiarrhythmic medications, RFCA has become the treatment of choice for some forms of arrhythmias in children.

Pediatric indications for RFCA vary from those for adults not only because of the smaller size of the child and the immaturity of the myocardium, but also because of the mechanism of the arrhythmia and the possible presence of structural congenital heart defects. Candidates for RFCA should be at least 3 years old. The smaller size of the child presents challenges in the size of the catheters to be used as well as limiting the amount of maneuverable space within the heart.

Spontaneous resolution of tachycardia can be expected in some cases, but if tachycardia is present after the age of 5, the chances for it to resolve decrease significantly.[15] Thus for infants and small children, it would be advisable to postpone RFCA if the tachycardia can be treated effectively with medication. Catheter ablation risks for children are similar to those for adults.

SUMMARY

From diagnostic to interventional catheterization, from newborns to young adults, pediatric cardiac catheterization procedures offer a wide range of experiences and opportunities for the nursing staff. Staff must be prepared to meet the emotional needs of the sedated child and their families, as well as to assess and react to the changing physical status of the critically ill child in the catheterization laboratory.

REFERENCES

1. Neches WH, Park SC, Zuberbuhler JR. *Pediatric Cardiac Catheterization: Perspectives in Pediatric Cardiology*, Vol. 3. Mount Kisco, NY: Futura; 1991.
2. Pederson C, Harbaugh BL. Children's and adolescents' experiences while undergoing cardiac catheterization. *Matern Child Nurs J* 1995; 23:15–25.

3. Monett ZJ, Roberts PJ. Patient care for interventional cardiac catheterization. *Nurs Clin North Am* 1995;30:333–345.

4. Gerdes JE. An ambulatory approach to outpatient pediatric cardiac catheterization. *J Post Anesth Nurs* 1990;5:407–410.

5. Agamalian B. Pediatric cardiac catheterization. *J Pediatr Nurs* 1986;1:73–79.

6. Radtke W. Interventional pediatric cardiology: state of the art and future perspectives. *Eur J Pediatr* 1994;153:542–547.

7. Allen HD, Beekman RH 3rd, Garson A Jr, et al. Pediatric therapeutic cardiac catheterization: a statement for healthcare professionals from the Council on Cardiovascular Disease in the Young, American Heart Association. *Circulation* 1998;97:609–625.

8. Moss AJ, Adams FH, Emmanouilides GC. *Moss and Adams Heart Disease in Infants, Children, and Adolescents,* 5th ed. Baltimore, MD: Williams & Wilkins; 1995.

9. Landzberg MJ, Lock JE. Interventional catheter procedures used in congenital heart disease. *Cardiol Clin* 1993;11:569–587.

10. Lock JE. Cardiac catheterization. In: Keane JL. *Nadas' Pediatric Cardiology* (pp. 213–250). Philadelphia: Saunders; 2006.

11. Baim DS, Grossman W. *Cardiac Catheterisation, Angiography and Intervention*, 5th ed. Baltimore, MD: Williams & Wilkins; 1996.

12. McCrindle BW. Independent predictors of immediate results of percutaneous balloon aortic valvotomy in children: Valvuloplasty and Angio- plasty of Congenital Anomalies (VACA) registry investigators. *Am J Cardiol* 1996;77:286–293.

13. Callow LB. Nursing implications of interventional device placement in pediatric cardiology and pediatric cardiac surgery. *Crit Care Nurs Clin North Am* 1994;6:133–151.

14. Rao PS, Wilson AD, Chopra PS. Transcatheter closure of atrial septal defect by "buttoned" devices. *Am J Cardiol* 1992;69:1056–1061.

15. Van Hare GF. Indications for radiofrequency ablation in the pediatric population. *J Cardiovasc Electrophysiol* 1997;8:952–962.

SUGGESTED READING

ACC/AHA guidelines for cardiac catheterization and cardiac catheterization laboratories: American College of Cardiology/American Heart Association Ad Hoc Task Force on Cardiac Catheterization. *J Am Coll Card* 1991;18:1149–1182.

Bubien RS, Knotts SM, McLaughlin S, George P. What you need to know about radiofrequency ablation. *Am J Nurs* 1993;July:30–36.

Park MK. *Pediatric Cardiology Handbook*, 3rd ed. St. Louis, MO: Mosby; 2003.

Perry SB, Keane JF, Lock JE. Pediatric interventions. In: Baim DS, Grossman W. *Cardiac Catheterization, Angiography and Intervention*, 5th ed. Baltimore, MD: Williams & Wilkins, 1996; 713–734.

Saul JP, Walsh EP, Triedman JK. Mechanisms and therapy of complex arrhythmias in pediatric patients. *J Cardiovasc Electrophysiol* 1995;6:1129–1148.

Chapter 28

PERCUTANEOUS CAROTID ANGIOGRAPHY AND INTERVENTION

Daniel Walsh, RT
Stephanie Ray, RN
Sharon Holloway, RN, MSN, ACNP-CS, CCRN

INTRODUCTION

Stroke, also known as cerebrovascular accident, or assault, (CVA) is a leading cause of morbidity and mortality worldwide. Within the United States, it is estimated that there are 700,000 new strokes diagnosed each year and 4.7 million stroke survivors.[1] With longer life expectancies, the incidence and prevalence of stroke will continue to rise, as will its debilitating sequelae.

Stroke can either be ischemic or hemorrhagic (bleeding) in origin. Similar to what occurs in the heart, with an ischemic stroke, plaque development in a cranial or extracranial artery leads to disruption of cerebral blood flow and ultimately tissue infarction. In a hemorrhagic stroke, a weakening of the vessel wall leads to bleeding and infarction of brain tissue. Hemorrhagic strokes are more difficult to treat and often more lethal than ischemic strokes.

In order to appreciate carotid angiography and stenting, one must first understand stroke and its relationship to the carotid arteries. In this chapter, we will review cerebrovascular anatomy as well as the etiology of stroke. This will be followed by a detailed discussion of carotid angiography and stenting including patient selection, diagnostic and interventional techniques, nursing considerations, and postprocedural care.

CEREBROVASCULAR ANATOMY AND PATHOLOGY

Most people have four extracranial arteries: two carotid arteries and two vertebral arteries. The carotid arteries form what is referred to as the anterior circulation, while the vertebrals form the posterior circulation. In the majority of patients, the right carotid artery arises from the brachiocephalic (innominate) artery, and the left carotid arises directly from the aortic arch with the vertebral arteries arising from the subclavian arteries (see Figure 28-1), although there can be some variances in the aortic arch anatomy.

Figure 28-1. Arch of the aorta and great vessels. BCA = brachiocephalic (innominate) artery; LCCA = left common carotid artery; LSA = left subclavian artery; RSA = right subclavian artery; RCCA = right common carotid artery; ICA = internal carotid artery; ECA = external carotid artery; VA = vertebral artery; IMA = internal mammary artery; TCT = thyrocervical trunk.

Figure 28-2. Extracranial and intracranial circulation. ACA = anterior communicating artery; BA = basilar artery; R/L ACA = right/left anterior cerebral artery; R/L CCA = right/left common carotid artery; R/L ECA = right/left external carotid artery; R/L ICA = right/leftinternal carotid artery; R/L MCA = right/left middle cerebral artery; R/L PCA = right/left posterior cerebralartery; R/L SA = right/left subclavian artery; R/L VA = right/left verterbal artery.

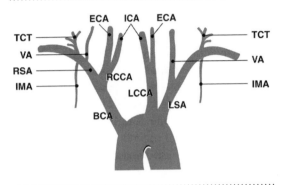

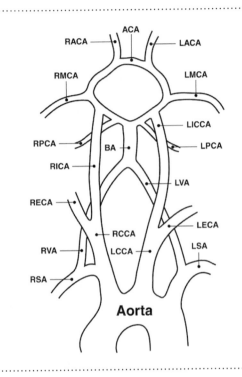

Each carotid artery runs cephalad in the anterior neck and divides near the level of the mandible, giving rise to an internal and external carotid artery. This is where the carotid pulse is palpated and/or ausculated for the presence of bruits. At this division, there is a natural widening of the vessel known as the carotid bulb. The external carotid arteries immediately divide into a myriad of branches that provide blood to the thyroid, face, and skull.

The internal carotids continue on as a direct conduit to the brain, giving rise only to the ophthalmic arteries just before they join in forming the circle of Willis (see Figure 28-2). The vessel then divides into anterior and middle cerebral arteries. The right and left vertebral arteries supply blood to the cerebellum and brainstem. The vertebral arteries flow in the posterior neck within the vertebrae, and join together to form the basilar artery. Posteriorly, the basilar artery feeds into the circle of Willis, which is the confluence of tributaries to the brain, and provides circulatory redundancy. This vessel redundancy provides some degree of cerebral protection by maintaining cerebral blood flow in the pres-

ence of a carotid or vertebral artery stenosis or occlusion.

Stroke

There are several ways in which ischemic stroke can occur. Atherosclerotic plaque (cholesterol and inflammatory cells) build up beneath the endothelium of the artery. This plaque can rupture similar to coronary plaques, causing instant unfavorable anatomical changes, and sometimes arterial occlusion. As angina is to heart disease, transient ischemic attacks (TIAs) are the result of a temporary decrease in blood flow to the brain.

Symptoms of a TIA include visual and speech disturbances or motor dysfunction. Generally, these symptoms last a few moments to a few hours. TIAs often signal an impending stroke. Alternatively, a clot can travel in the bloodstream to the neck or brain, causing occlusion of a cranial or extracranial artery. This is known as a cerebral embolism. The most common origins of these emboli are the heart and the carotid bulb. For this reason, plaque development within the extracranial carotid artery has been identified as a significant risk factor for stroke.[2] The more severe the stenosis, the higher is the risk for stroke.

Surgical revascularization with a carotid endarterectomy, performed in the operating room under general anesthesia, has long been the treatment of choice.[3,4] With the development of newer percutaneous techniques, carotid artery stenting (CAS) has become a proven treatment option for appropriately selected patients comparing favorably to conventional surgical revascularization.[5-9] Treatment of symptomatic and asymptomatic carotid artery disease can be achieved with carotid artery stenting, theoretically decreasing the risk to the patient seen with surgical endarterectomy.

DIAGNOSIS AND PATIENT SELECTION

Atherosclerotic plaque development is a slow process. Asymptomatic carotid artery disease is often found on routine physical examination, when a practitioner auscultates the carotid arteries on either side of the neck and hears a bruit. A carotid bruit is audible due to blood flowing through a narrowed vessel producing turbulence. This narrowing is verified and quantified with duplex ultrasound and/or CT angiography.

After a significant carotid stenosis has been confirmed by noninvasive testing, the patient may be referred for carotid angiography. Generally, the patient is referred when the stenosis is greater than 70% and/or shows signs of in-

stability. A patient may also be referred for angiography if there is conflicting or confusing noninvasive data. In the case of inconclusive noninvasive data, CT angiography can be performed to further delineate the carotid anatomy prior to proceeding with invasive angiography. Also, patients are more confident of the need to proceed with the invasive procedure if the CT angiography data confirms the diagnosis of a significant carotid lesion.

PATIENT PREPARATION

Prior to the procedure, the patient undergoes a neurologic evaluation. A neurologist should perform an independent exam to identify any preexisting deficit, establish the patient's suitability for the procedure, and the timing of the procedure in relation to any recent neurologic event. After the procedure, the patient is examined again by the neurologist to evaluate the patient for any change from baseline.

Routine precatheterization blood work and diagnostic testing is performed. Routine testing includes a complete blood count, chemistry panel, coagulation panel, ECG, and CXR. The test results are reviewed, and any abnormalities that require further evaluation should be addressed prior to the procedure. The presence of extracranial carotid artery disease places the patient at high risk for having other occult cardiovascular disease. A complete cardiovascular work-up should be considered to evaluate for the presence of concomitant disease.

Patients are admitted to the catheterization holding area the morning of the procedure after maintaining NPO (nothing by mouth) status since midnight. Patients are informed again about the procedure, and general instructions are reviewed. The most frequently asked questions pertain to hospital stay, procedure length, and permanence of the stent. Patients are reminded that they will be required to stay overnight, that the procedure itself takes about 2 hours, and that the stent is permanent. The physician reviews the risk and benefits with the patient and family and consent is obtained from the patient or surrogate.

The patient is brought into the catheterization suite and prepped and draped in the same fashion as for coronary angiography.

DIAGNOSTIC PROCEDURE

Access is obtained by the physician using the Seldinger technique, and a sheath or introducer set is inserted into the artery, usually the femoral artery. The procedure can be successfully performed via the brachial or radial arteries, although these approaches lend less support during the interventional portion of the procedure than femoral access.

After the sheath is safely in place, most physicians give a small dose of heparin for the diagnostic procedure (2000 to 2500 units).

A pigtail or flush catheter is inserted into the ascending aorta in preparation for aortic arch angiography. The position of the camera should be LAO (left anterior oblique) 40°; this angle elongates the aortic arch and demonstrates the origin of the great vessels. The pigtail or flush catheter is then connected to the power injector loaded with contrast media. A commonly used contrast injection rate is 20 ml for 2 seconds for a total of 40 ml. Digital subtraction angiography is also recommended.

After performing aortic arch angiography, the physician evaluates the image and decides which catheter is best suited for selective angiography of the carotid and/or vertebral arteries. The most common catheters are the Simmons, Headhunter, Bentson, and Mani catheters. After inserting the selective catheter, it is advanced past the origin of the great vessels and pulled back. This should allow the catheter to smoothly engage the origin of the right brachiocephalic artery (innominate artery). Many physicians prefer to use an angled hydrophilic guide wire (i.e., Glidewire) to assist

the catheter past the innominate bifurcation and selectively into the right carotid.

Once the catheter is placed in the carotid artery, angiography can be performed. Some physicians choose to perform one cine run of the innominate bifurcation in the RAO 40 projection to excluded ostial carotid disease prior to engaging the carotid. The usual camera angle of the right carotid system is RAO 30° to 40° and RAO 90°; this will provide clear visual separation of the bifurcation of the right internal and right external carotid artery. For anterior cerebral circulation, RAO 90° and AP cranial 30° (known as Townes View), are taken of the whole skull. Take care to record a prolonged cine to ensure capture of the venous phase as well.

After all images of the right carotid system have been successfully recorded, the catheter is disengaged and inserted into the left common carotid artery. This can often be achieved without the reinsertion of the wire.

Most often, the ostium of the left common carotid artery originates between the right brachiocephalic artery and the left subclavian artery in a standard Type 1 aortic arch as seen in Figure 28-3. In a Bovine arch, the left common carotid artery originates from the right brachiocephalic artery as seen in Figure 28-4.

The usual angles for imaging the left carotid system are LAO 30° to 40°, and LAO 90°; this allows separation of the bifurcation of the left internal and left external carotid artery.

For anterior cerebral circulation, LAO 90° and AP cranial 30° are taken of the entire skull, making sure to visualize the venous phase. If the suspected target of intervention is the right carotid artery, it is recommended to perform the angiography of the left carotid first to avoid cannulating the right carotid artery twice.

The circulating nurse continuously evaluates and ensures patient safety and notes any deviation from the baseline neurologic and hemodynamic assessment. After completion of the diagnostic imaging and identification of a significant carotid

Figure 28-3. Normal Type 1 aortic arch. 1: aortic arch, 2: rt brachio-cephalic artery, 3: left common carotid artery, 4: left subclavian artery, 5: left vertebral artery, 6: rt subclavian artery, 7: right common carotid artery, 8: right vertebral artery.

Figure 28-4. A Bovine arch: the left common carotid artery originates from the right brachiocephalic artery.

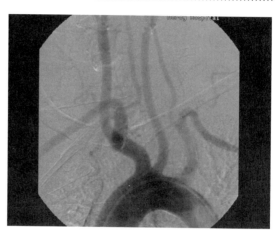

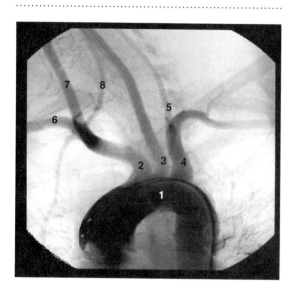

artery stenosis, if all parameters remain within normal limits, the interventional portion of the procedure may commence. Most often the diagnostic and interventional procedures are performed in the same setting.

INTERVENTION

The additional equipment needed for the interventional portion of the procedure includes a guiding catheter or 90 cm guide sheath, embolic protection device, a self-expanding stent, and an angioplasty balloon.

Depending on physician preference, a guide catheter or 90 cm guide sheath long enough to extend from the common femoral artery to the proximal portion of the common carotid is used. The use of traditional guide catheter techniques has fallen as companies have developed specialty guide sheaths with integrated hemostasis valves

for CAS procedures. The diagnostic catheter is exchanged for the guiding catheter or sheath with the use of a stiff exchange wire with a very soft tip.

Next, the embolic protection device is inserted. Devices for embolic protection may have an occlusive distal balloon, a basket filter, or a proximal occlusive balloon that is designed temporarily halt proximal flow. Distal protection is the most accepted technique currently. The most commonly used devices are usually a steerable .014-inch guide wire with a self-expanding filter basket at the end, designed to capture any debris that may become dislodged from the lesion during the intervention. Distal embolization of plaque debris places the patient at risk for development of a procedure-related neurologic event. Placement and use of the distal protection device does not hinder cerebral blood flow or perfusion. The distal protection device must be sized accurately. If the device is sized too small for the carotid artery, the risk of debris flowing past the basket resulting in transient cerebral ischemia or infarction exists. Correct placement of the basket is well distal to the target lesion, preferably in a straight portion of the artery, allowing room to safely pass the balloon and stent without the basket or wire moving during exchanges. Distal protection devices are discussed in greater depth in Chapter 17.

Predilatation can be performed to ensure that a stent delivery system can safely pass through the stenosis. Safe predilatation is done by undersizing the artery; if the lumen of the artery is 6 mm in diameter, the predilatation balloon should measure about 4 mm. The balloon is inserted over the distal protection device wire. Once the balloon is in position, the inflation device is attached, and the balloon is inflated to a nominal pressure. This should provide enough artery dilatation to safely pass the stent through the lesion. After predilatation, the balloon is removed from the patient.

The most common self-expanding stents are made of nitinol self-tapering and prefabricated tapered stents. When choosing the stent, the size of the common carotid artery proximal to the lesion, as well as the internal carotid artery distal to the lesion, must be determined. If the internal carotid artery appears to be the same size as the common carotid artery, a self-tapering stent is best. If the internal carotid artery is smaller than the common carotid artery, then a prefabricated tapered stent is preferable.

In regards to stent diameter, it is usually best to oversize the stent. Oversizing by 1–2 mm compared to the vessel size allows the stent to expand after postdilatation, decreasing the risk of migration. For example, if the vessel is 6 mm, an 8 mm stent is appropriate. The length of the stent is chosen in the same way; if the lesion length is 20 mm, a 30 or 40 mm stent is chosen. The stent should extend past both the proximal and distal portion of the lesion. When the stent is ready for deployment, it is optimal to initially deploy only one-third of the stent, and double check placement due to the fact most self-expanding stents tend to jump forward during deployment. If the physician is satisfied with stent placement,

the stent is then fully deployed, and the delivery system is removed.

Postdilatation is performed to ensure proper expansion of the stent and effectively dilate any remaining plaque against the wall of the artery. The size of the postdilatation balloon should be the size of the vessel at the distal deployment edge of the stent. Before inflating the balloon, make sure that the staff are ready and alert.

At this juncture, intravenous atropine sulfate can be given prophylactically to maintain the heart rate and counter the blood pressure drop normally seen during high-pressure balloon inflation. Intravenous fluids are open to the patient and prepped with a pressure bag. The balloon should be inflated quickly, monitoring both the patient's vital signs and the size of the balloon. Once full expansion of the stent has been achieved, the balloon is deflated immediately.

Before removing the balloon, angiography should be performed to ensure that no perforation or dissection of the vessel has occurred. The balloon is then carefully removed, followed by the distal protection device. With all devices removed, a final set of angiograms is performed in a minimum of two views. Poststent cerebral angiography should also be performed to ensure the patency of all vessels.

TEAM CONSIDERATIONS

The circulator performs a critical role during the procedure, responsible for the constant assessment of the patient. This assessment includes the patient's vital signs, neurological status, and identification of any procedural complications. The circulator also facilitates the smooth flow of the procedure, providing the physician and the scrub assistant with any needed equipment and communicating any pertinent patient information.

The circulator is also responsible for monitoring the patient's anticoagulation. Once the decision is made to proceed with carotid stenting, intravenous anticoagulation is given. Angiomax

(Bivalirudin) and unfractionated heparin are most commonly used. If heparin is used, the medication should be administered to achieve an activated clotting time (ACT) greater than 200 seconds. In one laboratory, the staff routinely use the IIb/IIIa antiplatelet medication Eptifibatide (Integrelin) in conjunction with heparin. Based on the patient's weight, a loading dose of Eptifibatide is given, followed by initiation of a 12-hour continuous infusion. Therefore, it is important to assess the patient continuously for signs of abnormal bleeding, such as hematoma at the insertion site. The ACT is tested 5 minutes after heparin has been administered, and every half hour thereafter, until the interventional portion of the procedure has been completed. Additional heparin may be needed to maintain the ACT.

Constant monitoring of the patient's heart rate and blood pressure during the procedure is imperative. The monitoring nurse or tech must be especially vigilant during stent implantation and postdilatation due to the sensitivity of the carotid baroreceptors. Stretching of the carotid baroreceptors during stent deployment commonly causes bradycardia or transient episodes of asystole. The circulator should be on alert and ready to administer intravenous atropine sulfate 0.6 mg to 1 mg for the treatment of bradyarrhythmias. Atropine is sometimes administered prophylactically to prevent severe bradycardia. The circulator should also be prepared to assist with transvenous or external pacemaker placement if necessary.

Blood pressure management is critical during carotid artery stenting. Extreme fluctuations in blood pressure increase the patient's risk of complications, so aggressive monitoring and maintenance of systemic blood pressure control is essential. Patients normally maintain an elevated blood pressure as a compensatory mechanism to deliver blood flow to brain tissue beyond the stenosis, thereby preventing ischemia. As the carotid baroreceptors get stretched and become irritated during the procedure, a reflex lowering of blood pressure (hypotension) can occur. At times, intravenous pressor support is instituted to maintain a systolic blood pressure greater than or equal to 80 mmHg. Swings from high to low blood pressure should be avoided. A sudden sharp rise in blood pressure once the stenosis is treated may cause cerebral hyperperfusion, resulting in seizures, cerebral infarction, and hemorrhage.[10] The goal postprocedure is to maintain a systolic blood pressure between 80 mmHg to 110 mmHg. Intravenous medication is given to maintain systemic blood pressure in this range.

POSTPROCEDURE CARE

Following the procedure, patients are monitored for 24 hours in a dedicated interventional unit or CCU. Patients receive oral antiplatelet therapy with aspirin (162 mg or 325 mg), clopidogrel (75 mg), and may receive continued intravenous therapy with Eptifibatide, for 12 hours postprocedure.

The sheath is usually removed immediately after the procedure, and when appropriate, a closure device is inserted into the common femoral artery. Otherwise, hemostasis is achieved via manual pressure or an alternative such as Femostop or C-clamp. Postsheath removal, the site should be thoroughly cleaned with a chlorahexidine or betadine solution and covered with a bandage (preferably a transparent dressing). If a pressure dressing is applied, it should allow the nursing staff to easily visualize the access site to quickly identify bleeding or a growing hematoma. Standard postcatheterization assessment of the procedure site and extremity is performed to identify and prevent any vascular complications.

After successful completion of the bed-rest restriction, patient can walk with supervision. The patient is still carefully monitored for any procedure site complications with ambulation. If bleeding or a hematoma is observed, the patient should return to bed, and manual pressure applied until hemostasis is again achieved. An ultrasound of the puncture site is performed to assess for the development of an arteriovenous fistula or pseudoaneurysm as a cause for any bleeding.

A neurologic assessment is added to the postprocedure observation regimen to evaluate for any signs and symptoms of neurologic impairment. Any variations from baseline are reported to the physician as well as the neurologist immediately.

Prior to discharge, the patient will receive information about their medication regimen and activity restrictions. For the first 2 weeks, the patient should refrain from moving his or her neck too quickly or too often, and refrain from heavy lifting > 5 lbs (2 kg). The procedure site should be monitored for signs of bleeding or infection. Also, the importance of blood pressure control, medication compliance, and signs and symptoms of neurologic impairment are reviewed. The importance of reporting any abnormalities to the physician is emphasized.

The patient will continue aspirin 162–325 mg and clopidogrel 75 mg for a minimum of 4 weeks along with statin therapy. Occasionally, aggrenox is used in place of clopidogrel for patients who have a documented history of recurrent TIA. Other medications are continued as appropriate. If the blood pressure remains low at discharge, the patient is told to hold their antihypertensive medications for 1 or 2 days.

If there are no complications, the patient is discharged the morning following the procedure.

Patients are seen within 2 weeks after the procedure and undergo routine carotid ultrasound surveillance at 6 months, 1 year, and then yearly thereafter. Rarely, in-stent restenosis occurs due to neointimal hyperplasia, and is most likely to occur within the first 6 months after carotid artery stenting.

SUMMARY

Carotid artery stenting is still in its infancy with rapid technique and device refinement. It is a safe and effective treatment option for appropriately selected patients.

REFERENCES

1. American Heart Association. *Heart Disease and Stroke Statistics—2006 Update*. Dallas, TX: American Heart Association; 2006.
2. Inzitar, D, Eliasziw M, Gates P, et al. The causes and risk of stroke in patients with asymptomatic internal carotid artery stenosis. *N Engl J Med* 2003;342:1693–1700.
3. Zarins CK. Carotid endarterectomy: the gold standard. *J Endovasc Surgery* 1996;3:10–15.
4. North American Symptomatic Carotid Endarterectomy Trial Collaborators. Beneficial effect of carotid endarterectomy in symptomatic patients with high grade carotid stenosis. *N Engl J Med* 1991;325:445–453.
5. Endovascular Versus Surgical Treatment in Patients with Carotid Stenosis in the Carotid and Vertebral Artery Transluminal Angioplasty Study (CAVATAS): a randomized trial. *Lancet* 2001;357:1729–1737.
6. Brooks WH, McCure RR, Jones MR, et al. Carotid angioplasty and stents verses carotid endarterectomy: a randomized trial in a community hospital. *J Am Coll Cardiol* 2001;38:1589–1595.
7. Wholey MH, Wholey M, Bergeron P, et al. Current global statistics of carotid artery stent placement. *Cathet Cardiovasc Diagn* 1998;44:1–6.
8. Yadav JS, Wholey MH, Kuntz RE, et al. Protected carotid-artery stenting versus endarterectomy in high-risk patients. *N Engl J Med* 2004;351:1493–1501.
9. Gurm HS, Yadav JS, Fayad P, et al. Long-term results of carotid stenting versus endarterectomy in high-risk patients (Sapphire Study). *N Engl J Med* 2008;358:1572–1579.
10. Al-Mubarak N, Iyer S, Roubin G. Procedural complications. In: *Carotid Artery Stenting: Current Practice and Techniques* (pp. 137–115). CITY, ST: Lippincott Williams & Wilkins; 2004.

Chapter 29

RENAL ARTERY INTERVENTIONS

Brenda McCulloch, RN, MSN, CNS

RENAL ARTERY STENOSIS

There are primarily two disorders that cause renal artery stenoses (RAS fibromuscular dysplasia (FMD) and atherosclerotic renal artery stenosis (AS-RAS). FMD accounts for about 10% of RAS, and is more common in females between the ages of 15 and 50. AS-RAS accounts for up to 90% of cases of RAS. The prevalence of AS-RAS increases with age, in patients with diabetes, aorto-iliac occlusive disease, coronary artery disease or hypertension. Renal artery stenosis may lead to systemic hypertension and kidney dysfunction. There is no observed gender difference. Patients can present with both FMD and AS-RAS but it is rare.

Other, less common, causes of RAS include renal artery aneurysm, arteriovenous malformations, neurofibromatosis, renal artery dissections, renal artery trauma, Takayasu's arteritis, and renal arteriovenous fistula.

Catheter-based interventions, such as renal artery balloon angioplasty and/or stenting, may be performed for patients with occlusive RAS.

Fibromuscular Dysplasia

FMD is a non-inflammatory, non-atherosclerotic disease involving the main renal artery and its branches. Its etiology is unknown. It may involve the intimal, medial, or adventitial layer of the vessel, but medial FMD is most common and accounts for the majority of cases.[1,2] It typically involves the middle and distal two-thirds of the main renal artery. It may involve the renal artery branches and it can occur bilaterally. The angiographic findings of medial FMD demonstrate a very characteristic "string of beads" appearance in the lumen of the artery (Figure 29-1). In FMD, complete occlusion is extremely rare.

FMD may also affect other arteries, including the carotid and vertebral arteries, and less

Figure 29-1. Fibromuscular dysplasia of the renal artery.

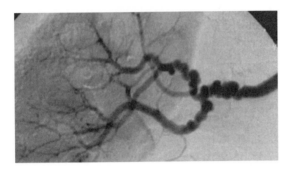

Figure 29-2. CT image of right renal artery stenosis. *Source:* Image courtesy of Siemens Healthcare.

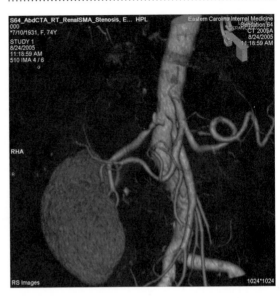

commonly, the iliac and mesenteric arteries. The cause of FMD is unknown; a genetic predisposition, smoking, hormonal factors, and disorders of the blood supply to the renal artery itself are some of the casual theories associated with the disease. Angioplasty alone should be performed for FMD. Technical success occurs in more than 90% of patients with medial FMD, and angioplasty results are usually long lasting.[3]

Atherosclerotic Renal Artery Stenosis

Atherosclerosis is by far the most common cause of RAS. Unlike FMD, AS-RAS is a progressive disease that can lead to a total occlusion of blood flow to the kidney. Most RAS lesions are aorto-ostial in nature, and bilateral RAS is common.[2] (see Figure 29-2). It is estimated to be the cause of end-stage renal disease in about 15% of the patients over age 50 who begin dialysis each year.[1] Patients older than 65 years of age and patients with documented lower extremity peripheral artery disease are more likely to have RAS. It remains controversial which lesions are associated with important clinical sequelae. With angioplasty alone, long-term improvement in blood pressure can be expected in only about 50%–60% of patients. AS-RAS requires stent

placement for optimal results, and the technical success for this is between 75%–95%.[1,2,3]

Clinical Manifestations

Patients with symptomatic renovascular disease present with significantly elevated blood pressure that is difficult to control, although it is not readily distinguishable from other forms of hypertension. Certain classic features, such as no known family history of hypertension, recent onset of hypertension, or the onset of hypertension before the age of 50, are more suggestive of renovascular hypertension than other forms of high blood pressure (see Table 29-1).[4] Blood pressure is frequently higher than 180/100 and may be resistant to multiple medications. Hypertension caused by renovascular disease is believed to affect 5%–10% of all hypertensive patients in the United States.[5]

Table 29-1. When to Suspect Renovascular Hypertension[1,6,7]

- Onset of hypertension is ≤ 30 or ≥ 55 years of age
- HTN is accelerated, resistant to treatment or difficult to control
- Unexplained renal dysfunction; kidney is atrophic or there is discrepancy in renal size (≥ 1.5 cm between kidneys)
- Patient developed elevated BUN and creatinine during ACE inhibitor therapy
- Epigastric bruit is detected
- Atherosclerosis is generalized; multivessel (≥ 2) coronary artery disease
- There is recurrent pulmonary edema; flash pulmonary edema

Diagnostic Assessment

Several diagnostic studies may be used to assess perfusion to the kidneys.

- Renal duplex ultrasonography (2-D imaging and Doppler) is a widely available screening test. While cost effective, it is technologist dependent. It provides important information about stenosis severity and kidney size.
- Renal angiography, comprised of both flush aortogram and selective renal angiography (see Figure 29-3), has been considered the gold standard for diagnosing renal artery stenosis, but is being replaced by the noninvasive modalities of magnetic resonance angiography (MRA) and computerized tomography angiography (CTA). For patients at high risk of contrast-induced nephropathy, the use of CO_2 or gadolinium rather than iodine-based contrast media may be an option for some patients undergoing renal angiography.
- Magnetic resonance angiography (MRA) is increasingly useful, but costly. It cannot

Figure 29-3. Selective right renal angiography demonstrating a 90% ostial lesion.

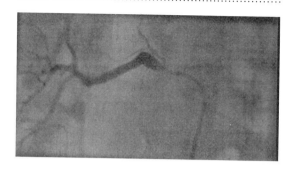

be performed on patients with ferromagnetic implants, which makes it difficult to image inside a stent to detect restenosis. Contrast-enhanced MRA (see Figure 29-4) is performed with gadolinium, which is a less nephrotoxic than conventional contrast media.

Figure 29-4. MRA image—normal renal arteries.

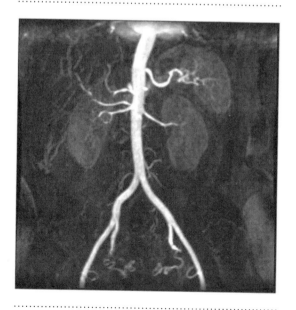

• CTA uses computerized X-ray images to construct 3-D images of the aorta and renal arteries (see Figure 29-5). It is less available and more expensive than duplex ultrasonography, and requires exposure to ionizing radiation and iodine-based contrast media, but metal images can be scanned.

• Renal nuclear scanning may be performed to assess overall glomerular filtration rate (GFR), and the differential GFR of each kidney; it is not recommended as a routine screening test.

Anatomy

The bilateral renal arteries (see Figure 29-6) arise from the lateral aspect of the descending aorta at the level of the first and second lumbar vertebrae. They lie just inferior to the origin of the superior mesenteric artery. The origin of the right renal artery is often slightly higher than the origin of

Figure 29-5. CTA 3-D reconstruction image of the aorta and renal arteries.

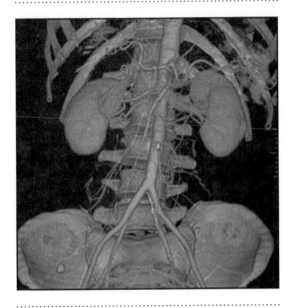

Figure 29-6. MRA showing normal renal arteries.

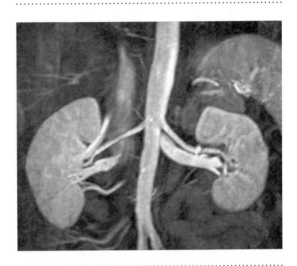

the left renal artery, and a number of variations in renal artery anatomy are regularly seen. The most common renal artery variant is the presence of an accessory renal artery (see Figure 29-7), which is a second and generally smaller artery that arises inferior to the main renal artery. More than one-third of patients have more than one renal artery supplying each kidney.[3] Occasionally, the accessory renal artery is as large as or larger than the main renal artery. Another renal artery variant is early subdivision of the main renal artery. Most accessory renal arteries supply the lower pole of the kidney and may arise anywhere from the suprarenal aorta to the iliac artery.

Treatment Options

Medical Therapy

Medical treatment of atherosclerotic renal artery disease is directed toward close follow-up, careful blood pressure control, antiplatelet therapy, and risk-factor management through careful control of blood sugar in diabetic patients, smoking cessation, lipid management, and weight reduction.

Figure 29-7. CT of aorta and renal arteries demonstrating an accessory renal artery to the right kidney. *Source:* Image courtesy of Siemens Healthcare. Sutter Medical Center, Sacramento CA.

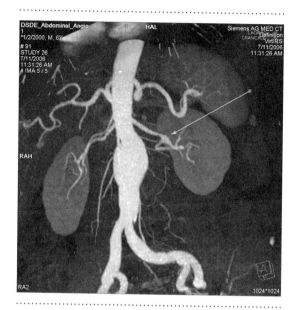

Angiotensin-converting enzyme (ACE) inhibitors may be indicated in the presence of renal stenosis. More aggressive management is required for patients with poorly controlled hypertension, heart failure, or renal insufficiency.

Surgery

Surgical management of RAS is limited to those patients who present with severe hypertension in spite of maximal medical therapy and ischemic nephropathy. Procedures that may be performed include endarterectomy, aortorenal bypass (the most common surgery performed for patients with renovascular disease), renal artery thromboendarterectomy, or renal artery reimplantation and nephrectomy.

Endovascular Therapy

Angioplasty of the renal artery was introduced in 1978 by Gruntzig and has continued to advance and surpass surgical revascularization. See Table 29-2 for indications for endovascular repair and revascularization.

Patients with FMD have good outcomes with renal angioplasty, with improvements or cure in most patients. In AS-RAS, percutaneous ballooning and stenting of renal artery atherosclerotic lesions have success rates of near 100% when performed by an experienced physician. Stents have become the favored mode of revascularization for ostial AS-RAS. Following stenting, the restenosis rate is $\leq$ 20%.[1] The optimal treatment of renal artery in-stent restenosis is still uncertain.

ENDOVASCULAR PROCEDURE

Preprocedure antiplatelet therapy with aspirin 325 mg and clopidogrel 300 mg may be administered to decrease the risk of platelet aggregation during the procedure, although there is little evidence that clopidogrel has short or long term benefit in renal intervention.[2] Many physicians continue the patient's blood pressure medication until the procedure is completed.[4] Vigorous periprocedural hydration should be administered

Table 29-2. Indications for Endovascular Repair/Revascularization of RAS[2,6]

Percutaneous revascularization is reasonable for patients with:
- Hemodynamically significant RAS and accelerated hypertension, resistant hypertension, malignant hypertension, hypertension with an unexpected unilateral small kidney, and hypertension with intolerance to medication.
- RAS and progressive kidney disease with bilateral RAS or RAS to a solitary functioning kidney.
- RAS and chronic renal insufficiency with unilateral RAS.
- Hemodynamically significant RAS and recurrent, unexplained congestive heart failure or sudden, unexplained pulmonary edema.
- Hemodynamically significant RAS and unstable angina.

and *N*-acetylcysteine may be administered in patients with documented renal insufficiency. A sodium bicarbonate infusion may also be beneficial in some patients with renal insufficiency.[2,3] The volume of contrast media administered should be monitored carefully.

Arterial access is generally obtained retrograde via the common femoral artery. If there is severe bilateral aortoiliac disease or if an abdominal aortic aneurysm is present, an antegrade approach, via the brachial artery, may be selected. The antegrade approach may provide better support for the guiding catheter for ostial lesions that are more inferior and posterior. 6F to 8F sheaths are most commonly used in renal interventions. Sheath selection depends on the site of vascular access (femoral, radial, or brachial), the size of the renal artery, use of adjunctive distal protection devices, and the balloon/stent profile. Because many patients with RAS also have aortic and/or aortoiliac disease, a longer sheath (25 to 45 cm) may be needed to minimize potential wire and catheter trauma during guide wire advancement and catheter exchanges.

After arterial access has been obtained, the patient is anticoagulated with unfractionated heparin (70 units/kg) or bivalirudin to achieve an ACT of 250–300 seconds. The routine use of IIb/IIIa inhibitors is not recommended in renal interventions, although they may be helpful in cases complicated by acute thrombus or distal embolization. Because renal arteries and their branches are prone to vasospasm and dissection, guide wires and catheters should be manipulated carefully. Some operators may opt to administer intra-arterial nitroglycerin into the renal artery before advancing the guide wire to decrease the risk of spasm.

Angiography

Prior to renal intervention, the patient should have a flush abdominal aortogram to obtain anatomic information about the location of renal artery ostia, the presence of high-grade ostial lesions, the presence of accessory renal arteries, the degree of aortic calcification, and the degree of aneurismal dilation of the abdominal aorta. An ostial or proximal lesion of the renal artery is better visualized by aortogram than by selective arteriography.[2] An aortogram will help the physician to decide what shape catheter to use and what supplies and equipment will be necessary for the procedure. A flush abdominal aortography, using digital subtraction angiography (DSA) and a large field of view image intensifier, can be performed by placing a pigtail catheter at the level of the first lumbar vertebra and injecting contrast material at a rate of 20 ml/second for a total volume of 6 to 12 ml. The left renal artery is often best visualized in AP orientation, while 15°–30° LAO orientation is best to visualize the right renal artery. Cineangiography should be performed long enough to allow visualization of contrast in the renal cortex to obtain information about kidney size and regional function. One disadvantage of flush aortography is the increased volume of iodinated contrast administered to the patient. Some operators may choose to dilute the iodinated contrast with heparinized saline to decrease the total volume of contrast to the patient.

Contrast medium choices include low-ionic or nonionic contrast media, gadolinium, or CO_2 imaging in place of contrast for those patients at high risk of contrast-induced renal failure.

Hemodynamic Assessment

Visual assessment of the stenoses may not be reliable in assessing the severity of the lesion. Pressure gradient measurements are often invaluable in determining the physiologic severity of renal artery stenoses. In the angiographically intermediate (50%–70%) stenoses, a translesional peak systolic pressure gradient of > 10–20 mmHg demonstrates renal parenchymal flow limitation.[2] Renal artery pull-back gradients are often inconsistent and nonre-producible, so they are not a true reflection of the translesional gradient. Accurate intra-arterial measurement of translesional pressure gradients can be performed using a dual-lumen catheter and two calibrated transducers to measure the gradient, or a proximal catheter and micro-manometer 0.014-inch pressure wire placed distal to the stenosis to measure the gradient.[2]

Material

Guiding Catheters

The choice of a guiding catheter depends on the anatomy of the aorta and the angle of the renal artery take-off, as well as operator preference. A 6F guiding catheter is commonly used, although 7F and 8F are not uncommon. A wide assortment of guiding catheter shapes may be used, including the IMA, JR4, renal standard curve (RSC), renal double curve (RDC), Simmons, visceral hook, Cobra, Cobra-2, Sos Omni Selective, and hockey stick shapes. Tight stenoses may be easier to cross with a reverse curve shape. Some operators may use a shuttle sheath or multipurpose catheter positioned just outside the ostium.[3] To prevent trauma to the aorta, the guiding catheter should always be advanced and removed over a guide wire.

Guide Wires

In renal interventions, 0.014- and 0.035-inch guide wires can be used, although many operators use 0.014-inch wires because most stent platforms, pressure wires, and distal protection devices take 0.014-inch guide wires. Wires should be nonhydrophilic to prevent renal branch vessel perforation and hematomas. Avoid stiff guide wires whenever possible, and be very conscious of the tip of the wire at all times to prevent injury to the kidney. Changes in the patient's respiration

can alter the angle of the renal arteries' take-off, so asking a patient to breathe in deeply may help the wire to negotiate the lesion.

Balloons

Optimal results are often obtained with angioplasty alone for FMD, but stenting is usually performed in AS-RAS. The average angioplasty balloon size is from 5 mm to 7 mm, and many operators use an initial balloon with a diameter that is 1 mm less than the measured diameter of the vessel for predilatation. Predilatation is commonly performed to decrease the inflation pressure necessary to fully deploy the stent. If the patient complains of severe pain in the ipsilateral flank during balloon inflation, the vessel may be overstretched, and the balloon should be immediately deflated.

Stents

Balloon-expandable stents are most commonly used in renal intervention. Stents placed in aorto-ostial lesions should cover the entire lesion with 1 to 2 mm extending into the abdominal aorta to completely cover any overhanging plaque.[2,3] The operator should confirm the stent placement in two views before deployment to avoid missing the ostium. Off-label use of various stainless steel and nitinol devices is common practice.

Typical stent sizes used in the renal artery range from 5 mm to 8 mm in diameter and 10 mm to 20 mm in length. Stenting the distal renal artery can make future surgical revascularization difficult or can damage branch vessels. High pressures of 10 to 14 Atm for poststenting dilatation pressures may be required. For patients with bilateral AS-RAS, a staged procedure may be planned or the operator may choose to intervene upon each lesion during the same procedure. Drug-eluting stents may play a future role in renal artery intervention; additional research is needed to elucidate their role (see Figures 29-8 to 29-11).

Figure 29-8. Initial angiographic image prior to renal intervention demonstrating bilateral renal artery stenosis. The patient's serum creatinine was 3.4 mg/dl. *Source:* Courtesy of Sutter Medical Center, Sacramento, CA.

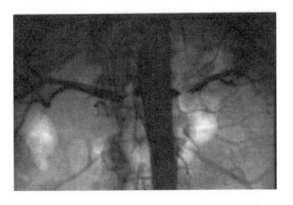

Figure 29-9. Balloon inflation proximal left renal artery.

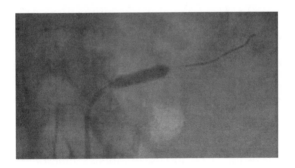

Figure 29-10. Stent deployed in proximal left renal artery.

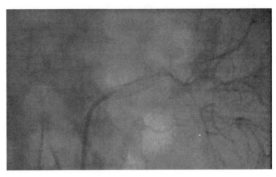

Figure 29-11. Renal ostium following stent deployment. After successful treatment of both renal arteries, the patient's serum creatinine stabilized at 1.7 mg/dl.

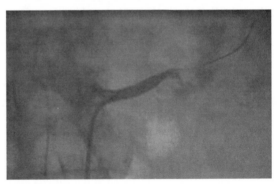

Postintervention Assessment

Angiographic success is defined as more than 30% stenosis reduction, or less than 50% residual stenosis, with normal brisk renal parenchymal arterial flow. Hemodynamic success has been defined as a post-intervention gradient of less than 10 mmHg.[8] Postprocedure angiographic assessment should include checking for distal embolization, residual thrombus, vessel perforation, and renal hematoma.

Intravascular Ultrasound

Intravascular ultrasound (IVUS) can be used in renal intervention. Pre-intervention, it is used to evaluate of lesion morphology, thrombus, atheroma burden, and vessel sizing. IVUS is useful for stenosis assessment, evaluation of in-stent restenosis, and stent thrombosis. After the intervention, it can be used for stent analysis (stent apposition, expansion, lesion coverage, confirmation of 1 mm to 2 mm extension into abdominal aorta for ostial lesions), and to detect dissection, thrombus, hematoma, perforation, and rupture.

Complications

Procedural complications have been reported in 5%–15% of cases (see Table 29-3). Access site bleeding and vascular complications (including hematoma, vessel injury, retroperitoneal bleed, pseudoaneurysm, arteriovenous fistula, and nerve injury) are the most common.

Periprocedural complications of renal artery angioplasty and stenting may include atheroma embolization or atheroemboli (cholesterol embolization), vessel rupture, and renal infarction. Atheroma embolization is more likely to occur following aggressive catheter or guide wire manipulation. Atheremboli can affect the kidney as well as the skin, intestine, myocardium, retina, and brain.

Distal embolization to the kidney may result in worsening renal function. Transient renal failure affects 2% of patients who undergo renal intervention, which may also be partially caused by the use of iodinated contrast media and occurs within 48 hours of procedure. Supportive care with adequate hydration may reverse the renal failure, and short-term hemodialysis may

be necessary in 1% of patients. The onset of cholesterol embolization may be insidious. Secondary livedo reticularis, or a red, blue, or mottled discoloration in the flank area, and splinter hemorrhages in the toes may be seen along with an elevated erythrocyte sedimentation rate and eosinophilia.[2]

Distal protective devices may be used in renal interventions and have been shown to collect significant amounts of embolic debris (small atheroma, cholesterol crystals, acute or chronic clots) in most cases. The embolic protection devices that are currently available were not specifically designed for renal arteries, and the use of the currently approved coronary devices may lead to undersizing of the filter.

Dissection or renal artery perforation is rare, but can occur with aggressive manipulation of guides and guide wire or oversizing of the balloon or stent. It may be more common in aneurysmal arteries. Artery dissection should be managed by repeated inflations of the balloon to control bleeding and reversing anticoagulation. If this does not stop the bleeding, a covered stent may be used. If attempts to control the perforation are unsuccessful, a vascular surgeon should be contacted and emergency nephrectomy or aortorenal bypass may be necessary.

Table 29-3. Complications of Renal Artery Interventions[1,2,3,4,9]

- Access site bleeding and vascular complications
- Distal embolization to renal artery
- Deterioration in renal function
- Cholesterol embolization to lower extremity circulation or to mesenteric circulation
- Renal artery dissection
- Renal artery/aortic perforation
- Renal infarction
- Occlusion or thrombosis of renal artery
- Perinephric hematoma
- Stent embolization
- Restenosis

Contrast-Induced Nephropathy

Contrast-induced nephropathy (CIN) is the worsening of renal function, typically with serum creatinine increases $\geq 25\%$ above baseline within 24–48 hours following contrast administration. The serum creatinine usually peaks within 3–5 days generally, and then returns to baseline within 7–10 days. CIN is the third leading cause of hospital-acquired renal failure; the risk of CIN ranges from 2%–30% and has significant impact on patient morbidity and mortality.[9] Short-term dialysis may be needed for some patients; rarely is long-term hemodialysis required.

The major risk factor for CIN is preexisting renal insufficiency, including diabetic nephropathy. Historically, serum creatinine has been used to assess the severity of renal impairment. The estimated creatinine clearance (eCrCl) or GFR are more accurate indicators of renal function than serum creatinine and may be used as a screening tool to assess risk. Patients at the highest risk are those with an eCrCl of < 60 mL. One equation commonly used to determine eCrCl is the Cockcroft-Gault formula in which the patient's gender, body weight, and serum creatinine is taken into consideration. Another formula, the Modification of Diet in Renal Disease (MDRD) formula, also factors in the patient's race and serum albumin and may be more accurate in the elderly or the obese patient.[9]

Various strategies used to decrease the risk of CIN include the use of low-osmolar or iso-osmolar contrast media, minimizing contrast volume, and intravenous hydration. The administration of N-acetylcysteine and sodium bicarbonate may be helpful also. Discontinuing certain medications, if possible, such as nonsteroidal antiinflammatory drugs (NSAIDS), aminoglycoside antibiotics, and antirejection agents is recommended. Additional strategies that may be beneficial include the use of theophylline, calcium channel blockers, ascorbic acid, prostaglandins, and hemofiltration, although additional clinical research is needed to determine their efficacy. Strategies found not to be of benefit to reduce the risk of CIN include the use of mannitol, furosemide, dopamine, atrial natriuretic factor, fenoldopam, and hemodialysis (see Table 29-3).[10]

Postprocedure Care

The care of the patient who has undergone renal artery stenting is similar to the care of the patient who has undergone other types of peripheral angioplasty. Because renal stenting is performed by

Table 29-4. Recommendations for Prevention of CIN[9,10,11]

- Identify patients at high risk.
- Withhold, if possible, NSAIDS and potentially nephrotoxic medications, such as aminoglycoside antibiotics and antirejection agents.
- N-acetylcysteine 600 mg orally every 12 hours × 4 doses, beginning precontrast administration.
- Avoid dehydration. Administer at least 1 L of normal saline beginning 3 hours before and continuing 6–8 hours after contrast administration.
- Sodium bicarbonate 154 mEq/L at 3 mL/kg/min starting 1 hour before and decreasing to 1 mL/kg/min following contrast administration.
- Use low or iso-osmolar contrast media and minimize volume of contrast media.
- Reassess serum creatinine 48 hours after contrast administration and consider holding medications such as NSAIDS and metformin, until serum creatinine normalizes.

percutaneous arterial access, careful monitoring of the access site is needed, along with regular assessment of distal pulses and circulation to the affected extremity.

The patient's blood pressure should be monitored carefully in the period immediately after the procedure, because significant hypotension can occur. Some operators may withhold all or some of the antihypertensive medications to prevent inadvertent hypotension which may be caused by renormalization of renal blood flow. Changes to the patient's antihypertensive medication regime will probably be necessary following the intervention.

Monitoring of urinary output is important, and follow-up testing of blood urea nitrogen (BUN) and creatinine levels is important to assess renal function.

Life-long aspirin therapy is prescribed at discharge and many operators may also choose to prescribe clopidogrel 75 mg daily for 1 month.

Patients need to be instructed on the importance of regular and continuing medical follow-up;

close monitoring of blood pressure is mandatory. Patients should be taught about risk factor reduction, including smoking cessation, if applicable.

Patients must be monitored for progression of renovascular disease and decline in renal function. Complications of untreated renovascular disease can include severely elevated blood pressure, stroke, renal insufficiency and failure, heart failure, retinopathy, and death.

SUMMARY

Renal artery intervention, including balloon angioplasty and stenting, may be an excellent option for many patients who suffer from hypertension and renal dysfunction due to fibromuscular dysplasia or renal artery stenosis. While procedural success is high and long-term results are good, attention to detail during the procedure is needed to prevent potential complications. Cath lab staff members play an important role in caring for these patients by ensuring administration of adequate hydration and anticoagulation/antiplatelet therapy, and meticulous monitoring of blood pressure, and maintaining optimal distal guide wire position during the procedure. Careful postprocedure assessment and monitoring is needed to detect hypotension, worsening renal function, or vascular complications.

REFERENCES

1. Guttormsen B and Gimelli G. Renal artery disease. In Dieter RS, Dieter RA, and Dieter RS, *eds. Peripheral Arterial Disease,* New York, McGraw Hill, 2009.
2. Hirsch AT, Haskal ZJ, Hertzer NR, et al. ACC/AHA guidelines for the management of patients with peripheral arterial disease (lower extremity, renal, mesenteric, and abdominal aortic). *J Am Coll Cardiol* 2005;47(6):1239–1312.
3. *Interventional Radiology Grand Rounds: Renovascular Hypertension.* Society of Interventional Radiology. Available at http://www.sirWEB.org. Accessed December 7, 2007.
4. Lin PH, Safaya R, Bohannon T. *Renal artery occlusive disease.* In Lumsden AB, Lin PH, Bush RL, and Chen C, *ed. Endovascular Therapy: Principles of Peripheral Interventions.* Malden, MA: Blackwell Publishing, 2006.
5. Reddy BK. Renal artery angioplasty and stenting. In: King SB, Yeung AC, eds. *Interventional Cardiology.* New York: McGraw Hill Medical; 2007.
6. Reginelli JP, Cooper CJ. Renal artery intervention. In: Casserly IP, Sachar R, Yadav JS, eds. *Manual of Peripheral Vascular Intervention.* Philadelphia: Lippincott Williams & Wilkins; 2005.
7. Rudnick MR, Kesselheim A, Goldfarb S. Contrast-induced nephropathy: How it develops, how to prevent it. *Cleve Clin J Med* 2006; 73(1):75–87.
8. Schweiger MJ, Chambers CE, Davidson CJ, et al. Prevention of contrast induced nephropathy: recommendations for the high risk patient undergoing cardiovascular procedures. *Catheter Cardiovasc Interv* 2007;69:135–140.
9. Sos, TA and Trost DW. Renal angioplasty and stenting. In Kandarpa, K, ed. *Peripheral Vascular Interventions.* Philadelphia: Lippincott Williams & Wilkins; 2007.
10. Valji K. *Vascular and Interventional Radiology,* 2nd ed. St. Louis, MO: Elsivier, Inc.; 2006.
11. White CJ. Renal artery stenosis: when and how to treat it. In: Heurser RR, et Henry M, eds. *Textbook of Peripheral Interventions.* London: Informa Health Care; 2004.

Acknowledgments
The author appreciates the contributions of Sutter Medical Center, Sacramento, California; Michael Fugit, MD; Sacramento Heart and Vascular Medical Associates; and Leslie Ferrini of Siemens Medical Solutions to this manuscript.

Chapter 30

LOWER EXTREMITY ANGIOGRAPHY AND INTERVENTION

Charles C. Barbiere, RN, CCRN, RCIS, CCT, CRT, EMT, FSICP

PERIPHERAL ARTERY DISEASE

Peripheral artery disease (PAD) can be defined as the obstruction of blood flow into an arterial tree excluding the coronary and intracranial circulations. Patients with PAD have obstructing plaques caused by atherosclerotic disease. These plaques frequently induce symptoms by obstructing blood flow or by breaking apart and embolizing atherosclerotic and/or thrombotic debris into more distal blood vessels.

This chapter is concerned with PAD in the legs (see Figure 30-1). Atherosclerotic disease in this part of the body leads to pain on walking, and, if untreated, may lead to amputation.

The treatment goals are to stop the progression of the disease, its associated morbidity, prevent the loss of limbs, and improve the functional capacity of symptomatic patients. This includes risk reduction through behavior modification, exercise prescriptions, and medical therapies.

In patients who are sedentary and where the plaque deposits accumulate slowly over time, there may be no (or minimal) symptoms despite complete occlusion. Due to collateral flow, many patients with PAD have no symptoms.

Diagnosis

By the time a patient has been referred for angiography, he or she should have undergone a series of noninvasive tests.

An ankle-brachial index (ABI) is performed by measuring the patient's blood pressure at the ankles and the arms while a person is at rest. Measurements are usually repeated on both sites after 5 minutes of walking on a treadmill. The ABI is calculated by dividing each ankle systolic pressure by the brachial systolic pressure. The patient is considered to have PAD if the value is less than 0.8 (see Table 30-1). Patients with scores

Figure 30-1. Arterial circulation of the lower extremity.

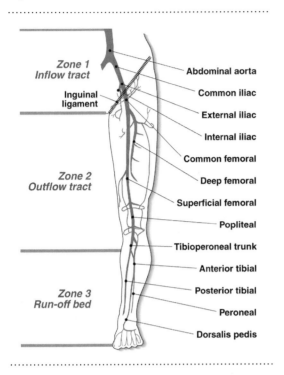

of less than 0.5 generally have rest pain, and a score of less than 0.3 is when tissue loss begins to occur. Scores greater than or equal to 1.0 are considered normal.

Doppler ultrasound gives accurate images of the structure of the blood vessels and measures the speed that the blood is flowing. It is commonly used in locating obstructions in peripheral arteries.

Computerized tomography (CT) produces 3-D images that are as accurate as those of conventional catheter angiography and is used for planning operations or endovascular therapies. Magnetic resonance angiography (MRA) is also considered a choice for visualization of the vessels. If percutaneous revascularization is planned, however, an angiography is performed prior to the interventional procedure, so this is the diagnostic mode of choice in patients who clearly require intervention.

ILIAC ARTERY DISEASE

When plaques around the aortic bifurcation and the iliac arteries become large enough, they can

Table 30-1.

ABI value	Interpretation	Action	Symptoms
> 1.2	Suggestive of severe Vessel hardening/ calcification from PVD; common finding in patients with multiple risk factors (ie., diabetes, smoking, family history)	Referral for assessment and monitoring	
1.0–1.2	Normal range	None	
0.9–1.0	Low Normal / Acceptable		
0.8–0.9	Early developing arterial disease	Aggressive management of risk factors	Pain, intermittent claudication
0.5–0.8	Moderate arterial disease	Referral for assessment of percutaneous or surgical intervention	Venous ulcers— use full compression stockings Mixed ulcers — use reduced compression stockings/ bandaging
< 0.5	Severe arterial disease	Urgent referral for percutaneous or surgical intervention	Arterial ulcers no compression bandaging used

reduce the amount of blood flowing into the legs. When the blood flow is reduced so much that the muscles in the legs do not get enough oxygen, the result is cramping pain, known as claudication. This usually occurs first in the calf muscles, then the thigh, hip, and into the buttock muscles. Intermittent claudication refers to cramping pains in the legs that are relieved with rest from exercise.

Impotence may occur with more extensive proximal lesions, and if distal embolization occurs, patients may present with "blue toe" syndrome. Obstructive lesions may be present in the infrarenal aorta, common iliac, internal iliac (hypogastric), external iliac, or combinations of any or all of these vessels.

Treatment Options

The traditional means of surgically treating occlusive iliac disease are aortoiliac thromboendarterectomy (TEA) and aortobifemoral bypass (AFB), with AFB being the more common procedure. Although highly effective, these surgical interventions are associated with a substantial procedure-related risk for the patient.

Balloon angioplasty and stenting is a less-invasive treatment option than surgery and has proven to be effective for short, focal, concentric stenosis of the common or external iliac artery. Patients with bilateral, long, severely stenotic, and/or occlusive disease are generally considered better candidates for aortofemoral bypass surgery. The use of stents in the iliac arteries has improved patency compared to angioplasty for focal disease, so many interventionists routinely implant stents during most, if not all, iliac interventions.

Most iliac balloon catheters and stent delivery systems are over-the-wire (OTW) systems, although rapid exchange (RX) systems are also available. OTW systems give added back-up support, which is very important with crossover procedures.

Endovascular Procedure

The procedure is performed in the angiographic cath lab after the patient has been assessed, informed, and prepared. Iliac artery lesions are approached from an ipsilateral approach, or from a contralateral retrograde approach, with the decision typically based on lesion location and physician preference (see Figure 30-2). Arterial

Figure 30-2. Arterial approach. (a) Right contralateral retrograde femoral puncture with a left femoral target; (b) Left ipsilateral antegrade femoral puncture; (c) Left axillary puncture with left femoral target; (d) Right ipsilateral retrograde popliteal puncture; (p) Puncture site.

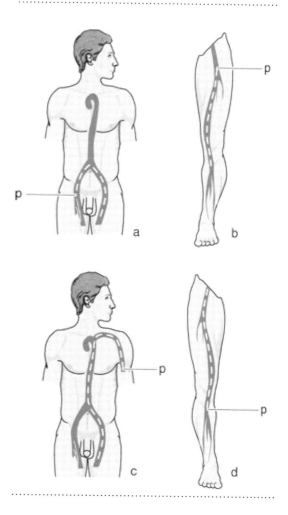

puncture is often performed with a micropuncture needle with ultrasound guidance.

Unlike coronary interventions, guiding catheters are typically not used; specialized sheaths with radiopaque marker bands, hemostatic valves, and "side-arm" tubing with stopcocks are used for iliac interventions. Angiography is performed through the sheath's side arm, and a roadmap is created. The operator will also look for a natural marker, such as a bone, that is visible without contrast media injection, to indicate the position of the lesion. Some operators will use radiopaque rulers or measuring tape for guidance. Semitransparent roadmaps (trace subtraction) may be superimposed on the live fluoroscopic image for guidance as well. The radiopacity of this roadmap may be adjusted to the operator's preference.

Balloon angioplasty is seldom used as a stand-alone procedure in the iliac arteries, but it is often used to pre- and postdilate stenting. Iliac stenting may be performed with either self-expanding or balloon-expandable stents. Self-expanding stents are preferred in most instances to avoid "crush injury" of the stents due to natural body movements.

Successful treatment of iliac lesions often requires the use of special techniques, such as the crossover and the kissing-balloon techniques. A crossover procedure is performed in many cases due to the proximity of the lesion to a possible ipsilateral access site. A crossover sheath reduces the procedure time and it allows for direct angiographic injections via the sheath. It is basically a long introducer sheath (about 40 cm in length) with a dilator and a curved tip to help cross the aortic bifurcation.

As with coronary bifurcation lesions, dilating an iliac bifurcation lesion with one balloon often partially shifts plaque material from the ballooned side into the other iliac artery. To prevent plaque shifting, iliac bifurcation lesions are usually treated using the kissing-balloon technique. Both sides of the groin are accessed with an intro-

ducer sheath, and two guide wires are advanced in a retrograde fashion, one from each side, crossed through the lesion(s), and positioned deep in the aorta. Two balloon catheters are positioned in the lesion(s), with their tips in the aorta. Both balloons are then inflated simultaneously, with their distal balloon sections touching ("kissing") each other (see Figure 30-3). Two stents can also be implanted in a similar fashion.

Following successful lesion treatment, final angiographic images are made including the distal runoff to exclude distal embolization caused by the procedure.

Complication rates after intervention are low, around 7%, and major complications at 3.4%. As with coronary arteries, larger plaque burden and total occlusions have poorer long-term outcomes. Restenosis rates vary and are dependent on patient lifestyle choices, in particular smoking cessation. Five-year patency rates of 90% are comparable to those of open surgical reconstruction.[1-4]

LOWER LEG DISEASE

Patients with acute ischemia present with a sudden onset of limb-threatening ischemia. Most are due a thrombotic or embolic process and are an exacerbation of preexisting disease. Patients with chronic ischemia may be asymptomatic, or the

Figure 30-3. Kissing balloons.

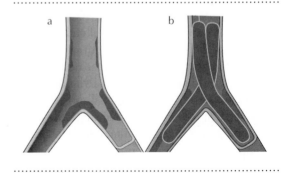

Figure 30-4. Example of peripheral arterial collateralization: occluded L popliteal artery revascularized by collateral vessels.

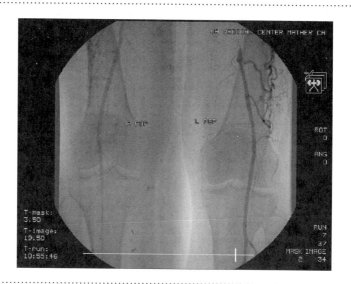

ischemia may threaten limbs, and gangrene may be present. As with all atherosclerotic diseases, the incidence and severity increase over time.

Patients are defined as having critical limb ischemia (CLI) if they have chronic ischemic pain at rest, ulcers, or gangrene that can be directly attributed to arterial occlusive disease. A large number of patients with documented occlusive disease remain without significant complaints (only 19%–22% with symptoms), due to collateralization.[5–7]

Findings from the patients' history and physical examination are confirmed by noninvasive studies, ultrasound, and sequential ABIs and are helpful in determining the level of involvement. Although other newer imaging modalities are gaining in popularity, however, contrast angiography remains the gold standard diagnostic technique.

Treatment Options

Treatment options include surgery or peripheral vascular intervention (PVI). Both options have advantages, but surgery is now more commonly reserved for patients for whom a PVI is not an option. When the decision has been made to treat, the first step is to obtain diagnostic angiograms to determine the best approach for the lesion: endovascular intervention or open surgical repair. All patients should be evaluated for their medical comorbidities, because a planned endovascular repair may convert to open technique after determining the extent of disease, technical difficulties, or due to complications.

Patients with PAD have a high occurrence of concomitant atherosclerotic coronary artery disease, and as a result have increased risk for major acute coronary events.

Endovascular Procedure

After consent has been obtained, the patient is made comfortable on the table. The use of cushions and rubber supports is common to keep the patient's legs stationary during the procedure. The patient is attached to an ECG, and other monitoring equipment as is deemed appropriate. The usual sterile table and catheter preparation is then carried out.

Using the optimal approach to SFA and infrapopliteal lesions is crucial to the success of the procedure. Choices include ipsilateral antegrade femoral puncture, contralateral retrograde femoral puncture, left axillary puncture, and ipsilateral retrograde popliteal puncture. Each has advantages and disadvantages. The choice is determined by the location of lesion, the vascular structures involved, patency of the various access sites, the tools available, and the operator's experience.

After arterial access has been obtained and a decision has been made to proceed with an intervention, an anticoagulant (commonly unfractionated heparin) should be administered to obtain and maintain an ACT above 250.

The following steps are the same as with a coronary procedure. The first goal is to cross the lesion with a guide wire. Guide wires with diameters 0.035 inch, 0.018 inch, and 0.014 inch are commonly used in these interventions. Once the wire is through the lesion, balloon angioplasty, stenting, cryoplasty, subintimal angioplasty, cutting balloon, or atherectomy is carried out.

Stents

Stenting is indicated for residual restenosis > 30 percent, as well as angioplasty complications including dissection and perforation. Primary stenting is commonly used for restenosis, ulcerative lesions, and occlusive lesions. Both self-expanding and balloon expandable stents can be used, although the more flexible self-expanding stents are favored in the SFA. Drug-eluting stents (DES) have been placed in BTK arteries, but their effectiveness has yet to be proven. It appears as though the restenosic mechanism is different to that of coronary arteries.

These systems are usually over-the-wire and come with a large selection of shaft lengths, as well as balloon (and stent) diameters and lengths.

Covered Stents/Stentgrafts

Covered vascular stents are metal stents that are covered with a microporous material. They are used to treat inadvertent punctures, traumatic atriovenous fistulae, vessel ruptures, and to exclude aneurysms of smaller vessels (iliac and infrapopliteal arteries). These are an essential item to have present in the laboratory for treatment of these procedural complications.

Cutting Balloons

The cutting balloon has longitudinally mounted microsurgical blades (atherotomes). As the balloon is inflated, the atherotomes are deployed into the vessel wall. When the balloon is deflated, the atherotomes are folded back into the balloon. Using the cutting balloon is thought to reduce elastic recoil, improve compliance of the diseased segment, and allow for lower balloon pressures, which is believed to reduce balloon trauma.

Subintimal Angioplasty

With this technique, the guide wire is passed around the lesion, between the vessel's intima and medial layers, and back into the "true" lumen distal to the lesion. After an angiogram has been obtained, angioplasty is then performed in this new subintimal track. It is not uncommon to stent any residual stenosis greater than 30% that resists angioplasty.[8,9] Subintimal angioplasty has wide acceptance for flush occlusions (no stump to start in), calcific lesions, chronic occlusions, and long lesions.

Atherectomy

Atherectomy is indicated for fibrocalcific lesions, where stent malexpansion and fractures are more common, diabetics with small vessels, and challenging femoropopliteal segments in which stenting is undesirable. Atherectomy in peripheral vessels has been performed with excellent short-term technical results, but long-term restenosis rates are not optimal.

Rotational Atherectomy

The Rotablator (from Boston Scientific of Natick, Massachusetts) uses a concentrically rotating diamond-dust–coated burr rotating at 150,000–200,000 rpm. The vessel lumen is as large as the burr size after the procedure. The Diamondback (from Cardiovascular Systems, Inc. of St. Paul, Minnesota) has an eccentric diamond-coated crown, and the debulking area grows larger as the speed of rotation is increased.

Cryotherapy

The PolarCath System (from Boston Scientific of Natick, Massachusetts) uses nitrous oxide to fill an angioplasty balloon. The nitrous oxide evaporates into a gas on entering the balloon, and the balloon expands, causing the vessel to dilate and cool to −10°C. This causes several physiological reactions that open the artery with less medial barotrauma than standard balloon therapies. The plaque cracks when it freezes, allowing for a more uniform dilation of the blood vessel than in standard balloon angioplasty. The rapid cooling also causes apoptosis, or programmed cell death, which minimizes the growth of new scar tissue that occurs during conventional angioplasty.

Superficial Femoral Artery Disease

The superficial femoral artery (SFA) is the longest artery in the body. It has two major flexion points where the artery is bent and twisted with every step we take, and the distal artery lies within a major muscle group, which compresses and stretches the artery whenever the leg is flexed. It is an area that attracts atherosclerotic deposits, particularly in patients with activity deficits.

Chronic atherosclerotic obstructions of the SFA can cause lifestyle-limiting claudication. Patients typically complain of exercise-induced pain in the calf, which resolves itself after a few minutes of rest. Ischemic pain at rest, or nonhealing ulcers occur only seldom. If present, significant infrapopliteal obstructions can usually be found as well.

The SFA is approached in a retrograde or antegrade fashion. It is common to use a micropuncture system to make the initial access on patients with poor pulses.

The staff should communicate with the operator prior to any procedure to ensure that the correct puncture site is indentified; it is not uncommon to approach complex femoral lesions from an upper extremity. The location of the lesion and the vascular structures will determine the therapeutic approach. The staff should be familiar with the laboratory's selection of sheaths wires and diagnostic catheters that are necessary for both antegrade and the more common retrograde approach (see Figure 30-5).

The contralateral retrograde femoral puncture is the most commonly used approach, and the preferred approach for common femoral artery, and high SFA lesions. The advantage is the low puncture-site complication rates and an uncompromised blood flow in the treated leg during postprocedural compression of the puncture site. The disadvantage is the need to "work around" the bifurcation.

The ipsilateral antegrade femoral approach provides a short, straight path to distal SFA lesions, but it is often difficult in obese patients. The left axillary, or brachial, puncture approach is possible for proximal femoral lesions if the contralateral iliac-femoral system is occluded. However, working from the arm is cumbersome and requires especially long wires, angiographic catheters, and balloon catheters. Such an approach also brings with it a risk of cerebral embolization, especially if conducted from the right side.

The ipsilateral retrograde popliteal approach provides a short and direct access to proximal SFA lesions, can facilitate recanalization of total occlusions, and can be also used in obese patients. However, the patient must be prone (lying on

Figure 30-5a and b. Arterial puncture technique.

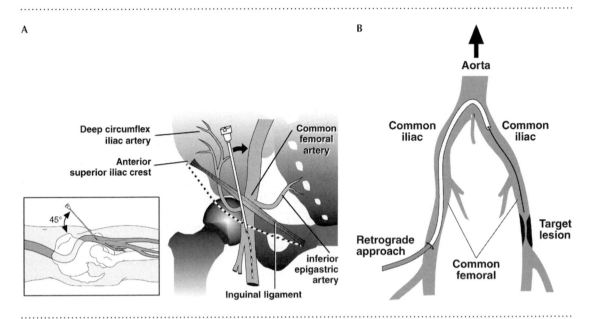

A

Deep circumflex
iliac artery

Anterior
superior iliac crest

45°

Common
femoral
artery

inferior
epigastric
artery

Inguinal ligament

B

Aorta

Common
iliac

Common
iliac

Retrograde
approach

Target
lesion

Common
femoral

his or her stomach), and arterial puncture is not always easy because of the close vicinity of the popliteal vein and nerve; it should be performed under ultrasound guidance.

Balloon angioplasty is a well-established treatment modality, with 90% technical successes rates for patients with lesions in the femoropopliteal segments with a 5-year patency rate between 38% and 58%.[10,11] As with coronary artery lesions, longer lesions, nonconcentric lesions, complex lesions, lesions with large plaque burdens, and total occlusions have lower technical success rates and lower 5-year patency rates.

A new generation of super-flexible, self-expanding stents have been used in the SFA with good results,[12] but it will take some years until it can be determined whether they bring long-term results superior to that of balloon angioplasty.

Infrapopliteal Artery Disease

This area includes all the arteries inferior to the popliteal artery, and is also known as below the knee (BTK). The current recommendations for balloon angioplasty are for limb salvage only. Angioplasty can permit enough blood to get to the lower leg and foot, allowing ischemic wounds to heal, and allowing the patient to ambulate to some extent. Cutting balloons, atherectomy devices, and new stents show some promise in improving clinical outcomes. As with femoropopliteal segments, the severity of the lesion greatly affects technical results and long-term outcomes.

Infrapopliteal lesions are rarely found in isolation; they are most commonly accompanied by lesions in the SFA and iliac arteries. Treatment is therefore a multilevel approach, with the more proximal lesions being treated first, followed by the more distal, infrapopliteal lesions.

Good flow in the BTK arteries is important for preservation of the lower extremities, and a good run-off supports the long-term patency and the clinical outcome after intervention in the upper leg arteries; an initially successful iliac artery revascularization will be quickly jeopardized if distal run-off is not ensured.

Complications

The type and nature of periprocedural and post-procedural complications are similar to those associated with coronary interventions. The staff should constantly observe for and be prepared to intervene by having the necessary drugs and devices readily at hand. One major difference is that failed peripheral interventions are much more easily converted to open surgical procedure than a failed coronary intervention. They are generally not immediately life or limb threatening, allowing additional time to consider other options.

Vessel spasm can occur during interventions in small vessels; nifedipine and nitroglycerin are used to prevent and treat it.

POSTPROCEDURE

After a satisfactory result has been reached, the guide wire, catheters, and sheath are removed from the patient. The puncture site is closed with manual compression or a closure device. Patients are typically placed on aspirin for life, and those who have received at least one stent are placed on additional antiplatelet agents (clopidogrel) for at least 6 weeks.

STAFFING

Experienced staff who have worked in a cardiac catheterization laboratory will have little difficulty acquiring the necessary knowledge and skills to ensure excellent technical outcomes and provide safe care to patients. Although the approaches and complications are similar, the devices can be used differently, and staff should become familiar with these differences prior to assisting in a peripheral procedure.

Currently, physicians from three different disciplines perform various peripheral diagnostic and interventional procedures: interventional radiologists, vascular surgeons, and cardiologists. As a result, each physician specialty has independently developed training, credentialing, quality assurance, and educational guidelines. The guidelines for each specialty should be benchmarks for physicians and laboratories in determining the appropriateness of individuals in each specialty to safely and effectively perform endovascular procedures.

REFERENCES

1. Onal B, Ilgit ET, Yucel C, et al. Primary stenting for complex atherosclerotic plaques in aortic and iliac stenosis. *Cardiovasc Intervent Radiol* 1998;21:386–392.
2. Treiman GS, Schneider PA, Lawrence PF, et al. Does stent placement improve the results of ineffective or complicated iliac angioplasty? *J Vasc Surg* 1998;28:104–112; discussion 113–114.
3. Bosch JL, Hunink MG. Meta-analysis of the results of percutaneous transluminal angioplasty and stent placement for aortic occlusive disease. *Radiology* 1997;204:87–96.
4. Timaran CH, Ohki T, Gargiulo NJ III, et al. Iliac artery stenting in patients with poor distal runoff: influence of concomitant arterial reconstruction. *J Vasc Surg* 2003;38:479–484; discussion 484–485.
5. Stoffers HE, Rinkens PE, Kester AD, et al. The prevalence of asymptomatic and unrecognized peripheral arterial occlusive disease. *Int J Epidemiol* 1996;25:282–290.
6. Dormandy JA, Rutherford RB. Management of peripheral artery disease (PAD). TASC Working Group. Trans-Atlantic Inter-Society Consensus (TASC). *J Vasc Interv Radiol* 1999; 10:723–731.
7. Rutherford RB, Becker GJ. Standards for evaluating results of interventional therapy for peripheral vascular disease. *Circulation* 1991;83(suppl 2):S6–S11
8. Lipsitz EC, Ohki T, et al. Does subintimal angioplasty have a role in the treatment of severe lower extremity ischemia? *J Vasc Surg* 2003;37:386–391.
9. Treiman GS, Whiting JH, Treimal RL et al. Treatment of limb-threatening ischemia with percutaneous intentional extraluminal

recanalization: a preliminary evaluation. *J Vasc Surg* 2003;38:29–35.

10. Johnston KW. Femoral and popliteal arteries: re-analysis of results of balloon angioplasty. *Radiology* 1992;183:767–771.

11. Hunink MG, Donaldson MC, et al. Risks and benefits of femoropopliteal percutaneous balloon angioplasty. *J Vasc Surg* 1993;17:183–194.

12. Mewissen MW. Self-expanding nitinol stents in the femoropopliteal segment: technique and mid-term results. *Tech Vasc Interv Radiol* 2004;7:2–5.

SUGGESTED READING

Hertzer NR, Beven EG, Young JR, et al. Coronary artery disease in peripheral vascular patients. A classification of 1000 coronary angiograms and results of surgical management. *Ann Surg* 1984;199:223–233.

Heuser RR, Henry M, eds. *Textbook of Peripheral Vascular Interventions.* New York: Informa Health Care; 2004.

Bonnett R, Heuser RR, Biamino G. *Peripheral Vascular Stenting,* 2nd ed. New York: Taylor & Francis; 2005.

Lumsden AB, Lin PH, Bush RL, Chen C. *Endovascular Therapy Principles of Peripheral Interventions.* Malden, MA: Blackwell Futura; 2006.

Norgren L, Hiatt WR, Dormandy JA, et al. Inter-Society Consensus for the Management of Peripheral Arterial Disease (TASC II) on behalf of the TASC II Working Group. *Eur J Vasc Endovasc Surg* 2007;33:(Suppl 1): S1-75.

Chapter 31

Abdominal Aortic Aneurysm Repair

Matin Ghorbati, MS, RN

ABDOMINAL AORTIC ANEURYSM

An abdominal aortic aneurysm (AAA) is a common, potentially life-threatening condition. The majority of AAAs are believed to be due to a degenerative process of the abdominal aorta which is often attributed to atherosclerosis. The incidence of AAA in the adult population is 2%–4%, and it is five times more common in men than in women and more than three-fourths of patients with AAA are older than 60.[1]

An aneurysm is a focal dilatation of a blood vessel with the cross-sectional vessel diameter measuring at ≥ 50% than the normal adjacent arterial diameter. The abdominal aorta is aneurismal when the aortic diameter measures ≥ 3 cm. Generally, an AAA enlarges gradually at a rate of 0.2 mm to 0.8 mm/year. If untreated, AAAs will eventually rupture.[2]

The aortic wall contains smooth muscle, elastin, and collagen, which are arranged in concentric layers. This combination helps to withstand the high arterial pressure. A gradual reduction in collagen and elastin content is noted in the aorta from the proximal to the distal aorta. Elastin fragmentation and degeneration, mainly caused by atherosclerosis, is thought to be responsible for the structural weakening of the aortic wall and the loss of recoil capability.

Degenerative aneurysms account for more than 90% of all infrarenal AAAs.[2] Other causes of aortic aneurysms include infection, cystic medial necrosis, arteritis, trauma, inherited connective tissue disorders, and anastomotic disruption.

Diagnosis

The majority of AAAs present without symptoms. Frequently, an AAA is discovered as an incidental finding during diagnostic testing for an unrelated problem. Physical examination for the detection of an AAA can be limited by patient obesity. A large AAA may be discovered by the patient because they may notice a pulsatile mass in their abdomen, and seek medical consultation.

When an AAA becomes symptomatic, it can have catastrophic results. Constant back, flank, or groin pain due to pressure on adjacent organs and structures may signal the presence of an abdominal aortic aneurysm. Distal embolization from the debris within the AAA can result in the development of cyanosis and mottling of the lower extremities with leg rest pain and gangrene. Total thrombosis of the AAA, although rare, results in acute lower extremity ischemia. Rarely, large AAAs may cause gastrointestinal symptoms such as indigestion, early satiety, abdominal distension, and constipation. An AAA near the aorta's renal branch can cause signs and symptoms like those of renal colic. An AAA may erode into the vena cava, causing a large arteriovenous fistula resulting in tachycardia, congestive heart failure, leg swelling, renal failure, and peripheral ischemia.

An aortic aneurysm is best identified with a variety of imaging tests:

- A chest X-ray or ultrasound is commonly used for screening patients.
- CT scanning with 3-D reconstruction can be useful for planning an intervention.
- Contrast medium-enhanced aortography may be ordered if embolization of accessory renal or internal iliac arteries will be done prior to the procedure.

Treatment

A stable asymptomatic AAA with a diameter less than 5 cm is usually monitored with periodic imaging such as abdominal ultrasound or CT scanning. Conservative measures such as smoking cessation and blood pressure control are also included in the treatment plan.

Rapid growth of an abdominal aortic aneurysm is an increase in diameter of ≥ 1 cm/year[3]

warrants elective repair. The risk/benefit ration of a rapidly enlarging increasing AAA favors repair. Abdominal aortic aneurysms are generally repaired once they reach 5 cm.

Surgical Repair

Surgical repair of an aortic aneurysm involves either a transperitoneal incision or a retroperitoneal approach. The surgeon cross-clamps the aorta and opens the aneurysm sac securing a synthetic PTFE or Dacron graft proximally and distally. The proximal anastomosis is placed near the renal arteries to avoid subsequent aneurismal dilation of the residual infrarenal aorta. The distal anastomosis is sewn into either the iliac or femoral arteries. The aneurysm sac is then wrapped around the graft to isolate it from the small intestine, to prevent the development of an aortoenteric fistula.

Complications of surgical AAA repair include pneumonia (2%–5%), myocardial infarction (2%–5%), groin infection (less than 5%), and graft infection (less than 1%).[2] Cross-clamping the aorta may result in distal embolization, renal or bowel ischemia, or hemodynamic changes. During the operation, cardiac workload and myocardial oxygen demands are increased. Releasing the clamp restores perfusion but also triggers release of toxins such as oxygen-free radicals into the systemic circulation which may result in reperfusion injury.

Elective surgical repair of AAA has a mortality rate of approximately 8%, however, repair of a ruptured AAA has a high mortality rate, approaching 50%.[2]

Endovascular Repair

Endovascular aneurysm repair (EVAR) is an alternative to open surgery for the treatment of AAA. The stent grafts have evolved from simple tubular endografts to more complex bifurcated designs with a variety of proximal and distal fixation designs. The safety, efficacy, and utility of this technique continue to be under investigation.

EVAR does not require cross-clamping of the aorta, and therefore reduces cardiac complications. Blood loss is minimal with EVAR, and it results in a decrease in the length of hospitalization, and a shortened postoperative EVAR recovery period for the patient.

Contraindications

EVAR is an alternative to open surgical repair for patients considered to be a high perioperative risk or who have multiple comorbidities. Unfortunately, EVAR is not always feasible due to the anatomical characteristics of the aneurysm or its proximity to the renal arteries. An adequate length of healthy, nonaneurismal aorta must exist for secure proximal attachment of the endograft. Excessive torturosity or angulations of the aorta may affect the ability to deploy the endograft successfully. Small or occluded femoral or iliac arteries may prevent passage of the stent delivery system. Some of these anatomic challenges can be overcome using a hybrid approach to AAA repair, combining both open and endovascular techniques.

Complications

Complications of EVAR can include distal embolization from plaque or thrombus dislodged by the use of guide wires and graft delivery systems. Vessel injuries at the access sites may also occur.

Endoleaks are a frequent finding after EVAR. An endoleak is blood flowing into the aneurysm sac after exclusion of the aneurysm sac with an endovascular stent graft.

Endoleaks

Exclusion of the aneurysm sac is the main goal of the stent-graft treatment, and clinical success is defined by the "total exclusion" of the aneurysm.

However, at times, failure of the stent-graft to totally exclude blood flow to the aneurysm sac may occur. Sources of endoleaks include blood flow from the lumbar arteries and inadequate proximal or distal fixation of the stent graft, allowing blood to flow into the aneurysm sac rather than through the stent graft, modular limb disconnection, or graft porosity (10% to 44%). Endoleaks are the major cause of complications, and thus failure of the endoluminal treatment of AAA. When an endoleak occurs, it causes continued pressurization of the aneurysm sac and may leave the patient at risk of an AAA rupture.

An endoleak is defined as a persistent blood flow outside the lumen of the endoluminal graft, but within an aneurysm sac or adjacent vascular segment being treated by the device. Endoleaks that are identified on follow-up CT scanning are initially monitored with additional CT scans and usually resolve without intervention. A persistent endoleak with aneurysm sac volume increasing will usually require an intervention to rectify it.

Endoleaks are classified in four types:

Type I: Blood flow into the aneurysm sac due to incomplete seal or ineffective seal at the end of the graft. This type of endoleak usually occurs in the early course of treatment, but may also occur later.

Type II: Blood flow into the aneurysm sac due to opposing blood flow from collateral vessels.

Type III: Blood flow into the aneurysm sac due to inadequate or ineffective sealing of overlapping graft joints or rupture of the graft fabric.

Type IV: Blood flow into the aneurysm sac due to the porosity of the graft fabric, causing blood to pass through from the graft and into the aneurysm sac.

The nurse should watch the patient's hemodynamic and mental status carefully. The symptoms of a large endoleak are basically those of shock from blood loss. Careful and frequent assessment of patient's abdomen for sudden pain, distension, and pulsatile mass are also essential if an endoleak is to be diagnosed in a timely fashion.

Postimplantation syndrome is an ill-defined noninfectious phenomenon following EVAR, occurring in up to 50% of patients.[4] It is considered to be an inflammatory reaction to the stent graft. It usually manifests as an increase in the white blood cell count accompanied by fever and can persist up to 10 days.

Additional complications include stent graft occlusion (3%–19%) and stent graft infection (0.4%). Although rare, colon necrosis or renal failure may occur as well as aortic dissection and infection.[4] The mortality rate of endovascular repair of AAA is about 8%.[2]

ENDOVASCULAR ANEURYSM REPAIR

Material

Fluoroscopy equipment with a mobile C-arm image intensifier is required for the procedure. EVAR can be performed in the operating room or CCL.

Endovascular AAA stent-graft systems have a two piece design including a catheter with the trunk and one graft limb, and another with the contralateral graft limb. Aortic endovascular stents are predominantly made of self-expandable Nitinol, which is characterized by elasticity and thermal shape memory. Nitinol stents are MRI safe.

The material covering the stent must be rigid enough to resist kinking, yet flexible enough to follow arterial angulations. The graft material is usually a combination of conventional polyester and polytetrafluoroethylene (PTFE).

Stent grafts are delivered into the vascular tree using introducer sheaths, trocars, deployment capsules, and retractable covers. Other essential accessories for the procedure are floppy to superstiff guide wires, angiographic and guiding catheters, dilatation balloons, a snare, and a power injector.

Preprocedure Care

Preprocedure care focuses on the physical, emotional, and psychosocial preparation of a patient. Explanations of the procedure and what the patient may experience must use language targeted to the patient's educational level and degree of anxiety. Concise explanations of the procedure delivered in a calm and organized manner may help reduce the patient's level of fear and anxiety. The patient's expectations should be discussed and all questions answered.

Preoperative diagnostic evaluation should include a baseline electrocardiogram, chest X-ray, and blood tests. Preprocedural baseline BUN and creatinine are essential. Contrast dye is used during the EVAR procedure, and protective measures should be taken to prevent further renal damage in patients with compromised renal function.

Nursing assessment includes a thorough physical examination including peripheral pulse examination. Appropriate measures to maintain a normal blood pressure should be instituted.

Procedure

The patient is prepared as if for a bilateral diagnostic cardiac catheterization. The patient's EGC and blood pressure are monitored continuously. Oxygen saturation is measured via pulse oxymetry during the procedure.

The procedure requires constant assessment of the patient's vital signs, neurological status, peripheral pulses, neck veins, sensation and motor activity of the extremities, and cardiac rhythm. It is also necessary to assess the patient for clinical manifestations of cardiac tamponade: tachypnea, dyspnea progressing to air hunger, oliguria, hypotension, leading to symptoms of poor perfusion, pulsus paradoxus, and elevated jugular vein pressure.

According to the strategy of the center and the patient's general condition, premedication with mild sedatives may be given. The procedure can be performed under general, regional, or local anesthesia. An anesthetist is usually present for the procedure, and they will monitor the patient's hemodynamic status.

The EVAR procedure (see Figure 31-1) begins with bilateral femoral artery access being established with introducer sheaths, usually 18F. An angiogram is performed above the renal ostium with a pigtail catheter to define the aortic anatomy.

Before insertion of the stent graft, and under sterile conditions, the device is flushed to prevent air bubbles in the system. All material is prepared following strict aseptic technique (Figure 31-1).

A guide wire is passed through the contralateral femoral site into the aortic arch.

The compressed stent graft inside the delivery catheter is passed over the guide wire and posi-tioned in the aorta. Angiography is performed to ensure that the proximal part of the stent graft is just distal to the lowest renal artery after which the pigtail catheter is removed. The main body of the stent graft and its ipsilateral limb are deployed. The stent-graft delivery catheter is withdrawn from the sheath.

Most stent grafts are self-expandable. In some cases, balloon catheters are positioned and inflated at either end of the stent graft to ensure attachment of the stent and reduce the occurrence of endoleaks.

A guide wire is passed from the other femoral sheath through the stump in the stent graft. The contralateral limb of the stent graft is compressed inside the delivery catheter and is passed over the guide wire and positioned so its distal end is within the stump. The contralateral limb of the stent graft is deployed. Balloon inflation of this limb may be also be performed.

Figure 31-1. AAA stent graft procedure. *Source:* Adapted from Euro PCR 04, Marco, Jean et al. The Paris Course of Revascularization, 2004, p.378.

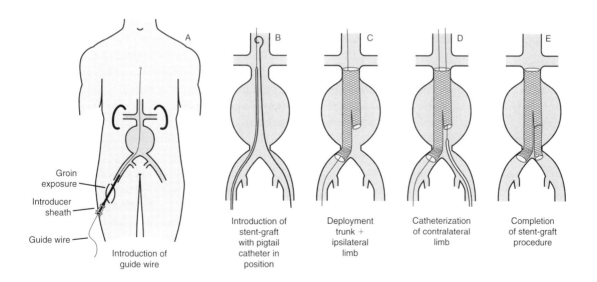

An aortogram is performed on completion of the procedure to document successful deployment of the endovascular stent graft and to identify the presence of immediate endoleaks.

Postprocedure

After successful deployment of the stent graft, the introducer sheaths are removed, and manual compression or vascular closure devices are used to achieve homeostasis. Complications occur in about 5% of cases when closure devices are used; they include leg ischemia, infection, and bleeding.[5] After achieving homeostasis, the patient may be transferred to the surgical ward or to an intensive care unit.

The postprocedure nursing assessment includes vital signs, inspection of insertion sites, peripheral pulse examination, and neurovascular assessment. This assessment is performed every 15 minutes for 1 hour, followed by every 30 minutes for 1 hour, and then hourly for 4 hours. If the patient remains stable after this initial postprocedural assessment, the nursing assessment should be performed at a minimum of once every shift until discharge.

A change in peripheral pulse examination from the patient's preprocedure assessment suggests peripheral circulation compromise and the surgeon must be alerted immediately. The patient may suddenly experience pain in the lower abdomen or both lower extremities with signs of poor perfusion. Prolonged peripheral ischemia may lead to limb loss.

Monitoring the patient's blood pressure and maintaining a minimum mean pressure of 70 mmHg ensures adequate perfusion to the major organs. Careful infusion of IV fluids such as lactated Ringer's, 0.9% sodium chloride solution, or blood products can help stabilize blood pressure.

Maintain a calm patient environment. Environmental stressors increase myocardial oxygen demand and can trigger catecholamine release, leading to hemodynamic changes.

Precise positioning of the stent graft below the renal arteries is determined during the completion angiogram; however, if the stent graft occludes renal blood flow acute tubular necrosis and renal failure will occur. Also, the contrast medium used during the endovascular AAA repair may result in renal damage, so accurate measurement and recording of the patient's intake and output is critical. Blood tests including BUN and creatinine are important indicators of glomerular filtration. Urine output of 50 ml/hr indicates adequate renal perfusion.

Postprocedure pain may be experienced by the patient at the insertion sites. Some patients may describe a vague, general abdominal discomfort that may be due to postdilatation syndrome. Pain self-report tools are useful to assess the patient's pain level. All complaints of pain should be evaluated thoroughly to determine its cause before treatment.

Opioids are often used for postprocedural pain management. These drugs may cause respiratory depression, therefore, respiratory rate and effort in addition to oxygen saturation should be closely monitored.

The risk of myocardial infarction following EVAR is about 2%–5%,[2] so continuous ECG monitoring, serial 12-lead ECGs, and lab tests including cardiac biomarkers are prescribed postprocedure. Preoperative cardiac medications should be resumed as soon as possible.

Any sign or symptom suggestive of infection needs to be thoroughly evaluated. If an infection is confirmed, appropriate antibiotic therapy should be prescribed.

Hematoma formation, retroperitoneal bleeding, arterial thrombosis, arteriovenous fistula, and pseudoaneurysm can all occur during an EVAR. The patient should be assessed for lumbar or groin pain, a significant drop in hematocrit, hypotension, pulsatile mass in the groin, bruit, decreased temperature of the extremity, loss of pulse, color changes, decreased sensation, and motor function.

Anticoagulation is monitored with ACT. Heparin is administered at 100 iU per kilogram IV. The goal indices are about 275 to 300 seconds. ACT levels below 250 seconds have been associated with thrombotic complications.[5]

Patients are discharged with their usual medications, along with a prescription for pain medication and stool softener. If some other event occurred during their hospitalization and additional medications were prescribed, they are to be included in their discharge prescription.

Follow-Up

A comprehensive follow-up program is important after EVAR to detect complications. Periodic imaging studies including CT scans and abdominal X-rays are important to assess for endoleaks, graft migration, and graft integrity. These studies are typically obtained at 1, 6, 12, and 18 month intervals and then annually.

SUMMARY

Tremendous technological advances have been made in endovascular repair of AAA, but a successful procedure is highly dependent on careful, detailed imaging for both treatment and execution, an ethical patient selection, a strictly sterile procedure, and thorough nursing care plan. Awareness and understanding of possible complications should help ensure a safe, successful procedure. The nurse's alertness to these clues and early intervention with reassurance or appropriate treatment may help to prevent more serious events for this promising new catheter-based approach.

REFERENCES

1. O'Connor RE. *Aneurysm, Abdominal*. 2009. Available at: http://www.emedicine.com/article/756735-overview. Accessed November 13, 2009

2. Pearce WH. *Abdominal Aortic Aneurysm*. 2009. Available at: http://www.emedicine.com/MED/topic3443.htm. Accessed November 13, 2009.

3. Dean RH, Yao JST, Brewater DC. Current diagnosis and treatment in vascular surgery. *Lange* 1995;(507).

4. Mita T, Arita T, Matsunaga N, et al. Complications of endovascular repair for thoracic and abdominal aortic aneurysm: an imaging spectrum. *Radiographics* 2000;20(5):1263–1278.

5. Woods SL. Sivarajan Froelicher ES, Underhill Motzer S, Bridges EJ *Cardiac Nursing*, 6th ed. Baltimore Lippincott Williams & Wilkins; 2005.

SUGGESTED READING

Irwin GH. How to protect a patient with aortic aneurysm. *Nursing* 2007;37(2):1–13.

Kalman P G. Stent-graft repair for abdominal aortic aneurysm. *MNAJ* 1999;2:1133.

Chapter 32

FOREIGN BODY RETRIEVAL

Sandy Watson, RN, BN, NFESC

The retrieval of foreign bodies from a patient's vascular system is, thankfully, a procedure that seldom needs to be performed. The materials used in the manufacture of modern intravascular equipment are strong and have been subjected to stringent testing. All the same, stents do occasionally slide off the balloon before placement, and guide wires do get caught and unravel. This chapter will give a brief state-of-the-market overview of the commonly available object-retrieval equipment and the few nursing considerations that accompany their use.

The techniques involved in intravascular foreign body retrieval are as varied as the objects to be retrieved and the vascular spaces in which they can be found. Literature describes the retrieval of objects as varied as embolization coils,[1] Swan-Ganz catheters,[2] laparotomy sponges,[3] ruptured balloons,[4] a TEC cutter head,[5] guide wire coating[6] and, of course, many stents.[7] In fact, just about anything that can be placed in the vascular

system has the potential to come loose and require retrieval.

A few points concerning how not to leave objects in a patient's vascular system are worth making.

- If a catheter becomes twisted or knotted during manipulation, pull it out and begin again with a new one. Today's thin-walled catheters are strong, but their limits can be reached. The cost and time associated with catheter replacement is nothing compared to retrieval of its distal end from the aorta or a coronary artery.
- If a crimp-on stent is being used, ensure that it is firmly in place. Premounted stents should also be checked before insertion.
- Insert guide wires through needles; do not advance needles over guide wires. This can lead to shearing off the guide wire's coating.

- If a guide wire becomes caught in a distal branch, try to free it using the (uninflated) balloon catheter. If this does not work, try to free the distal end with one of the devices described in this chapter before it becomes disengaged from the main body. Pull on it to its limit, but do not cause the wire to unravel, as this makes it much more difficult to remove than if it is still intact.

Despite good technique and the best intentions, objects do become disengaged. If the following points are observed, the retrieval procedure and the patient's recovery will be somewhat easier.

- Always follow strict aseptic technique in the lab. Then if an object cannot be removed and poses no danger to the patient, it should not be responsible for an infection.
- When choosing a stent, select one that is at least moderately radio-opaque. Looking for a lost stent can be very frustrating, and this is made more so if it is practically transparent.
- If an object becomes disengaged, try to stabilize it immediately with whatever material is already in the vessel. This may mean just sliding the guide wire through the stent, or inflating the balloon to a low pressure to trap the end of a guide wire against the vessel wall. Another sheath can be inserted if it is then necessary to position a retrieval device. Once an object is loose in the vascular system it can be very difficult to find, and may lodge in a less accessible place than where it first became loose.
- If the proximal end of a guide wire has been grasped with a device, be gentle while trying to dislodge it. Rough treatment may result in further breaking up

of the object, requiring several retrieval procedures.
- If possible, use the X-ray equipment with the best resolution to lessen frustration while searching for the object. Biplane equipment is recommended where available, as catching small objects with these small devices can be very tricky, especially if only two dimensions are available.
- Know your team's limitations and be prepared to call for surgical assistance before the patient is in danger. Much interventional material is thrombogenic in a disengaged state, and thrombus formation can be life-threatening.
- Catching an object and bringing it to the periphery is one thing, but it is often not possible to bring it out through the sheath. It is sometimes necessary to resort to surgery for this last stage of removal. Ensure that the surgical team is informed beforehand for a smooth conclusion to the procedure.

INSTRUMENTS

Due to the infrequency of foreign object retrieval, the range of products to perform this procedure is quite limited. The following are all widely available and have been extensively used in a wide variety of situations.

Amplatz Goose Neck Snare

As the name suggests, the Amplatz goose neck snare (ev3, Inc.) is a snare-like loop attached to the end of a wire (see Figure 32-1). This is mounted in a flexible tube, and the snare is deployed by pushing it out through the distal end of the tube. The snare has a fold in it, enabling effective withdrawal back into the tube. The distal end of the device is very radio-opaque, enabling good visualization of the procedure.

Figure 32-1. Amplatz goose neck snare. *Source:* ev3, Inc., Plymouth, MN.

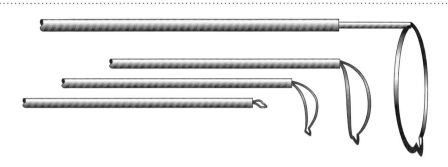

This retrieval device is particularly good for free-floating objects. It can also be used to grab the proximal end of broken guide wires. Once the object has been captured, withdrawal of the loop back into the tube will secure it, and the object can be withdrawn from the vascular system. If the object cannot be removed despite its being grasped firmly, a surgical procedure should be considered. Biplane fluoroscopy is recommended, although not essential, for effective deployment of the snare.

Curry Intravascular Retriever

The Curry intravascular retriever, manufactured by Cook Vascular, is similar in design and function to the goose neck snare. It comes complete with an introducer and guide wire (see Figure 32-2).

Figure 32-2. Curry intravascular retrieval set. *Source:* Adapted from Cook Vascular, Vandergrift, PA.

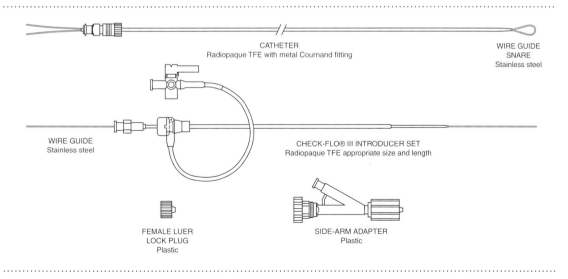

Dotter Intravascular Retriever

The Dotter tntravascular retriever (Cook Vascular) has a helical loop basket that emerges from the tip of the catheter (see Figure 32-3). Its design allows for the capture of guide wire tips and stents, which can be difficult to "lasso" with the snare of the previous two products. Another advantage is that it is not always necessary to actually loop the device over the object, which can be a very frustrating exercise on this scale. If the "basket" is placed on the object, it will often be drawn in when the device is retracted. This retriever may be too bulky to use in small vessels, however.

Vascular Retrieval Forceps

As the name implies, the Vascular retrieval forceps (Cook Vascular) consists of a small (3F) forceps attached to a flexible catheter (see Figure 32-4). The very tip of the forceps is a spring coil designed in the same fashion as guide wires, ensuring that the vessel wall is not damaged during placement. It can be used effectively on a variety of objects, but it is especially good for dislocated guide wires when their position is such that the loops of the previously described devices cannot be placed over them.

Figure 32-3. Dotter intravascular retrieval set. *Source:* Adapted from Cook Vascular, Vandergrift, PA.

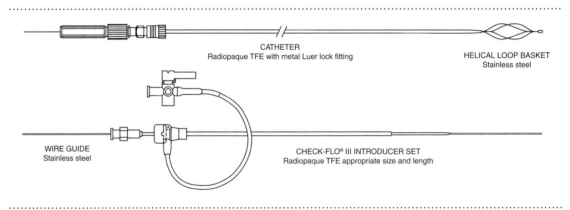

Figure 32-4. Vascular retrieval forceps. *Source:* Adapted from Cook Vascular, Vandergrift, PA.

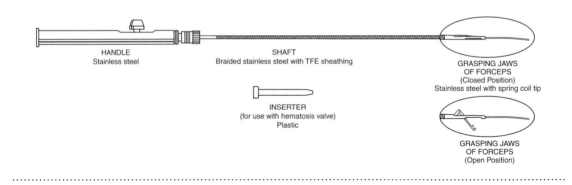

Welter Retrieval Loop

The Welter retrieval loop (Cook Vascular) has a loop at its distal end, but the loop is wound around the shaft of the catheter (Figure 32-5). This design makes free-floating objects easier to grasp, as the catheter has only to be side-on to the object, rather than having its tip touching it. Controlling the exact movement of the loop, however, is not as straightforward as with the goose neck or Curry catheters.

Biopsy Forceps

These come in a variety of sizes, and are manufactured for the removal of myocardial tissue (see Chapter 18). They have also been used successfully in a number of object retrieval procedures. The jaws are smaller than those of the retrieval forceps (see Figure 32-6), but this can be an advantage in small vessels.

Figure 32-5. Welter retrieval loop catheter. *Source:* Adapted from Cook Vascular, Vandergrift, PA.

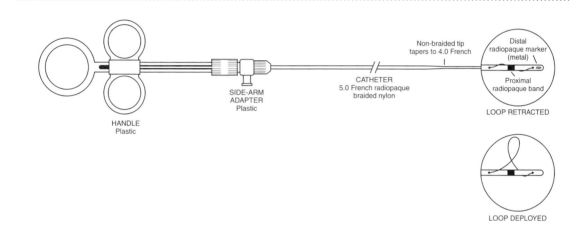

Figure 32-6. Myocardial biopsy forceps. *Source:* Adapted from Cook Vascular, Vandergrift, PA.

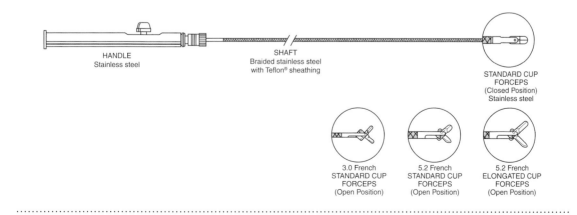

REFERENCES

1. Cekirge S, Saatci I, Firat MM, Balkanci F. Retrieval of an embolization coil from the internal carotid artery using the Amplatz microsnare retrieval system. *Cardiovasc Intervent Radiol* 1995;18:262–264.

2. Matzko J, Matsumoto AH, Tegtmeyer CJ, Spotnitz WD. Percutaneous removal of a Swan-Ganz catheter sutured to the superior vena cava. *J Vasc Interv Radiol* 1994;5(4):653–656.

3. Cekirge S, Weiss JP, McLean GK. Percutaneous removal of a surgical laparotomy sponge from the peritoneal cavity. *Cardiovasc Intervent Radiol* 1995;18:59–61.

4. Kirsch MJ, Ellwood RA. Removal of a ruptured angioplasty balloon catheter with use of a nitinol goose neck snare. *J Vasc Interv Radiol* 1995;6:537–538.

5. Mishra JP, Bemis CE, McCormick DJ. Detachment of transluminal extraction catheter cutter head from shaft and successful retrieval. *Cathet Cardiovasc Diagn* 1997;42:325–327.

6. Gibson M, Foale R, Spyrou N, Al-Kutoubi A. Retrieval of detached coating of a hydrophilic guidewire from the profunda femoris artery using an Amplatz gooseneck snare. *Cathet Cardiovasc Diagn* 1997;42:310–312.

7. Linnemeier TJ. Stent stranded in left main coronary artery. *Cathet Cardiovasc Diagn* 1996;38(4):405.

Chapter 33

EMERGENCIES IN THE CARDIAC CATHETERIZATION LABORATORY

Charles C. Barbiere, RN, CCRN, RCIS, CCT, CRT, EMT, FSICP

INTRODUCTION

With the introduction of coronary angiography by Dr. Sones, somatic complications associated with the procedure were bound to occur and did with infrequent regularity. Early experience with coronary angiography resulted in minor complications such as hypotension, dysrhythmias, contrast reactions, retroperitoneal bleeding, loss of pulse in the affected limb, and hematoma. Major complications such as coronary artery dissection, coronary artery spasm, myocardial infarction (MI), embolizations, perforations, cerebral vascular accident (CVA), and death also occurred.

The incidence of many of these complications, in particular dissection and spasm, were reduced with the development of smaller devices, the advent of soft-tipped catheters, and the greater experience of operators. The introduction of improved contrast media also reduced the severity and incidence of reactions also. Safer approaches to diagnostic procedures were developed, and these led to further reductions in complications. Then, with the advent of percutaneous coronary interventions (PCI), the process of refining devices and increasing experience of operators began again. The introduction of stents and devices for removing plaque and clot burden started the cycle once more.

Percutaneous interventions are now being performed on new subsets of patients with increasingly grave conditions.[1–5] It is to be expected, therefore, that complications will occur during diagnostic and interventional procedures. When these procedures are performed on patients at high risk for major acute coronary events, it also follows that an increase in complications will be observed. It is imperative that the laboratory staff anticipates, recognizes, and promptly treats all complications. The CCL should contain all the equipment and drugs necessary, and the staff should be competent in their use. An effort should be made to identify patients at high risk for complications so that, by modifying the procedure, complications may be avoided or their severity reduced.[6]

MINOR COMPLICATIONS

Anaphylactic Reactions

Anaphylaxis is an acute, systemic, and severe allergic reaction. It can be triggered when contrast medium, medication, or allergens enter the patient's body. The following are the recommendations of the Society for Cardiac Angiography and Interventions for the treatment of anaphylactic reactions in the CCL.[7]

Urticaria

For urticaria and skin itching, the therapy is:

1. No treatment
2. Diphenhydramine 25 to 50 mg IV

   If there is no response, then the therapy is:

1. Epinephrine 0.3 cc of 1:1000 solution sub-Q q 15 minutes up to 1 cc
2. Cimetidine 300mg or ranitidine 50 mg in 20 cc NS IV over 15 minutes

Bronchospasm

For bronchospasm, the recommended treatments are:

1. Oxygen by mask
2. Depending on the severity of the bronchospasm:
   - *Mild:* 2 puffs Albuterol inhaler
   - *Moderate:* Epinephrine 0.3 cc of 1:1000 solution sub-Q q 15 minutes, up to 1 cc
   - *Severe:* Epinephrine IV as a bolus of 10 µg/min and then infusion of 1 to 4 µg/min;

observe for desired effect with BP and ECG monitoring. Bolus epinephrine dose: (0.1 cc of 1:1000 solution, or 1 cc of 1:10,000) diluted to 10 cc (10µg/cc). Infusion epinephrine dose: (1 cc of 1:1000 or 10 cc of 1:10,000) in 250cc NS (4µg/cc)
3. Diphenhydramine 50 mg IV
4. Hydrocortisone 20 mg to 400 mg IV
5. Optional: H_2 blocker as outlined

Edema

Facial edema and laryngeal edema are treated by the following steps:

1. Call anesthesia
2. Assess airway, then do the following:
   - Oxygen by mask
   - Intubation
   - Prepare tracheotomy tray if necessary
3. *Mild:* Epinephrine sub-Q as outlined
4. *Moderate/Severe:* Epinephrine IV as outlined
5. Diphenhydramine 50 mg IV
6. Oximetry/arterial blood gases (ABG)
7. Optional: H_2 blocker if indicated

Hypotension and Shock

The recommended treatment for hypotension is:

1. Simultaneous administration of:
   - Epinephrine IV; bolus(es) 10 µg/min IV until desired BP response is obtained, then infuse 4 µg/min to maintain desired BP.
   - Large volume of 0.9% NS (3 liters in the first hour)
2. Depending on degree of hypotension:
   - Oxygen by mask
   - Intubation
3. Diphenhydramine 50 mg to 100 mg IV
4. Hydrocortisone 400 mg IV
5. CVP/Swan-Ganz
6. Oximetry/ABG

If there is no response:

1. H_2 blocker as outlined
2. Dopamine 2 to 15 μg/Kg/min IV
3. Advanced cardiac life support

Bradycardia

Patients may present with hypotension, bradycardia, or both on arrival in the lab, and this may be a result of the patient's underlying medical condition or it may be caused by medication. However, these conditions are more commonly seen in the CCL in association with the injection of intracoronary contrast medium.

Bradycardia may also be observed with manipulation of the femoral artery for access, for placement of transfemoral devices, or to achieve hemostasis. If bradycardia occurs during these manipulations, it is most likely part of a vasovagal response. In rare cases, malignant vasovagal syncope may occur with profound bradycardia and hypotension, and full resuscitative efforts may be required.[8]

All patients should have at least one peripheral IV line as an access for fluid resuscitation and for administration of drugs. As in any acute care setting, emergency drugs, notably atropine, epinephrine, lidocaine, and oxygen, should be immediately available. If a bradycardia proves refractory to a full dose of atropine (2 mg IV push), then a transvenous pacemaker should be promptly placed.[8]

If possible, all patients should be instructed in cough cardiopulmonary resuscitation prior to starting the procedure. When the patient coughs, his or her intrathoracic pump mechanism generates an increase in cardiac output, which may help to stabilize the patient until more definitive resuscitative measures can be employed.

Vascular Incidents

Most vascular incidents occur near the sites of sheath or catheter insertions, but these complications may also result from the embolic debris that enters the patient's circulation due to the manipulation of catheters and wires. In addition, new coronary revascularization technology often requires larger bore sheaths and catheters. This has resulted in an increase in reported vascular complications.[9] Vascular complications are reported to occur in less than 1% of cases.[10]

Vascular complications away from the insertion site are infrequent when compared to those reported for femoral and brachial sites. Major incidents are thrombosis, local obstructions from flaps, dissections, and subintimal hemorrhage. When these complications occur at the brachial site, they can usually be treated by localized revision in the CCL. When hemorrhage occurs as a result of percutaneous femoral artery puncture, open surgical correction may become necessary.[10] Arteriovenous fistula, pseudoaneurysms, local nerve damage, infection, persistent pain, and loss of limb may occur with either method.

Alternative treatments have been explored for patients who are at high risk for adverse outcomes from general anesthesia. High-risk patients who have an arteriovenous fistula or pseudoaneurysms have been successfully treated using ultrasound-guided pressure via mechanical compression devices.[11] With major vascular complications, early consultation with vascular surgeons is advisable. Serial measurements of vital signs, hematocrit/hemoglobin, limb diameter, size of hematoma, and the presence and quality of distal pulses should be maintained until surgery can be undertaken.

MAJOR COMPLICATIONS

Cardiac Tamponade

Cardiac tamponade occurs when fluid accumulates between the two layers of the pericardium. Cardiac tamponade may occur due to a neoplastic or infectious process, connective tissue disorder, after an MI, or because of chest trauma. It can also be seen as a complication following surgery and percutaneous cardiac procedures. Typically, patients present with:

- Distended neck veins
- Decreased arterial pressure
- Narrowing pulse pressure
- Muffled heart sounds
- Pulsus paradox
- Pressure plateau
- Sinus tachycardia
- Electrical alternans

In the CCL, hemodynamic measurements of the right heart may reveal a pressure plateau. This occurs when sufficient fluid accumulates inside the pericardial sack to cause diastolic pressure equalization in all chambers of the heart. When enough fluid accumulates, it can severely restrict cardiac function and become life threatening. Echocardiography is the best method for the definitive diagnosis of tamponade when time permits.

Development of cardiac tamponade in the CCL is generally due to aortic dissection, vessel perforation, cardiac perforation, coronary artery rupture, or cardiac rupture. During procedures, if a perforation is suspected, contrast is noted in the pericardial space or a stain associated with a dissection is seen, the staff should assess the patient for signs and symptoms of cardiac tamponade.[12]

In nonemergent presentations, performing a balloon pericardotomy, pericardial window, or both can drain the fluid that has accumulated within the pericardial space. Balloon pericardotomy is described in detail in Chapter 36.

Acute Coronary Syndrome

MI should be treated aggressively in the CCL.[13,14] MI may be the result of air or thrombus embolism or arterial damage from the catheter manipulation, resulting in spasm or dissection. If signs and symptoms of severe ischemia are observed, both coronary arteries should be promptly vi-

sualized in an effort to identify and quantify the presence of the obstruction. After diagnostic angiograms have been obtained, and if indicated, reperfusion should be attempted, starting with intracoronary nitroglycerin and moving to percutaneous coronary intervention (PCI) or coronary artery bypass surgery as indicated.

In facilities that provide primary PCI for acute coronary syndrome, a complete report of the treatments the patient received prior to arrival in the catheterization laboratory is essential. This should include any prehospital and emergency room interventions, results from diagnostic studies already performed, and any medications that may have been given. Departments involved with the treatment of these patients need to function as a system that moves the patient to the catheterization laboratory as rapidly as possible. Prehospital systems, emergency departments, and catheterization laboratory should all have in place protocols that facilitate this movement and there should be systematic monitoring of the "door-to-balloon time" process, with a goal of less than 90 minutes.[13-15] The longer the patient remains ischemic, the greater the loss of viable myocardium.

It is critical to monitor patients undergoing diagnostic and interventional procedures for signs and symptoms of new or ongoing myocardial ischemia. Vital signs and a baseline multilead ECG should be obtained and recorded on arrival in the CCL as a reference. The patient should be instructed to report any chest pain, shortness of breath, other pain, or unusual sensations. Most newer hemodynamic recorders display and record multiple ECG channels, and the display should be observed continuously. The staff should be diligent in monitoring the ECG for any changes that are suggestive of MI. If changes are observed, they should be recorded and promptly brought to the attention of the team.

Ischemia in the absence of MI is characterized by symmetrical changes in the T waves, which may vary from a slightly flattened depression to deep inversion. The ST-segment should be scrutinized for elevation. Elevation of the ST-segment may be only slight, or it may increase as much as 10 mm above baseline. If the ST-segment is elevated without associated Q waves, this may represent a non-Q wave infarction and may be the precursor of a larger infarct. The presence of ST-elevation signifies acute MI. With subendocardial ischemia and with some patients receiving digitalis, the ST-segment may be depressed. Any significant ST-segment depression should cause suspicion as to the presence of ongoing ischemia.

The diagnosis of MI is usually made by the presence of significant Q waves. A significant Q wave is at least 0.04 sec in duration and 25 percent of the R wave amplitude, provided the R wave is 5 mm. By observing which ECG leads have significant Q waves, it is possible to determine the location of infarct and the culprit artery (see Table 33-1). In an acute posterior infarct, a large R wave and ST-segment depression are present in V1 and V2. The right coronary artery is the affected artery. The 2007 ACC/AHA focused update of the practice guidelines for the management of patients with ST-elevation myocardium infarction provide the most recent recommendations for treatment of these patients.[14]

Depending upon the size of the ischemic or infarcted area, complications ranging from hypotension to cardiac arrest may occur, and the staff should be prepared to intervene promptly. Treatment should include oxygen, IV access, pain relief, nitrates, and ECG monitoring. Ef-

forts should be made to limit the infarct size with antiplatelet, antithrombin therapy, or primary percutaneous intervention. Other considerations include administration of aspirin, IV heparin, antidysrhythmic drugs, atropine, epinephrine, inotropic agents, beta and calcium blockade, correction of electrolyte abnormalities, temporary transvenous or transcutaneous pacing, volume correction, basic life support, and, if necessary, advanced life support as required. It is vital that every CCL contains all of these just-mentioned equipment, that it is checked frequently, and that all the CCL staff are instructed in its use.

Life-Threatening Dysrhythmias

When certain dysrhythmias occur, treatment must be immediate. An inability to terminate these dysrhythmias portends grave consequences for the patient. Treatment requires a rapid determination of the cause of the dysrhythmia. In the CCL, these dysrhythmias can result from a wide range of causes. The most common are the following:

- Irritation from devices in the left or right ventricle
- Ischemia
- Electrolyte imbalance
- Contrast injection
- Air or thrombus embolism
- Hypoxia
- Dissection/abrupt closure
- Spasm
- Accidental electrical shock
- Drug poisoning/overdose

Table 33-1. Q Wave Correlations

ECG Lead	Location of Infarct	Coronary Artery
V1, V2, V3, V4	Anterior infarct	Left anterior descending
I and AVL	Lateral infarct	Circumflex or diagonal
II, III, AVF	Inferior infarct	Right coronary artery

Ventricular tachycardia is produced by a single ventricular ectopic focus that discharges at a frequency of 150 to 250/min (see Figure 33-1). This dysrhythmia is sometimes called atrioventricular dissociation. The atria and ventricles depolarize at different rates and, as a result, distinct P waves are only occasionally observed depending on ventricular frequency. The patient loses his or her "atrial kick" and, in addition, the rapid depolarization of the ventricles results in a shorter filling time, which leads to decreased cardiac output.

Ventricular flutter is produced by a single ventricular ectopic focus discharging at a frequency of 250 to 350/min. Because of this rapid frequency,

the ventricles cannot fill and there is no flow out of the ventricle. As the heart attempts to compensate, ventricular fibrillation almost invariably occurs.

Ventricular fibrillation is an erratic rhythm caused by continuous rapid discharges from numerous ectopic foci in the ventricle (see Figure 33-2). The result is totally erratic and uncoordinated electric and mechanical activity, which results in waveforms that are indistinguishable.

Asystole occurs when there is no detectable cardiac activity. This results in a flat baseline (see Figure 33-3).

The American Heart Association 2005 Guidelines for Cardiopulmonary Resuscitation and

Figure 33-1. Ventricular tachycardia.

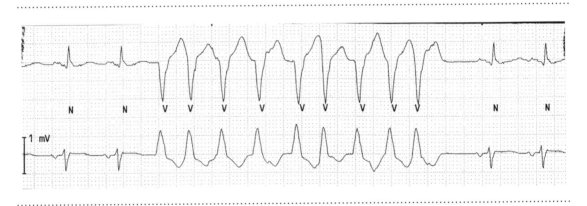

Figure 33-2. Ventricular fibrillation.

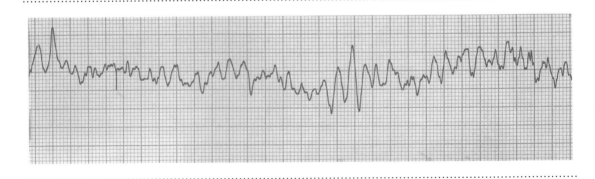

Figure 33-3. Asystole.

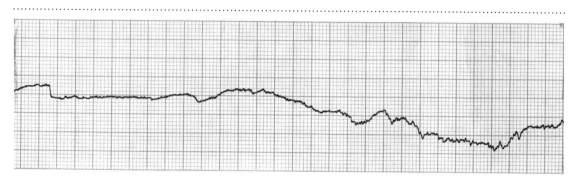

Emergency Cardiac Care[15] address treatment options and sequences. The Comprehensive ECC Algorithm serves as a starting point for problem solving and interventions (see Figure 33-4). Differential diagnosis of the dysrhythmia indicates the appropriate algorithm by which the situation should be managed (see Figures 33-5 and 33-6). Special attention should be paid to iatrogenic causes for these rhythms, such as embolism or dissection.

With rotating gantries, it is not uncommon to inadvertently disconnect an ECG lead, IV tubing, or other piece of equipment. If ventricular tachycardia, ventricular fibrillation, or asystole are observed, always confirm that the patient is pulseless and that the ECG leads are in place. If arterial access is in place, the arterial waveform can be used to confirm loss of, or decreased, cardiac function.

Cerebrovascular Accident

CVAs vary widely in occurrence, duration, and etiology, depending on the size and location of the affected area of the brain. Most emboli are probably atheromatous or composed of thrombotic particles. However, air and foreign bodies from catheters and wires have been reported as causative agents.

The administration of contrast medium may result in seizures, neurologic deficits, or transient blindness. Several large patient registries report that the incidence of CVAs is lower than any other complication related to cardiac catheterization, ranging from 0.03%–0.13%.[16,17]

Staff should be instructed in the proper techniques for the injection of contrast medium, with an emphasis on ensuring that the delivery system is clear of any air, and that the hub of the syringe be held up at 30°–45°. This will ensure that any inadvertent air is retained in the distal part of the syringe. Also, the use of a spacer or similar device (see Figure 33-7) on the barrel of the syringe is helpful in ensuring that the last few cc's of contrast medium will not be injected, further minimizing the possibility of the introduction of air.

The treatment for embolic stroke usually includes systemic heparinization while air emboli are best treated with hyperbaric oxygenation.

Patients with existing signs and symptoms of cerebrovascular disease and those with hypertension are at greatest risk for CVA. Extra care should be taken to observe these patients' neurological status throughout the stay in the CCL. In the hypertensive patient, efforts should be made to control the patient's blood pressure prior to the procedure.

Figure 33-4. Comprehensive ECC algorithm.[15]

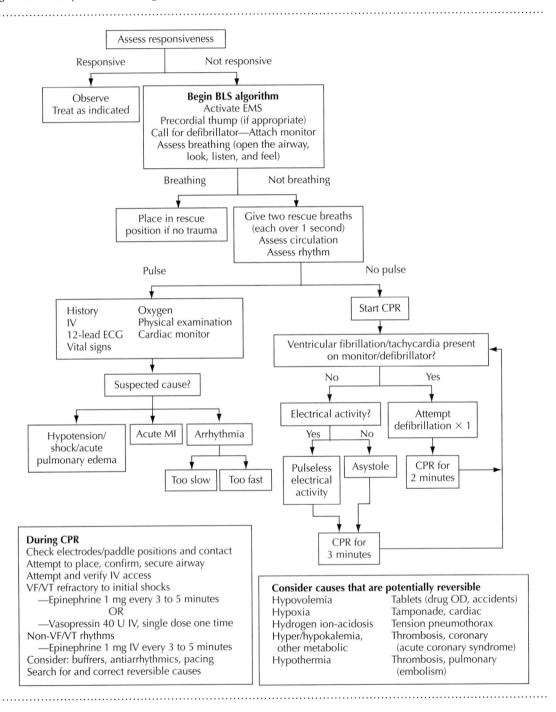

Figure 33-5. Ventricular fibrillation/pulseless ventricular tachycardia algorithm.[15]

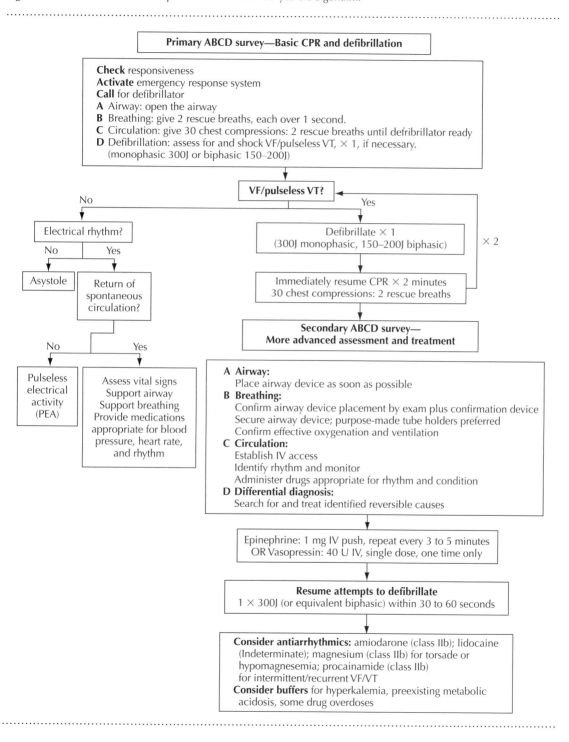

Figure 33-6. Pulseless electrical activity algorithm.[15]

```
┌─────────────────────────────────────────────────────┐
│ Pulseless Electrical Activity (PEA)                   │
│ (rhythm on monitor, without detectable pulse)         │
│ Includes:                                             │
│ Electromechanical dissociation (EMD)                  │
│ Pseudo-EMD                                            │
│ Idioventricular rhythms                               │
│ Ventricular escape rhythms                            │
│ Bradyasystolic rhythms                                │
│ Postdefibrillation idioventricular rhythms            │
└─────────────────────────────────────────────────────┘
                          │
                          ▼
┌─────────────────────────────────────────────────────┐
│ Primary ABCD survey—Basic CPR and defibrillation      │
│ Check responsiveness                                  │
│ Activate emergency response system                    │
│ Call for defibrillator                                │
│ A Airway: open the airway                             │
│ B Breathing: give 2 rescue breaths, each over 1 second│
│ C Circulation: give 30 chest compressions: 2 rescue   │
│   breaths                                             │
│ D Defibrillation: assess for VF/pulseless VT, shock   │
│   if indicated                                        │
└─────────────────────────────────────────────────────┘
                          │
                          ▼
┌─────────────────────────────────────────────────────┐
│ Secondary ABCD survey—More advanced assessments and   │
│   treatment                                           │
│ A Airway: Place airway device as soon as possible     │
│ B Breathing:                                          │
│    Confirm airway device placement by exam plus       │
│    confirmation device                                │
│    Secure airway device; purpose-made tube hilders    │
│    preferred                                          │
│    Confirm effective oxygenation and ventilation      │
│ C Circulation:                                        │
│    Establish IV access                                │
│    Identify rhythm and monitor                        │
│    Give medications appropriate for rhythm and        │
│    condition                                          │
│    Assess for occult blood flow (pseudo-EMT)          │
│ D Differential diagnosis: Search for and treat        │
│   identified reversible causes                        │
└─────────────────────────────────────────────────────┘
                          │
                          ▼
┌─────────────────────────────────────────────────────┐
│ Review for most frequent causes (treatment in         │
│   parenthesis)                                        │
│ Hypovolemia (volume infusion)                         │
│ Hypoxia (ventilation)                                 │
│ Cardiac tamponade (pericardiocentesis)                │
│ Tension pneumothorax (needle decompression)           │
│ Hypothermia                                           │
│ Massive pulmonary emobism (surgery, thrombolytics)    │
│ Drug overdoses such as tricyclics, digitalis,         │
│   beta-blockers, calcium channel blockers             │
│ Hyper/hypokalemia                                     │
│ Acidosis                                              │
│ Massive acute myocardial infarction                   │
└─────────────────────────────────────────────────────┘
                          │
                          ▼
          ┌───────────────────────────────────┐
          │ Epinephrine 1 mg IV push          │
          │ Repeat every 3–5 minutes          │
          └───────────────────────────────────┘
                          │
                          ▼
       ┌───────────────────────────────────────┐
       │ Atropine 1 mg IV (if PEA rate is slow) │
       │ Repeat every 3–5 minutes to a total of │
       │ 0.04 mg/kg                             │
       └───────────────────────────────────────┘
```

Figure 33-7. Contrast syringe with spacer (arrow) on barrel/plunger.

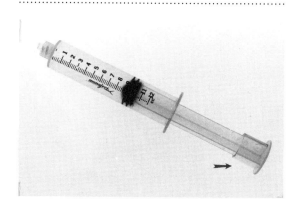

OTHER COMPLICATIONS

The variety of complications that can occur as a result of cardiac catheterization are enormous. Taken as a group these complications occur very seldom, but can be a challenge to manage.

Acute (Flash) Pulmonary Edema

Pulmonary edema is a clinical syndrome characterized by the sudden development of respiratory distress associated with a rapid accumulation of fluid within the lung interstitial space, as a result of acutely elevated cardiac filling pressures. Initial treatments are directed at ensuring adequate oxygenation and maintaining hemodynamic stability while attempting to reduce myocardial stress. Treatment may include oxygen, noninvasive positive-pressure ventilation, mechanical ventilation, diuretics, vasodilators inotropic agents, and ACE inhibitors.

Endocarditis and Infection

Although PCI is performed under sterile conditions, bacteremia and sepsis can occur. Septic complications can manifest as femoral artery mycotic aneurysm, arthritis, and thrombosis.

Risk factors for PCI-related bacteremia are long procedures, repeated catheterizations at the same access site, difficult vascular access, and having the arterial sheath in place for more than 1 day.[18] Treatment is the same as for any infection, and is based on antibiotic therapy.

Vascular Spasm

Vascular spasm is seen in the CCL most frequently as a sequela of the deep seating of a catheter. Often retraction of the catheter will alleviate the spasm, and if necessary, intracoronary nitroglycerine may be administered.

Acute Renal Failure

The most common causes of acute renal failure in the CCL are hemodynamic instability, radiocontrast toxicity, atheroembolism, and drug toxicity. Acute renal failure is most likely in patients with diabetes mellitus who have a baseline plasma creatinine concentration > 1.5 mg/dl (132 µmol/l). Treatments may include hydration, mannitol, diuretics, and acetylcysteine.

Patients at higher risk for developing or worsening renal failure should be considered for noninvasive testing if possible. If invasive studies are necessary, pretreatment may be indicated and a nonionic, low-osmolality contrast media should be selected, and the amount injected should be kept to a minimum. The use of a biplane imaging system, with proper positioning, may reduce the total number of contrast injections, because two exposures are obtained with each injection.

The prevention and treatment of contrast medium induced nephropathy are discussed in Chapter 5.

Pulmonary Infarct

In the CCL, pulmonary infarcts are generally due to migration of the catheter tip or a balloon left inflated in the wedge position for an extended period of time. This is a potentially avoidable complication. If a pulmonary artery catheter is required for patient management after the patient leaves the laboratory, confirmation of placement by waveform should be promptly performed at the receiving unit. When small, these infarcts may be asymptomatic and diagnosed only by chest X-ray.

Vascular and Coronary Rupture

These types of complications, although rare, can be life-threatening. As an example, pulmonary artery perforation has a mortality rate in excess of 30% and usually requires thoracotomy for management. This complication may occur during insertion, but more often results from balloon inflation of a catheter that has inadvertently migrated into a distal position in the pulmonary artery. Self-limited pulmonary hemorrhage following perforation may result in a pulmonary artery pseudoaneurysm.[19,20] The diagnosis of pulmonary artery pseudoaneurysm is usually made on the basis of a contrast-enhanced CT scan.

If perforation of a coronary vessel occurs as a complication of a PCI and tamponade is suspected, several courses of action can be taken. Any antiplatelet and antithrombin therapies should be terminated and possibly reversed. If the perforation is self-limiting, and there is no immediate danger of significant tamponade, the patient may be closely observed in the intensive care unit with a pericardiocentesis tray at the bedside. It may be possible to deploy, in approximation to the perforation, a coronary stent, which may seal the perforation. As the technology develops, covered endovascular stents are becoming the treatment of choice for coronary artery perforation.

If there is danger of continued hemorrhage into the pericardial space, and the perforated artery can be sacrificed, a balloon may be advanced over a wire at the perforation and inflated to block the artery for a prolonged period of time. If the artery cannot be sacrificed, covered stent implantation can be attempted, or the patient must be sent for emergency coronary bypass.[12]

Cholesterol Emboli

Aortic atherosclerotic plaques are an important source of emboli in patients with unexplained stroke, transient ischemic attack, and arterial embolization. Embolic events in the setting of aortic atherosclerosis may occur spontaneously or as result of interventions such as cardiac catheterization, intra-aortic balloon pumping, and cardiac surgery. Treatment is specific to the system affected and the severity of symptoms.[21]

SUMMARY

Diagnostic cardiac catheterization has evolved into a relatively safe procedure. The composite rate for all complications is low at between 1% and 2%,[22,23] being higher for PCI than for diagnostic procedures. It is essential to have surveillance mechanisms in place to identify the frequency and type of complications in every CCL. After major complications occur, a review of the case, interventions, and outcomes is helpful in identifying problems and finding solutions.

When complications occur, it is imperative that staff work together as a group to promptly intervene and, if necessary, apply resuscitative measures for the patient. Adequate equipment, staff trained annually in the use of this equipment, anticipation of complications, and diligent monitoring of the patient will all serve to facilitate the best possible outcome when complications arise.

REFERENCES

1. Ritchie JL, Nissen SE, Douglas JS, et al. Nonionic or low-osmolar contrast agents in cardiovascular procedures, use of: position statement. *Am J Coll Cardiol* 1993;21:269–273.

2. Barbiere CC. Percutaneous transluminal coronary angioplasty (PTCA) in high-risk patients. *Crit Care Nurs* 1990;10:66–69.

3. Morrison DA, Sethi G, Sacks J, et al. Percutaneous coronary intervention versus coronary bypass graft surgery for patients with medically refractory myocardial ischemia and risk factors for adverse outcomes with bypass: The VA AWESOME multicenter registry: comparison with the randomized clinical trial. *Am J Cardiol* 2002;39(2):266–273.

4. Morrison DA, Sethi G, Sacks J, et al. Percutaneous coronary intervention versus coronary artery bypass graft surgery for patients with medically refractory myocardial ischemia and risk factors for adverse outcomes with bypass: a multicenter, randomized trial. Investigators of the Department of Veterans Affairs Cooperative Study #385, the Angina with Extremely Serious Operative Mortality Evaluation (AWESOME). *J Am Coll Cardiol* 2001;38(1):143–149.

5. Krone RJ, Johnson L, Noto T. Five year trends in cardiac catheterization: a report from the Registry of the Society for Cardiac Angiography and Interventions. *Cathet Cardiovasc Diag* 1996;39;31–35.

6. Kimmel SE, Berlin JA, Strom BL, Laskey WK. Development and validation of simplified predictive index for major complications in contemporary percutaneous transluminal coronary angioplasty practice. The Registry Committee of the Society for Cardiac Angiography and Interventions. *J Am Coll Cardiol* 1995;26: 931–938.

7. Goss JE, Chambers CE, Heupler FA Jr. Systemic anaphylactoid reactions to iodinated contrast media during cardiac catheterization procedures: guidelines for prevention, diagnosis and treatment. *Cathet Cardiovasc Diagn* 1995;34:99–104.

8. Barbiere CC. Malignant vasovagal syncope after PTCA: a potential for disaster. *Crit Care Nurse* 1994;14:90–93.

9. Kaufman J, Moglia R, Lacy C, et al. Peripheral vascular complications from percutaneous transluminal coronary angioplasty: a comparison with transfemoral cardiac catheterization. *Am J Med Sci* 1989;297:22–25.

10. Messina LM, Brothers TE, Wakefield TW, et al. Clinical characteristics and surgical management of vascular complications in patients undergoing cardiac catheterization: interventional versus diagnostic procedures. *J Vasc Surg* 1991;13:593–600.

11. Fellmeth BD, Roberts AC, Bookstein JJ, et al. Post angiographic femoral artery injuries: nonsurgical repair with US-guided compression. *Radiology* 1991;178:671–675.

12. Barbiere CC. Cardiac tamponade: diagnosis and emergency intervention. *Critical Care Nurse* 1990 April 10;(4):20–22.

13. Anderson J. ACC/AHA 2007 guidelines for the management of patients with unstable angina/non ST-elevation myocardial infarction. *Circulation* 2007;116;803–877.

14. Antman E, Hand M. 2007 focused update of the ACC/AHA 2004 guidelines for the management of patients with ST-elevation myocardial infarction. *Circulation* 2008;117:296–329.

15. 2005 American Heart Association guidelines for cardiopulmonary resuscitation and emergency cardiovascular care. *Circulation* 2005;112:IV1–IV5.

16. Dunitz M, Morrison D, Serruys P. *High Risk Cardiac Revascularization.* London: Informa Health Care; 2002.

17. Kennedy JW, Baxley WA, Bunnel IL, et al. Mortality related to cardiac catheterization and angiography. *Cathet Cardiovasc Diagn* 1982;8: 323–340.

18. Kennedy JW. Complications associated with cardiac catheterization and arteriography. *Cathet Cardiovasc Diagn* 1982;8:5–11.

19. Samore MH, Wessolossky MA, Lewis SM, et al. Frequency, risk factors, and outcome for bacteremia after percutaneous transluminal coronary angioplasty. *Am J Cardiol* 1997;79(7):873–877.

20. Coulter TD, Wiedemann HP. Complications of hemodynamic monitoring. *Clin Chest Med* 1999;20(2):249–267.

21. Kearney TJ, Shabot MM. Pulmonary artery rupture associated with the Swan-Ganz catheter. *Chest* 1995;108(5):1349–1352.

22. Scanlon PJ, Faxon DP, Audet AM, et al. ACC/AHA guidelines for coronary angiography: a report of the American College of Cardiology/American Heart Association Task Force on Practice Guidelines (Committee on Coronary Angiography). Developed in collaboration with the Society for Cardiac Angiography and Interventions. *J Am Coll Cardiol* 1999;33:1756–1824.

23. Bashmore TM, Bates ER, Berger PB, et al. American College of Cardiology/Society for Cardiac Angiography and Interventions clinical expert consensus document on cardiac catheterization laboratory standards. *J Am Coll Cardiol* 2001;37(8):2170–2214.

Chapter 34

DEFIBRILLATION AND RESYNCHRONIZATION

Ilcias G. Vargas, RCES, RCIS, HM2

DEFIBRILLATION

Ventricular fibrillation (VF) is the most lethal of all cardiac arrhythmias. It generally starts as ventricular tachycardia from a single, tornado-like focus, and propagates throughout the heart. The ventricle contracts in a rapid, uncoordinated, quivering manner, effectively ceasing blood flow to the body. The patient loses consciousness, and death occurs within minutes unless defibrillation shock therapy is applied. Conditions which may initiate VF include trauma, myocardial infarction, congestive heart failure/cardiomyopathy, or electrolyte imbalance.

Ventricular fibrillation was first witnessed and documented in 1849 by M. Hoffa, a student of Carl Ludwig.[1] While studying vagal influences on the hearts of dogs and cats, Hoffa induced ventricular fibrillation by electrical stimulus, resulting in cardiac arrest; some of the animals recovered and some did not.

In 1899 J. L. Prevost and F. Battelli, also working with animals, discovered that, whereas VF can be initiated by a weak electrical stimulus, a much stronger stimulus applied to the heart can stop it, restoring normal sinus rhythm.[2] In spite of the evidence, defibrillation did not enjoy a lot of attention from the scientific community. The first successful defibrillation of a human heart wasn't performed until nearly half a century later, by thoracic surgeon Claude S Beck in 1947.[3] Dr. Beck applied AC current directly to the heart during surgery, saving the patient's life.

Indications

Defibrillation is indicated for the treatment of ventricular fibrillation and pulseless ventricular tachycardia. In the case of stable ventricular tachycardia with a pulse and stable supraventricular tachycardias, synchronized cardioversion is the treatment of choice.

According to the American Heart Association,[4] the chances of survival from cardiac arrest due to VF or pulseless VT decreases by 7% to 10% for each minute that passes without defibrillation. The best chance for survival is for defibrillation to be delivered within the first 4 minutes of the arrhythmia onset.

Preparation

Every defibrillator must be checked at least once every day, usually as part of the morning lab preparation. Every defibrillator has a test mode wherein the apparatus gives itself a shock, and checks the amount of current that it receives. The unit should then be left such that it is readily accessible to use at all times.

Conductive gel is applied to the paddles before defibrillation to ensure good electrical conduction, and minimizes skin burning during the shock. Some cath labs regularly apply gel to the paddles at the beginning of the day, ensuring that they are ready quickly in an emergency. However, if the gel remains on the paddles and they are not regularly and properly cleaned, the gel can damage the paddles. Alternately, Gel Pads may be used.

Hands-free defibrillator pads are available for use with most defibrillators. Standard hands-free pads will obstruct angiographic views, but radiolucent pads are available. When dealing with a patient with an ST segment Elevation Myocardial Infarction (STEMI) or Acute Myocardial Infarction (AMI), it is good practice to place hands-free defibrillator pads on the patient at the beginning of the procedure. This can save valuable time if defibrillation is needed. Defibrillator pads are also recommended for critically ill patients.

Procedure

As soon as ventricular fibrillation or ventricular tachycardia is evidenced on the patient's ECG, the first action is to check the patient's verbal response. If the patient is feeling well, check the ECG electrodes to ensure they are all connected. If the patient is in the catheterization laboratory and has an arterial line in place, a rapid uniform loss of the waveform will be witnessed (see Figures 34-1 and 34-2).

When the patient's VT or VF has been confirmed, speak to him until he loses consciousness; defibrillation is very painful.

Charge the defibrillator and set the amount of power to be given. Biphasic defibrillators vary by

Figure 34-1. Ventricular Tachycardia.`

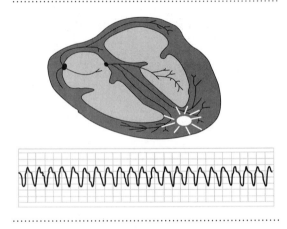

Figure 34-2. Ventricular Fibrillation.

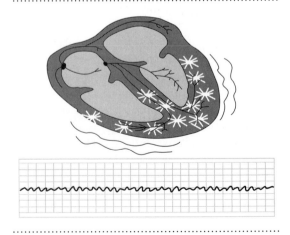

manufacturers; follow your institutional guide-lines for delivering the initial shock. When using a monophasic defibrillator, the first shock should be at least 200 joules.

The most common placement for the defibril-lator paddles is the anterior and lateral place-ment. Place one paddle on the patient's upper right torso and the other one at the bottom of the left pectoral muscle, at the apical region. For female patients, place under the left breast (see Figure 34-3).

After placing the paddles and getting the ready signal from the defibrillator, shout "every-one clear," and make sure that no one is touch-ing the patient. Deliver the shock by pressing on the shock bottom located on the side of the paddles.

Once the first therapy has been delivered, be prepared to begin CPR (and to continue it for 2 minutes) if the first shock is not successful before attempting a second shock (unless the physician orders a second shock right after the first one). According to the American Heart Association 2005 Guidelines for Cardiopulmonary Resus-citation and Emergency Cardiovascular Care,[4] chest compressions are vital to reviving a pa-tient before and after defibrillation has been at-tempted. CPR helps to ensure blood flow to the body and primes the heart muscle, increasing the chances of successful defibrillation on the second attempt.

In most cath labs, the circulator is responsible for the use of the defibrillator. The physician operator or scrub assistant pulls back the sterile drape and maintains control of the equipment to continue the procedure once the emergency has been resolved.

Post Resuscitation Care

Post defibrillation, patients should receive con-tinuous ECG monitoring, and vital signs should be assessed frequently after resuscitation. Refer to your institution guidelines for the frequency. Temporary pacing and pharmacological inter-vention may be necessary if the patient continues to be hemodynamically unstable.

Medicate as needed for pain and discomfort related to the procedure. In some situations, the patient may have a minor burn from the defibril-lation. Apply a topical cream to the areas where the pads were placed to help healing. Hydrocorti-sone, bacitracin, and silver sulphadiazine creams are often used.

SYNCHRONIZED CARDIOVERSION

Indications

Synchronized cardioversion (or resynchro-nization), is indicated for the treatment of supraventricular tachycardias on the stable pa-tient with signs and symptoms related to the arrhythmia. These tachycardias include atrial fibrillation, atrial flutter, and narrow complex atrial tachycardias. Resynchronization is most commonly used to treat new onset atrial fibrilla-tion and atrial flutter. The goal of cardioversion is to convert the tachycardia into normal sinus rhythm (see Figures 34-4 and 34-5).

Figure 34-3. Defibrillation Electrode Placement: Anterior-lateral placement.

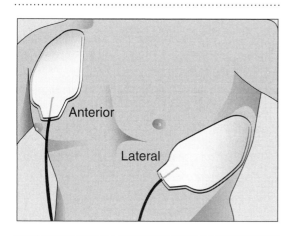

Figure 34-4. Atrial fibrillation.

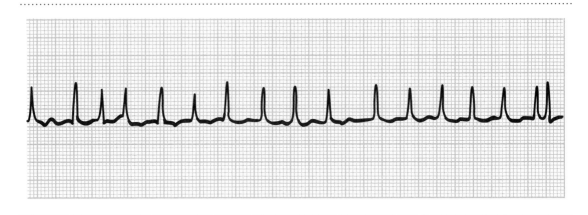

Preprocedure Care

Both the patient and the family should be educated regarding what to expect before, during, and after the procedure, as well as the risks involved.

An echocardiogram is performed preprocedure to rule out any blood clots or thrombus build-up in the atria, due to the potential of dislodgement during resynchronization. Transesophageal echocardiograms (TEE) are generally preferred because of the higher diagnostic quality the images.

Before the procedure begins, the patient must have a stable and well functioning intravenous (IV) line.

Monitor vital signs per institutional guidelines, which should include ECG (from the defibrillator monitor), noninvasive blood pressure, respiration, and pulse oximetry.

Figure 34-5. Atrial flutter.

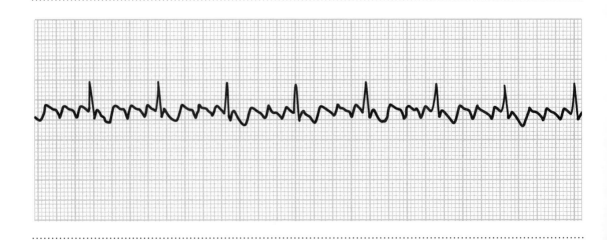

Make sure that the synchronized function is selected on the defibrillator. The energy delivered during cardioversion is synchronized with the QRS signal on the patient's ECG to prevent shocking the patient during the T wave portion of the cardiac cycle (which can put the patient into ventricular fibrillation).

It is important to have a fully functioning crash cart on hand in case of complications.

Medication

Electrical Cardioversion may be performed with conscious, or with deep sedation. Conscious sedaton drugs commonly used include Versed (midazolam) and Fentanyl (sublimaze). Versed is administered via IV push over 2 minutes using 1 to 2mg at a time, until the desired effect has been achieved. Fentanyl is given IV, pushed over 1 to 2 minutes using 25 to 50mcg at a time.

Before administering any sedatives or narcotics, the physician should evaluate the patient's health status, including airway assessment, according to the guidelines of the American Society of Anesthesiologists.[5]

Always make sure the drug's reversal agent is available, and have airway and suction equipment available. Romazicon is used to reverse Versed, and Narcan to reverse Fentanyl. In some situations, an anesthesiologist or certified registered nurse anesthetist (CRNA) may use propofol (diprivan) to induce momentary deep sedation for cardioversion.

Antiarrhythmic drugs such as adenosine, amiodarone, cardizem, and metoprolol are frequently given before cardioversion to decrease the heart rate, stabilize the patient, and increase the chance that electrical cardioversion is successful. Administered first, these medicines may stabilize the irritable myocardium and allow the heart to resume normal function on its own without electrical cardioversion. These agents are also often prescribed to maintain normal rhythm after a cardioversion.

Procedure

Pads should be used instead of paddles whenever possible, due to their better conduction, and ease of use. Place the pads using the right parasternal-posterior placement. Place the right parasternal pad on the upper right torso at midclavicular line, between nipple and clavicle. Place the posterior pad below the left shoulder blade between the left subscapular area and the left midaxillary line (see Figure 34-6).

Verify that the patient has reached the desired state of sedation, checking the level of consciousness, paying special attention to verbal response. Also make sure that patient's heart rate, blood pressure, respiratory rate and oxygen saturation are stable. If appropriate, record the patient's ECG during the procedure for the procedural documentation.

Make sure, again, that the synchronized function is selected on the defibrillator. Select the appropriate energy level, usually 70 to 200 joules for biphasic, or between 100 and 360 joules for monophasic defibrillators.

Ensure that no one is touching the patient. Deliver the shock once and check the patient's ECG. Also check the patient's response or state of sedation. One shock is usually adequate to convert the patient to sinus rhythm.

Figure 34-6. Defibrillator pad placement. Right parasternal-posterior placement .

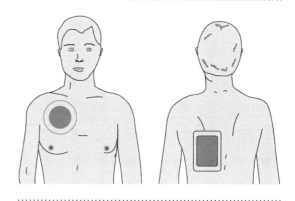

Postprocedure Care

After the procedure, check and document heart rate, blood pressure, respiratory rate, and oxygen saturation. Make sure that the patient has fully recovered from the sedation, checking verbal responses to access the level of consciousness in relation to self, time, and place.

Postprocedure instructions to the patient and family after the recovery period include any medication changes, and making sure the patient does not drive for the following 24 hours. Most institutions recommend 2 days of rest before returning back to work.

REFERENCES

1. Hoffa M, Ludwig C. Einig neue Versuche uber Herzbewegung. *Zeitschrift Rationelle Medizin* 1850.

2. Prevost J-L, & Battelli F. La mort par les descharges electriques. *Journ. De Physiol* 1899.

3. Beck CS, Pritchard WH, Feil HS. Ventricular fibrillation of long duration abolished by electric shock. *Jour Amer Med Assoc* 135:985, 1947.

4. 2005 American Heart Association guidelines for cardiopulmonary resuscitation and emergency cardiovascular care. *Circulation* 2005.

5. *American Society of Anesthesiologist Relative Value Guide.* ASA Publications, 2009.

Chapter 35

INTRA-AORTIC BALLOON PUMP AND OTHER CARDIAC ASSIST DEVICES

Brenda McCulloch, RN, MSN, CNS

INTRODUCTION

When the myocardium becomes damaged, cardiac output is insufficient to meet the oxygenation demands of the body. Blood pressure falls, and the myocardium continues to get weaker as it struggles to provide vital organs with oxygenated blood. Pharmacologic intervention may not be enough, and oftentimes places further demands on the myocardium. In situations such as acute myocardial infarction, cardiogenic shock, septic shock, and cardiac surgery, mechanical myocardial support can be the solution.

INTRA-AORTIC BALLOON PUMP

Intra-aortic ballooning pumping (IABP) is a short-term, cardiac support modality available for patients who are hemodynamically unstable or for those who are undergoing high-risk procedures in the CCL. This technology works on the basis of counterpulsation; inflating a balloon catheter within the aorta during diastole to augment coronary perfusion and improve hemodynamics.

Staff members in the cardiac catheterization laboratory must be able to assist with the insertion of the balloon catheter and the operation of the balloon pump console. Knowledge of the electromechanical events of the cardiac cycle and troubleshooting skills are essential when caring for hemodynamically compromised patients who require intra-aortic balloon pump support.

The IABP device was pioneered at the Grace-Sinai Hospital in Detroit, Michigan, during the early 1960s by Dr. Adrian Kantrowitz and developed for use in heart surgery by Dr. David Bregman in 1976. The first intra-aortic balloon catheters were surgically placed, via cutdown of the femoral artery. In 1979, the first percutaneous balloon was introduced and placement techniques in the femoral artery were refined. Less-common alternatives for catheter placement include surgical placement via a transthoracic or translumbar approach, or through the iliac, subclavian, or axillary artery. While the percutaneous procedure can be performed at the bedside, it is most commonly done in the CCL or cardiac surgery suite using fluoroscopy.

The intra-aortic balloon catheter is a polyurethane prewrapped balloon mounted on a flexible shaft. Depending on the manufacturer, balloon volumes range from 25 ml to 50 ml and 7 to 9.5F in diameter. The balloon catheter has a double lumen. The inner lumen is designed for guide wire passage and pressure monitoring, and the outer lumen is designed for helium transport. Helium is used to inflate and deflate the intra-aortic balloon because its low molecular weight allows for fast shuttling of gas. Recently, intra-aortic balloon catheters have been introduced with high-fidelity fiber optic sensors for monitoring pressure and timing of the balloon inflation and deflation.

Selecting proper volume intra-aortic balloon catheters is related to patient height; lower volume balloons are designed for shorter patients,

while the higher volume balloons are for taller patients. The "standard" catheter is 40 ml, which should adequately support patients ranging in height from 5′4″ to 6′. Some manufacturers have convenient sizing charts on their exterior packaging. Optimally sized and positioned, the balloon should sit in the aorta 1 to 3 cm below the origin of the left subclavian artery, superior to the origins of the right and left renal arteries (see Figure 35-1). The balloon is designed to inflate at the beginning of diastole and deflate at the beginning of systole (see Figures 35-2 and 35-3). If the balloon is placed too high, blood flow to the left subclavian is compromised; if too low, blood flow to the renal arteries may be impeded. When looking at a chest X-ray of a patient with an intra-aortic balloon catheter, the distal catheter tip should sit between the second and the third intercostal spaces, at the level of the carina.[1] When fully inflated, the intra-aortic balloon catheter should occupy 80% to 90% of the aorta to prevent trauma to the aortic wall.

Figure 35-1. Correct placement of balloon pump catheter. *Source:* Courtesy of Teleflex Incorporated.

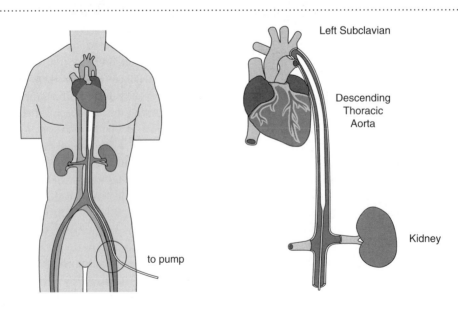

Figure 35-2. Balloon inflation. *Source:* Courtesy of Teleflex Incorporated.

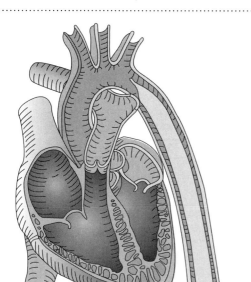

Figure 35-3. Balloon deflation. *Source:* Courtesy of Teleflex Incorporated.

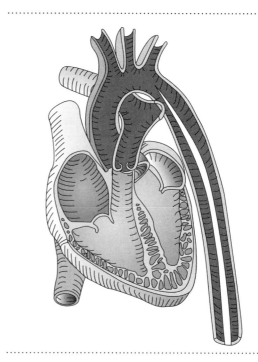

A "trigger" is required so that the console can properly time inflation and deflation of the balloon. The electrocardiogram and the arterial pressure waveform are the most commonly used. To meet the many clinical situations that may be encountered, multiple trigger options exist. Examples of triggers available (depending upon manufacturer) include ECG, arterial, and pacer (usually atrial and ventricular). Additional options include trigger software algorithms that compensate for patients in atrial fibrillation. A fixed rate, internal trigger mode may be used during open heart surgery or cardiac arrest (see Table 35-1).

A variety of operational modes for balloon pump consoles exist. A manual operator mode may be used to allow the clinician freedom to choose the ECG input source, select displayed ECG lead(s), the trigger, and fully automatic, semiautomatic, or fully manual timing. In contrast, modern pumps have a fully automatic operation mode (autopilot, auto) which selects the ECG source, AP source, trigger, and timing for the clinician simply by turning the pump on.

The balloon can be set to inflate at different frequencies. In 1:1 pumping, diastolic augmentation occurs with each cardiac cycle. Other frequencies available on different consoles allow for augmentation every second (1:2), third (1:3), fourth (1:4), or eighth (1:8) diastole (see Figure 35-4).

Physiologic Principles of Counterpulsation

The predominant physiologic effect of properly timed intra-aortic balloon pump therapy is afterload reduction. Inflation of the balloon during diastole increases arterial pressure and increases

Table 35-1. Trigger Modes

Trigger Type	Description
ECG	Most commonly used trigger; console looks at the positively or negatively deflected QRS complex; the peak of the R wave corresponds to the beginning of systole—the balloon deflates. The middle of the T wave corresponds to the middle of the T wave—the balloon inflates. ECG may not work well if heart rate $>$ 130 or QRS is wide.
Arterial pressure	Uses the dicrotic notch for inflation and systolic upslope of the arterial waveform as the trigger for deflation when the ECG is inconsistent; best used with regular rhythms.
Atrial fibrillation	Use this, when available, for irregular rhythms. The balloon will automatically deflate when an R wave is sensed.
Pacer	Uses the ventricular or atrial pacing spike as the trigger. This mode can only be used when the patient is 100% paced.
Internal	Infrequently used. Inflates and deflates at a regular preset rate. Used when there is no cardiac output, such as coming off cardiopulmonary bypass or in ventricular standstill, although Internal is not the trigger of choice in a code situation. Typically, it is preset at 80 BPM, but may be able to be adjusted, depending on the manufacturer.

Figure 35-4. Landmarks for optimal timing. *Source:* Courtesy of Teleflex Incorporated.

Landmarks for timing include:

- **PAEDP/UEDP**: Patient End-Diagnostic Pressure or Unassisted End Diastolic Pressure–determines afterload

- **PSP**: Peak Systolic Pressure–unassisted; beginning of systole

- **DN**: Dicrotic Notch–indicates the beginning of diastole when the aortic valve closes. Balloon inflation occurs just prior to the onset of the dicrotic notch, or beginning of diastole. A sharp "V" should be seen.

- **PDP/DA**: Peak Diastolic Pressure or diastolic augmentation– should be greater than the patient's systolic pressure

- **BAEDP**: Balloon Assisted End Diastolic Pressure–lowest aortic pressure produced by the deflation of the balloon. Optimally, BAEDP $<$ PAEDP.

- **APSP**: Assisted Patient Systolic Pressure–systole following IAB deflation. The APSP $<$ PSP

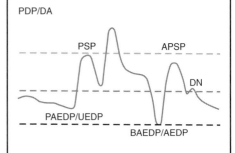

coronary blood flow. Balloon deflation, just prior to the onset of systole, rapidly reduces aortic volume and pressure, decreasing the resistance against which the left ventricle ejects its stroke volume. Cardiac output may be improved by as much as 40 percent with IABP therapy.[2]

Indications

Cardiogenic shock is the most common reason that intra-aortic balloon pumping is initiated (see Table 35-2).

Contraindications

Aortic valve insufficiency/regurgitation of 2+ or greater is an absolute contraindication for intra-aortic balloon pump therapy.[3] The displacement of blood during diastole would force additional blood volume through the incompetent aortic valve, increasing the severity of the insufficiency/regurgitation (see Table 35-3).

Insertion

For insertion of intra-aortic balloon catheters in the CCL or cardiac operating room setting:

1. Gather all necessary supplies and equipment, including balloon pump catheter kit

Table 35-2. Indications for Intra-Aortic Balloon Pumping

- Cardiogenic shock
- Hemodynamic support for high risk cardiac catheterization laboratory procedures
- Acute myocardial infarction complicated by papillary muscle dysfunction, severe mitral regurgitation, ventricular septal defect, continuing ischemia
- Intractable ventricular arrhythmias
- Hemodynamic support for high risk cardiac surgery; inability to wean from cardiopulmonary bypass following cardiac surgery
- Bridge to transplant

Table 35-3. Contraindications to Intra-Aortic Balloon Pumping

---

- Aortic insufficiency/regurgitation > 2+
- Aortic dissection
- Abdominal aortic aneurysm
- Severe peripheral arterial disease, bilateral femoral-popliteal bypass grafts
- Uncontrolled sepsis
- Severe coagulopathy

---

and pump console. Verify adequate helium supply. Obtain all necessary patient cables (slave, direct, or combination of both).

2. Position pump console and plug into electrical outlet.

3. Set up the pressure tubing, transducer, and continuous pressurized saline* flush solution set-up for balloon catheter central lumen.

4. If the arterial pressure is "slaved" into the console from the hemodynamic monitor, connect the appropriate cable from the hemodynamic monitoring system to the balloon console and verify the waveform.

5. Assess the patient's circulation to their legs and feet by evaluating pedal pulses and skin color and temperature. Mark pulses.

6. Place the skin leads on the patient. Select the lead with the best R wave.

7. Prepare the bilateral femoral artery access sites and place sterile drapes.

8. Using a sterile technique, assist the physician as needed with the infiltration of local anesthetic and obtaining arterial access.

9. Assist with guide wire advancement and sheath placement as needed.

10. Prepare the intra-aortic balloon catheter for insertion. Leaving the balloon catheter in the tray, attach the enclosed one-way valve to the catheter and pull the vacuum using a 60 ml syringe. Do not remove the one-way valve until after the balloon catheter is in place in the aorta.

11. Rinse the outside of the balloon catheter with sterile saline.*
12. Flush the central lumen of the catheter with sterile saline. Do not remove the balloon catheter from tray until ready to insert.
13. Advance the IAB catheter into position over the guide wire and assist as directed.
14. Administer anticoagulation per your institution policy.
15. After the balloon is advanced and positioned, the central lumen is gently aspirated and flushed with saline.
16. Connect the pressurized saline* flush to the central lumen, level, and zero the transducer and initiate arterial pressure monitoring.
17. Remove the one-way valve from the gas line and connect the gas line to the pump.
18. Purge the balloon catheter of air and replace it with helium. See the manufacturer's recommendations for pump-specific information on purging.
19. Initiate 1:1 pumping. See the manufacturer's recommendations for pump-specific information on initiating pumping.
20. Under fluoroscopic guidance, ensure that the balloon is fully unwrapped and remains properly positioned in the aorta distal to the left subclavian and superior to the renal arteries.
21. Secure the catheter securely in place, apply sterile dressing, and tape the pressure tubing and gas line to prevent migration and dislodgment.
22. Assess circulation to the affected leg and foot by checking pedal pulses and evaluating skin color and temperature. Notify the physician of significant changes from preballoon insertion.

---

*Heparinized saline can be used to prep the catheter and pressurized flush. Some hospitals have discontinued using heparin-flush solutions due to concerns over heparin-induced thrombocytopenia. Consult your hospital protocol for practice guidelines.

Prior to transporting the patient from the CCL to the critical care setting, obtain the supplies and equipment that might be needed during transport, such as a portable monitor/defibrillator, resuscitation medications, oxygen tank and cannula/mask, and a bag-valve mask. Many facilities have adopted the practice of having a pre-assembled "transport kit" containing these items. Know the most direct route to the receiving unit and be familiar with optimal placement of the bed/gurney, pump console, infusion pumps, and ventilators in any elevator that may be required during the transfer.

Bedside insertion of an intra-aortic balloon catheter may be occasionally required, particularly for the highly unstable patient who is too ill to safely transport to the CCL. The steps listed will be the same for bedside insertion. Special attention must be paid to maintaining sterile technique during preparation and insertion of the balloon catheter. At the bedside, it is helpful to have two staff members in the room; one to assist the physician with the procedure and one to connect the pump, initiate pumping, and monitor the patient. In these situations, proper catheter placement may be confirmed by a portable chest X-ray.

Timing

To achieve optimal hemodynamics, precise timing is required. Select an ECG lead that optimizes the R-wave. The peak of the R wave corresponds to the beginning of systole, signaling the balloon to deflate. The middle of the T wave corresponds to the middle of diastole, signaling the balloon to inflate. The timing of balloon inflation and deflation is best assessed by examining the arterial waveform when the pump is in the 1:2 (IAB catheter inflates every other cardiac cycle) mode so that a comparison can be made between assisted and unassisted waveforms. Timing is adjusted by separate controls for inflation and deflation. Timing methods vary depending upon the manufacturer. It is important to refer to the instructions for use (IFU) specific to the pump console being used for additional details.

To set inflation, identify the dicrotic notch in the unassisted aortic waveform, which represents closure of the aortic valve. Adjust the balloon inflation so that it inflates at the dicrotic notch on the aortic waveform. The goal of therapy is to produce a rapid rise in the aortic pressure, which should produce a sharp "V" in most patients. This should result in an augmented diastolic pressure > peak systolic pressure (PDP/DA > PSP). Deflation is set by identifying the aortic end-diastolic pressure on the unassisted beat. The goal is to reduce the afterload by reducing the aortic end diastolic pressure. This should result in the balloon augmented end diastolic pressure < the patients aortic end diastolic pressure (BAED/ AEDP < PAEDP/UEDP) and an assisted patient systolic pressure < the patient systolic pressure (APSP < PSP).

When optimal inflation and deflation have been determined, timing should be reassessed hourly and whenever significant changes in the heart rate or rhythm occur. Atrial fibrillation and other irregular rhythms, especially when rapid, can make inflation and deflation difficult to maintain. An option available on some balloon pump consoles is to change the trigger to the atrial fibrillation trigger. Newly available options are intra-aortic balloon catheters and consoles with high-fidelity fiber optic pressure sensors for monitoring and timing. The fiber optic waveform is a high-fidelity, real-time signal that enhances the ability of the balloon pump console to compensate for dysrhythmias and inflate and deflate as needed.

Timing Errors

Four major timing errors can occur and they include early or late inflation and early or late deflation (see Figure 35-5). Poorly timed balloon

Figure 35-5. Example of timing errors. *Source:* Courtesy of Teleflex Incorporated.

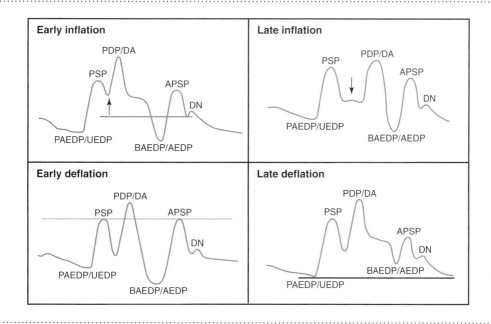

inflation and deflation do not optimize the patient's hemodynamic status and can be detrimental to the patient.

Early inflation: The intra-aortic balloon inflates before the aortic valve has closed, causing premature closing of the valve and reduction of stroke volume.
Late inflation: This causes displacement of less blood, resulting in lower arterial pressure increase.
Early deflation: The intra-aortic balloon deflates before the interventricular contraction phase of systole. There is no afterload reduction and the workload of the heart is not decreased.
Late deflation: The intra-aortic balloon is inflated at the beginning of ventricular systole, causing the left ventricle to eject its stroke volume against the inflated balloon. This increases the workload of the left ventricle. In late deflation, the BAEDP > PAEDP.

Balloon Pressure Waveforms

Additional information about the function of the balloon can be determined by examining the balloon pressure waveform (see Figure 35-6). This waveform reflects the movement of helium between the catheter and the console. A normal balloon pressure waveform has a baseline pressure slightly above zero. This is followed by a sharp upstroke that occurs as the helium quickly inflates the balloon. There is a normal peak inflation artifact and pressure plateau. The plateau is created by the balloon inflation, and approximates the time the balloon is inflated. This plateau pressure should be plus or minus 20 mmHg of the peak-augmented diastolic pressure. This is followed by rapid descent of the waveform as the helium is shuttled out of the balloon. A normal negative deflection is seen as the helium stabilizes within the system. Abnormal balloon pressure waveforms may indicate problems with the intra-

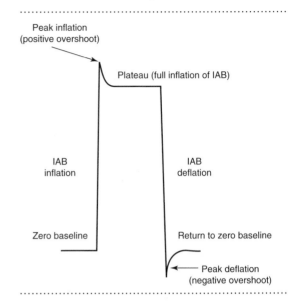

Figure 35-6. Balloon pressure waveform landmarks. *Source:* Courtesy of Datascope Corporation, Cardiac Assist Division, Fairfield, New Jersey.

aortic balloon catheter or the intra-aortic balloon pump console.

Troubleshooting

There are multiple alarms that may be activated during intra-aortic balloon pumping. Some alarms may cause the pump to stop pumping. The console screen will display the type of alarm. Alarms can be triggered by a loss of trigger, gas leak, kinked line, battery disconnect, poor ECG, low battery, and low helium. Refer to the instructions for use specific to the pump console being used for detailed information on managing and troubleshooting alarms.

Arrhythmias, especially those that are irregular or rapid, can be problematic for the balloon pump. If the patient develops atrial fibrillation, change to the atrial fibrillation trigger if the pump has one. If a patient becomes tachycardic, it may be necessary to decrease the frequency to 1:2. If the patient develops asystole and is undergoing CPR, change to the arterial trigger. If CPR does not generate enough pressure to trigger the balloon, change to the internal trigger. If the patient develops ventricular tachycardia or ventricular fibrillation, cardiovert or defibrillate as necessary. The console is electrically isolated and will not be damaged.

Intra-aortic balloon failure or loss of vacuum can occur. Assess all connections on the tubing and tighten if needed. Assess the power supply; change to another AC outlet if possible. Change to a new balloon console if needed. The balloon should not be dormant in the aorta. If automatic pumping fails, hand inflate and deflate the balloon with air. Use one-half the volume of the balloon (20 ml of air for a 40 ml balloon) and rapidly inflate/deflate every 5 minutes to prevent thrombus formation around the catheter.

Rarely, balloon perforation can occur, causing helium to leak from the catheter. Assess the gas line for blood. The blood may appear as brown flecks. Blood in the gas line indicates that the balloon has perforated. Assess the balloon pressure waveform, if present. The pressure plateau may gradually decrease if gas is leaking from the catheter. If the balloon is perforated, it should be clamped to prevent more blood from entering the gas line and potentially the pump. The catheter should be disconnected from the pump. The catheter will need to be removed within 30 minutes to prevent thrombus formation. If the patient remains hemodynamically unstable, another intra-aortic balloon catheter will need to be placed.

Patient Care

Frequent assessment of the patient on an intra-aortic balloon pump is essential. Regular assessment of the patient's cardiovascular, neurological, renal, and peripheral vascular system is necessary. Vital signs, including pulmonary artery

pressures, cardiac output, assisted pressures, and peak-augmented diastolic pressure, should be monitored regularly to assess the effectiveness of intra-aortic balloon pumping therapy. The left radial pulse should be assessed regularly to ensure that the balloon has not migrated superiorly and is obstructing flow to the left subclavian artery. Circulation to the foot of the affected leg can be affected by the balloon pump catheter, causing diminished or absent pulses and/or pale, mottled, or cyanotic toes or feet. Distal pulses, skin temperature, and color should be assessed frequently while the patient is receiving intra-aortic balloon pump support.

Changes in level of consciousness, transient ischemic attack, cerebrovascular accident, or myocardial infarction may occur if thrombus forms on the balloon catheter, becomes dislodged, and embolizes. Decreased urine output may indicate inadequate perfusion to the kidneys caused when the balloon is obstructing flow to the renal arteries. A urinary catheter is generally placed in the patient receiving intra-aortic balloon pump therapy.

The central lumen of the balloon catheter is connected to a continuous pressurized (to 300 mmHg) saline flush that delivers 3 ml/hour (see Figure 35-7). The central lumen was designed only for guide wire passage and arterial pressure monitoring, and should not be used for blood sampling (particularly with 7F or 8F catheters). Manual flushing using a syringe is contraindicated.[4] Regular assessment of the femoral dressing and the surrounding area is required to monitor for signs of bleeding and/or hematoma formation. If the patient receives heparin, anticoagulation parameters are monitored frequently and adjustments are made in the heparin infusion rate to maintain the PTT within the desired range of 50 to 70 seconds.

Daily labs, including complete blood count and basic metabolic profile, should be ordered. The hemoglobin and hematocrit often decrease because

Figure 35-7. Continuous pressurized flush. *Source:* Courtesy of Maquet, Cardiac Assist Division, San Jose, CA.

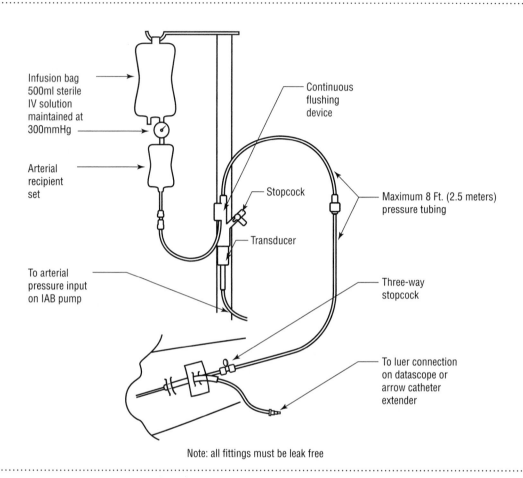

Note: all fittings must be leak free

of hemolysis related to mechanical damage to erythrocytes, as well as bleeding at the vascular access site. Thrombocytopenia may also occur because of the mechanical destruction of platelets and/or heparin administration.[1] A daily portable chest X-ray is recommended to assess the position of the intra-aortic balloon catheter.

Patients on intra-aortic balloon pump therapy are on bed rest. The head of bed should not be elevated more than 30° to prevent kinking or upward migration of the balloon catheter. Analgesia and sedation may be required to maintain patient comfort. Movement of the affected leg and foot is restricted and immobilization or restraint of the leg/foot may be required. Regular turning, using the log-rolling technique, and repositioning is required to maintain comfort. Pressure-reducing or pressure-relieving devices may be beneficial for patients on prolonged bed rest. Passive and active range of motion exercises may help prevent muscle atrophy.

In the rare event that the balloon becomes nonfunctional, it should be removed promptly or thrombosis may occur. Intra-aortic balloons that have been immobile for 30 minutes or more should be removed immediately.[1]

Interfacility Transport

When transferring the patient via ground or air ambulance to another facility for a higher level of care or services, additional planning is required. The patient may be disconnected from the intra-aortic balloon pump and be placed on a smaller transport pump. Many ambulances are equipped with an AC power inverter that can be used as the primary power source. Check the available battery time to ensure that there is enough power to last the time of the transport as back-up. An additional helium canister should be available for longer transports. Patients being transferred via ground or air ambulance must be accompanied by a registered nurse, perfusionist, or cardiovascular technologist who is well trained and fully competent in the care of unstable patients and the operation and troubleshooting of the intra-aortic balloon pump.

For air transport, there are additional special requirements. Changes in barometric pressure affect the volume of helium, which expands with increases in altitude. The volume of helium may be increased by 25%–62.5% with an altitude change from sea level to 10,500 feet. Depending on the manufacturer, the pump may have an automatic altitude correction feature. The amount of helium should be equalized every 1000–2000 feet. Refer to the manufacturer's recommendation for specific information regarding air transport.

Notify the receiving hospital of the estimated time of arrival. Determine the type of pump console that is used at the receiving hospital. Special adapters may be required to connect differing brands of balloon catheters and balloon consoles.

Weaning and Balloon Removal

As the patient's condition improves, weaning from the intra-aortic balloon pump can be initiated. Prior to weaning, the patient should be free of chest pain, have a normal heart rate, no unstable arrhythmias, have adequate blood pressure with minimal or no vasopressors, normal wedge pressure, and cardiac index > 2.4.

There are several methods for weaning from the intra-aortic balloon pump. Refer to your institution's policy on weaning or follow the physician's orders. Weaning is frequently accomplished by decreasing the assist ratio (1:2, 1:3, 1:4) over time and monitoring the patient's response to these changes. Some balloon pumps have an assist ratio as low as 1:8. An alternative approach to weaning is to slowly decrease the amount of diastolic augmentation while maintaining the balloon pump at a 1:1 frequency.

Removal of the balloon pump catheter may be performed by properly trained personnel including physicians, physician assistants (PAs), advanced practice nurses (APNs), registered nurses, or cath lab technician. Anticoagulation should be stopped at least 2 hours before the anticipated time of removal to allow the PTT to decrease. To assist with balloon removal, turn the balloon pump console to standby or off to allow the balloon to deflate. It is not necessary to aspirate helium from the balloon. Remove all dressings, sutures, and/or ties covering and securing the catheter. Disconnect the balloon from the pump console.

The catheter should be pulled back slightly, until resistance is met, indicating that the balloon is within the sheath. While holding the sheath, the balloon and sheath are removed simultaneously as a unit. Do not withdraw the balloon through the sheath; this can severely damage the sheath and/or balloon, potentially causing vascular damage. Upon removal, allow some bleed-back both proximal and distal to the insertion site to expel any potential clots.

Firm pressure over the arteriotomy is required for at least 30 minutes to obtain hemostasis. This can be accomplished by manual pressure or mechanical pressure using a FemoStop or mechanical clamp device. Follow your institution's policies and procedures for the use of these devices. There are reports in the literature regarding the use of various vascular closure devices when intra-aortic balloon catheters are removed. After hemostasis is achieved, frequent assessment of the access site and distal pulses is required. The patient should remain on bed rest for at least 6 hours.

Complications

Like many percutaneous procedures, the most commonly seen complications of intra-aortic balloon pumping are vascular complications. During insertion, failure to advance the catheter because of severe peripheral arterial disease or aortic dissection and arterial perforation may also occur. While complications have decreased with the use of smaller diameter catheters, risks remain. In the Benchmark Counterpulsation Outcomes Registry, access site bleeding occurred in 4.3% of patients and acute limb ischemia occurred in 2.3% of patients; 1.4% of patients receiving intra-aortic balloon support required blood transfusion.[3]

Predictors for major vascular complications include age $\geq$ 75, peripheral arterial disease, diabetes mellitus, female gender, and small body surface area (<1.65 m²).[1] Ischemia to the left subclavian and renal arteries can be caused by improper balloon placement within the aorta. Though rare, mechanical complications, such as balloon rupture and helium emboli can occur (see Table 35-4).

Summary

Intra-aortic balloon pumping is frequently used to provide short-term hemodynamic support for patients in cardiogenic shock and those undergoing high-risk procedures in the CCL. It effectively enhances cardiac output by decreasing the afterload against which the heart must work. The primary complications of intra-aortic balloon pump therapy are vascular complications, requiring frequent assessment and monitoring of the patient. It is imperative that staff working in

Table 35-4. Complications of Intra-Aortic Balloon Pumping

- Vascular complications, both minor and major: bleeding, hematoma, thromboembolism, arterial dissection, limb ischemia, amputation
- Renal ischemia, spinal cord ischemia
- Hemolysis, thrombocytopenia
- Mechanical complications, including balloon leak/rupture, inadequate inflation, inadequate diastolic augmentation
- Infection, sepsis

the CCL be very familiar with the technique of balloon catheter insertion, setting up the pump and initiating balloon pumping, proper timing, and troubleshooting.

PERCUTANEOUS VENTRICULAR ASSIST DEVICES

Nonpulsatile ventricular-assist devices have been used in small numbers in emergent and nonemergent high-risk patients with varying success. Their use has been complicated in the past by complex technical setup and the requirement of large-bore access sheaths. One of advantages of left ventricular assist devices is that they provide perfusion regardless of the patients' intrinsic heart rate, and some are capable of perfusing the peripheries without forward flow out of the heart. Placing patients on these devices does not treat ischemic heart disease, and patients will remain ischemic until culprit lesions have been treated.

TandemHeart

TandemHeart is a percutaneous left ventricular assist device (see Figures 35-8 and 35-9). It removes blood from the left atrium via a 21F transseptal cannula, which inserted in the left femoral vein. The blood is then circulated through the Tandem-Heart system pump, then through a canulla into the distal aorta through 15F–17F arterial cannula.

This TandemHeart pump circulates the blood at up to 5 l/min at 7500 rpm. It is dual cham-

Figure 35-8. TandemHeart™ controller. *Source:* Courtesy of CardicAssist, Inc., Pittsburgh, PA.

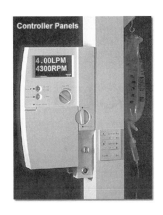

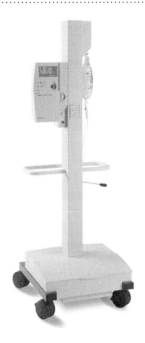

bered; one portion contains the impeller for in-flow and output of blood, the other contains a motor, communication line, and an infusate line. Heparinized saline cools and lubricates the pump bearing and provides local anticoagulation.

Figure 35-9. TandemHeart™ centrifugal pump. *Source:* Courtesy of CardicAssist, Inc.

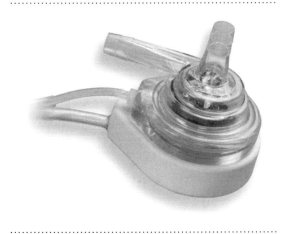

The advantages of this device are its portability, short extra-cardiac connections, and its ease of use; it can be implanted in the catheterization laboratory under just a local anesthetic.

TandemHeart has been successfully used as a back up in high-risk procedures and as a bridge to transplantation or implantation of a more permanent assist device.[5,6] The TandemHeart system cannot be coupled to an oxygenator, as can the percutaneous coronary bypass (PCB), so right heart failure is a contraindication to its use.

Impella

The Impella from Abiomed (of Danvers, Massachusetts) is a catheter designed to actively unload the ventricle, allowing the heart to rest and recover. The distal end of the catheter has a pigtail, which rests within the left ventricle. The pump itself is within the body of the catheter (see Figure 35-10). It draws blood through inlet ports in the pigtail segment, and the outlet ports lie within the aorta.

Figure 35-10. The Impella. *Source:* Courtesy of Abiomed.

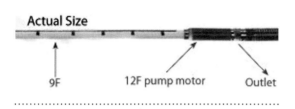

The LP2.5 can unload the left ventricle of 2.5 liters per minute of blood flow for up to 5 days. The Impella Mobile Console is compact, weighing only 3 kg, and can be easily mounted on an IV pole. Its simple design and ease of placement has many advantages over many support devices.

Percutaneous Coronary Bypass

The percutaneous coronary bypass (PCB) is a complex extracorporeal device that removes venous blood from the junction of the patient's inferior vena cava and right atrium, oxygenates this blood, and returns it via a heat exchanger to the patient's aorta (see Figure 35-11). This process generates an effective forward flow or an equivalent cardiac output of up to 5.5l/min, dependent on vascular volumes and size of cannulae (16F–21F). PCB, however, does not directly perfuse the myocardium.

PCB is fraught with potential technical difficulties and life-threatening complications. Specially trained personnel such as perfusionists should perform PCB setup, implementation, and monitoring. PCB can maintain hemodynamic stability

Figure 35-11. Percutaneous coronary bypass system.

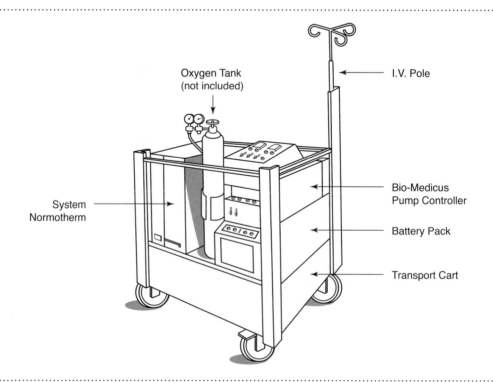

in the absence of an intrinsic cardiac rhythm or effective cardiac output and can improve tissue perfusion in cases of severe left ventricular failure. Survival rates after PCB have been reported to range from 16%–64%.[7,8,9]

PCB is rarely utilized for high-risk PCI and only available at a few specialized hospitals. With the availability of permanent surgical LVADs and other, less-complicated temporary devices, use of PCB in the catheterization laboratory has all but disappeared.

Summary

Devices to augment and sustain myocardial function are part of the equipment in every cath lab and this will continue to increase as technologic advancements with assist devices continue. The goal is to quickly support a patient's cardiac output when the heart's pump doesn't function as desired. Cath lab personnel play a key role in assisting with the set-up, insertion, and management of these devices.

REFERENCES

1. Trost JC, Hillis LD. Intra-aortic balloon counterpulsation. *Am J Cardiol* 2006;97:1391–1398.
2. Paul S, Vollano L. Care of patients with acute heart failure. In: Moser DK, Riegel B, eds. *Cardiac Nursing: A Companion to Braunwald's Heart Disease.* St Louis, MO: Saunders Elsevier; 2008.
3. Stone GW, Ohman EM, Miller MF, et al. Contemporary utilization and outcomes of intra-aortic balloon counterpulsation in acute myocardial infarction: the benchmark registry. *J Am Coll Cardiol* 2003;41:1940–1945.
4. Quaal SJ. Nursing care of the intraaortic balloon catheter's inner lumen. *Progress in Cardiovascular Nursing.* 2000;15(1):11–13.
5. Westaby S, Katsumata T, Pigott D, et al. Mechanical bridge to recovery in fulminant myocarditis. *Ann Thorac Surg* 2000;70:278–282.
6. Thiele H, Lauer B, Hambrecht R, et al. Reversal of cardiogenic shock by percutaneous left atrial-to-femoral arterial bypass assistance. *Circulation* 2001;104(24):2917–2922.
7. Grambow D, Deeb GM, Pavlides GS, et al. Emergent percutaneous cardiopulmonary bypass in patients having cardiovascular collapse in the cardiac catheterization laboratory. *Am J Cardiol* 1994;73:872–875.
8. Teirstein P, Vogel R, Dorros G, et al. Prophylactic versus standby cardiopulmonary support for high risk percutaneous transluminal coronary angioplasty. *J Am Coll Cardiol* 1993;21:590–596.
9. Shawl FA, Domanski MJ, Wish MH, Davis M. Percutaneous cardiopulmonary bypass support in the cardiac catheterization laboratory: technique and complications. *Am Heart J* 1990;120:195–203.

SUGGESTED READING

Burkoff, D. Intra-aortic balloon counterpulsation and other circulatory assist devices. In: Baim, DS. *Grossman's Cardiac Catheterization, Angiography, and Intervention,* 7th ed. Philadelphia: Lippincott Williams & Wilkins; 2006.
Diepenbrock, N. How do we mend a broken heart? *Nursing Critical Care* 2007;2(2):36–46.
Essebag V, Halabi AR, Churchill-Smith M, Lutchmedial S. Air medical transport of cardiac patients. *Chest* 2003;124;1937–1945
Jacobson C, Marzlin K, Webner C. *Cardiovascular Nursing Practice: A Comprehensive Resource Manual and Study Guide for Clinical Nurses.* Burien, WA: Cardiovascular Nursing Education Associates; 2007.
Quaal, SJ. Intraaortic balloon pump management. In: Lynn-McHale DJ, Carlson, KK, eds. *AACN Procedure Manual for Critical Care*, 4th ed. St. Louis, MO: W.B. Saunders; 2001.
Woods SL, Froelciher ES, Motzer SA, Bridges EJ. *Cardiac Nursing,* 5th ed. Philadelphia: Lippincott Williams & Wilkins; 2004.

Chapter 36

BALLOON PERICARDOTOMY

Sharon Holloway, RN, MSN, ACNP-CS, CCRN

BALLOON PERICARDIOTOMY

The pericardium is a membranous sac, comprised of a double layer of fibrous tissue, covering the heart. The inner layer, known as the *visceral pericardium* or *epicardium*, covers the heart and the great vessels, forming the outermost layer of the heart. The outer layer of the pericardium is a tough pouch known as the *parietal pericardium*, and it is attached to structures within the chest. Between the two layers is a small amount of pericardial fluid, which absorbs shock and minimizes friction as the heart moves within the chest.

The pericardium itself can become inflamed, and this is known as *pericarditis*. The inflammation can become restrictive due to fibrin deposition, and this is known as *constrictive pericarditis*. The space between the two layers of pericardium can become filled with fluid, a condition that is called a *pericardial effusion*. The fluid may accumulate, causing the heart to be compressed. Compression of the heart by the pericardial fluid may prevent the heart from filling adequately with blood during diastole. Therefore, the amount of blood available for systole is reduced. As this condition worsens, cardiac tamponade may occur.

Cardiac tamponade causes a severe impairment of cardiac function and is considered a medical emergency. The rate of fluid accumulation usually determines whether a pericardial effusion results in cardiac tamponade. With a slow accumulation of fluid, the person is able to adjust to the hemodynamic changes, allowing time for a treatment plan to be instituted. With rapid accumulation the opposite is true.

Pericardial effusions are most often the result of a malignant etiology.[1] Other causes are uremia, traumatic injury, viral, bacterial, idiopathic and HIV-related conditions. Because of the existence of other comorbid illnesses, these patients are typically not considered good surgical candidates. The underlying condition, after drainage of the fluid, often results in reaccumulation of fluid. Most often, the goal is improvement of the patient's quality of life while minimizing procedural risk. With that in mind, percutaneous therapy offers a most advantageous treatment for this population of patients.

Balloon pericardiotomy was first introduced by Palacios and colleagues.[2] Since that time, there has been a slow and steady trend to offer percutaneous balloon pericardiotomy or balloon pericardial window as an alternative to surgery for relief of pericardial effusions or as emergency treatment for cardiac tamponade.[3-5]

Technique

The patient's upper body is positioned as high on the table as the X-ray equipment allows. The chest is prepped and draped in sterile fashion. A right-heart catheter may be inserted, and hemodynamic data is collected. The standard sub-xiphoid approach is used for the pericardial puncture. An 18-gauge needle is inserted into the pericardium approximately 1 cm below the inferior rib margin. A J-tipped guide wire is then advanced into the pericardial space.

Dilatation with an 8F or 9F dilator is usually necessary to enlarge the entry tract (see Figure 36-1). A drainage catheter is inserted, and the pericardial pressure is measured. The right-heart catheter placed prior to the puncture can then be used to make simultaneous right atrial and right ventricular measurements. The cardiac output can also be measured pre- and post-drainage. The pericardial fluid is removed with a large-bore syringe, and the fluid is sent for laboratory analysis. At least 100–200 mL of fluid is left within the pericardial space.

Once the fluid has been removed, patients experience symptomatic relief of their shortness of breath almost immediately. They then can be further prepared for the balloon portion of the procedure. They must be placed in a supine position to facilitate positioning of the balloon catheter. A J-tipped, extra-stiff guide wire is inserted and left looped in the pericardial space.

Figure 36-1. Balloon pericardiotomy. *A:* A schematic of the percutaneous balloon pericardiotomy. The balloon is positioned over the wire in the pericardial space and inflated, creating a drainage space in the pericardium. *B:* Inflation of the balloon with a waist visible, caused by the pericardium. *C:* Full inflation of the balloon in the pericardium. *Source:* Reprinted from Ziskind AA, Pearce AC, Lemmon CC, et al. Percutaneous bal-loon pericardiotomy for the treatment of cardiac tamponade and large pericardial effusions: description of technique and report of the first 50 cases. *J Am Coll Cardiol* 1993;21:1–5.

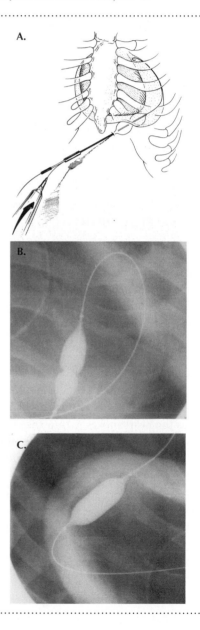

A.

B.

C.

The drainage catheter is removed, and a 20 mm balloon is inserted over the wire and under the ribs. An Inoue balloon may also be used.[6] An indentation in the balloon will confirm placement in the pericardium. Contrast may also be injected into the pericardial space to help visualize the pericardial membrane.

The balloon is then inflated by hand. Usually two or three inflations will suffice. This creates an exit from the pericardium to facilitate drainage via the body's own system. Once the procedure is completed, repeat hemodynamic measurements are performed. Initially, equalization of right atrial and pericardial diastolic pressures is seen (see Figure 36-2). After drainage is complete, right atrial pressure should return to 10 mmHg or less and pericardial pressure to 0 mmHg. The cardiac output should increase. The balloon is removed or replaced with a drainage catheter which is connected to a collection bag. The drainage catheter is sewn in place, and the patient is returned to the ward. The bag may be left in place for 24–48 hours.

Figure 36-2. Pericardial pressures. Simultaneous right atrial and pericardial pressures in a patient with cardiac tamponade. In the left panel, equalization of pressures is shown as well as systemic hypotension. After pericardiocentesis, the right panel shows return of the pericardial pressures and right atrial pressure to normal. In addition, the right atrial pressure tracing shows the return of the diastolic y descent, which is missing from the other tracing. This is the result of right atrial compression and impedance of diastolic right atrial emptying in cardiac tamponade. *Source:* Courtesy of T. Feldman, MD.

Risks of the procedure include cardiac perforation with the needle during placement and vagal reactions.[6] Sedation is often needed during the procedure because balloon manipulation may cause pain.

REFERENCES

1. Markiewicz W, Borovik R, Eckers S. Cardiac tamponade in medical patients: treatment and prognosis in the echocardiographic era. *Am Heart J* 1986;111:1138–1142.
2. Palacios IF, Tuzcu EM, Ziskind AA, Younger J, Block PC. Percutaneous balloon pericardial window for patients with malignant pericardial effusion and tamponade. *Cathet Cardiovasc Diagn* 1991;22:244–249.
3. Ziskind AA, Pearce AC, Lemmon CC, et al. Percutaneous balloon pericadiotomy for the treatment of cardiac tamponade and large pericardial effusions: description of technique and report of the first 50 cases. *J Am Coll Cardiol* 1993;21:1–5.
4. Kopecky SL, Callahan JA, Tajik A, Seward JB. Percutaneous pericardial catheter drainage: report of 42 consecutive cases. *Am J Cardiol* 1986; 58:633–635.
5. Chow LT, Chow WH. Mechanism of pericardial window creation by ballon pericardiotomy. *Am J Cardiol* 1983;72:1321–1322.
6. Chow WH, Chow TC, Cheung KL. Nonsurgical creation of a pericadial window using the Inoue balloon catheter. *Am Heart J* 1992;124:1100–1102.

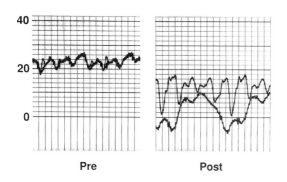

Chapter 37

TEMPORARY CARDIAC PACING

Patrick Hoier, BS, RCSA, RCIS, FSICP

In the early 1950s, a cardiologist, Paul M. Zoll, began to look at techniques that could be used to treat patients in high-grade atrioventricular blocks and asystole. His research led to the design of an external electrode and console system that allowed the user to administer small electrical charges to the patient's chest at set intervals. These electrical impulses would cause the cardiac muscle to depolarize and trigger the heart to contract. In 1952, Dr. Zoll published an article describing the successful use of this device on a 65-year-old cardiac patient suffering from angina and Adam-Stokes disease. His machine was able to sustain the patient's heart rate for a period of 50 hours at a time and allowed the patient to successfully recover from his ailments.[1] The new device rapidly began to revolutionize the way in which physicians treated bradycardia, dysrhythmias, and cardiac standstill.

Since the first temporary cardiac pacemaker, this technology has grown to be able to diagnose and treat patients suffering bradycardia-related emergencies. Today, symptomatic bradycardia can quickly be alleviated by the application of a temporary pacemaker and can improve the chances of resuscitating a patient in asystole. In the field of emergency cardiac care, the temporary pacemaker has become an essential tool in the treatment of cardiac dysrhythmias.

MYOCARDIAL CONDUCTION

In the normal heart, the cardiac electrical impulse is produced by the heart's natural pacemaker, the sinoatrial (SA) node, which is located in the superior aspect of the right atrium's posterior wall (see Figure 37-1). The electrical impulse is then released into the atrial muscle, where it is conducted through the rest of the atria, and down to the ventricles.

Between the atria and the ventricles lies a ring of connective tissue that acts to insulate the ventricles from the atrial impulse. The atrioventricular (AV) node is designed to slow down the

Figure 37-1. Anatomy of the cardiac conduction system.

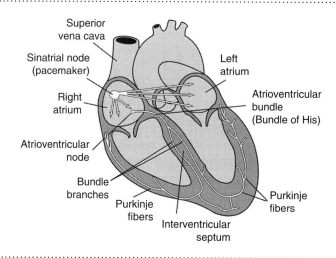

electrical impulse, allowing the ventricles to max-imally fill with blood. As the impulse leaves the AV node and enters the Bundle of His, it resumes normal conduction speed again.

From the Bundle of His, the impulse is con-ducted toward the right and left ventricles by the right and left bundle branches. The left bundle branch bifurcates again into the anterior and posterior fascicles, and the right bundle branch continues as one fascicle. A vast series of electrical conduction tissues, called the purkinje network, branch off from the fascicles, and deliver the elec-trical impulse into the ventricular muscle cells.

Bradycardia

Bradycardia/bradyarrhythmias are common and can be the result of a wide variety of disorders. Bradyarrhythmias can originate from either the SA or AV node, causing a wide variety of symptoms.

Sinus bradycardia is characterized as a normal sinus rhythm resting heart rate under 60 beats per minute, though it is seldom symptomatic until the rate drops below 50 beat/min. Bradycardic rhythms may be caused by a failure of the SA

node to create and release an electrical impulse at an adequate rate.

Another cause of ventricular bradycardia can be attributed to the loss of the impulse within the AV node or other conductive tissues due to injury of the cardiac structure. In either of these situations, the resulting patient's heart rate may not be fast enough to maintain sufficient sys-temic circulation, and the patient could suffer from symptoms associated with a decreased car-diac output.

- Dizziness, syncope, lightheadedness
- Difficulty concentrating/confusion
- Chest pain
- Shortness of breath
- Generalized weakness

Asystole

Asystole is defined as a complete lack of cardiac electrical activity. Ventricular asystole may be related to a number of problems within the car-diac conduction system. The SA node may be in-volved and fail to produce an electrical impulse; the AV node may be injured and become unable to conduct the electrical impulse to the ventricles; the Bundle of His or both bundle branches may be damaged, and become unable to conduct the electrical signals to either ventricle; or a combination of any of these. In these situations, the ventricles may not receive an electrical impulse to trigger depolarization. Without the electrical depolarization, the ventricle muscles will not be stimulated to contract.

PACEMAKER THERAPY

A temporary cardiac pacemaker is an electronic device that produces an electrical impulse in a controlled manner and then transmits the impulse to the cardiac tissues. It can sense the heart's intrinsic electrical activity (when there is any), so that inappropriate artificial stimulation does not occur. Although a temporary pacemaker has many of the same mechanical elements of a permanent pacemaker (a generator and lead system), its overall design and application is quite different.

Unlike a permanent cardiac pacemaker, a temporary device is only placed in emergent situations, or when it is determined that there is a high likelihood that the patient's cardiac rhythm will return to normal within a reasonable amount of time.

Indications for Temporary Pacing

The American College of Cardiology and the American Heart Association have developed a list of indications that may be successfully treated with temporary pacing (see Table 37-1).[2] Despite the fact that they may be of benefit to patients experiencing any of the listed indications, physicians should consider initial treatment with a pharmaceutical agent to avoid potential complications associated with temporary pacing. To avoid the possibility of infection, physicians may want to reconsider starting a temporary transvenous pacemaker on a patient that will likely require a permanent pacemaker implantation at a later date.

Some indications require rapid application of temporary pacing therapy in order to be successful. Patients presenting with asystole should have temporary pacing instituted quickly in an attempt to stimulate the cardiac muscle cells. Patients experiencing significant hemodynamic instability due to a slow heart rate, and who continue to be refractory to medical therapy, should also receive temporary pacing therapy.

Patients presenting with any of the elective indications noted may have a temporary pacemaker applied out of concern that their current dysrhythmia may worsen. In the early days of percutaneuous transluminal coronary angioplasty (PTCA), prophylactic insertion of a temporary pacemaker was common, particularly when treating the right coronary artery. Despite being listed as an indication, placement of a temporary pacemaker during coronary angioplasty is rarely necessary today, due to the use of low ionic and iso-osmolar contrast media.

Table 37-1. ACC / AHA Indications for Temporary Pacing

Emergent Indications	Elective Indications
• Asystole • Symptomatic Bradycardia refractory to medications • Bilateral bundle branch block • Mobits type II heart block • Symptomatic second or third degree heart block	• Cardiac surgeries (aortic, trisuspic valve, septal defect, bypass surgeries) • General anaesthesia administration (in the presence of second degree, third degree, or intermittent heart block) • Coronary angioplasty • Antitachycardia Pacing

Temporary pacemaker therapy may also be initiated to treat patients presenting with supraventricular tachyarrhythmias. The atrial conduction rate may be > 200 beats per minute, with a 1:1 ventricular response. Overdrive (antitachycardia) pacing is performed by programming the pacing generator to stimulate the heart faster than the patient's intrinsic rate. Once the pacemaker has the heart beating at the faster rate for a short period of time, the pacemaker is abruptly turned off. When the pacing is abruptly discontinued, the cardiac cellular depolarization pauses as the action potentials are forced to reset. This pause may allow the SA node time to regain control of cardiac depolarization before the ectopic pacemaker focus can recover.

Temporary Pacemaker Terminology

In order to understand how temporary pacemakers work, it is necessary to learn the terminology used to describe the devices and their functions.

A-V Interval

This setting is used only when both the atria and ventricles are being paced. The A-V interval setting is used to produce an artificial A-V interval that occurs in the natural cardiac cycle. This setting is seldom changed with temporary pacemaker therapy. This setting is measured in milliseconds (msec).

Bipolar

Bipolar is a term that can be used to refer to a pacing lead that that has both the positive and negative electrodes needed to create a pacing circuit.

Capture

The term capture is used to indicate successful cardiac muscle depolarization triggered by cardiac pacing. A "captured beat" can be identified on the ECG by noting a pacing spike that is followed by a P wave (if atrial paced) or QRS complex (if ventricular paced). Failure to note a cardiac depolarization following a pacer spike is referred to as a failure to capture.

Current (Output)

The strength of the electrical impulse created by the temporary pacemaker generator is defined as the pacing current (or output). In order to stimulate the cardiac muscles to depolarize, the electrical current produced by the pacemaker must be greater than the myocardial cells intrinsic threshold. A current that is not strong enough will result in a failure to trigger cardiac depolarization and contraction. The current of the electrical impulse produced is normally a setting that can be controlled by the operator. The amount of current that is used depends on the type of temporary pacing that is utilized. Current is measured in milliamps (mA).

Lead

The pacemaker lead refers to the electrode system that connects the patient to the external generator. There are many different types of electrode systems that can be used to create the temporary pacing leads. The type of electrode system used depends on the indication for pacing, the type of temporary generator that will be utilized, and the patient's emergency status. The main functions of the pacing lead system are to deliver the electrical impulse created by generator to the patient's body and to deliver intrinsic cardiac electrical signals from the patient's body back to the generator for analysis and sensing.

Mode

Pacemakers can be utilized to sense and stimulate the atria, the ventricles, or both. The chambers that the pacemaker senses and paces determine the mode of the pacemaker. Pacing modes are often referred to by their three-letter-coded abbreviation that was developed by the Heart Rhythm Society (see Table 37-2). The first letter is the chambers that will receive the pacing therapy if necessary, the second code indicates the chambers sensed, and the final letter indicates what type of action the pacemaker will take if intrinsic activity is detected. Temporary pacing therapy usually focuses on single-chamber (AAI or VVI) or dual-chamber (DDD) pacing.

Pulse Generator

The term generator is used to describe the battery and control console of the pacemaker. This part of the pacing system creates and manipulates the electrical impulse that is to be delivered to the heart. The operator of the temporary pacemaker is able to control the strength and duration of the electrical impulse, as well as the cardiac rate by changing the control settings found on the generator. Most temporary pacemaker generators can also sense and analyze the intrinsic (natural) electrical activity of the heart, thus avoiding unnecessary and inappropriate pacing therapy. Unlike permanent pacemaker generators, temporary pacemaker generators are always found outside of the body. There are many different types of pacemaker generators that are available for clinical use.

Pulse Width

Pulse width is defined as the amount of time the electrical impulse is applied to the cardiac tissue. In order for the cardiac tissue to respond to the current generated by the pacemaker, the current must be applied for a specific duration. If the current is not applied to the heart long enough, the cardiac cells will not depolarize and chamber contraction will not occur. Prolonged pulse widths may decrease the necessary current required to capture the cardiac muscle; however, changing the pulse width may also drain the battery of pacemaker generators. Though some types of temporary pacemaker units allow pulse width to be changed, operators will seldom need to alter the setting. Pulse width is measured in milliseconds (msec).

Sensitivity

Sensitivity of the pacemaker refers to the ability of the generator system to detect and analyze the intrinsic electrical activity of the heart. In many cases of symptomatic bradycardia, a patient may have some natural electrical activity present. Most temporary pacemakers are able to detect that electrical activity and inhibit a pacing impulse being released unnecessarily. Although sensitivity is not always a setting that can be altered on a temporary pacemaker, most devices do allow this factor to be changed. If a pacemaker is not sensing the patient's intrinsic electrical activity, this setting should be decreased until proper sensing is noted. Sensitivity is measured in millivolts (mV).

Synchronous / Asynchronous

These terms are used to differentiate a pacemaker setting that allows the pulse generator to sense

Table 37-2. Heart Rhythm Society pacing codes

Position I (Chamber Paced)	Position II (Chamber Sensed)	Position III (Response to Sensing)
O = None	O = None	O = None
A = Atria	A = Atria	T = Trigger
V = Ventricle	V = Ventricle	I = Inhibit
D = Atria and Ventricle (Dual)	D = Atria and Ventricle (Dual)	D = Dual (I + T)

the intrinsic electrical activity of the heart. A pacemaker that is set to sense an intrinsic underlying rhythm is said to be "synchronized" pacing, a pacemaker that is not set to sense the rhythm is said to be "asynchronized" pacing.

Threshold

Threshold is defined as the minimum energy required to stimulate cardiac muscle depolarization.

Unipolar

The term unipolar can be used to describe to a pacing lead that has only one electrode connection. The second electrode is a remote patch or wire that grounds the electrical impulse, completing the pacing circuit.

TYPES OF TEMPORARY PACEMAKERS

There are four main methods for performing temporary cardiac pacing: external (transcutaneous) pacing, transesophageal pacing, transthoracic epicardial pacing, and internal transvenous pacing. The type of temporary pacemaker system that is utilized is dependent on the patient's presentation, emergency status, and the length of time that temporary pacing therapy may be required.

External Transcutaneous Pacing

The external transcutaneous pacemaker is an ideal choice for treating the emergent patient presenting (or suddenly developing) bradycardia dysrhythmias or asystole. This type of pacemaker can be initiated quickly, is very easy to apply to the patient in the emergency setting, and is fairly easy to operate. The operator of this device has limited control of the pacing activity, and thus does not require a lot of excessive training.

Components

As discussed earlier, all pacemaker systems have two main components: the electrode lead and the pulse generator. Modern external transcutaneous pacemakers use a lead system that is composed of two self-adhesive patches that have a coating of conductive gel on the side that is attached to the patient. The pacing patches are the same patches that are used for hands-free cardiac defibrillation and cardioversion and allow for the possibility of multiple therapies to be available from one system.

The generator for a transcutaneous pacemaker is a specially modified external defibrillator that contains pacemaker controls and software. Activation of the control unit's pacemaker software typically deactivates the defibrillation controls. This type of programming set-up decreases the chances of accidental defibrillation or cardioversion during pacing therapy.

Function

The external transcutaneous temporary pacemaker works by delivering a timed electrical impulse to the chest wall of the patient through the pacing electrode patches. This impulse travels through the chest wall, stimulating all muscle tissues within the chest to depolarize and contract (including the heart). Because the electrical impulse is not delivered directly to the heart (and is dispersed throughout the chest), its output needs to be fairly large to ensure that enough of the current reaches the cardiac tissues.

Placement Procedure

For pacing therapies, the electrode patches can be placed on the right pectoral and left lateral position that is typically used for defibrillation (see Figure 37-2). An alternative placement of a left anterior patch and a left posterior patch (placed on the cardiac region of the chest and back) may also be used (see Figures 37-3 and 37-4). Place-

Figure 37-2. Right pectoral/left lateral placement of transcutaneous pacing patches.

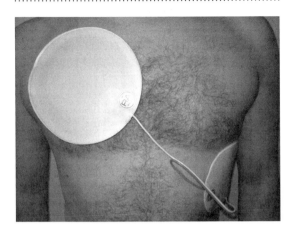

Figure 37-3. Posterior placement of transcutaneous pacing patches.

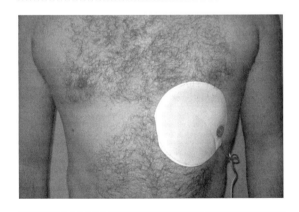

ment of the patches in the anterior and posterior positions may decrease the amount of patient discomfort that is often associated with this type of pacing therapy. In addition to the pacing electrodes, external cardiac pacing devices also require the patient to be connected to surface ECG electrodes. The transcutaneous pacing system uses the surface ECG electrodes to sense the patient's intrinsic rhythm.

Figure 37-4. Anterior placement of transcutaneous pacing patches.

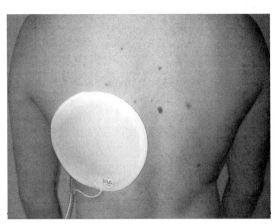

Pulse Generator Settings

The external transcutaneous pacemaker is a fairly simple device and has few control settings that the operator can change. Because the electrical impulse will stimulate the atria and ventricles simultaneously, the pacemaker mode cannot be altered. The atrial and ventricles will depolarize and be stimulated to contract at the same time.

The pulse width is also a set factor on most external pacing system. As stated earlier, the electrical impulse created needs to be quite large and must be applied to the chest for a set period of time to ensure cardiac depolarization. To increase the ease of programming, this setting is predetermined by the manufacturer, and is generally not changed. Typical preset pulse widths are 20 to 40 msec.[3]

Pacing output is a setting that can be altered on most transcutaneous external pacemakers. Most patients can be successfully paced by the external system using a current of 50 to 100 mA.[4] The exact setting to be used depends on the actual patient receiving the pacing therapy. The operator should program the pacing unit to the lowest current level that successfully triggers cardiac depolarization. Programming the system using in this way will decrease patient discomfort.

Sensitivity is not normally a setting that will be altered by the operator. Cardiac sensing is typically performed through the surface ECG electrodes connected to the transcutaneous pacing generator. If failure to sense is noted by the operator, increasing the gain setting for the ECG monitor usually will correct this problem.

The operator will be most concerned with programming an adequate pacing rate. Because transcutaneous external pacing is rather uncomfortable for the patient, the rate of pacing should be very carefully programmed so that the patient is not receiving unnecessary therapy. The pacing rate should be set to the point where the patient's symptoms are alleviated. For most patients, the suggested pacing rate is 80 beats per minute.

Complications

Despite the benefits that transcutaneous external pacing may have for the emergent cardiac patient, the technique does have significant drawbacks. First, transcutaneous pacing impulses trigger the ventricle chambers of the heart to depolarize without triggering atrial depolarization. This is because the atrial electrical threshold is significantly higher than the ventricular threshold when pacing transcutaneously.[5] With the use of the transcutaneous pacemaker, the patient loses the normal atrial-ventricular conduction relationship. The loss of the atrial and ventricular synchrony can have a negative hemodynamic effect (a loss of approximately 20% of the atria contribution to ventricular filling). The loss of the atrial contribution can further exacerbate the patient's preexisting symptoms caused by the bradycardia. If the loss of the A-V synchrony seems to trigger symptoms of hemodynamic instability, pacing the patient at a faster rate may help.

A second drawback with the transcutaneous pacing system is that the electrical impulse that is created and released by the generator enters the patient's body through the chest wall. As the electrical charge crosses through the chest, the electrical impulse will also trigger the chest skeletal muscles to contract. This creates a very uncomfortable sensation and usually requires the patient to be sedated if this form of pacing will be utilized for any length of time. Most patients are able to tolerate 15 to 20 minutes of transcutaneous external pacing, but longer periods may become very unpleasant. Placing the patches in the anterior and posterior positions and programming the lowest electrical stimulus that will trigger cardiac depolarization will decrease this sensation slightly. This method of temporary pacing should only be used for short periods of time and should be replaced by an intravenous temporary pacemaker, or a permanent implantable pacemaker (if indicated), as soon as possible.

A third drawback is that there is an increased risk of failure to capture the cardiac muscle cells. Because the cardiac muscle is indirectly stimulated by an electrical impulse that is passing through the chest wall, failure to capture is a significant possibility. If external pacing is not successful in capturing the cardiac muscle tissues, a temporary intravenous pacemaker implantation is suggested.

Transesophageal Pacing

Transesophageal pacing is a noninvasive approach to the temporary treatment of cardiac bradycardias. This method of pacing is performed by inserting an electrode into the patient's esophagus, and then transmitting an electrical impulse through the esophagus into the cardiac muscle. It is typically utilized for treatment of patients suffering from atrial focused bradycardias and in patients with functioning AV node and ventricular conduction pathways. Though direct ventricular pacing can be performed by this method,[6] the higher pacing thresholds required may cause patient discomfort. Transesophageal pacing has been found to be as effective in short-term treatment of bradyarrhythmias when compared to transcutaneous and transvenous pacing methods.[6,7] Transesophageal pacing is less complicated to insert than transvenous pacing, and it is more efficient than transcutaneous pacing.

Components

There are currently two basic lead designs for transesophageal pacing. The first is a bipolar pacing catheter that can be inserted into the esophagus through the mouth or nasal passages. This catheter is similar in appearance to intravascular temporary pacemaker leads; however, the transesophageal lead has a unique connector to ensure it is used with the proper pulse generator. The pacing leads are currently available in 5 or 10 French diameters, and have a length between 93 and 100 cm. Each catheter has depth of insertion (DOI) markings on the catheter body to help the physician with proper electrode placement. There are esophageal stethoscope leads also available that allow for concurrent recording of the patient's temperature. These leads are a bit more sophisticated than would be necessary for an emergent pacemaker therapy and are generally larger in diameter. The lead system requires manual advancement of the catheter into the esophagus by a physician. Once the lead is in the proper place and at the proper DOI, it is held in place by being taped to the patient's cheek.

The second lead design is an electrode pill. This lead design has a thin electrode wire attached to the small pacing electrode, which is then covered by a disposable gelatin capsule. The lead is placed into the esophagus by having the patient voluntarily swallowing the gelatin capsule. Once swallowed, the electrode is held in the proper position within the esophagus by taping the electrode wire to the patient's cheek.

The transesophageal pulse generator (see Figure 37-5) is an external control system that is designed specifically for this type of therapy.

Figure 37-5. Transesophageal pulse generator.

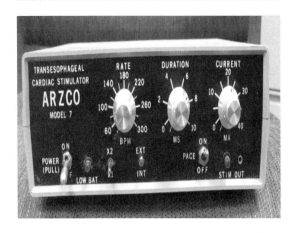

The more advanced generators allow for operator control of pacing current, pulse width, and stimulated heart rate. Transesophageal pulse generators are designed to always function in an asynchronous mode and do not allow for inhibition of pacing if an intrinsic cardiac rhythm is present. Some generators do allow for concurrent recording of the cardiac electrogram through the pacing catheter. The recording ability is used to ensure proper electrode placement and successful pacing therapy; it cannot be used to provide synchronous pacing.

Function

As the esophagus travels toward the stomach, it travels just posterior to the left atrium of the heart. By inserting a pacing electrode into the esophagus and applying a large enough electrical current, it is possible to capture the atrial muscle tissue and trigger depolarization. This method of temporary pacing does not have the same negative effect of causing chest muscle depolarization that the transcutaneous system has and thus is generally better tolerated by the patient. There is some risk of esophageal mucosal damage with prolonged transesophageal pacing. Temporary pacing by this method should only be used for short periods of time to avoid this complication.

Placement Procedure

One of the primary detractions of the transesophageal pacing method is that insertion of the catheter into the esophagus may cause the patient to gag and cough. To alleviate this occurrence, most physicians will numb the throat using a lidocaine oral spray or lubricating the pacing electrode with a lidocaine-based gel. Once the patient is anaesthetized in this fashion, the physician will begin advancing the catheter into the patient's esophagus through either the mouth or nasal passages (both being equally sufficient for placement and maintenance of the pacing catheter).

In order for transesophageal pacing to be successful, it must be in the correct position behind the cardiac structure (left atria or left ventricle). There are several methods for determining proper electrode placement.

Placement procedures for primary atrial pacing:

Patient's Height

The DOI for the transesophageal pacing catheter can be determined by utilizing the patient's height (in centimeters or inches). If the patient's height is known, then the following equations may be utilized to calculate proper DOI:[7]

$$DOI = Height\ in\ cm/5$$
$$or\ Height\ in\ inches/2$$

Add 3 to 4 centimeters if the catheter is to be inserted through the nasal passages.

Esophageal ECG Tracing

Proper electrode placement for atrial pacing can also be verified by utilizing the ECG tracing that can be recorded from the tip of the transesophageal catheter. To optimize electrode placement using the ECG tracing, the physician inserts the pacing lead to an initial level determined by using the method just described; however, an additional 5 cm should be added to the DOI that is calculated. When the electrode is in place, the physician will then begin to draw the catheter back slowly, watching the ECG signal that is displayed on the monitor. The physician will continue to draw the electrode catheter back until the recorded P wave is at the maximum amplitude for the patient. The catheter is then secured in place.[8]

Pacing Stimulus

Another way to determine proper transesophageal electrode placement is to evaluate the pacing threshold required to successfully capture the atrial muscle tissue. Utilizing the placement equations outlined in the first method described, place the catheter at the level calculated (adding 5 cm to the initial result). Pacing should begin utilizing 20 mA of current. The catheter should slowly be pulled back until atrial capture is achieved (which can be determined by noting successful atrial pacing on the ECG monitor). Once atrial capture is achieved and maintained, the catheter should be secured in place.[9]

Transesophageal pacing of the ventricle can be performed by placing the catheter electrodes within the fundus of the stomach. This position has proven to allow for consistent ventricular pacing with lower current requirements. In this position, research has indicated that transesophageal pacing may have better ventricular capture success than traditional transcutaneous pacing methods.[5]

Pulse Generator Settings

The operator of the transesophageal pacemaker generator is only able to alter three basic pacing parameters: pacing rate; pacing current; and pulse width.

Since the transesophageal temporary pacemaker is only able to stimulate the heart in an asynchronous mode, it is important to set the pacing rate a minimum of 12 beats per minute above the patient's intrinsic heart rate. In patients suffering from hemodynamically unstable bradycardia, research has indicated that transesophageal pacing at rates greater than 60 beats per minute resulted in increase arterial blood pressures.[8] The resulting hemodynamic improvement utilizing the transesophageal pacemaker was comparable to the increase achieved utilizing transvenous pacing methods.[6] Based on these findings, the suggested rate settings for the transesophageal pacemaker is dependent on the patient's hemodynamic stability. Several studies have suggested that a base rate of 80 beats per minute is a sufficient rate to provide treatment for most patients.[10,11]

Complications/Contraindications

Transesophageal pacing is more tolerable for the patient compared to transcutaneous pacing; however, there are several complications associated with this therapy. Most of these complications are minor and can be tolerated for the short period of time that this type of pacemaker therapy is utilized.

The primary complication associated with transesophageal pacing is the unwanted stimulation of the patient's gag reflex. As the pacing electrode is advanced into the esophagus, many patients may cough and gag. Utilizing a spray anesthesia prior to insertion may decrease this reflex; however, some patients may still have significant coughing spells during catheter advancement. If patient emesis occurs during catheter advancement, there is a risk of aspirating of the stomach contents. The physician and staff should be prepared to respond to a respiratory emergency if this would occur.

During transesophageal pacing, some patients will experience chest discomfort that may be described as heartburn. This chest pain is typically mild to moderate when experienced and will cease when pacing is stopped. In most situations, slight sedation is all that is necessary to alleviate this symptom. If possible, reducing the pacing current may also alleviate this pain. Pacing therapy will rarely need to be discontinued because of this sensation.

One of the more serious complications that may occur during transesophageal pacing is the formation of mucosal burns within the esophagus. Results in animal studies showed that current levels above 75 mA applied for 30 minutes, or currents above 60 mA over 4 hours, produced this type of injury.[12] These settings are significantly higher than the average currents necessary for atrial or ventricular pacing. Despite the lack of evidence that prolonged therapy at lower currents causes esophageal burns, current guidelines do not suggest constant transesophageal pacing therapy for periods longer than 1 hour.

Finally, this type of pacemaker is contraindicated in several situations. Patients with pre-existing esophageal injury should not receive this therapy. Transesophageal pacing has not been found beneficial for treating asystolic rhythms. Finally, transesophageal atrial pacing will not successfully treat bradycardia that is caused by AV nodal or ventricular conduction problems.

Transthoracic Epicardial Pacing

Transthoracic temporary pacemaker implantation is not typically used to treat acute bradycardia arrhythmias. Although emergent placement of transthoracic pacing leads is possible, it is considered a risky procedure associated with significant complications and low success rates.[13] In most cases, transthoracic epicardial pacemakers are inserted during cardiac surgeries to treat any postsurgical bradyarrhythmias that may develop.

Components

The leads for transthoracic pacemaker systems are normally teflon-coated stainless steel wires that are directly sutured to the epicardial tissue (surgical implantation) or placed adjacent to the epicardial tissues within the pericardial space (emergent implantation). During surgical implantation, the epicardial wires are typically attached to the right atria and right ventricle to allow for dual-chamber pacing if necessary. In the emergent situation, only one wire is advanced into the pericardial space. This wire is generally placed for right ventricular pacing therapy.

The pulse generator that is used during transthoracic epicardial pacing is generally the same pulse generator that is used for transvenous pacemakers. This type of pulse generator allows for control of cardiac rate, pacing current, and pulse width. Furthermore, unlike the previous types of generators discussed, this type of pulse generator allows for atria and ventricular sequential pacing.

Function

The transthoracic epicardial lead system allows for the electrical impulse produced by the pulse generator to be directly transmitted to the ventricular and atrial muscle tissues. Because of the direct cardiac stimulation, the transthoracic pacing therapy is much better tolerated by the patient than the previously discussed methods. Skeletal muscle and diaphragm stimulation is an uncommon occurrence with this system.

In the postsurgical setting, the atrial thransthoracic pacing electrode can also be used to record an atrial electrocardiogram. The exposed portion of the atrial wires can be connected to an ECG with alligator clips, allowing for the interpretation of the intrinsic atrial impulse. This atrial recording can be very helpful in determining the origin of narrow-complex tachycardias.

Placement Procedure

Temporary surgical implantation of epicardial leads is commonly performed during coronary artery bypass and other cardiac surgical procedures. During surgical implantation, the epicardial leads are typically applied to both the right atria and right ventricle. Having epicardial leads on both the atria and the ventricle allows the pulse generator to sense and pace the heart in a more natural sequence (atrial-ventricular sequential pacing). This type of pacing is hemodynamically similar to the intrinsic activity of the heart and usually results in increased cardiac output and stroke volume.

In most cases, a set of two insulated stainless steel wires are lightly sutured to epicardium of each chamber. Attaching two wires to each of the chambers allows for bipolar pacing (which generally decreases current required to obtain capture). To distinguish the two sets of wires from each other, the surgeon will create separate exit points out of the chest for each of the chamber electrodes. The pair of atrial electrodes usually exits from the right side of the sternum while the ventricular pair of electrodes usually exits from the left side of the sternum.

Direct Transthoracic Epicardial Lead Placement

Direct transthoracic lead placement involves inserting a large-lumen needle through the left chest wall and into the pericardial space. Once the needle's position within the pericardial space is confirmed, an epicardial pacing wire is advanced into the pericardial cavity. This wire is then connected to an external pulse generator to act as the negative pole for the pacing circuit. The other pacing pole is created by connecting the needle, or another electrode placed on the patient's skin, to the pulse generator. Using two separate poles in this manner creates a unipolar lead system.

Direct transthoracic lead placement is not a suggested method for providing temporary pacing therapy. This method of pacing has relatively low success rates in the bradycardia and asystolic patient.[14] Furthermore, this method of temporary pacemaker placement is also associated with significant complications such as pneumothorax, coronary artery perforation, cardiac tamponade, and perforation of the ventricular chamber.[15]

Pulse Generator Settings

Settings for atrial and ventricular temporary epicardial pacing systems are dependent on where the electrodes are placed on the heart and can vary considerably between patients. Because of this, recent studies have not identified specific normal values for temporary epicardial pacing.

The pacing current should be set at two times the threshold value achieved during initial epicardial lead implantation. The normal threshold values of both chambers differ greatly depending on the position of the electrode. Atrial thresholds may measure anywhere between 4.96 and 8.59 mA depending on electrode placement.[16] The average pulse width setting for epicardial pacing is between 0.5 msec to 1.0 msec. The majority of epicardial pulse generators are also designed to sense the heart's intrinsic electrical activity, decreasing the occurrences of inappropriate cardiac pacing. Because of this ability, these generators usually allow for manipulation of the atrial and ventricular sensitivity settings. The normal sensitivity settings for an epicardial lead system are between 2 and 5 mV.

The pacing rate should be set higher than 60 beats per minute and at a rate that is sufficient to alleviate patient symptoms. Because transthoracic epicardial systems allow for sequential atrial-ventricular depolarization, this method of pacing will generally require lower paced rates to achieve hemodynamic stability. The typical setting for the epicardial paced rate is between 70 and 90 beats per minute.

Complications

Most complications occur during the removal of the epicardial pacing leads. Because the epicardial leads are lightly sutured onto the cardiac structure, removal requires the use of gentle traction applied to the external portion of the wire to pull them out of the chest cavity. Complications that may occur are ventricular or atrial lacerations with bleeding, cardiac tamponade, laceration of bypass grafts, laceration of the superior epigastric artery, and wire breakage resulting in the retention of the distal portion of the epicardial lead.[17]

Many of these complications may be avoided by proper placement of the leads during surgery; however, there are steps that can be taken during the time of removal that will also decrease the likelihood of problems occurring during extraction. Be aware of the patient's coagulation status. The patient's INR should be less than 1.5 before the epicardial lead is removed to avoid bleeding complications. Pull out only one wire at a time to ensure control of the lead during extraction. Finally, if you feel excessive resistance, immediately contact the surgeon to discuss how the lead should be removed.

Transvenous Endocardial Pacing

Transvenous endocardial pacing for bradycardia has become the preferred method of treatment for patients that are refractory to appropriate medical therapy. Transvenous pacing is better tolerated by patients than transcutaneous and transesophageal pacing and is safer to perform than direct thoracic epicardial pacemaker insertion. Despite these benefits, the transvenous pacemaker insertion requires more operator skill and training than the transcutaneous and transesophageal methods.

Components

Transvenous pacemakers utilize a lead-based electrode system to deliver the electrical impulse to the endocardium. The transvenous pacemaker can be set up to provide therapy to the right atrium, right ventricle, or to both. The leads that are used may be guided through the vascular system under direct fluoroscopy or by noting the hemodynamic tracings that are recorded from the catheter during advancement. The type of pacing lead that is utilized depends on how the catheter will be advanced through the vasculature and what cardiac chambers will be paced.

Balloon flow-assisted pacing catheters have a balloon on the distal tip that can be inflated with air after it is advanced past the end of the sheath. Once the balloon is inflated, the physician advances the catheter through the venous system, allowing the antegrade blood flow to help guide the catheter into the cardiac chambers. This type of pacing catheter usually has a dedicated port to allow for hemodynamic monitoring through the distal tip (much like a pulmonary artery pressure catheter). The position of the catheter within the body and cardiac chambers is determined by evaluating the hemodynamic waveform that is being recorded. When the atrial or ventricular pressure waveform is noted, the pacing lead can be connected to the pulse generator and pacing therapy can be initiated. Because the balloon tip may inhibit the pacing electrode from obtaining maximum contact with the endocardial tissues, the pacing thresholds for this type of lead may be higher than with other transvenous lead systems.[2]

Another type of transvenous pacing catheter that can be used is a stiffer, polyethylene catheter. This catheter is advanced through the vasculature using a fluoroscopic X-ray imaging system. The physician manipulates the catheter through the venous system until visual confirmation is made that the pacing electrodes are in the right atrial or ventricular chambers. This type of lead has better pacing thresholds and long-term stability than the balloon assisted design; however, the stiffer catheter material is also associated with more complications.

Finally, a very special J-tipped pacing catheter has been developed to assist with right atrial pacing. The J-tipped catheter is designed to obtain catheter placement within the right atrial appendage. This specific placement helps improve atrial pacing thresholds and lead stability.

There are several different pulse generators that can be used for transvenous endocardial pacing (see Figure 37-6), and most pulse generators are designed to allow manipulation of the same pacing parameters. Transvenous generators typically allow the operator to alter the pacing rate, rhythm, pacing current, and pacing pulse width. If the pacing generator is a dual-chamber design (meaning that it is capable of simultaneously pacing the right atrium and right ventricle), then the operator may also be able to alter the atrioventricular interval. By changing this setting, the operator can manipulate the time between atrial and ventricular depolarization, allowing for maximum ventricular filling and stroke volume.

Function

Transvenous pacing is performed by advancing electrode catheters into the heart and delivering the pacing impulse directly into the endocardial tissues. Transvenous endocardial pacing can be utilized to obtain right atrial, right ventricle, or dual-chamber pacing. In the setting of a bradycar-

Figure 37-6. Examples of dual chamber transvenous pulse generators.

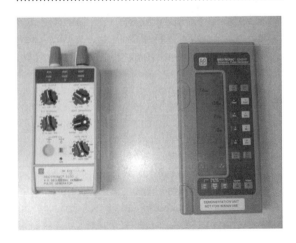

dia emergency, single-chamber ventricular pacing is usually performed due to the ease of lead placement and concern over the health of the AV node. Pacing from the right ventricle may be faster and easier, however, it will cause the loss of atrioventricular synchrony, which will result in a lower paced cardiac output and blood pressure.[18]

Placement Procedure

Placement of the transvenous pacing lead requires access to a large systemic vein. This access is usually obtained utilizing a modified Seldinger percutaneous approach, although a cutdown procedure can be performed to access the brachial vein. There are several veins that are commonly used as an access point for transvenous lead insertion: internal jugular; external jugular; left or right subclavian, brachial, or femoral veins. Though access through each of these vessels is possible, there are advantages and disadvantages to each of them. A recent study suggests that access through the internal jugular vessel has the highest success rates for experienced and inexperienced operators and is associated with the lowest number of complications. Furthermore, access through the internal jugular offers an easier, more direct route of advancement into the right atria and ventricle.[19]

Femoral vein insertion is the most practical route for inserting a transvenous lead during the cardiac catheterization procedure. However, this method results in suboptimal performance, particularly when balloon-tipped or "pacing swans" are utilized. Lead stability from the femoral approach is less secure, there is an increased risk of infection, and the patient needs to be immobilized the entire time that pacing therapy is being delivered, unless the patient is already undergoing a catheter procedure.[18]

Brachial venous insertion requires less immobilization of the patient than the femoral approach and may be a better choice of access for a patient that will be receiving thrombolytic therapy. The concern with brachial access is that even if the arm is adequately immobilized, the patient may still be able to move the arm enough to dislodge the electrode from the cardiac chamber. This possibility decreases the suitability of the brachial vein for temporary endocardial lead placement.

Internal jugular or subclavian venous access allows for a more stable lead placement and requires less patient immobilization. Percutaneous access of the subclavian vessels is a bit more difficult and is associated with significant complications (such as a potential pneumothorax or hemothorax).[18] If a permanent pacemaker insertion is required, the preexisting placement of the temporary pacing lead in one of the subclavian veins may become problematic. The subclavian vessels are not typically used for temporary pacing because of the difficulty of the insertion technique, and the potential that the emergently paced patient may later require a permanent pacemaker insertion.

Internal jugular access is suitable for the experienced and inexperienced operator because it offers the most direct route to the right atria and ventricle, and it is associated with the lowest complication rates.[19] Despite this, the operator must take care to identify the jugular vein and avoid accessing the carotid artery by mistake. This precaution is especially necessary if the patient has been receiving thrombolytic therapy or has been placed on any anticoagulant medications.

Placement of the ventricular pacing lead is typically performed by advancing the electrode catheter into the right ventricular apex. Atrial pacing is best performed by utilizing a J-shaped atrial lead that is positioned within the right atrial appendage. Though most temporary atrial and ventricular endocardial leads are passively placed within the chamber, there are temporary active fixation leads available. These leads have a screw that can be advanced into the endocardial muscle tissue. Though the active fixation lead increases stability, there may be increased difficulty in removing the lead from the cardiac chamber if it is left in place for prolonged periods of time. Once properly placed within the cardiac chamber the electrode catheter and the venous sheath should be sutured to the skin to decrease the chance of accidentally pulling the catheter out of position.

Pulse Generator Settings

Transvenous endocardial pulse generators typically allow the operator to program chamber current, sensitivity, pulse width, and pacing rate. A dual-chamber generator will allow programming of these parameters for both the atria and the ventricle as well as programming of the A-V interval to better simulate the patient's intrinsic atrioventricular interval.

To set the pulse generator current for ventricular pacing, the operator must first determine the ventricular pacing threshold. The average threshold for the right ventricle varies depending on the type of catheter utilized. Balloon-flow-assisted leads are generally associated with higher thresholds, while bipolar catheters generally resulted in achieving ventricular capture with lower currents.[2] To determine the ventricular threshold, the pulse generator is set to pace at a rate faster than the patient's intrinsic rate (usually 80 bpm) with an output of 5.0 mA. The current is then decreased until ventricular capture is lost. Once loss of ventricular capture is noted, the current is then increased until ventricular pacing returns. The current at which ventricular pacing is achieved is the ventricular threshold. To ensure consistent pacing of the ventricle, the pulse generator current should be set at two to three times the threshold value. If the pacing current that would be required to ensure ventricular pacing exceeds 10 mA, the operator should consider repositioning the pacing lead.[19]

Programming the right atrial current setting is very similar to the method utilized for the right ventricle; however, the threshold levels achieved vary greatly depending on the position of the atrial pacing lead. To determine the necessary pacing current, the steps utilized to determine ventricular threshold are used. Once threshold is determined, the atrial pacing current should be programmed at a level two to three times this value to ensure consistent atrial pacing.

Pulse width setting for the pacing of the right atrium and the right ventricle are typically the same. The starting pulse width for both of these chambers is normally 1.0 msec. Though increasing the pulse width may decrease the current that is necessary to trigger depolarization, very little benefit seems to be gained from decreasing the output current during endocardial pacing.

Atrial and ventricular sensitivity settings should be tested if the transvenous pacemaker is expected to remain in use for a prolonged period of time. To test the sensitivity settings; the pacing rate should be programmed below the intrinsic cardiac rate, and the cardiac rhythm should be evaluated for inappropriate pacing. If inappropriate pacing is noted, the sensitivity should be decreased until the pacemaker inhibits pacing when intrinsic activity is present. Normal ventricular sensitivity settings are 2.0 mV, atrial sensitivity settings are typically around 0.5 mV.

The atrial-ventricular interval setting is designed to allow dual-chamber pacing to simulate intrinsic atrial-ventricular synchrony as much as is possible. Although the physician may request the A-V interval setting to be reprogrammed based upon the target heart rate (slower rates assigned longer intervals, faster rates shorter intervals), most A-V interval values will be between 150–250 msec.

As with all temporary pacemaker devices, the programmed cardiac rate should be above 60 beats per minute, and at a rate that establishes hemodynamic stability. Single-chamber, ventricular pacing will require a higher pacing rate due to the loss of the A-V synchrony. A single-chamber, ventricular paced rhythm of 80 beats per minute was found not to offer any more hemodynamic benefit to the patient than the intrinsic bradycardia rhythm.[18] Dual-chamber temporary pacing will produced the best cardiac output and resulting blood pressure at any programmed rate.

Complications

Although temporary pacing via the transvenous pacing approach is better tolerated by the patient than many of the other methods described, this procedure is associated with unusually high rates of complications. Experience is a determining factor in the types and number of complications and transvenous pacemakers require significant training and preparation in order to be effective and beneficial to the patient.

The most common complication encountered with transvenous endocardial pacing is the dislodgement of the lead from the cardiac chamber. Lead dislodgment is often caused by the patient's movement (especially if the site of access for lead insertion was the brachial or femoral vein). In these situations, better immobilization of the limb may have prevented many of these occurrences. Utilizing a more stable access site (such as the internal jugular or subclavian veins) may also improve the likelihood of the pacing leads remaining in their original positions.

The second most common complication is local and systemic infection. Pacemaker leads left in place for more than 48 hours have higher infection rates than those that remain in place for shorter periods of time.[18] To decrease infection rates, proper sterile technique should be observed during the transvenous pacing lead insertion. Applying a sterile pacing lead sheath over the exposed part of the pacing catheter may also help in decreasing the infection risk.

CHOOSING A TEMPORARY PACING SYSTEM

Although all of the temporary pacing systems discussed can be utilized for treating patients with bradycardia, the difficulty of implementing and maintaining pacing therapy needs to be consid-

ered when determining which method should be used in a given scenario. In the emergent cardiac patient, there are two methods that are most commonly used due to the empirical evidence of success and due to their ease of use (see Table 37-3).

During the acute phase of a cardiac bradycardia or asystolic emergency, the transcutaneous pacemaker may be the best system to use. This system can be applied very quickly and easily to the patient and generally does not interfere with any other resuscitation efforts that may be occurring simultaneously. The anterior-posterior patch placement is currently being suggested for delivering acute pacing therapy; however, the right anterior and left lateral patch placement is also successful (and does not require the patient to be moved if CPR is being performed). Furthermore, this type of pacing therapy does not require a lot of extra operator training or extra procedural preparation. Although there is more discomfort experienced by the conscious patient utilizing this method of pacing, it is usually tolerable during the acute phase of the emergency.

For prolonged temporary pacemaker therapy, the transvenous system is the suggested method of pacing delivery. Transvenous pacing is much easier to maintain for long periods of time (when compared to transesophageal pacing) and is better tolerated by the patient. Although transvenous pacing does require significant operator training for it to be successful, it does not require surgical implantation like epicardial leads. Transvenous pacemakers are not indicated for the emergent asystolic patient due to the fact that it takes far too long to prepare, insert, and stabilize the

Table 37-3. Selecting an Appropriate Pacemaker System

Emergent Bradycardia	Emergent Asystole	Emergent Anitachycardia	Anesthesia and Perisurgical
Transcutaneous	Transcutaneous	Transvenous	Transvenous
Transvenous	Transvenous	Transesophageal	Transesophageal
Transesophageal			Transthoracic epicardial

catheter in the acute setting. Transvenous pacing systems should be considered the preferred method to provide temporary pacing therapy for a patient that is refractory to medical therapies.

The pacing system choice for antitachycardia pacing is less clear. Several studies have shown the benefits of utilizing transvenous or transesophageal pacing to treat supraventricular tachycardias (SVT). SVTs occurring following cardiac surgeries have also been successfully treated utilizing the implanted epicardial leads. The appropriate pacing system to use for treating SVT in the emergent setting depends on the equipment available, and the operator's experience.

REFERENCES

1. Nelson GD. Brief history of cardiac pacing. *Tex Heart I J* 20(1):12–18; 1993.
2. Gammage MD. Electrophysiology: temporary cardiac pacing. *Heart* 2000;83:715–720.
3. Bocka JJ. External pacemakers. February 5, 2008. Available at: www.emedicine.com/emerg/TOPIC699.HTM. Accessed April 10, 2008.
4. McEneaney DJ, Cochrane DJ, Anderson JA, Adgey AA. Ventricular pacing with a novel gastroesophageal electrode: a comparison with external pacing. *Am Heart J* 1997;133(6):674–680.
5. Rotter SJ, Koehler D. A comparison of transesophageal and transvenous pacing. *Anesthesia Analg* 1995;80:SCA78.
6. Roth JV, Brody JD, Denham EJ. Implications for transesophageal ventricular pacing. *Anesthesia Analg* 1996;83(1):48–54.
7. Pattison CZ, Atlee JL, Mathews EL, et al. Atrial pacing thresholds measured in anesthetized patients with the use of an esophageal stethoscope modified for pacing. *Anesthesiology* 1991; 75(5):854–859.
8. Benson DW, Snaford M, Dunnigan A, Benditt DG. Transesophageal atrial pacing threshold: role of interelectrode spacing, pulse width, and catheter insertion depth. *Am J Cardiol* 1984;53(1):63–67.
9. Atlee JL, Pattison CZ, Mathews EL, Hedman AG. Transesophageal atrial pacing for intraoperative sinus bradycardia or AV junctional rhythm: feasibility as prophylaxis in 200 anesthetized adults anddhemodynamic effects of treatment. *J Cardiothor Vasc An* 1993;7(4):436–441.
10. Hogue CW, Davila-Roman VG, Pond C, et al. Transesophageal atrial pacing in anesthetized patients with coronary artery disease. Hemodynamic benefits versus risk of myocardial ischemia. *Anesthesiology* 1996;85(1):69–76.
11. Dick M, Campbell RM, Jenkins JM. Thresholds for transesophageal atrial pacing. *Catheter Cardio Diag* 1984;10(5):507–513.
12. Nishimura M, Katoh T, Hanai S, Watanabe Y. Optimal mode of transesophageal atrial pacing. *Am J Cardiol* 1986; 57(10):791–796.
13. Brown CG, Gurley HT. Injuries associated with percutaneous placement of transthoracic pacemakers. *Ann Emerg Med* 1985;14(3):223–228.
14. Kern MJ. *Agiographic Data. The Cardiac Catheterization Handbook*, 4th ed. Philadelphia: Mosby; 2003; 324.
15. Samuels LE, Samuels FL, Kaufman MS, et al. Temporary epicardial atrial pacing electrodes: duration of effectiveness based on position. *Am J Med Sci* 1998;315(4):248–250.
16. McClurken JB. Minimizing complications from temporary epicardial pacing wires after cardiac surgery. Patient safety advisory: Pennsylvania patient safety reporting system. 2006; 1–2.
17. Killeavy ES, Ferguson JJ. The use of temporary transvenous pacing catheters. *Tex Heart I J* 1990;17(1):37–41.
18. Betts TR. Regional survey of temporary transvenous pacing procedures and complications. *Postgrad Med J* 2003;79:463–465.
19. Hynes JK, Holmes DR, Harrison CE. Five-year experience with temporary pacemaker therapy in the coronary care unit. *Mayo Clin Proc* 1983;58:122–126.

Chapter 38

CARDIAC PHARMACOLOGY

John E. Hawk, PharmD, BCPS
Sherri L. Derstine-Hawk, BSPharm, BCPS
Ryan Bickel, PharmD

INTRODUCTION

As new technology and devices such as drug-eluting coronary stents are developed and put into clinical practice, an ever-increasing number of patients can now be treated with catheter-based therapies. A broad palette of medication is used in cardiovascular catheter laboratories to decrease both acute and long-term complications. This makes medication use in PCI a very dynamic field. This chapter is an introduction and an overview of cardiac pharmacology and its applications in the catheterization laboratory; it is not exhaustive.

LOCAL ANESTHETICS

Local anesthetics provide anesthesia (blocking the sensation of pain) by preventing both the generation and the conduction of the nerve impulse. They block conduction by decreasing or preventing the large transient increase in the permeability of the membrane to sodium ion. The threshold for electrical excitability gradually increases and produces a block of conduction.[1]

There are two classifications of local anesthetics: the amide group and the ester group (see Table 38-1). The ester group includes cocaine, procaine, chloroprocaine, and tetracaine. The amide group includes lidocaine (the most common local anesthetic used), mepivacaine, prilocaine, bupivacaine, etidocaine, and ropivacaine.[1,2] Local anesthetics are manufactured in many different strengths/concentrations, with or without epinephrine (to increase the duration of the effect), and with or without preservative.

The incidence of allergy to lidocaine, other local anesthetics, or all "cains," is less than 1%.[3] Most claims of allergy are really adverse reactions, such as vasovagal or anxiety episodes. Other adverse reactions common with local anesthetics are neurotoxic (seizure, disorientation, tremors, restlessness, depression, and coma), cardiotoxic (myocardial depression, hypotension,

Table 38.1. Properties of Commonly Used Local Anesthetics[3]

Agent	Trade Name	Local Class Anesthetic	Concentration (%)	Maximal Safe Dose (mg/kg)	Onset (min)	Duration (h)
Procaine	Novocaine	Ester	0.5–1.0	7	2–5	0.25–0.75
Procaine with epinephrine				9		0.5–1.5
Lidocaine	Xylocaine	Amide	0.5–2.0	4.5	2–5	1–2
Lidocaine with epinephrine				7		2–4
Bupivacaine	Marcaine	Amide	0.125–0.25	2	2–5	4–8
Bupivacaine with epinephrine				3		8–16

cardiac arrest), idiosyncratic/metabolic, local delayed hypersensitivity, local urticaria, and local maculopapular eruption. These are all extremely rare reactions.

Another reason for allergic reactions to local anesthetics is the preservative used for both the local anesthetic and the epinephrine. Most, if not all, multidose vials of local anesthetic contain methylparaben, and preparations with epinephrine contain sodium metabisulfite as a preservative. Methylparaben-free local anesthetic solutions are commonly used for spinal or epidural anesthesia. If the offending agent is the metabisulfite, use nonepinephrine-containing local anesthetic if at all possible; just be aware that the duration of effect will be much shorter.

ANALGESICS AND SEDATIVES

Opioids

Morphine, meperidine, fentanyl, and others are analgesics derived from opium, from the poppy plant. Opioids can be naturally made, semisynthetically made, or totally synthetically made. These medications mimic the actions of other agents made by the body, such as endorphins, enkephalins, and dysmorphins. Opioids are classified according to their actions on the opioid receptors: agonist, agonist-antagonist, or antagonist.[4]

Table 38-2 lists equivalent dosing of some widely used opioids. Keep in mind that these are only equivalents and not dosing recommendations.

Morphine

Morphine is an opiate agonist and is the most commonly used opiate. Morphine is available in many dosage forms including intravenous, intramuscular, oral immediate release tablet, oral sustained release (or long-acting) tablet, oral liquid, sublingual concentrated liquid, rectal, and epidural/intratheacal injection.

Morphine not only relieves pain, but also decreases sympathetic discharge and catecholamine release. Morphine is frequently used as a frontline agent (along with supplemental oxygen, nitroglycerin, and aspirin) when a patient presents to the hospital with chest pain.

Morphine doses are largely dependent on the type of pain being treated, the patient's history of taking opioid medications, route of administration, and overall health and age of the patient. The typical dosage range of intravenous morphine is 1–10 mg. In the catheterization laboratory, 2–5 mg IV are generally administered per

Table 38-2. Opioid Analgesics Commonly Used for Moderate to Severe Pain[5]

Narcotic Agonists	Parenteral (mg)	Oral (mg)	Half-Life (hr)	Comment
Morphine	10	30	2–4	Standard of comparison for opioid analgesics; start lower dose for patients with respiratory insufficiency.
Hydromorphone (Dilaudid)	1.5	7.5	2–3	Slightly shorter acting.
Fentanyl (Sublimaze)	100 mcg		1–2	Short half-life; transdermal and transmucosal preparations available.
Meperidine (Demerol)	75	300	2–3	Not recommended for chronic cancer pain, impaired renal function, or if receiving monoamine oxidase inhibitors because of toxic metabolites.

dose and may be repeated as necessary. Lower doses can be given every 5–30 minutes to get pain under control.[5] The duration of action will be 3–4 hours.

The most common side effects of morphine administration are respiratory depression, nausea, hypotension, and bradycardia.[6]

Meperidine

Meperidine (Demerol) doses are largely dependent on the type of pain being treated, the patient's history of taking opioid medications, the route of administration, and overall health and age of the patient. Caution should be used when giving Meperidine to older patients and those with renal failure.

Meperidine can be given via intravascular injection, intramuscular injection, and orally. The usual dosage is around 50–150 mg, given IM, IV, SQ, or orally, and the action duration is 3–4 hours. For cath lab applications, typical dosing is 25–100mg IV.

The metabolite, normeperidine, has half the analgesic potency, but twice the neuroexcitatory effect of the parent drug, meperidine, and can cause seizures. Aside from the increased risk of neurologic toxicity from the normeperidine

metabolite, meperidine has a side-effect profile much like morphine.[7]

Fentanyl

Fentanyl is a synthetic opioid with a quicker onset and a much shorter duration of action than morphine. Fentanyl is approximately100 times more potent than morphine, largely due to its lipid solubility and its ability to cross the blood-brain barrier more rapidly. Fentanyl has traditionally been given via intravenous injection or infusion, but more recently, it has been manufactured as transmucosal, transdermal, spinal, and epidural formulations. Fentanyl is more cardiac stable, and therefore will not cause as severe hypotension as morphine.[4]

Like all other opioid analgesics, the dosing is patient-specific, but caution should be used when administering fentanyl. Due to its potency and narrow therapeutic index, fentanyl can quickly cause sedation and severe respiratory depression. A dose of 100 mcg of fentanyl is approximately equal to 4 mg of morphine, and usual doses for sedation are 25–100 mcg, with a duration of action from 30 minutes to 60 minutes. Adverse effects are much the same as with other opiates.

Reversing Opioids

Naloxone is a pure opioid receptor antagonist and will reverse the effects of opioid receptor agonists such as morphine, meperidine, and fentanyl. The dose commonly used is 0.4 mg to 2 mg, either IV, IM, or SQ. Caution should be used when administering to patients with opioid dependence, because naloxone can precipitate withdrawal syndrome.

Naloxone acts as a competitive inhibitor on the receptor and can completely remove all opioid from the receptor and block the receptor for a period of time. If intravenous administration is an option, consider diluting 0.4 mg in 10 ml sodium chloride, and administer 2 ml every few seconds until the patient can be awakened and is breathing spontaneously. When administering naloxone to a patient with underlying pain or in whom you may need to give more opioid, administer only the dose that reverses the symptoms that need to be reversed.

Benzodiazepines

Benzodiazepines are a class of medications that can cause anxiolysis, hypnosis, amnesia, and sedation. Benzodiazepines also have muscle relaxant and anticonvulsant properties, however, they do not have analgesic properties. Benzodiazepines cause a dose-dependent respiratory depression effect and at moderate to high doses cause vasodilation and hypotension.[8]

Diazepam

Diazepam, also known as valium, is a benzodiazepine that has been used for many years. Diazepam is metabolized in the liver to many active metabolites. These metabolites have half-lives of hundreds of hours, and caution should be used when administering this medication to elderly patients or when giving multiple or large doses. The metabolism of diazepam can be inhibited by many agents such as amiodarone, cimetidine, fluconazole, omeprazole, and valproic acid, causing the half-life to be increased.

Diazepam can be given by either the intravenous or the oral route. The usual doses for diazepam are 2 to 10 mg as a slow (no more than 5 mg/min) IV push, or 2 to 10 mg orally.[7] In the cath lab setting, diazepam is typically administered in dosages of 2.5 to 5 mg IV.

Midazolam

Midazolam (Versed) is a benzodiazepine that has a much faster onset of action and much shorter duration of action than diazepam. Midazolam is also metabolized by the liver, but by a different pathway, so older patients and patients with liver insufficiencies may experience prolonged effects of this medication. Also, the metabolism of midazolam can be inhibited by cimetidine, diltiazem, erythromycin, indinavir, ketoconazole, and verapamil. Unlike diazepam, certain medications can induce or quicken the metabolism of midazolam: barbiturates, phenytoin, rifampin, and carbamazepine. Midazolam, as with all other benzodiazepines, can cause a dose-related respiratory depression, and at moderate to large doses can cause vasodilation and hypotension.[8]

Midazolam is commonly given intravenously, but can be given IM and orally. The dose can range from as low as 0.25 mg up to about 2.5 mg at one time. Generally, midazolam is administered in the cath lab setting in doses of 0.5 to 1 mg. Allow at least 2 minutes before giving additional doses. Onset can range from 3 to 5 minutes, and duration can range from 30 to 80 minutes.

Lorazepam

Lorazepam (Ativan) is one of the most potent benzodiazepines. Lorazepam is metabolized in the liver by glucuronidation to only inactive metabolites. Lorazepam has a slower onset and a longer duration of action than midazolam.

Lorazepam can be given intravenously, intramuscularly, and orally. When giving lorazepam via the IV route, dilute the solution with equal parts D5W or 0.9% NACL solution. The usual dose is 0.25 to 2 mg IV. The onset of action takes about 15 to 20 minutes when given IV, and the duration is 6 to 8 hours. Lorazepam is less commonly utilized in the cath lab setting than diazepam or midazolam.

Reversing Benzodiazepines

Flumazenil acts on the benzodiazepine site of the GABA receptor and antagonizes the effects of benzodiazepines in much the same way as naloxone works on the opioid receptors to antagonize opioids. The half-life of flumazenil is only about 1 hour, much shorter than most benzodiazepines. Because of its short half-life, the reversal effects of flumazenil may wear off before significant amounts of the benzodiazepine can be cleared from the body. Therefore, the patient needs to be monitored for the time period that the benzodiazepine would be expected to still be present.

Flumazenil must be administered intravenously. The dose is 0.2 mg IV over 15 seconds. After 1 minute, if the reversal does not achieve the desired effects, another 0.2 mg may be given and repeated at 1-minute intervals up to a total of 1 mg.

Flumazenil is associated with precipitating seizures, especially in patients who are on chronic benzodiazepines or who have a history of seizures. Strong caution should be used in these patients. The ability to manage seizures should always be available when this medication is administered. Anxiety, cognitive impairment, confusion, psychotic disorder, and panic attacks have all been reported during treatment with flumazenil, especially if the sedation is reversed too quickly or with higher-than-recommended doses.

VASODILATORS

Nitroglycerine

Nitrates are indicated for angina and for suspected myocardial ischemia. Nitroglycerin is a nitrate that is routinely used to treat angina. Nitroglycerin produces venous vasodilation, causing a reduction in venous return and preload. At higher doses, nitroglycerin also produces arterial vasodilation, reducing afterload.[9] Nitroglycerin improves myocardial oxygen delivery and decreases myocardial oxygen demand. Nitroglycerin will dilate large coronary arteries, promote collateral flow, and the redistribution of coronary blood flow to ischemic areas.

Nitroglycerin can be given intravenously, sublingually (tablet), translingually (spray), orally (sustained release capsule), topically (ointment), transdermally (patch), and intranasally (spray). The infusion rate for intravenous nitroglycerin is 5 mcg/min, and may be titrated in 5 mcg/min intervals to target effects. If 20 mcg/min is reached with no effects, titrate at 10 to 20 mcg/min intervals. The sublingual dose range from 150 mcg to 600 mcg and can be repeated every 5 minutes for up to three doses.[7]

Nitroglycerin may be administered by direct intracoronary (IC) injection during catheterization procedures. Intracoronary nitroglycerin may be used in quanitified angiographic or IVUS studies, during PCI procedures to facilitate device placement, or to treat catheter-induced vasospasm. Doses of IC nitroglycerin are generally 200 to 400 mcg.

Nitroglycerin should be avoided in patients who are hypotensive, have taken sildenafil (Viagra) within the last 24 hours, and in patients who have had a right ventricular infarction.

Nitrate tolerance can occur with continual exposure to nitrates and is believed to be caused by the depletion of sulfhydryl groups by the nitroglycerin. Nitrate tolerance leads to decreased hemodynamic and antianginal effects and can be avoided by giving the patient an 8–12 hour nitrate-free period where no nitrates are administered.[9–11]

Sodium Nitroprusside

Sodium nitroprusside decreases afterload and preload by dilating both arterial and venous vessels.

Nitroprusside is very potent and care should be taken when using this agent. In patients with coronary artery disease, it can produce "coronary steal" syndrome; when there is a significant reduction in regional blood flow, causing a decrease in blood flow to the coronary arteries. Caution should be taken when using this agent on older patients and patients with impaired renal function, because nitroprusside converts to cyanide at a rate controlled by the dose. The elimination of cyanide needs a well-functioning liver, well-functioning kidneys, and available thiosulfate.[12]

The dosage range for nitroprusside is 0.3 to 10 mcg/kg/min with an average of 3 mcg/kg/min. The onset of action is 30 to 60 seconds, and the duration of action is 1 to 10 minutes. It is recommended that if sufficient effects are not seen after treatment at 10 mcg/kg/min after 10 minutes to stop nitroprusside. It is also recommended that a maximum dose of 70 mg/kg not be exceeded in a 14-day period. To avoid rapid and severe increases in blood pressure, nitroprusside should be titrated or weaned down gradually.[7]

As with nitroglycerin, intracoronary nitroprusside may be administered in the catheterization laboratory in dosages of 200 to 400 mcg. Nitroprusside IC administration is most commonly used during PCI procedures involving saphenous vein bypass grafts, vasospasm resistant to IC nitroglycerin injections, and with no-reflow phenomenon.

BETA RECEPTOR BLOCKERS

Beta receptor blockers (beta-blockers) are categorized as beta$_1$ and beta$_2$ (see Table 38-3). The beta$_1$ receptors affect the heart by increasing contractility and increasing the heart rate when stimulated. When blocked, the opposite effect occurs. Beta$_2$ receptors cause vasodilation and bronchodilation when stimulated and vasoconstriction and bronchoconstriction when blocked.[13]

Beta-blockers can be further classified into different groups based on specific actions of that agent. Cardioselective beta-blockers block predominately the beta$_1$ (cardiac) beta-receptor, while noncardioselective beta-blockers block beta$_1$ and beta$_2$ (bronchial) receptors equally. The noncardioselective beta-blockers are more likely to produce bronchospasms in patients at risk. Some beta-blockers are more lipid soluble than other beta-blockers, and therefore may be grouped together. These beta-blockers may be less bioavailable than beta-blockers that are less lipid soluble, thereby requiring larger oral doses.[14]

Table 38-3. Receptor Actions[14]

Receptor	Distribution	Response
Alpha^1	Smooth muscle	Constriction
Alpha^2	Presynaptic	Inhibit norepinephrine release
Beta^1	Heart	Inotropy
		Chronotropy
Beta^2	Smooth muscle	Dilation
		Relaxation
Dopamine (DA^1)	Renal, mesenteric, splenic, and coronary vascular smooth muscle	Vasodilatation (strongest in the renal arteries)
		Natriuresis
Dopamine (DA^2)	Presynaptic	Inhibit norepinephrine and perhaps acetylcholine release

Lipid soluble beta-blockers may also cross the blood brain barrier easier, giving increased incidence of CNS side effects.

The intrinsic sympathomimetic activity (ISA) also separates the different beta-blockers. Agents with ISA are thought to slightly stimulate the beta-receptors, making them less likely to depress cardiac output or cause bronchial reactivity.[14] Some beta-blockers have membrane-stabilizing activity and can act like a local anesthetic.[15]

Patients who take beta-blockers over a long time period should not have their therapy abruptly stopped. This can cause rebound tachycardia or hypertension and may precipitate angina in patients with coronary artery disease.[14]

Metoprolol

Metoprolol (Lopressor) is a cardioselective beta-blocker with weak MSA, no ISA, and is moderately lipid soluble. Metoprolol may be given by slow IV push at 2 to 20 mg doses. When a patient presents to the hospital with chest pain (if hemodynamically stable), metoprolol 5 mg IV may be given: 5 mg intravenously every 5 minutes for three doses, then oral therapy is started after 15 minutes. Metoprolol IV may also be used in the hospital or cath lab to control hypertension and sinus tachycardia in stable patients with angina. Oral metoprolol is commonly given as 25 to 200 mg twice daily, although many different regimens may be followed.[7]

Propranolol

Propranolol (Inderal) is a noncardioselective beta-blocker with no ISA, lipid soluble, and a moderate to high amount of MSA. Propranolol may be given intravenously or, more commonly, orally. The intravenous dose is 1 to 3 mg while the oral dose is 80 mg to 240 mg per day. The oral formulations can be sustained release or immediate release.

Esmolol

Esmolol (Brevivloc) is a cardioselective beta-blocker without either ISA or MSA and has low lipid solubility properties. Esmolol is utilized for the treatment of sinus and supraventricular tachydysrhythmias. Esmolol may only be administered intravenously and a loading dose should be given prior to the continuous infusion. Esmolol is metabolized by red blood cell esterases and its elimination is not dependant on either the liver or the kidneys. Esmolol is very rapid acting (almost immediately) and has a very short duration of action (10 to 30 minutes) with a half-life of approximately 9 minutes.

The standard dosing regimen is 500 mcg/kg over 1 minute, then 50 mcg/kg/min. After 4 more minutes (a total of 5 minutes counting the loading dose), if the heart rate is still not under control, another loading dose of 500 mcg/kg over 1 minute may be given, and the rate then increased to 100 mcg/kg/min. This upward titration may continue in this manner until heart rate control is achieved, or a maximum recommended rate of 200 mcg/kg/min is reached. If loading doses are not given, it will take 30 minutes for esmolol to obtain a steady state.

Labetalol

Labetalol is a beta-blocker with alpha-receptor blocking activity. Labetalol is predominantly a beta-blocking agent with some alpha-blocking activity that assists in vasodilatation. Labetalol's beta-blockade is noncardioselective and has equal beta$_1$ and beta$_2$ activity. Labetalol has weak ISA, no MSA, and is moderately lipid soluble.

Labetalol can be given orally at 100 to 400 mg twice a day, and intravenously at 20 mg over 2 minutes, up to 80 mg at 10-minute intervals. The onset of intravenous labetalol takes 5 to 20 minutes, and its duration is 3 to 6 hours.

CALCIUM CHANNEL BLOCKERS

There are three types of calcium channel blockers (see Table 38-4): phenylalkylamine, benzothiazepine, and dihydropyridine. Calcium channel blockers (CCBs) can also be separated into "heart rate accelerating" (dihydropyridine) and "heart rate limiting" (phenylalkylamine and benzothiazepine) drugs. In general, CCBs inhibit calcium ion movement from plasma into cells through calcium channels, thereby limiting vascular smooth-muscle contraction.

Side effects of calcium channel blockers include dizziness, asthenia, flushing, and ankle edema for diltiazem. Verapamil's side effects are the same as with diltiazem but also include constipation. The dihydropyridine CCBs, being different in action, have side effects that include headache, palpitations, tachycardia, ankle edema, flushing, gastrointestinal symptoms, gingival hyperplasia, weakness, nausea, heartburn, and dizziness.[16,17]

Diltiazem

Diltiazem (Cardizem) is a benzothiazepine calcium channel blocker with actions similar to the phenylalkylamine CCBs, with some vasodilation properties, but mostly negative chronotropic (slows the heart rate) properties. Diltiazem may also decrease myocardial contractility.

The intravenous dose of diltiazem is 0.25 mg/kg over 2 minutes, then 5 mg/hr infusion. The maximum single bolus dose is 0.35 mg/kg, or 25 mg bolus, and the maximum recommended rate is 15 mg/hr for less than 24 hours.[7]

Verapamil

Verapamil is a phenylalkylamine CCB that will slow the heart rate, cause some vasodilation, and will decrease myocardial contractility. The intravenous dose range is 2.5 to 10 mg over 2 minutes, with a maximum recommended dose of 20 mg.[7] Verapamil may also be given IC in the catheterization laboratory, most commonly in dosages of 50 to 200 mcg. Verapamil IC is most commonly administered during PCI procedures where there is vasospasm and/or no-reflow phenomenon resistant to IC nitroglycerin injections.

Nicardipine

Nicardipine (Cardene) is a dihydroperidine CCB much like nifedipine, although it may be given intravenously as a continuous infusion or as an IV push. This initial dose is generally 5 mg/hr and titrated in 2.5 mg/hr increments every 5 to 15 minutes to a maximum recommended dose of 15 mg/hr, or until the desired effect is achieved.

VASOPRESSOR/INOTROPIC AGENTS

Vasopressors raise blood pressure by constricting the vasculature. Inotropes increase cardiac output by increasing the contractility of the heart, which in turn, raises blood pressure. Table 38-5 shows the actions of alpha, beta, and dopaminergic receptors, different vasopressors/inotropes, and the receptors they activate.

Table 38-6 shows the dosing range and actions of common vasopressors and inotropes.

Table 38-4. Action of Calcium Channel Blockers

Type of CCB	CCB	Heart rate	Vasodilation	Contractility
Phenylalkylamine	Verapamil	Slow	Some	Decrease
Benzothiazepine	Diltiazem	Slow	Some	Decrease
Dihydroperidine	Nifedipine Nicardipine Others	May increase	Yes	Promote

Table 38-5. Receptor Pharmacology of Selected Inotropic and Vasopressors[16]

Agent	Alpha$_1$	Alpha$_2$	Beta$_1$	Beta$_2$	Dopaminergic
			Activity at Receptors		
Dobutamine	+	+	+ + + +	+ +	0
Dopamine	+ +/+ + +	?	+ + + +	+ +	+ + + +
Epinephrine	+ + + +	+ + + +	+ + + +	+ + +	0
Norepinephrine	+ + +	+ + +	+ + +	+/+ +	0
Phenylephrine	+ +/+ + +	+	?	0	0

Activity ranges from no activity (0) to maximal (+ + + +) activity or ? when activity is not known.

Table 38-6. Vasopressors[17]

Pressor	Dose	Cardiac Stimulation	Vasoconstriction	Vasodilatation	Dopaminergic
Dopamine	1–10 mcg/kg/minute	++	+	++	+++
	10–20 mcg/kg/minute	+++	+++	+	0
Norepinephrine	2–100 mcg/minute	+++	++++	0	0
Phenylephrine	20–200 mcg/minute	0	++++	0	0
Epinephrine	1–8 mcg/minute	++++	++++	++	0
Dobutamine	1–10 mcg/kg/minute	++++	+	++	0

0 = no significant change; + = mild increase; ++ = moderate increase; +++ = large increase; ++++ = very large increase.

ANTICOAGULATION AGENTS

Anticoagulation is very important in the cath lab. It minimizes clot formation on intravascular devices and in the vasculature during the procedure. It is also important in the long term, reducing patient's thrombotic response to the presence of a foreign body.

Platelet Aggregation Inhibitors

Drugs which impair blood platelet aggregation are used in most PCI procedures. Table 38-7 lists their indications and dosing.

Aspirin

Aspirin is used for prophylaxis of ischemic complications in patients undergoing PCI proce-

dures. Aspirin should be administered as soon as possible when a patient presents to the hospital with chest pain. Aspirin prevents platelet aggregation by inhibiting platelet cyclooxygenase. The inhibition of platelet function lasts for the lifetime of a platelet (5 to 7 days).

Aspirin is usually administered in doses ranging from 81 mg to 325 mg, and optimally given at least 2 hours prior to PCI.[18] Aspirin is also used to reduce the risk of death or nonfatal myocardial infarction in patients with previous infarctions or patients with unstable angina. Aspirin should be continued daily, in a dose ranging from 81 mg to 325 mg, for platelet aggregation inhibition. Cardiac patients may need to be educated that acetaminophen (Tylenol) and ibuprofen (Motrin) are not aspirin and cannot be used as a substitute. If a patient has gastrointestinal

Table 38-7. Indications and Dosing of Antiplatelet Medication used in Percutaneous Coronary Interventions[7, 29, 30, 31]

Medication	Description and Indication	Dose in PCI	Comments
Abciximab (Reopro®)	Glycoprotein IIb/IIIa inhibitor Adjunctive therapy with heparin, aspirin, ADP inhibitor (+/− bivalirudin)	0.25 mg/kg IV bolus 10–60 minutes before start of PCI + 0.125mcg/kg/min (maximum of 10 mcg/min) × 12 hrs	Risk of bleeding Monitor PLTs Must filter bolus and infusion through 0.2–0.22 micron filter
Eptifibatide (Integrilin®)	Small molecule glycoprotein IIb/IIIa inhibitor Adjunctive therapy with heparin, aspirin, ADP inhibitor (+/− bivalirudin)	180 mcg/kg IV double-bolus (give each 10 minutes apart) + 2mcg/kg/min for 18–24 hrs or until hospital discharge (whichever comes first) minimum of 12 hours.	Risk of bleeding Monitor PLTs Avoid if Scr > 4mg/dL or in hemodialysis patients
Tirofiban (Aggrastat®)	Small molecule glycoprotein IIb/IIIa inhibitor Adjunctive therapy with heparin, aspirin, ADP inhibitor	0.4 mcg/kg/min × 30 min. + 0.1mcg/kg/min × 12–24 hrs post-PCI Patients with a CrCl < 30 ml/min use 0.2 mcg/kg/min × 30 minutes + 0.05mcg/kg/min × 12–24 hrs post-PCI	Risk of bleeding Monitor PLTs Renal dosing adjustment needed Avoid if Scr > 2.5mg/dL
Clopidogrel (Plavix®)	ADP inhibitor Adjunctive therapy with heparin, aspirin, and glycoprotein IIb/IIIa inhibitor	Oral loading dose between 150mg−600mg. Given anywhere from 24 hours to immediately prior to PCI followed by 75mg PO daily.	Risk of bleeding Monitor PLTs
Ticlipodine (Ticlid®)	ADP inhibitor Adjunctive therapy with heparin, aspirin, and glycoprotein IIb/IIIa inhibitor	Oral loading dose of 500mg. Given anywhere from 24 hours to immediately prior to PCI followed by 250mg PO twice a day.	Risk of bleeding Monitor PLTs

distress with aspirin, lower dose therapy (81 mg), buffered, or enteric-coated aspirin may be considered.

Aspirin can increase the mean bleeding time by several minutes and should be used with caution in patients with platelet and bleeding disorders, renal dysfunction, erosive gastritis, or peptic ulcer disease. Some adverse reactions to aspirin include nausea, vomiting, gastrointestinal distress, bleeding, ulcers, bronchospasm, hepatotoxicity, and tinnitus.

Adenosin Diphosphate Inhibitors

Platelet activation is a primary factor in the development of in-stent thrombosis. Clopidogrel (Plavix) and Ticlopidine (Ticlid) inhibit platelet aggregation induced by adenosine diphosphate (ADP).[19] The combination of an ADP inhibitor and aspirin provides greater protection from thrombotic complications than aspirin alone.[20]

Ticlopidine

Ticlopidine dosage in PCI patients is a 500 mg loading dose followed by 250 mg twice a day for 2 to 6 weeks. Ticlopidine has a number of side effects, including GI upset, dizziness, increased serum cholesterol levels, renal failure, thrombocytopenia, purpura, abnormal liver function tests, and skin rashes. The most serious side effect, severe neutropenia, has been reported in up to 1% of patients. Ticlopidine should be discontinued if a patient's absolute neutrophil counts fall below 1200/mm or if the platelet counts fall below 80,000/mm.[21]

Clopidogrel

Clopidogrel demonstrates dose-related inhibition of platelet aggregation and with the traditional daily doses of 75 mg, it may take 3 to 7 days until maximal platelet inhibition is achieved. However, rapid ADP-induced platelet inhibition can be achieved within 2 to 5 hours if loading doses are initiated. Since most cases of thrombotic stent occlusion occur shortly after stent implantation, a clopidogrel-loading dose is usually given prior to PCI. The most widely accepted dosing strategy is to administer a 300 mg loading dose of clopidogrel with 325 mg of aspirin in the morning on the day of PCI or immediately after the procedure. These patients should receive clopidogrel 75 mg daily starting the day after PCI for at least 1 month and up to 12 months.[22–24]

Several trials have shown no difference in the clinical outcomes among patients treated with ticlopidine or clopidogrel after stent placement.[25–27] Due to similar efficacy, its once daily dosing, and a more favorable side effect profile,

clopidogrel has replaced ticlopidine in virtually all practice settings.

Despite its superior safety profile to ticlopidine, clopidogrel use is not without risks. Both the ADP inhibitors should be used with caution in patients who are predisposed to bleeding (such as those with gastric or duodenal ulcers) and patients receiving oral anticoagulants. Coronary artery bypass surgery patients recently treated with clopidogrel appear to have an increased risk of hemorrhagic complications. This increased risk in bleeding appears to be greater in patients that received a clopidogrel-loading dose prior to PCI. There have been several cases of thrombotic thrombocytopenia purpura (TTP) reported in patients treated with clopidogrel.[28] It is recommended that complete blood counts, bleeding time, and liver function tests should be monitored during treatment.

Glycoprotein IIb/IIIa Inhibitors

The glycoprotein (GP) IIb/IIIa receptor is the final common pathway of platelet aggregation that is necessary for platelet binding to fibrinogen. When the GP IIb/IIIa receptor is stimulated, it leads to the formation of a platelet plug that can lead to the formation of an intracoronary thrombus.

There are three types of GP IIb/IIIa-receptor inhibitors: monoclonal antibodies (i.e., abciximab), reversible small-molecule IV inhibitors (i.e., eptifibatide and tirofiban), and oral inhibitors (i.e., orbofiban, sibrafiban, xemilofiban).[29] There are important differences in the pharmacokinetics, pharmacodynamics, and mechanisms of action of the three intravenous GP IIb/IIIa-receptor inhibitors (see Table 38-8).

GP IIb/IIIa-receptor inhibitors are indicated as adjunctive therapy (with heparin and aspirin) for the prevention of ischemic complications in patients undergoing PCI. GP IIb/IIIa-receptor inhibitors have had a significant impact on outcomes of PCI patients by reducing the rate of

Table 38-8. Antiplatelet and Antithrombin Agents Used in Percutaneous Coronary Interventions[7]

Antiplatelet Agents	
Aspirin	
Adenosine diphosphate inhibitors (ADP inhibitors)	Clopidogrel (Plavix) Ticlopidine (Ticlid)
Glycoprotein IIb/IIIa inhibitors (intravenous)	Abciximab (Reopro) Eptifibatide (Integrilin) Tirofiban (Aggrastat)
Antithrombin Agents	
Unfractionated heparin (UFH)	
Low molecular weight heparin (LMWH)	Dalteparin (Fragmin) Enoxaparin (Lovenox) Nadroparin (Fraxiparine) Reviparin
Direct thrombin inhibitors	Argatroban Bivalirudin (Angiomax) Lepirudin (Refludan)

short-term and long-term postprocedure ischemic complications.

Bleeding is the most common adverse effect from glycoprotein IIb/IIIa-receptor inhibitors. Careful management of the catheter insertion site, early sheath removal, and the use of low-dose weight adjusted heparin can decrease bleeding complications. Mild, severe, and profound thrombocytopenia (platelet counts less than 100,000/mcL, less than 50,000/mcL, and less than 20,000/mcL, respectively) have been reported, with a 1%–5% incidence of thrombocytopenia overall.[7] When thrombocytopenia occurs, it is within 1 to 24 hours of receiving the agent, and the most severe form usually occurs within 1 hour. Platelet counts should recover rapidly after discontinuation of the GP IIb/IIIa-receptor inhibitor. Platelet counts should be measured 2 hrs after starting the infusion and 12 hours later then daily.

GP IIb/IIIa-receptor inhibitors are contraindicated in patients who are actively bleeding. They are not recommended for use in patients who have had major surgery within the past 3 months, stroke in the past 6 months, or a history of recent trauma, uncontrolled hypertension, severe anemia, and thrombocytopenia.

Abciximab

Abciximab (Reopro), a monoclonal antibody fragment, was the first agent developed to bind to, and inhibit, GP IIb/IIIa receptors. Abciximab is a large molecule that irreversibly binds to platelets, which results in inhibition of platelet function for the life of the platelet (5 to 7 days). Platelet aggregation is almost completely inhibited 2 hours after initiation of abciximab therapy, and recovery of platelet function may be seen 48 hours after discontinuation of the infusion. It is also the most expensive GP IIb/IIIa-receptor inhibitor.

Abciximab is administered 10–60 minutes before the start of a PCI as an IV bolus of 0.25 mg/kg, followed by an infusion of 0.125 mcg/kg/min (up to a maximum of 10 mcg/min) for 12 hours post-PCI. Abciximab is approved for use in acute coronary syndrome (ACS) for up to 24 hours, but only if there is a plan for eventual PCI.

In the catheterization laboratory, GP IIb/IIIa inhibitors are usually given as an initial bolus after the arterial sheath has been placed, prior to balloon inflation, although some operators only give these agents if they encounter technical problems during the procedure. Use of abciximab as an adjunct to aspirin and heparin decreases the incidence of death, MI, and urgent target vessel revascularization.[21,29]

Patients with unstable angina not responding to conventional medical therapy and who are planned to undergo PCI within 24 hours may be treated with an abciximag 0.25 mg/kg intravenous bolus followed by an 18– to 24–hour intravenous infusion of 10 mcg/min, concluding 1 hour after the PCI.[29]

If a patient develops severe thrombocytopenia, platelet transfusions may be needed. Because abciximab was developed using monoclonal antibody technology, it may cause allergic reactions.

Eptifibatide

Eptifibatide (Integrilin) and tirofiban (Aggrastat) are small-molecule, GP IIb/IIIa inhibitors that reversibly bind to platelets. This results in short-term inhibition of platelet function, with significant inhibition of platelet function observed 1 hour after administration. Normal platelet function returns approximately 4 to 6 hours after stopping the infusion.

Eptifibatide is administered as an IV bolus of 180 mcg/kg over 1 to 2 minutes, followed by an infusion of 2 mcg/kg/min. A second 180 mcg/kg bolus is given 10 minutes after the first bolus, and the infusion is continued for 12 to 24 hours post-PCI. Eptifibatide infusion should be reduced for patients with CrCl < 50 ml/min to 1 mcg/kg/min and should be avoided in patients undergoing hemodialysis.[7,29]

Tirofiban

Tirofiban is given at the initial rate of 0.4 mcg/kg/min for 30 minutes, followed by a continuous infusion of 0.1 mcg/kg/min. The infusion is contin-

ued for 12 to 24 hours post-PCI. In patients with renal insufficiency (creatinine clearance < 30 mL/min), the dosage is reduced by 50% to the initial rate of 0.2 mcg/kg/min for 30 min, followed by a continuous infusion of 0.05 mcg/kg/min. The infusion is continued for 12 to 24 hours post-PCI. Tirofiban should be avoided in patients with severe renal failure (serum creatinine > 2.5 mg/dL).

Both eptifibatide and tirofiban are excreted renally, and dosing adjustments may be needed for patients with renal insufficiency. Bleeding is the primary complication of eptifibatide or tirofiban therapy.

Antithrombin Agents

Thrombin plays an important role in the cascade of reactions causing thrombus formation at the site of injury, contributing to post-PCI thrombotic events. Table 38-9 shows the indications and dosing of antithrombin medications used in PCI.

Unfractionated Heparin

Unfractionated heparin (UFH) has long been the standard antithrombin agent used in PCI to prevent thrombus formation at the site of arterial injury and to reduce the thrombogenic effects of guide wires and other catheter equipment used to dilate the coronary arteries. UFH potentiates the action of antithrombin III, which inactivates thrombin, plasmin, and activated coagulation factors IX, X, XI, XII. Heparin also prevents the conversion of fibrinogen to fibrin. Heparin preserves coagulation factors, so that normal clotting will occur when heparin administration is stopped and cleared from the body.

Heparin's effect on coagulation is usually determined by measuring activated partial thromboplastin time (aPTT). The aPTT is not particularly useful during PCI procedures, however, because the test cannot be performed on site. Activated

Table 38-9. Indications and Dosing of Antithrombin Medications used in PCI[7, 29, 32]

	Description and Indication	Dose in PCI	Medication
Unfractionated heparin	Traditionally the anti-thrombin agent of choice in PCI. Adjunctive therapy with aspirin, ADP inhibitor, and IIb/IIIa inhibitor	Fixed standard dose bolus: 5000–10,000 units Fixed low-dose bolus: 2500–5000 units Weight adjusted standard dose heparin bolus: 100 units/kg Weight adjusted low-dose heparin bolus: 50–70 units/kg	Adjust dose to desired activated clotting time (ACT) Risk of bleeding Monitor PLTs 5%–30% incidence of heparin induced thrombocytopenia (HIT)
Dalteparin (Fragmin®)	Low molecular weight heparin (LWMH) An alternative to heparin as adjunctive therapy	60 IU/kg IV bolus	Risk of bleeding Monitor PLTs 1% incidence of HIT
Enoxaparin (Lovenox®)	Low molecular weight heparin (LWMH) An alternative to heparin as adjunctive therapy with aspirin, ADP inhibitor, and IIb/IIIa inhibitor	0.75 mg/kg IV bolus OR 1 mg/kg IV bolus	Risk of bleeding Monitor PLTs 1% incidence of HIT
Reviparin	Low molecular weight heparin (LWMH) An alternative to heparin as adjunctive therapy	7000 IU IV bolus followed by infusion for 16 hours	Risk of bleeding Monitor PLTs 1% incidence of HIT
Argatroban	Direct thrombin inhibitor An alternative to heparin for patients with HIT as adjunctive therapy	350 mcg/kg IV bolus then infuse 15–40 mcg/kg/min Adjusted to ACT	Risk of bleeding Useful in patients with HIT and/or renal failure
Bivalirudin (Angiomax®)	Direct thrombin inhibitor An alternative to heparin in PCI as adjunctive therapy OR alternative to heparin and IIb/IIIa inhibitor in PCI	1 mg/kg bolus + 2.5 mg/kg/hr for 4 hours. An additional infusion may be given after PCI of 0.2mg/kg/hr for up to 18 hours if indicated. OR 0.75 mg/kg IV bolus followed by an infusion of 1.75 mg/kg/hr through the end of the procedure	Risk of bleeding Useful in patients with HIT NOTE: Reduce doses for patients with impaired renal function.

continues

Table 38-9. Indications and Dosing of Antithrombin Medications used in PCI[7, 29, 32] *continued*

	Description and Indication	Dose in PCI	Medication
Lepirudin (Refludan®)	Direct thrombin inhibitor An alternative to heparin in PCI for patients with HIT as adjunctive therapy	0.3 mg/kg IV bolus followed by an infusion of 0.12 mg/kg/hr titrated to a target aPTT of 2- to 4-fold prolongation of the reference aPTT with an additional 0.3 mg/kg bolus as necessary OR 0.5 mg/kg IV bolus followed by an infusion of 0.24 mg/kg/hr titrated to a target aPTT of 2- to 4-fold prolongation of the reference aPTT with an additional 0.3 mg/kg bolus as necessary.	Risk of bleeding Useful in patients with HIT NOTE: Reduce doses for patients with impaired renal function. Do not use in patients with severe renal dysfunction (CrCl < 15 ml/min).

clotting time (ACT) responds linearly to heparin concentration and can be measured easily in the cath lab. An ACT of between 250 and 350 seconds is necessary before a PCI can be safely carried out. Higher ACT levels may reduce the frequency of ischemic complications, however, higher levels of periprocedural anticoagulation have been shown to increase the risk of bleeding.

Patients are generally given a bolus dose of heparin at the start of PCI. Weight-adjusted doses are often used in efforts to avoid excessive anticoagulation, and lower ACT levels can be expected. Lower weight-adjusted doses of heparin are used when adjunctive GP IIb/IIIa inhibitors are administered to minimize the incidence of serious bleeding.

Heparin bolus dosing for PCI patients include:

Fixed standard dose bolus: 5000 to 10,000 units
Fixed low-dose bolus: 2500 to 5000 units
Weight-adjusted standard dose heparin bolus: 100 units/kg
Weight-adjusted low-dose heparin bolus: 50 to 70 units/kg

If the target ACT value is not realized after administration of the heparin bolus, additional boluses of 2000 to 5000 units can be administered until the target value has been reached. The routine use of postprocedure UFH or LMWH is not recommended because of the significant increase in the risk of bleeding.

Adverse affects of heparin include bruising, bleeding, increased liver enzymes, and thrombocytopenia. Heparin-induced thrombocytopenia (HIT) is a serious side effect that occurs to some extent in 5%–30% of patients receiving heparin.[7] HIT is an immune reaction involving the development of antibodies to heparin. It typically manifests itself 5 to 10 days after heparin administration, but it may appear earlier if there was a recent previous exposure to heparin. The clinical signs of HIT are petechiae, purpura, melena, and profound thrombocytopenia. Other major features of this disorder include an increase in heparin tolerance, and recurrent myocardial, cerebral, pulmonary, and/or peripheral arterial thromboembolism. There is no relationship between the amount of heparin administered and the severity of thrombocytopenia. When the heparin is discontinued, the platelet count will increase rapidly within 48 to 72 hours.

There is also a less-serious form of thrombocytopenia known as heparin-associated thrombocytopenia (HAT). HAT usually appears within 48 to 72 hours of heparin administration and is associated with smaller declines in platelet count than HIT.

Heparin Reversal

Protamine binds ionically with heparin and rapidly inactivates it. Protamine reverses heparin, but when used alone, it has mild anticoagulant properties,[30] so it is important to give no more protamine than is necessary to reverse the heparin effects. Protamine inhibits unfractionated (conventional) heparin at doses listed in Table 38-10. An easy-to-remember "rule of thumb" is that 1 mg of protamine will neutralize 100 units of heparin. Therefore, 50 mg of protamine will neutralize 5000 unit bolus of heparin.

The half-life of heparin is approximately 60 to 90 minutes, so if 1 hour has past since the heparin was last given, about half the amount of protamine needs to be given; if 2 hours have past, give a quarter of the protamine dose. In the event that the heparin has been continuously infusing, calculate the dose per hour for the last hour, half the dose per hour for the hour before, and quarter dose per hour for the hour before that. Add these up and calculate your dose of protamine based on that number. Subsequent doses of protamine should be guided by the APTT or ACT.[31]

The major adverse effects of protamine are hypotension, bradycardia, and pulmonary hypertension and edema. These can usually be avoided by its slow administration intravenously over 1 to 3 minutes, and not more than 50 mg in any 10-minute period.

Allergic responses, including anaphylaxis have occurred, and are associated with previous exposure to neutral protamine hagedorn (NPH) insulin, vasectomy, and allergies to fish. If a patient is at risk of having an allergic reaction to protamine, they may be pretreated with corticosteroids and histamine blockers if no other option is available.

Low Molecular-Weight Heparin

Low molecular-weight heparin (LMWH) is made up of fragments of unfractionated heparin (UFH) that have higher ratios of anti-Xa to anti-IIa activity than UFH. LMWH can be used as an alternative to unfractionated heparin during PCI.[32]

The advantages of LMWHs are that they have longer half-lives, require less frequent laboratory monitoring, and have a more predictable anticoagulant effect with a lower incidence of thrombocytopenia. The disadvantages of LMWHs are that they are significantly more expensive than heparin, have longer half-lives, are only partially reversed by protamine, and the cath lab staff are unable to use the ACT to determine the level of anticoagulation.

Adverse affects of LMWH include bruising, bleeding, increased liver enzymes, and thrombo-

Table 38-10. Protamine Neutralization of Heparin By Heparin Source[7]

Protamine	Heparin source	Heparin Neutralized
1 mg	Heparin sodium (bovine lung)	90 units
1 mg	Heparin sodium (porcine intestinal mucosa)	115 units
1 mg	Heparin calcium (porcine intestinal mucosa)	100 units

cytopenia.[7] LMWHs can also cause HIT (but at a lower incidence than unfractionated heparin), and should not be given to patients with a history of HIT.

Direct Thrombin Inhibitors

This class of agents was developed from hirudin (a substance isolated from the salivary gland of the leech), which is a potent, irreversible inhibitor of thrombin. The direct thrombin inhibitors are not structurally related to unfractionated heparin, so these agents are the antithrombin

agents of choice for the prophylaxis or treatment of thrombosis in patients with HIT. Table 38-11 lists the different classes of direct thrombin inhibitors.

Bivalirudin

Bivalirudin is a safe and effective alternative to heparin in the PCI setting. Compared with unfractionated heparin, bivalirudin reduces the rate of death, myocardial infarction, or revascularization, with a concurrent reduction in bleeding.[33]

Table 38-11. Pharmacologic and Clinical Properties of Direct Thrombin Inhibitors[36]

Properties	Lepirudin	Desirudin	Bivalirudin	Argatroban
Route of administration	IV or SC (bid)	IV or SC (bid)	IV	IV
Indication	Prophylaxis or treatment of thrombosis in patients with HIT	DVT prevention after THA (not available in the United States)	Patients with UA undergoing PTCA; PCI with provisional use of GPI; Patients with or at risk of HIT/HITTS undergoing PCI	Prophylaxis or treatment of thrombosis in patients with HIT; patients at risk for HIT undergoing PCI
Binding to thrombin	Irreversible catalytic site and exosite-1	Irreversible catalytic site and exosite-1	Partially reversible catalytic site and exosite-1	Reversible catalytic site
Half-life in healthy subjects	1.3–2 h	2–3 h	25 min	40–50 min
Monitoring	aPTT (IV)	aPTT (IV)	aPTT/ACT	aPTT/ACT
	SCr/CrCL	SCr/CrCL	SCr/CrCL	Liver function
Clearance	Renal	Renal	Proteolytic and renal	Hepatic
Dose	0.3 mg/kg IV bolus then infusion of 0.12mg/kg/hr then titrate	Not reported	May cross-react with antihirudin antibodies	No
Effect on INR	Slight increase	Slight increase	Slight increase	Increase

Abbreviations: ACT, activated clotting time; AF, atrial fibrillation; aPTT, activated partial thromboplastin time; bid, twice daily; CrCL, creatine clearance; DVT, deep vein thrombosis; GPI, glycoprotein IIb-IIIa inhibitor; HIT, heparin-induced thrombocytopenia; HITTS, heparin-induced thrombocytopenia and thrombosis syndrome; IV, intravenous; PCI, percutaneous coronary intervention; PTCA, percutaneous transluminal coronary angioplasty; qd, daily; SC, subcutaneous; SCr, serum creatinine; THA, total hip arthroplasty; UA, unstable angina; VTE, venous thromboembolism.

Warfarin

The routine use of warfarin is no longer recommended after PCI, unless there are other indications for its use, such as a poor LV function, atrial fibrillation, or mechanical heart valves. The only thing that can quickly reverse warfarin is fresh frozen plasma (FFP). Vitamin K can reverse the effects of warfarin, but it takes too long to work if the patient is an emergency admission. Generally, warfarin won't affect the heparin dosage.

Thrombolytics

Thrombolytics, also called fibrinolytics, are agents that are used to dissolve clots in patients with deep vein thrombosis (DVT), pulmonary embolism (PE), acute ischemic strokes, and in the setting of acute myocardial infarction (AMI). These agents act by converting plasminogen to plasmin, a proteolytic enzyme, that has the ability to break down fibrin, fibrinogen, and other coagulation factors. All thrombolytics activate plasminogen, but differ with respect to mechanisms of plasminogen activation and fibrin specificity.

Thrombolytics must not be used in patients with active internal bleeding, aortic dissection, acute pericarditis, or who have had a cerebrovascular process, procedure, or disease within the past 2 months. Risks and benefits must be weighed carefully in patients who have had recent major surgery or trauma (within 2 to 4 weeks), uncontrolled coagulation defects, pregnancy, or uncontrolled hypertension.[7]

Thrombolytic therapy is a reperfusion strategy commonly used to treat acute myocardial infarction patients in facilities where primary PCI is either unavailable or may not be available on a 24-hour basis. In most large medical centers with cardiac cath lab facilities, primary PCI is usually the preferred reperfusion strategy.

Many factors influence the decision to administer thrombolytic therapy. These include time since onset of symptoms, patient's age, hemodynamic status, and coexisting medical illnesses.

The ability to prevent ongoing myocardial damage and establish reperfusion increases with early administration of thrombolytic therapy (ideally within an hour of the onset of the symptoms of ischemic chest pain). However, a reduction in mortality may still be seen in patients treated up to at least 12 hours from onset of symptoms. Some communities employ a prehospital thrombolytic therapy strategy, which is beneficial when the transport time of AMI patients from their home to the hospital is 60 minutes or longer.

Streptokinase

Streptokinase (Streptase) is a nonselective thrombolytic agent. It is a nonenzymatic protein that forms a complex with plasminogen. This complex then converts additional circulating plasminogen to plasmin that degrades fibrin and fibrinogen causing clot lysis. This agent is indicated for use in patients with evolving AMI, DVT, and PE. The dose in the setting is typically 1.5 million IU infused intravenously over 60 minutes.

It should not be used in AMI patients with the following characteristics: age over 75 years with inferior MI or those in whom thrombolytic therapy is started more that 6 hours after the onset of symptoms. Adverse reactions to this agent include bleeding, hypotension, fever, and allergic reactions.

Anistreplase

Anistreplase (Eminase) is a nonselective thrombolytic agent. It is a nonenzymatic protein that forms a complex with plasminogen. This complex then converts additional circulating plasminogen to plasmin that degrades fibrin and fibrinogen causing clot lysis. This agent is indicated for use in acute myocardial infarction. The recommended dose following myocardial infarction is 30 units by IV bolus over 5 minutes. Adverse reactions include allergic reactions, bleeding complications, and reperfusion arrhythmias; reinfarction are the primary complications of therapy.

Urokinase

Urokinase (Abbokinase) is a nonselective thrombolytic agent. It is a direct plasminogen activator that is isolated from human cells grown in culture. Urokinase is significantly less antigenic than streptokinase. It is approved for use in patients with PE, coronary artery thrombosis, and MI, and to restore patency to IV catheters. Possible adverse reactions include bleeding, fever, and rare minor allergic reactions.

rTPA

rTPA (Alteplase or Activase) is a biosynthetic form of human tissue–type plasminogen activator, that converts plasminogen to plasmin. It is a fibrin-specific thrombolytic that causes clot lysis by activating plasminogen associated with thrombi in preference to circulating plasminogen. It is approved for use in patients with AMI, acute ischemic stroke, and PE. When used in the setting of AMI, it is recommended for use in patients who meet all the following criteria: age less than 75, anterior MI or bad-prognosis inferior MI, and who will be receiving thrombolytic treatment less than 6 hours after onset of AMI. Alteplase is also an alternative to using streptokinase in patients having a documented allergic reaction to that agent or who have received it 5 days to 12 months prior.

The dose use for AMI is a 15 mg intravenous bolus injection followed by a 0.75 mg/kg infusion over the following 30 minutes. This is then followed by an additional 0.5 mg/kg infusion over 60 minutes. The total dose is not to exceed 100 mg. These patients must also receive concurrent heparin therapy for 48 hours. Possible adverse reactions include bleeding, as well as rare hypersensitivity reactions and reperfusion arrhythmias.

Reteplase

Reteplase (Retavase) is a form of tissue plasminogen activator produced by recombinant DNA technology. It is fibrin specific and is approved for use in the treatment of AMI. The dose in this setting is a 10-unit bolus IV over 2 minutes followed by an additional 10-unit bolus, also over 2 minutes, given 30 minutes later. These patients must also receive concurrent heparin therapy for 48 hours. Bleeding is the most common adverse effect, but rare hypotension and rare hypersensitivity reactions have also been reported.

Tenectlepase

Tenectlepase (TNK-tPA or TNKase) is a form of tissue plasminogen activator produced by recombinant DNA technology. It is approved for use in the treatment of AMI. Tenectlepase is more fibrin specific than Alteplase, and this allows it to be given as a weight-based single-bolus dose (See Table 38-12). These patients must also receive concurrent heparin therapy for 48 hours. Adverse affects are similar

Table 38-12. Tenectlepase Dosing for AMI[7]

Patient weight (kg)	Tenecteplase (mg) Given as a single IV bolus over 5 seconds
Less than 60 kg	30mg
60 kg or more but less than 70 kg	35mg
70 kg or more but less than 80 kg	40mg
80 kg or more but less than 90 kg	45mg
90 kg or more	50mg

to Alteplase; bleeding (including intracranial hemorrhage) is the main complication. Tenecteplase appears more fibrin specific than Alteplase, which may account for its lower rate of noncerebral bleeding compared with Alteplase. Some patients have developed antibodies to tenecteplase.

Tenectlepase and reteplase, are bolus-only thrombolytic agents, so the have advantages over bolus-plus-infusion thrombolytic agents such as Altepase. Bolus-only agents are easier to administer which can aid in more rapid treatment of AMI and bolus-only agents can reduce the rate of medication errors.

Thrombolytics and Adjunctive Agents

All AMI patients who receive thrombolytic therapy should receive aspirin (165 to 325 mg) on arrival to the hospital, and daily thereafter. Heparin dosing will depend on the thrombolytic agent selected. Streptokinase, anistreplase, and urokinase have anticoagulant properties, so there is less need for heparin, however, heparin should be administered concomitantly with the fibrin-specific thrombolytics: Alteplase, reteplase, or tenecteplase.

For patients receiving nonselective thrombolytic agents (streptokinase, anistreplase, or urokinase):

With patients at high risk for systemic emboli (large or anterior MI, AF, previous embolus, or known LV thrombus), it is recommended that heparin be withheld for 6 hours and that aPTT testing begin at that time. Heparin should be started when the aPTT returns to less than two times control (about 70 seconds), then infused to keep aPTT 1.5 to 2.0 times control (initial infusion rate about 1000 units/hr). After 48 hours, a change to subcutaneous heparin, warfarin, or aspirin alone should be considered. With patients who are not at high risk, administer subcutaneous heparin, 7500 units to 12,500 units twice a day until completely ambulatory.

For patients receiving fibrin-specific thrombolytic agents (Alteplase, reteplase or tenecteplase):

Administer IV unfractionated heparin for 48 hrs. Administer weight-adjusted dosing; 60-unit/kg bolus (4000 unit maximum) followed by 12 units/kg/hr (1000 units/hr maximum), both adjusted to maintain an APTT 1.5 to 2.0 times control (50 to 70 seconds) for 48 hours. Continuation of heparin infusion beyond 48 hours should be considered in patients at high risk for systemic or venous thromboembolism.

REFERENCES

1. *Micromedex Healthcare Series*. www.pharmacorama.com/en/sections/sodium-5.php. Version 5.1. Greenwood Village, CO: Thomson Healthcare. Accessed January 29, 2010.
2. Soto-Aguilar M, deShazo R, Dawson E. Approach to the patient with suspected local anesthetic sensitivity. *Immunol Allergy Clin North Am* 1998; 18(4):851–865.
3. Hollander J, Singer A., Laceration management. *Ann Emerg Med* 1999;34:356–367.
4. Li JM. Pain management in the hospitalized patient. *Med Clin North Am* 2002;86(4):771–795.
5. Carver AC, Foley KM. Palliative care in neurology. *Neurol Clin* 2001;19(4):789–799.
6. Shannon AW, Harrigan RA. General pharmacologic treatment of acute myocardial infarction. General pharmacologic treatment of acute myocardial infarction. *Emerg Med Clin North Am* 2001;19(2):417–431.
7. Hutchison TA, Shahan DR, eds. DRUGDEX system. Vol. 116. Greenwood Village, CO: Micromedex; 2003.
8. Young CC, Prielipp RC. Benzodiazepines in the intensive care unit. *Crit Care Clin* 2001; 17(4):843–862.

9. Munk KM, Mortensen UM, Nielsen-Kudsk JE, Sorensen KE. Noninvasive assessment of nitrate tolerance using mitral Doppler and brachial artery ultrasonography. *Am J Cardiol* 2003;91(1):111–113.

10. Littrell KA, Kern KB. Acute ischemic syndromes. Adjunctive therapy. *Cardiol Clin* 2002;20(1): 159–175, ix–x.

11. Varon J, Marik PE. The diagnosis and management of hypertensive crises. *Chest* 2000; 118(1):214–227.

12. Packer M. Current role of beta-adrenergic blockers in the management of chronic heart failure. *Am J Med* 2001;110 Suppl 7A:81S–94S.

13. Vukmir RB. Cardiac arrhythmia therapy. *Am J Emerg Med* 1995;13(4):459–470.

14. Miller RD. *Anesthesia*. 5th ed. London: Churchill Livingston, Inc.; 2000.

15. Ram CV, Fenves A. Clinical pharmacology of antihypertensive drugs. *Cardiol Clin* 2002; 20(2):265–280.

16. Ognibene FP. The sepsis syndrome: hemodynamic support during sepsis. *Clin Chest Med* 1996;17(2):297–287.

17. Moussa I, Oetgen M, Roubin G, et al. Effectiveness of clopidogrel and aspirin versus ticlopidine and aspirin in preventing stent thrombosis after coronary stent implantation. *Circulation* 1999;99(18):2364–2366.

18. Quinn MJ, Fitzgerald DJ. Ticlopidine and clopidogrel. *Circulation* 1999;100(15):1667–1672.

19. Schomig A, Neumann FJ, Kastrati A, et al. A randomized comparison of antiplatelet and anticoagulant therapy after the placement of coronary-artery stents. *N Engl J Med* 1996;334(17):1084–1089.

20. Karvouni E, Katritsis DG, Ioannidis JP. Intravenous glycoprotein IIb/IIIa receptor antagonists reduce mortality after percutaneous coronary interventions. *J Am Coll Cardiol* 2003;41(1): 26–32.

21. Mitka M. Results of CURE trial for acute coronary syndrome. JAMA 2001;285(14):1828–1829.

22. Yusuf S, Zhao F, Mehta SR, et al. Effects of clopidogrel in addition to aspirin in patients with acute coronary syndromes without ST-segment elevation. *N Engl J Med* 2001;345(7):494–502.

23. Steinhubl SR. Early and sustained dual oral antiplatelet therapy following percutaneous coronary intervention. *JAMA* 2002;288(19):2411–2420.

24. Bertrand ME, Rupprecht HJ, Urban P, Gershlick AH, Investigators FT. Double-blind study of the safety of clopidogrel with and without a loading dose in combination with aspirin compared with ticlopidine in combination with aspirin after coronary stenting: the clopidogrel aspirin stent international cooperative study (CLASSICS). *Circulation* 2000;102(6):624–629.

25. Berger PB, Bell MR, Rihal CS, et al. Clopidogrel versus ticlopidine after intracoronary stent placement. *J Am Coll Cardiol* 1999;34(7): 1891–1894.

26. Muller C, Buttner HJ, Petersen J, Roskamm H. A randomized comparison of clopidogrel and aspirin versus ticlopidine and aspirin after the placement of coronary-artery stents. *Circulation* 2000;101(6):590–593.

27. Smith SC Jr, Dove JT, Jacobs AK. ACC/AHA guidelines for percutaneous coronary intervention (revision of the 1993 PTCA guidelines)—executive summary: a report of the American College of Cardiology/American Heart Association task force on practice guidelines (Committee to revise the 1993 guidelines for percutaneous transluminal coronary angioplasty) endorsed by the Society for Cardiac Angiography and Interventions. *Circulation* 2001;103(24):3019–3041.

28. Bhatt DL, Topol EJ. Current role of platelet glycoprotein IIb/IIIa inhibitors in acute coronary syndromes. *JAMA* 2000;284(12):1549–1558.

29. Butterworth J, Lin YA, Prielipp R, et al. The pharmacokinetics and cardiovascular effects of a single intravenous dose of protamine in normal volunteers. *Anesth Analg* 2002;94(3): 514–522.

30. Franck M, Sladen RN. Perioperative use of anticoagulants and thrombolytics: drugs to prevent and reverse anticoagulation. *Anesthesiol Clin North Am* 1999;17(4):799–881.

31. Kleinschmidt K, Charles R. Pharmacology of low molecular weight heparins. *Emerg Med Clin North Am* 2001;19(4):1025–1049.

32. Magnus OE. Intravenous thrombolysis in acute myocardial infarction. *Chest* 2001;119(1 Suppl): 253S–277S.

33. Ryan TJ, Antman EM, Brooks NH. 1999 update: ACC/AHA Guidelines for the Management of Patients with Acute Myocardial Infarction: Executive Summary and Recommendations: A report of the American College of Cardiology/ American Heart Association Task Force on Practice Guidelines (Committee on Management of Acute Myocardial Infarction). *Circulation* 1999;100(9):1016–1030.

SUGGESTED READING

Brunton L, Lazo J, Parker K. *Goodman & Gilman's The Pharmacological Basis of Therapeutics*. McGraw-Hill; 2006.

Chapter 39

CARDIOVASCULAR RESEARCH

Regina Deible, RN, BSN
Leslie C. Sweet, RN, BSN

INTRODUCTION

The impact of research affects all facets of cardiovascular (CV) medicine, especially in the cardiac catheterization laboratory (CCL). The fact that CV disease is listed as one of the leading causes of death around the world has fueled development and research aimed at prevention and treatment of this disease. Couple this with the growing demand for "evidenced-based medicine" and the necessity to perpetuate the research process is clear. The ingenuity associated with drug-eluting stents (DES), biodegradable stents, PFO closure devices, valvular clips, and new antiplatelet options has all been made possible by meticulous medical research.

Medical research is the gathering of clinical data in organized studies that evaluate treatment options aimed at improving patient care. Understanding basic types of research and outcomes is essential at a time when new treatment devices and medical regimens are being utilized to treat CV disease.

A brief look at the role the Food and Drug Administration, physicians, and CV staff play in bringing medical devices and pharmaceutical agents to the clinical arena highlights the importance of hospital participation in performing research. This chapter will provide an explanation of some basic guidelines an institution must follow to conduct research, showing how the CV staff can actively participate in research efforts.

CLINICAL TRIALS IN THE CCL

The types of ongoing CV research vary depending on the project's goals and how they relate to treatment and prevention of CV disease. There are typically four types of clinical trials: treatment, prevention, screening, and quality-of-life trials.[1] Treatment trials typically evaluate new devices and pharmaceuticals. Prevention trials are designed to evaluate the ability of how well medications and devices prevent diseases. Screening trials evaluate ways to detect or diagnose disease processes. Quality-of-life trials evaluate the patient's perceived effects of treatment strategies on his or her quality of life.[1]

The majority of research conducted in the CCL is clinical in nature and usually consists of trials testing medications and devices that can be used for therapeutic or preventive treatment of cardiovascular disease. These trials are often externally funded by pharmaceutical or device companies that sponsor the trial. In these trials, the sponsor is responsible for the oversight and compliance dictated by FDA regulations. However, investigator-initiated trials are becoming more prominent. These trials are internally sponsored, requiring the institution or research center to assume full responsibility for the funding and conduct of the trial.[2] Although equally important as industry-sponsored research, assurance that the outcome of the clinical trial is accurate and has not been manipulated by the researcher is imperative in the investigator-initiated trial. This is accomplished by using well-established research guidelines that delineate regulations regarding the study process, adverse event occurrence reporting, and data analysis.

The nature of the clinical trial dictates whether FDA approval is mandated prior to initiating the trial. The ultimate goal of an FDA-approved clinical trial is to obtain a new label or indication of use for a current FDA-approved drug or device, as well as to provide commercial availability of an investigational device. Investigator-initiated trials may not fall into either or these categories and may therefore not require FDA approval prior to trial initiation. Regardless of whether a clinical trial requires FDA review and approval, all clinical research does require the institution's investigational research board (IRB) review and approval prior to initiation and must uphold the FDA standards of performing clinical research on human subjects.

GOOD CLINICAL PRACTICE

The International Conference on Harmonization (ICH) was established with input from both international governmental bodies and industry representatives of the United States, the European Union, and Japan in 1990. Good Clinical Practice (GCP) is an international quality standard for research that is provided by the ICH.[3,4] These standards are observed internationally.

GCP guidelines include the protection of human rights of subjects in clinical trials, and they provide an assurance of the safety and efficacy of the devices and drugs used in the trial. They include standards on how clinical trials should be conducted and define the roles and responsibilities of trial sponsors, clinical research investigators, and monitors. The GCP guidelines provide a standard for design, conduct, monitoring, auditing, recordkeeping, and analysis of a trial.[5] Importantly, this standard provides assurance that not only are the data reported credible and accurate, but they also protect the rights, integrity, and confidentiality of the subjects. The FDA and institutional review boards provide the same level of oversight, regardless of a trial's sponsor.

The standards of good clinical practice are integral in the day-to-day activities of the clinical trial staff. This consistency protects the integrity of the data collected and should be uniform between sites.

A collegial and respectful relationship among the research coordinators and CCL staff plays an important role in the research process. Identification of subjects from the patient pool, the opportunity to provide ample time for the consenting process, coordinating the collection of specimen samples (to prevent the duplication of venipuncture), and obtaining accurate data points collected during the procedure are all important variables of the research process.

While many roles are required to complete a successful trial, the most pivotal role is handled by the clinical research coordinator (CRC), who obtains, organizes, and implements the research protocol. While the principal investigator (physician) is medico-legally responsible for the management of the trial at their site, the CRC handles the lion's share of the trial activities.[6]

Stringent attention to detail is mandated, and the CRC will strive to collect all the elements required for the case report form (CRF) from the hospital records. Technically, if the data cannot be tracked to the patient's record, then it does not exist. Hence, requirements for specific documentation are often requested to track an important trial variable.

Documentation is very important in GCP. Standards directing the CRC regarding the capture of data are well established and include elements as simple as using a black pen for data capture, lining through incorrect data, circling and initialing corrected data, and creating source documentation for the charts to ensure the specific CRF elements can be cross-referenced. Although the CRC is responsible for capturing the data, he or she relies on the hospital staff to document specific information that will serve as a reliable source for the trial. Capturing data in a specific and consistent manner that is easily cross-referenced promotes clean, clear, and dependable information that will facilitate the entire research process and make a particular site a good candidate for future studies.

PROTOCOL

A protocol is a detailed plan of the research study and should consist of the following factors:

1. A comprehensive description of all prior studies involving the drug or device that is being studied.
2. A summary of why the research is being performed, including the targeted disease process, and the benefits and limitations of current treatment strategies, if appropriate.
3. Data handling, recordkeeping, data quality assurance, and/or monitoring procedures.
4. Description of the treatment procedures:
   a. For blinded studies, this would include specific instructions regarding how to maintain blinding and the extreme situations when unblinding is permitted.
   b. For device studies, this might include inflation pressures, wire and/or device sizing, need for intravascular ultrasound, etc.
   c. For drug studies, this might include the timing of the study agent administration relative to interventional procedure timeline.
5. Distribution, receipt, storage, and return of investigational drug and/or device.
6. Patient eligibility criteria, with specific inclusion and exclusion criteria to define the designated population of the study.
7. Sponsor contact information.
8. Statistical analysis methods.
9. Study purpose, with objectives, both primary and secondary, with well-defined primary and secondary endpoints to answer the study's proposed questions.
10. The evaluation procedures, including baseline, treatment, and follow-up assessments (e.g., lab work, physical assessment, quantitative coronary angiography [QCA], ECG, patient surveys, etc.).
11. Trial design: randomized, nonrandomized or registry, single site or multicenter, blinded or unblinded, single or multiarm, number of patients, number of sites, and anticipated duration.

TRIAL DESIGN

The development stage of a research study entails many variables that must be considered for a successful design. The institution and the researcher must ensure that the elements of the project follow GCP guidelines to uphold clinical quality and ethics. To establish the best approach to the study, the following questions should be asked right at the beginning:

- Will the study be prospective or retrospective?
- Will the study be a randomized trial, a registry, or a postmarketing surveillance?

- Will the study be single center or multi-centered?
- How many subjects will be necessary to provide the statistical power?
- Will it be a negative or positive study?
- Will the study be blinded? If so, single blind or double blind?

Prospective and Retrospective

Prospective trials involve identifying eligible patients prior to treatment, and following them *forward in time* to achieve the established objective. Conversely, retrospective trials generally have a cohesive population of subjects with a known disease who are followed *backward in time*, usually through a review of patients' medical records.[7]

When designing the trial, the method chosen would be the one that is best able to capture the data necessary to support the hypothesis. Often large centers with data repositories are logical sites to pursue a retrospective analysis, because these trials are composites of data that have already been collected. Another focus may be to compare matched data sets of a newly approved technology with an existing technology via a medical record review or data query (e.g., comparing the impact on target vessel revascularization in diabetic patients with new drug-eluting stents versus bare-metal stents). It is imperative that the study is well designed, with specific inclusion/exclusion criteria to limit the bias. While numerous trials can be performed comparing data on established practices, there are benefits to choosing a prospective trial to evaluate a new treatment strategy. There is limited bias involved with a prospective trial, because a specific study question is identified and the outcomes are evaluated over a period of time.[8]

Randomized Trials

Ideally, clinical trials should be performed in a way that isolates the effect of the treatment on the study outcome. A common approach to achieve this aim is through randomization, whereby patients are assigned to a treatment group by random selection. That means that they are just as likely to be placed in one cohort as the other.

The assignment ratio in a randomized trial is variable and dependent on the individual study design. For example, the ratio of patients randomized to the study agent versus control may be 1:1, 1:2, 1:3, etc. Randomized trials are often referred to as the "gold standard" in the research world because they are the most scientifically sound in that they involve real-time comparisons of two matched cohorts with the exact same inclusion and exclusion criteria.

Some randomized trials contain a crossover cohort, whereby the participants may ultimately receive both treatments. This design allows the control/placebo cohort access to the study treatment if the placebo/conventional treatment has been received and has failed. This crossover cohort must be part of the FDA-approved protocol in order to be an option.

Registries

Many advancements in medicine have resulted from research involving the collection and analysis of the medical record information of patients with certain diseases or conditions. These are research registries whereby data is obtained via chart review, surveys (either by phone, Internet, or mail), clinical visits or defined clinical research protocols and used to answer a question. Research registries, also referred to as observational studies, have made important contributions to an understanding of how health care is delivered, and what outcomes are achieved in the noninvestigational clinical arena.[9]

There are many situations where RCTs are not practical (rare diseases/high-risk subjects), or feasible (long-term outcomes). The observational registry provides an opportunity to incorporate these unique patient populations in a study treatment cohort for review of the effect of the study agent.

Observational registries also provide an avenue to evaluate subjects that may receive a study agent that is "off-label." Off-label usage of a drug or device is defined as the use of a product for an indication not in the approved labeling, whereby the investigator has the responsibility to be well informed about the product and to base use of the device or product on the following factors:[10]

- Firm scientific rationale
- Sound medical evidence
- Management of records of the product's use and effects.

Use of a marketed product in this manner when the intent is the "practice of medicine" does not require the submission of an investigational new drug (IND) application or investigational device exemption (IDE).[10] The use of DES stents in acute MI settings is a typical example of off-label usage.

Registries merely record the results of procedures that would be undertaken anyway, so there is no additional risk of any physical injury to the participants due to their participation. A specific method used to strengthen observational studies adapts principles of the design of RCTs to the design of an observational study as follows: It identifies a "zero time" for determining a patient's eligibility and baseline features, uses inclusion and exclusion criteria similar to those of clinical trials, adjusts for differences in baseline susceptibility to the outcome, and uses statistical methods (e.g., intention-to-treat analysis) similar to those of randomized, controlled trials.[7]

Single Center Versus Multicenter

Single-centered trials are usually investigator driven, where the population is well established and the conditions are well controlled. From a methodological perspective, this design is advantageous, because it limits the extraneous variables that may be present in multicenter trials. However, when it is difficult to recruit enough subjects in a reasonable time frame, there is a distinct advantage to having multiple centers participating in enrollment. Additionally, the results of multicenter trials are more generalizable than those of single-center studies. It could be said that the results of a single-center study may only be applicable to practice at that institution, whereas results from multicenter trials may be applicable to all institutions.

Postmarketing Surveillance

These studies are designed to gather additional information regarding the safety and efficacy of a drug or device in "real-world" situations. Because all possible side effects of a drug or device can't possibly be anticipated based on preapproval studies involving a limited number of patients with very specific clinical characteristics, the FDA maintains a system of postmarket surveillance and risk-assessment programs to identify adverse events that did not appear during the drug or device approval process. The agency uses this information to update drug or device labeling, and, on rare occasions, to reevaluate the approval or marketing decision. Additionally, these studies are intended to further detect any previously unforeseen problems and are often required for devices that:

- Are permanent implants (because failure may result in serious health problems or death)
- Are intended to support or sustain life
- Pose a potential serious risk to health

Postmarketing surveillance studies are critically important with regards to the continued safety and effectiveness of any approved drug or device.

Negative or Positive Outcome Trials

An outcome is defined as either a measurement (i.e., a specific lab result such as serum troponin or serum creatinine) or a clinical event (i.e., death or target lesion revascularization). Several criteria must be considered in the selection of outcome measures that include:

- Accuracy of the measurement
- Clinical importance
- Completion of ascertainment
- Precision of their definition
- Responsiveness to the drug or device

The choice of outcomes is critical and must be prospectively identified.[11]

A negative outcome trial is as important as a positive outcome trial, because it demonstrates the lack of safety or efficacy of the study agent or device. Historically, negative outcome trials were often not published. The research community has begun to recognize the importance of negative trials, whether to encourage repeat trials to confirm the reproducibility of the trial or to provide critical information to redesign a trial to further evaluate the product in a potentially more effective way. Remember, the point of a clinical trial is to demonstrate not only the utility of the agent or device, but more importantly, the fact that is safe.[12]

Blinding

Blinded trials are randomized trials in which one or more parties are kept unaware of the treatment assignment. Single-blinded studies refer to the study subject not knowing what treatment he or she has received. In a double-blinded design, neither the researcher nor the participant knows if the participant received the actual treatment or a placebo. Blinding of the treating physician and the study patient is fairly straightforward when dealing with pharmaceutical studies, but it is more complicated when dealing with interventional or procedural studies, because it may not be feasible to blind the treating physician. Instead, the patient may be followed by a blinded, nontreating physician so bias of the follow-up data is minimized. Hence, the treating physician and the CCL personnel may know the randomization assignment, but the patient and postprocedure team do not. Open-label trials are the opposite of blinded trials, in that both the researcher and the participant are aware of what actual treatment is being received.

Compassionate Use

Another unique clinical trial study is one in which a study agent is made available to a patient for use outside of the FDA-approved clinical trial or the FDA-approved label. The compassionate characteristic of this use may be that the product is investigational but the patient does not meet inclusion-exclusion criteria or the product may or may not be FDA approved, but its intended use is not consistent with the pending or approved indication. There may be a specific written protocol with FDA approval in place, or it may all arise emergently without such a protocol. In either case, an IRB-approved, compassionate-use consent must be signed by the appropriate parties. Reporting of this use to the FDA and IRB will be determined by the governing parties, but is typically less detailed than a structured CRT.

INFORMED CONSENT

The decision to participate in a clinical trial is a significant one, and one of the most important ingredients of a clinical trial is the informed consent form (ICF). There must be evidence that a subject has been provided a comprehensive, yet understandable overview of all that the trial will entail, with adequate time for all of the patient's questions to be answered satisfactorily. The informed consent therefore serves as a safeguard in protecting the safety, welfare, and rights of the subjects while providing written documentation of the process.

The FDA code of federal regulations and ICH GCP's provide the guidelines required for all informed consents.[13] The fundamental elements include:

- Diagnosis or clinical indication prompting consideration for participation
- Number of intended study participants and sites participating in the trial
- Explanation of the purpose of the proposed treatment and results of previous clinical use if possible
- Explanation of the course of the study, specifically pertinent to patient involvement in the study (e.g., what procedures will be performed, how patient care will be managed, any follow-up schedules, etc.)
- Expected duration of treatment and patient involvement in the clinical trial
- Statement that participation is voluntary
- Description of possible risks and benefits of proposed treatment
- Description of possible risks of *not* receiving treatment
- Disclosure of possible alternatives to proposed treatment
- Statement of confidentiality
- Explanation of compensation/treatment for injury/anticipated expenses
- Contact information
- Identification of significant conflict of interests of members of the research team
- Explanation of study patient's rights
- Signature and date lines for the study participant, a witness of the participant's signature, the individual responsible for obtaining consent, and the legally authorized representative if the participant is unable to sign

Given all the elements required in a thorough ICF, it is likely that the consent form will be rather lengthy, and the detail provided may be overwhelming for many subjects. Therefore, it is critical that the subjects are allotted sufficient time to review the ICF and have all their questions answered. Also, the consent language must be understandable. A well-accepted guideline is to write the consent at or below the eighth-grade level using as many lay terms as possible. It is also essential that there be no evidence or perception of coercion during the consenting process.

No study-related activity may be initiated until the subject has signed an informed consent. There are unique situations in which exceptions to consent may be made for patients using investigational products. These typically involve emergency situations where it is not feasible to obtain informed consent before the patient must be treated. Other unusual consenting scenarios involve patient's under 18 years of age, incarcerated patients, pregnant patients, confused or unconscious patients, and the like. Specific guidelines are available for these unusual patient populations to ensure that their rights are equally protected.[14]

STATISTICS

Statistics is a branch of mathematics that has its own terminology, which can be difficult to decipher for the uninitiated. It is usually adequate, however, to have a grasp of a few basic terms and leave the deep statistics to the experts.

p-Value

The p-value is used to determine if any differences between the cohorts' results were related to the study's variable(s) (drug, device, etc.) or due to chance. In statistics, a result is deemed statistically significant if it is unlikely to have occurred by chance. Because the concept of chance is so elusive, it is regarded in statistics in terms of probability, or the p-value. The p-value is the measure of probability that the results demonstrate a real difference between the groups. The results of a study are calculated, and a p-value of 0.05 or less is considered to be statistically significant. The smaller the p-value, the more significant is the result.

The p-value in a study is influenced by power calculation and confidence interval.

Power

A power calculation confirms that the sample size in a study is adequate for detecting a clinically relevant difference. Power refers to the probability that a clinical trial will have a significant (positive) result; that is, it will have a p-value of less than the specified significance level (usually 5%). This probability is computed under the assumption that the treatment difference, or strength of association, equals the minimal detectable difference.[15]

Statistical power is the probability that the study results will be significant ($p < 0.05$) and that the new treatment (or device) actually works. In simple terms, power is the study's chance of success; making sure that the study has adequate power is equivalent to making sure that it is successful.[16] Determining the power required for any given trial must take into account the estimated difference between the results of the treatment modalities. This will dictate the number of subjects needed to have a $p < 0.05$. Clearly, the smaller the difference between the treatment results, the larger sample size must be to show that the difference is significant.[17]

FOOD AND DRUG ADMINISTRATION

The FDA is a branch of the U.S. government under the umbrella of the Department of Health and Human Services, which oversees and determines the approval of many of the consumer goods that can be marketed for public use. Medi-

cal devices and pharmaceuticals are just some of the many goods this agency monitors. The FDA has set guidelines that institutions and investigators must meet before any medical research can be conducted. Once research has been initiated, the FDA monitors all components for policy and procedure compliance. The FDA has made efforts to increase its relationships with researchers and device companies by attempting to implement policies that will decrease review time and allow devices to be brought to clinical use quicker.[18]

Key regulations for quick reference:[19]

21 CFR, Part 50	Informed consent
21 CFR, Part 56	IRB regulations
21 CFR, Part 312	Investigational new drug
21 CFR, Part 812	Investigational device
21 CFR, Part 814	Premarket approval

Following FDA approval and commercialization of a new drug or device, the FDA continues to monitor the product for significant safety concerns that may ultimately require closer monitoring and reporting, if not actual reversal of the FDA approval. The FDA has a postmarketing branch whose sole purpose is to review all safety reports and facilitate further investigations into the reports if warranted.

CE Mark and FDA Approval

The FDA process for commercial approval in the United States is very rigorous and controlled. The equivalent of FDA approval of investigational devices in Europe is the CE Mark, which is an acronym for the French phrase Conformité Européene, also known as European Conformity. Obtaining the CE Mark signifies that the product has met the European standards for safety, health, and environmental protection and may be marketed in Europe accordingly. The regulatory process for the CE mark is somewhat simpler and usually quicker than FDA approval, so many new products receive CE Mark approval prior to initiation of FDA clinical trials in the United States. The FDA may consider clinical data from European trials as a complement to the U.S. trial data, but typically not as the primary contributor to the scientific review process.

INSTITUTIONAL RESPONSIBILITY

Institutions engaging in research projects should develop standard operating procedures (SOP) that cover all of the requirements of good clinical research to assure GCP compliance. Topics that should be included in the SOP are as follows:

- Billing
- Device/drug availability and accountability
- Device/drug control
- Informed consent
- Reporting of adverse events/serious adverse events
- Handling and shipping of blood and tissue specimens
- Monitoring/inspections
- Health insurance regulations

Institutional Review Board

One of the most important elements in the research process is the protection of the rights and welfare of research subjects. The IRB is a vital component of this process, serving to oversee the conduct of the study by providing guidance and support to the research staff. The IRB establishes and enforces institutional, federal, and ethical standards, which ensures patient safety and welfare.

A committee of independent board members associated with medical research must be established according to FDA regulations. Each IRB has members with different backgrounds, both scientific and nonscientific, to promote complete and unbiased review of potential clinical research

protocols. The IRB must contain no less than five members, with at least one member having scientific and/or clinical experience, and one member who is considered a "lay person." At least one member should not be affiliated with the institution conducting the research. The board must meet regularly and keep minutes of every meeting, which must be made available to the FDA on request.

The primary types of IRB submissions include:

- Initial protocol review
- Protocol amendments
- Requests for continuation
- Adverse event reporting
- Protocol deviation reports (related to patient safety issues)
- Requests for termination

Depending on an individual IRB program, a full board review is typically required for new submissions, request for continuations, and protocol amendments that affect the safety analysis of a study. Other submissions may be considered as expedited reviews, in which a component of the IRB committee members may review and approve the submission without waiting for a full board meeting.

Following a review and discussion of a submission, the committee may:

- Approve the study.
- Approve the trial with stipulations.
- Delay decision on the project until the next meeting.
- Request further information.
- Request further investigation into the protocol issues.

Data-Monitoring Committee

A data-monitoring committee (DMC), also known as the data safety monitoring board (DSMB), is a group of individuals with pertinent expertise that reviews accumulating data from an ongoing clinical trial on a regular basis. This team is comprised of independent experts who have the capacity to review the adjudicated data with regards to safety aspects of the trial without bias, because they are not at all involved in the trial themselves. The committee independently reviews data at designated points through the course of the trial. They can decide if the study continues or is terminated. This group of experts adds an important check-and-balance safety component to the ongoing trial. The list of the DMC members is usually submitted to the FDA for review and acknowledgement.

Clinical Events Committee

The clinical events committee (CEC) is a separate group of experts who review:

- adverse events
- serious adverse events
- unanticipated adverse events

The CEC prepares reports during the course of the clinical trial. Based on these reports, the events will be adjudicated by the CEC, confirming whether the events were related solely to the study agent, and whether the events warrant a safety profile change of the study agent. The adjudicated reports of the CEC are forwarded to the DMC for evaluation, and they determine whether to continue or discontinue the study.

DEVICE VERSUS PHARMACEUTICAL TRIALS

Clinical research is the study of the use of medications, biologics, or devices in human subjects with the intent to discover potential beneficial effects, as well as determine their safety and efficacy. Before any drug or device can be made commercially available for human use, companies must undertake extensive research to determine that their product is safe and effective. There is a stringent study process required before any device or drug may become commercially available in the catheterization lab.

A medical device is any healthcare product that does not achieve its primary intended purpose(s) by chemical action or by being metabolized. This definition is now becoming convoluted, because the new technological advances include devices that are coated with drug polymers or alloys, which now provide a blending of devices and pharmaceuticals.

Pharmaceutical research processes involve filing with the FDA for an IND to perform the clinical work, and an NDA, which represents the formal request for permission to market the product.

Device research involves filing for an IDE with the FDA, although it is important to note that some studies may be exempt from IDE regulations.

The IND contains the following fundamental information:

- Any previous clinical experience with the study of drugs in humans
- Clinical protocol and investigator information (including a detailed protocol that can describe potential or known risks to the subject)
- Manufacturing information
- Pharmacologic and toxicology studies that provide preclinical safety data

The IDE application must contain the following information:

- Certification that all investigators have signed the investigator agreement
- Complete report of prior investigations and summary of investigational plan
- Copies of all labeling for the investigational device, CRFs to be used, and any informational material to be given to the subject

- Environmental assessment or claim for exclusion
- If device is to be sold, a cost recovery justification
- Investigator agreement
- Manufacturing methods, facilities, and controls
- Names, addresses of participating institutions, list of IRBs, and chairpersons of each IRB

STAGES OF A CLINICAL TRIAL

The preliminary work required to determine the safety and efficacy of a new study agent or device is done in preclinical trials. Preclinical research can take years to complete, because there must be sufficient evidence to validate that the product is safe enough to proceed to human trials. Preclinical work may involve bench-testing or laboratory work or it may involve animal research.

When preclinical studies show that the product has promise and is not considered to be dangerous, it is then tried out on humans. These trials are divided into phases that are taken step by step. A successful phase I study is necessary before the device or treatment can be tested in a phase II study, and so on.

Phase I

The primary focus of a phase I (or feasibility) study is subject safety, with the intent to document that no significant harm is being caused to the study subjects. These are small studies (20 to 80 subjects), where the drug or device is given for the first time, and usually in healthy volunteers. The purpose is to evaluate the metabolic and pharmacologic action of the drug or device in humans, assess adverse effects, and evaluate early efficacy.

Phase II

These trials are more rigid and involve more subjects. They usually have a randomized double-blinded arm in which one group of subjects will receive the experimental drug or device, while a second "control" group will receive a standard treatment or placebo. There are some studies in which the control group may actually be a historical control. In this situation, there is an established "objective performance criteria" (OPC) to which the investigational agent is compared.

The goal of the phase II study is to demonstrate efficacy in the proposed indication subset of a group with fairly strict inclusion/exclusion criteria. The adverse effects and risks are assessed. If the data demonstrates strong evidence favoring safety and efficacy, the study will launch into the next phase.

Phase III

These are larger and more comprehensive "pivotal" studies that are the results of a strong safety profile and sufficient evidence of efficacy in the phase II trial. They are much larger (often with hundreds or thousands of subjects) and represent the specific population the drug or device is intended to treat. These trials aim to demonstrate a more thorough understanding of the drug or device's effectiveness, benefits, and range of possible adverse reactions. The phase III trial often involves multiple centers, and results in the NDA and PMA (premarket approval) process.

Phase IV

These studies are initiated following approval of the IND or IDE and are often designed to determine additional information regarding safety and efficacy, specifically in a more real-world environment of less limited inclusion and exclusion criteria. Phase IV trials are sometimes required as a condition of FDA approval. They may be conducted to evaluate drugs or devices in comparison with an already marketed product, may be designed to look at long-term safety as required by the FDA, or may be pursued to familiarize physicians with the compound or device or new indications for use.

REGULATORY COMPONENTS UNIQUE TO DEVICES

There are two avenues that may be pursued when a company's goal is obtaining approval to market an investigational device. The first option is called premarket approval (PMA) and the second is premarket notification, or 510(k).

Premarket Approval

PMA is a stringent scientific process in which the FDA reviews the safety and efficacy data from the class III device clinical trials. This class of devices must pass through the most stringent regulatory process, because they entail devices designed to support or sustain life for which insufficient information exists to assure safety and effectiveness.[20] Class III devices are considered to carry "significant risks," and thus, require a more thorough approval process.

Volumes of material are submitted to the FDA, including device description and intended use, nonclinical and clinical studies, case report forms, manufacturing methods, and labeling. Once the data has been analyzed, the FDA may conclude that the device has demonstrated sufficient evidence and is cleared for marketing and commercialization.

The PMA process entails four steps:

1. Initial review to determine completeness
2. In-depth scientific and regulatory review
3. Review and recommendation by an FDA advisory committee
4. FDA premarket quality system inspection

Once the PMA has been submitted, the FDA review panel will either issue an approval letter acknowledging that the device substantially meets the requirements or a denial letter citing deficiencies. Additionally, the FDA may impose postapproval requirements, which may impose restrictions on the sale and distribution of the device or may require postmarketing surveillance to evaluate long-term safety, effectiveness, and reliability.

Premarket Notification

Premarket notification, or 510(k), entails a submission made to the FDA to demonstrate that the device is as safe and effective or substantially equivalent to the legally marketed device. A 510(k) approval means that the device is similar to another device approved by the FDA and is not subject to PMA. The device is considered substantially equivalent if the following criteria are met:

- It is intended for the same use as the approved device.
- It has the same technological characteristics.
- It does not raise new questions regarding safety and efficacy.
- It demonstrates that the device is as safe and effective as the predicate device.

Humanitarian Device Exemption

There are rare occasions when a device is medically necessary to be utilized that can benefit patients in the treatment and diagnosis of diseases or conditions that affect or are manifested in fewer than 4000 individuals in the United States per year. These devices can be used if there is no comparable device that is available to treat or diagnose the condition. This is called a humanitarian device exemption (HDE). A request for an HDE is similar to a PMA application, however, it is not necessary to show that it is effective; only that it is safe. The investigator must request IRB approval and should supply the committee with FDA letter of approval for the HDE. It is up to the IRB to determine whether an informed consent document is needed. Sometimes, in lieu of an informed consent document, a patient information sheet can be created to be given to the prospective subjects.

DRUG/DEVICE ACCOUNTABILITY

Device accountability is essential in a clinical trial that involves a custom or investigational device, as is drug accountability for pharmaceutical trials. While the process involved seems simplistic, there are often studies involving an approved drug or device that may be used in an off-label clinical evaluation whereby the study product and the approved shelf product are exactly the same, so the need for stringent accountability is essential.

The basic elements include:

- Receipt and inventory of study drug/device
- Study drug/device labeling, specifically that this product is investigational
- Secure storage of the study drug/device
- Log depicting dispensing of the drug/device
- Copy of signed informed consent with research file when used
- Log of return/destruction of drug/device

There should be a prompt inventory of each investigational device. The inventory log should include:

- Date dispensed and to whom
- Date received
- Expiration dates for every item
- Labeled "Caution: Investigational Device"
- Method shipping and handling (e.g., shipping choice)
- Number received

- Serial/lot number
- Stored in a secured, limited-access storage area with appropriate temperature
- Type of device or drug label name
- Dates returned to the sponsor

Similarly, study drugs should be labeled and stored in secured, locked refrigerators when warranted. Typically, when study products need to be stored in a refrigerated container, detailed logs must be maintained documenting the actual temperatures during the storage period, as well as alarm procedures for extreme temperature readings.

If a drug or device is implanted in a patient who has signed an informed consent for the trial, the inventory log may also reflect the date of consent.

If the drug or device expires prior to use or has been contaminated or damaged, it must be returned to the sponsor. The protocol should have specific guidelines for returning study products, including obtaining authorization to return the product prior to shipment.

FINANCIAL IMPLICATIONS

The financial implications of participating in research ventures have become a major focus among investigators, hospital finance departments, and industry. The relationships between researchers and industry are becoming more complex and the visibility relating to the financial relationship must be disclosed. Medicare and private insurers will provide compensation for research-related care as long as these charges are consistent with the standard of care and Medicare guidelines. Many research centers employ clinical trial budget specialists to review the protocols to determine the budget components. The budget specialists may obtain pricing from the hospital and Medicare in advance, and then have the capacity to negotiate price-discounting arrangements.

When clinical trials involve devices, there are established guidelines with regards to reimbursement:

- Category A: experimental investigational devices that are so innovative they are dissimilar to current approved technologies or therapies and for which there is no Medicare coverage.
- Category B: experimental or investigational devices that are similar to current approved technologies or therapies and that may receive Medicare coverage.

It is important to clarify the category and reimbursement issues at the onset of the trial. For example, the costs associated with the use of the Category A device becomes the responsibility of either the patient, institution, or sponsor, whereas most Category B devices are reimbursable. However, a specific process involving specific documents must be submitted to Medicare in order to be eligible for reimbursement.

Additionally, prior to the initiation of any trial, it is important for the investigators involved in the trial to sign a financial disclosure form to prevent any conflict of interest regarding personal financial gain. These forms include, but are not limited to:

- Acknowledgment of equity holdings
- Board memberships
- Consulting fees
- Other forms of compensation
- Patents
- Research grants
- Royalties

SUMMARY

The key to performing successful clinical research involves a multidisciplinary team approach that consistently puts the patient's interests first. Each healthcare professional's role, whether extensive or simple, plays a vital role in the overall success of the program.

Participation in clinical research, whether in a large multicenter, industry-sponsored trial or a limited, investigator-initiated trial, is an invaluable opportunity for everyone from patients to healthcare providers, to institutions and industries. Efforts that provide a mechanism to advance clinical knowledge, perfect clinical therapies, and increase treatment strategies with improved outcomes is always a win-win situation. For the clinical team and the institution, it can serve as a segue to publishing and speaking opportunities. Though the pathway to successful clinical research requires significant financial and resource commitments, the net gain is long term and worthwhile.

REFERENCES

1. Available at: http://www.clinicaltrials.gov/ct2/info/understand#Q18. Accessed November 14, 2009.
2. International Conference of Harmonization. International Conference of Harmonization guidelines. Available at: http://www.ich.org/cache/compo/276-254-1.html. Accessed November 14, 2009.
3. Food and Drug Administration. Available at: http://www.fda.gov/oc/gcp/guidance.html Accessed November 14, 2009.
4. Available at: http://www.ich.org/LOB/media/MEDIA482.pdf. Accessed 14 Nov 2009.
5. U.S. Food and Drug Administration. Available at: http://www.ich.org/cache/compo/276-254-1.html. Accessed November 14, 2009.
6. Woodin, KE. *The CRC's Guide to Coordinating Clinical Research*. Boston: Thomson CenterWatch; 2004.
7. Concato J, Shah N, Horwitz RI. Randomized, controlled trials, observational studies, and the hierarchy of research designs. *NJEM* 2000; 342:1887–1892.
8. Kimball J. Epidemiology. Available at: http://users.rcn.com/jkimball.ma.ultranet/BiologyPages/E/Epidemiology.html#relative_risk. Accessed November 14, 2009.

9. Brooke EM. *The Current and Future Use of Registers in Health Information Systems.* Geneva, Switzerland: World Health Organization; 1974.

10. Available at: http://www.fda.gov/OC/OHRT/IRBS/offlabel.html. Accessed November 14, 2009.

11. Kellum JA, Ramakrishnan N, Angus D. Appraising and using evidence in critical care. In: Grenvik A, Ayers SM, Holbrook PR, Shoemaker WC, eds. *Textbook of Critical Care.* Philadelphia: WB Saunders; 2000.

12. Gliklich RE, Dreyer NA, eds. *Registries for Evaluating Patient Outcomes: A User's Guide.* AHRQ Publication No. 07-EHC001-1. Rockville, MD: Agency for Healthcare Research and Quality; 2007.

13. U.S. Food and Drug Administration Code of Federal Regulations. International Conference on Harmonization guidelines for good clinical practice. Available at: http://www.fda.gov/oc/gcp/guidance.html.

14. U.S. Department of Health and Human Services. Code of Federal Regulations Part 46, Subparts B, C, D, and E. Available at: http://www.hhs.gov/ohrp/humansubjects/guidance/45cfr46.htm. Accessed November 14, 2009.

15. Schoenfied, D. Statistical considerations for clinical trials and scientific experiments. Available at: http://www.hedwig.mgh.harvard.edu/sample_size/size.html. Accessed November 14, 2009.

16. Coleman WP. Inferential statistics. In: Lindberg S, ed. *Expediting Drugs and Biologics Development,* 2nd ed.; 1999. Available at: http://williampcoleman.wordpress.com/2007/12/14/chapter-14-inferential-statistics-descriptive-statistics/. Accessed November 14, 2009.

17. Goodman SN. Toward evidence-based medical statistics. 1: the P value fallacy. *Ann Intern Med* 1999; 130(12):15.

18. Medical Device Innovation Initiative. Available at: http://www.fda.gov/AboutFDA/CentersOffices/CDRH/CDRHInitiatives/ucm118252.htm. Accessed November 14, 2009.

19. Available at: http://www.accessdata.fda.gov/scripts/cdrh/cfdocs/cfcfr/CFRSearch.cfm?CFR Part. Accessed November 14, 2009.

20. Available at: http://www.fda.gov/MedicalDevices/DeviceRegulationandGuidance/HowtoMarketYourDevice/PremarketSubmissions/PremarketApprovalPMA/default.htm. Accessed November 14, 2009.

SUGGESTED READING

ICH Guidelines on Good Clinical Practice. Available at: http://www.ich.org.

Society of Clinical Research Associates. Available at: http://www.socra.org.

Association of Clinical Research Professionals. Available at: http://www.acrpnet.orp and www.centerwatch.com.

GLOSSARY

A

AAA	Abdominal aortic aneurysm
AAMI	Association for the Advancement of Medical Instrumentation
Abdominal aortic aneurysm	Localized dilatation of the abdominal aorta exceeding the normal diameter (about 2 cm) by more than 50 percent
ABI	Ankle-brachial index
Abrupt closure	Closure of a vessel, usually caused by thrombus or dissection, either during or immediately following an intervention
Absolute refractory period	When a sufficient number of the cells have repolarized to allow for another action potential to spread, regardless of the stimuli strength
ACC	American College of Cardiology
ACLS	Advanced cardiac life support
ACT	Activated clotting time
Activated clotting time	Blood test for monitoring high-dose heparin anticoagulation
Acute	Rapid onset; less than 24 hours
Acute gain	The change in minimum lumen diameter (MLD) from baseline to immediate postprocedure
Acute take-off	Vessel branch is at a sharp angle to the main vessel
Adventitia	Outer layer of a blood vessel

AF	Atrial fibrillation
Afterload	Pressure that the chamber has to generate to eject blood
AHA	American Heart Association
Allen test	Test of the patency of both arteries supplying the hand. A negative Allen test is a contraindication for transradial access.
Analysis segment	Vessel segment starting 5 mm proximal to a stent and 5 mm distal to it
Anaphylaxis	Acute, systemic, and severe allergic reaction
Anastomosis	Where two blood vessels are joined by a bypass graft
Anemia	Deficiency of hemoglobin
Aneurysm	Bulge (dilation) in the wall of a blood vessel caused by disease or weakening of the vessel wall
Angina	Painful constriction or tightness
Angina pectoris	Chest pain, or pressure, caused by ischemia of the myocardium
Angiogram	An X-ray image or film of the inner lumen of blood vessels using contrast media
Angiography	X-ray procedure in which contrast media is used to outline the inner lumen of a blood vessel
Angioplasty	Technique of mechanically widening a narrowed or obstructed blood vessel
Angioscope	A photographic device used within blood vessels
Ankle-brachial index	PAD diagnostic test comparing blood pressure at the ankle to that of the upper arm
Anode	The positive electrode in an electrical circuit
Antegrade	In the direction of the blood flow (downstream) in an artery or a vein
Anterioposterior	X-ray beam travels through the patient from front to back
Anterior	Toward the front of a structure or the body
Anterior tibial artery	An artery in the leg below the knee
Anticoagulation	Administering medication to prevent the formation of blood clots
Antiplatelet medication	A drug that stops platelets from adhering to each other and forming blood clots
Antitachycardia pacing	Controlled sequences of pacing pulses used to terminate tachycardias in the atria or ventricles
Antithrombotic	Prevents the formation of blood clots
Aorta	Largest artery in the body; originates from the left ventricle
Aortic valve	Cardiac valve between the left ventricle and the aorta

AP	Anterioposterior
ARP	Absolute refractory period
Arrhythmia	Abnormal electrical activity in the heart
Arterial bypass graft	Arteries and/or vein is grafted from the aorta to a coronary artery distal to a narrowing
Arteriosclerosis	Hardening of the walls of an artery
Artery	Vessel that carries blood away from the heart
AS-RAS	Atherosclerotic renal artery stenosis
Ascites	Accumulation of fluid in the peritoneal cavity
Asepsis	Practice to reduce or eliminate contaminants from entering an operative field to prevent infection
Aspirin	Trade name of a platelet aggregation inhibitor drug, acetylsalicylic acid (ASA)
Asystole	Absence of cardiac electrical activity; no myocardial contractions and no cardiac output
Atherectomy	Removal of plaque material from a vessel's wall
Atherosclerosis	A type of arteriosclerosis, caused by a build-up of plaque on the inside walls of the arteries
ATP	Antitachycardia pacing
Atresia	Condition in which a passage in the body is abnormally closed or absent
Atria	Plural form of atrium
Atrial fibrillation	Erratic and uncoordinated electrical discharge from the atrium
Atrial flutter	Rapid, regular, atrial contractions usually occurring at rates of 250 to 350 beats per minutes
Atrium	Receiving chamber(s) of the heart, from which blood is pumped into the ventricles
Auscultate	To listen to the sounds made by the internal organs of the body
Automaticity	The ability of a cell to depolarize spontaneously
AV	Atrioventricular
AV fistula/shunt	An abnormal communication between an artery and vein due to birth defect, injury, infection, aneurysm, or cancer. See "Dialysis fistula/shunt"
AV valve	Heart valve(s) between the atrium and ventricle: mitral (left) valve, and tricuspid (right) valve
AVNRT	Atrioventricular nodal reentrant tachycardia

B

Back-up support	Ability of a guiding catheter to remain seated in the coronary ostium, providing a stable platform for advancement of devices
Bail-out	PCI procedure to overcome an acute problem, such as stenting due to a dissection/flap caused by balloon angioplasty
Balloon angioplasty	A narrowed or blocked artery is opened with a catheter-mounted balloon
Balloon catheter	A catheter with an inflatable balloon attached to its tip
Balloon compliance	How a balloon material deforms, or stretches, under pressure. The less compliant a balloon's material, the more dilating force it transmits, and the more uniformly it expands.
Balloon rewrapping	A balloon's ability to refold after having been inflated
Balloon septostomy	Widening of a PFO or ASD using a balloon catheter. See Rushkind's procedure.
Balloon-expandable stent	The stent is introduced into the body mounted on a balloon catheter, and is expanded by inflating the balloon
Bare metal stent	A stent that carries no medication
BAS	Balloon atrial septostomy
Baseline	A normal or initial level of a measurable quantity; used for comparison with values measured after an intervention
Benign	A medical condition or anatomical malformation that will not become life threatening
Bicuspid valve	A valve that consists of two segments (cusps); mitral valve
Bifurcation	Segment where one blood vessel divides into two
Binary restenosis	A lesion that shows 50% or more lumen diameter restenosis at follow-up
Bioabsorbable	A material that will be entirely absorbed (metabolized) by the body
Biocompatible	A medical device/implant that has minimal effect, or causes a minimal reaction, in living tissues
Biodegradable	An implanted material that degrades into smaller pieces
Biphasic shock	Bidirectional, high-voltage waveform; part of the energy is delivered from anode to cathode, and the rest from cathode to anode
Biplane	X-ray equipment with two X-ray cameras mounted perpendicular to each other
Blinded study	The subject or the investigator (or both which constitutes "double blind") are unaware of what study product the subject is receiving
Blood pressure	Pressure of blood on the walls of an artery
BMS	Bare metal stent

Bolus	A single, large dose of medication
BPEG	British Pacing and Electrophysiology Group
BPM (bpm)	Beats per minute; a measure of heart rate
Brachytherapy	Radiation therapy in which the irradiation source is placed within the area to be treated
Bradycardia	Slow heart beat; a resting heart rate of less than 60 bpm
Braunwald Classification of Unstable Angina I	A classification scheme for patients with angina, to identify those who are at increased risk for adverse events so that the appropriate treatment can be initiated
Class 1	New onset of severe or accelerated angina. Patients with new onset ($<$ 2 months in duration) exertional angina pectoris that is severe or frequent ($>$ 3 episodes/day) or patients with chronic stable angina who develop accelerated angina (that is, angina is distinctly more frequent, severe, longer in duration, or precipitated by distinctly less exertion than previously) but who have not experienced pain at rest during the preceding 2 months.
Class 2	Angina at rest, subacute. Patients with one or more episodes of angina at rest during the preceding month but not within the preceding 48 hours.
Class 3	Angina at rest, acute. Patients with one or more episodes of angina at rest within the preceding 48 hours.
Braunwald Classification of Unstable Angina II	Clinical circumstances under which unstable angina occurs:
Class A	Secondary unstable angina. Patients in whom unstable angina develops secondary to a clearly identified condition extrinsic to the coronary vascular bed that has intensified myocardial ischemia. Such conditions reduce myocardial oxygen supply or increase myocardial oxygen demand and include anemia, fever, infection, hypotension, uncontrolled hypertension, tachyarrhythmia, unusual emotional stress, thyrotoxicosis, and hypoxemia secondary to respiratory failure.
Class B	Primary unstable angina. Patients who develop unstable angina pectoris in the absence of an extra-cardiac condition that have intensified ischemia, as in Class A.
Class C	Postinfarction unstable angina. Patients who develop unstable angina within the first 2 weeks after a documented acute myocardial infarction.
BSA	Body surface area
BTK	Below the knee
BUN	Blood urea nitrogen

C

C-arm	Moveable frame with an X-ray source at the end of one arm and a camera at the other
CABG	Coronary artery bypass graft
CAD	Coronary artery disease
Calcium channel blockers	Inhibit calcium ion movement from plasma into cells through calcium channels, limiting vascular smooth muscle contraction
Calcium score	The extent of calcium in the coronary arteries—measured with cardiac EBCT
Canadian Cardiovascular Society Classification (CCS)	Measurement/classification of angina symptoms
Class 1	Ordinary physical activity does not cause angina, such as walking and climbing stairs. Angina with strenuous, rapid, or prolonged exertion at work or during recreation.
Class 2	Slight limitation of ordinary activity. Walking or climbing stairs rapidly, walking uphill, walking or stair climbing after meals, or in cold or wind, under emotional stress, or any only during the first hours after awakening. Walking more than two blocks on the level and climbing more than one flight of ordinary stairs at a normal pace and in normal conditions.
Class 3	Marked limitations of ordinary physical activity. Walking one to two blocks on the level and climbing one flight of stairs in normal conditions and at a normal pace.
Class 4	Inability to carry on any physical activity without discomfort. Angina syndrome may be present at rest.
Capillary	Smallest blood vessels in the body, connecting arterioles and venules
Cardiac index	Parameter that relates the cardiac output (CO) to body surface area (BSA), relating heart performance to the size of the individual
Cardiac output	Volume of blood pumped by the heart in a minute
Cardiac tamponade	Collection of fluid (blood) between the myocardium and the pericardial sac
Cardiac technician	Specialist in recording and monitoring different parameters of the heart
Cardiologist	Physician specializing in the diagnosis and treatment of heart disease
Cardiology	Medical specialty dealing with disorders of the heart and blood vessels
Cardiovascular catheterization laboratory	Room where diagnostic angiograms and vascular interventions are performed

Cardiovascular system	Bodily system consisting of the heart, blood vessels, and blood
Cardioversion	A cardiac arrhythmia is terminated by a therapeutic dose of electric current delivered to the heart at a specific moment in the cardiac cycle
Carina	Where the trachea splits into the two primary bronchi
CAT scan	Computed axial tomography
Catecholamines	Group of chemical compounds including adrenaline, noradrenaline, and dopamine
Cath lab	Room where catheter-based procedures are performed with specialized X-ray, catheter-based devices, and emergency equipment
Catheter	A long tubular, flexible medical instrument that is inserted into a body cavity, duct, or vessel
Cathode	Negative electrode in an electrical circuit
Caudal	Toward the feet
CCL	Cardiovascular catheter laboratory
CE Mark	Conformité Européenne (European Conformity). Mandatory European marking to indicate conformity with the essential health and safety requirements set out in European Directives.
CEC	Clinical events committee
Central venous pressure	The pressure within the superior vena cava, directly outside the right atrium
Cerebrovascular	Blood supply to the brain
Cerebrovascular accident	Stroke; rapidly developing loss of brain functions due to a disruption of the blood supply to the brain
CHD	Coronary heart disease. See Coronary artery disease.
CHF	Congestive heart failure
Cholesterol	A fat (lipid) in the blood; essential component of cell membranes, brain and nerve cells, and bile
Chronaxie	The minimum time over which an electrical current, double the strength of the rheobase, needs to be applied, in order to stimulate muscle fiber or nerve cell.
Chronic	Of a long duration
CI	Cardiac index
CI	Coupling interval
CIN	Contrast (medium)-induced nephropathy
Cirrhosis	Hardening and shrinking of liver tissue
CK	Creatinine kinase
CK-MB	Cardiac muscle isoenzyme of creatine kinase

Claudication	Cramp-like pain in the calves caused by poor circulation to the leg muscles
CLI	Critical limb ischemia
CO	Cardiac output
Coagulation	Process by which blood forms into clots
Coarctation of the aorta	Congenital condition whereby the aorta narrows in the area of the ductus arteriosus
Coated stent	Stent with a surface coating on its struts
Coaxial	Two or more forms share a common axis
Cobalt chromium (CoCr)	A metal alloy containing cobalt, chrome, molybdenum, and other metals
Collateral circulation	Small vessels that develop around an occlusion, providing alternate blood flow
Collimation	X-ray imaging field can be reduced with lead leaves, or collimators, to limit the beam
Compliance (balloon)	Change in inflated balloon diameter corresponding to a change in pressure
Computed tomography (CT)	X-ray consisting of slices through the body taken from many different angles
Conductivity	The ability of a cell to allow electrical impulses to be transmitted
Congestive heart failure	Structural or functional cardiac disorder that impairs its ability to supply sufficient blood flow to meet the body's needs
Contractility	The inherent ability of myocardial sarcomeres to generate force and to shorten
Contraindication	Symptom or circumstance that renders a medication or a procedure inadvisable
Contralateral	At, or from, the other side
Contrast medium (CM)	Radiopaque fluid used to view vessels and chambers during X-ray studies
Contrast medium nephropathy	Acute decline in renal function after administration of a contrast medium
Control group	Subjects in a controlled study who receive no treatment, a standard treatment, or placebo
Coronary arteries	Arteries that supply the heart muscle (myocardium) with blood
Coronary artery bypass graft	Surgery that attaches part of an artery or vein to an artery, so that the blood has an alternate route around a narrowed or blocked area
Coronary artery disease	Disease in which the coronary arteries become hardened and narrowed due to build-up of plaque
Coronary ostium	Opening where a coronary artery joins the aorta
Coronary sinus	Where blood from the cardiac veins empties into the right atrium

Covered stent	Stent covered by a thin, tubular sheath; also referred to as stentgraft or endograft
Cranial	Toward the head
CRC	Clinical research coordinator
CRF	Case report form
Creatinine kinase	Enzyme found primarily in the heart and skeletal muscles; also known as creatine phosphokinase (CPK)
Critical limb ischemia	Severe obstruction of arteries that seriously decreases blood flow to the extremities (hands, feet, and legs) and has progressed to the point of severe pain, skin ulcers, or sores or gangrene
Crossability	Ease with which an interventional device can cross a lesion
Crossing profile	Diameter of an uninflated balloon or stent; a measure of how easily a device can pass through a lesion
Crossover procedure	An ilio-femoro-popliteal intervention, accessed from the groin of the other side by crossing the iliac bifurcation
Crossover sheath	A long introducer sheath with a curved tip to easily cross the iliac bifurcation
CS	Coronary sinus
CT	Computed tomography
CTA	Computerized tomography angiography
CVA	Cerebrovascular accident
CVP	Central venous pressure
CX	Circumflex artery
CXR	Chest X-ray
Cycle length	The length of a cycle, or the time between two events occurring repetitively; measured in milliseconds
D	
DCA	Directional coronary atherectomy
De novo lesion	A lesion that has not been previously treated
Death	End of life, marked by the full cessation of vital functions
Death—cardiac	Any death due to immediate cardiac cause (MI, low-output failure, fatal arrhythmia). Unwitnessed death and death of unknown cause will be classified as cardiac death.
Death—vascular	Death due to cerebrovascular disease, pulmonary embolism, ruptured aortic aneurysm, dissecting aneurysm, or other vascular cause
Deep seating	Technique that advances the tip of a guiding catheter "deep" into the coronary artery
Defibrillation	A therapeutic dose of electrical energy delivered to the heart

Defibrillation threshold	Lowest energy at which successful defibrillation occurs
Deflation time	Time needed to evacuate the fluid from an inflated balloon
Deliverability	Ability of a catheter to pass through a lesion
Depolarization	Causing contraction through a shift of the cell to a positive polarity
DES	Drug-eluting stent
Device success	The attainment of < 30% residual stenosis by QCA (or < 20% by visual assessment) AND either a TIMI flow 3 or a consistent TIMI flow 2 before and after the procedure, using the assigned device only
DFT	Defibrillation threshold
Diabetes	Diabetes mellitus
Diabetes mellitus	Metabolic disorder characterized by high blood sugar. Type 1 is usually due to autoimmune destruction of the pancreatic beta cells that produce insulin. Type 2 is characterized by tissue-wide insulin resistance.
Diagnostic catheter	A catheter for the delivery of contrast media to a vessel or structure for the purpose of performing an angiogram
Dialysis	Hemodialysis
Dialysis fistula/shunt	Surgically established communication between an artery and a vein, typically at the forearm, providing access to the bloodstream of patients receiving hemodialysis
Diameter stenosis (%)	Diameter of the reference vessel minus the minimal luminal diameter, divided by the reference diameter and multiplied by 100
Diastole	Relaxation phase of the cardiac cycle
Dichrotic notch	A "bump" in the downstroke of the PA and Ao waveforms signaling the closure of the pulmonic or aortic valves
Digital subtraction angiography	Special X-ray technique giving accurate images of CM-filled vessels by blocking out other structures
Direct stenting	Stent implantation performed without predilatation of the lesion with a balloon catheter
Directional coronary atherectomy	Cutting away plaque from the inside of a vessel using a device with a circular spinning blade
Disposable	Only intended for one time use, after which it has to be thrown away
Dissection	Rip or tear of the vessel lining (intima)
Distal	Further away from the center of the body, or a point of origin
Distal run-off	Angiographic assessment of the blood flow distally in iliac and/or femoropopliteal artery lesions. A good run-off includes quick flow in at least two tibial arteries
DMC	Data monitoring committee

Dominance	Side of the coronary circulation that supplies the inferior wall of the heart
Doppler effect	Change in frequency of sound or electromagnetic waves as the source moves away from (lower frequency) or toward (higher frequency) the observer
Doppler principle	When sound is reflected from a moving object, there is a change in frequency that can be used to calculate the speed at which the object is traveling
Double blind study	Neither the subject nor the investigator knows what treatment a subject is receiving
Drive train	Length of time between consecutive paced beats in a specific EP stimulation sequence
Drug-eluting stent	Stent that releases a drug
DSA	Digital subtraction angiography
DSMB	Data safety monitoring board
DSVR	Diastolic/systolic velocity ratio; Doppler lesion measurement method
Ductus arteriosus	Shunt connecting the pulmonary artery to the aortic arch; allows blood from the right ventricle to bypass the fetus' lungs; closes soon after birth
Duplex ultrasound	Ultrasound study that that incorporates a Doppler display to visualize the blood flow, the structure, and the hemodynamics within a vessel
Dyspnoea	Shortness of breath
Dysrhythmia	Abnormal electical activity in the heart

E

EBCT	Electron beam computed tomography
Echocardiography	Examination of the heart with ultrasound
ECG	Electrocardiogram
Edema	Abnormal accumulation of fluid in one or more cavities of the body or beneath the skin
EF	Ejection fraction
Effective refractory period	Longest interval that fails to result in the action potential in an electrophysiology
Efficacy	Capacity to produce a desired size of an effect under ideal or optimal conditions
EGM	Intracardiac electrogram
Ejection fraction	Proportion (percentage) of blood ejected from the left ventricle in a single heartbeat, compared with the total ventricular volume

Elastic recoil	Acute narrowing of an artery after balloon angioplasty; tendency of a vessel wall to retract after being expanded
ELCA	Excimer laser coronary angioplasty
Elective procedure	Procedure performed on a patient who is in a stable condition
Electrocardiogram	Graphic representation of the electrical activity of the heart
Emboli	Plural of embolus
Embolus	An object (often a blood clot) traveling through the circulatory system
Emergent procedure	Patient with unstable cardiac function requiring emergency intervention
Endocardium	Inner surface of the heart
Endoleak	Persistence of blood flow outside the lumen of the endograft (stent-graft), but within the aneurismal sac
Endoprosthesis	Artificial device (prosthesis) that is implanted in the body
Endothelium	Inner (intimal) layer of blood vessels
Endovascular aneurysm	Procedure that uses stent grafts to seal an AAA repair
EP	Electrophysiology
Epicardium	Serous lining on the heart's outer surface
Endovascular	Within a blood vessel (artery or vein)
EOL	End of life
ERP	Effective refractory period
Erythrocyte	Red blood cell
ESC	European Society of Cardiology
EVAR	Endovascular aneurysm repair
Excitability	Ability of a cell to depolarize and produce an action potential in response to a stimuli
Exercise (stress) ECG	Diagnostic test that measures electrical changes in the patient's CG during controlled exercise on a treadmill or pedaling a stationary bicycle
Extension/extension wire	Extra wire connected to the proximal end of a steerable guide wire to increase its length and allow for over-the-wire (OTW) device exchange
External	Outside, further from the center
Extracellular matrix	Connective tissue produced by transformed smooth muscle cells, forming the bulk of neointimal tissue
Extrastimulus	Electrical impulse delivered at a preset or programmed interval
F	
FDA	Food and Drug Administration
FFR	Fractional flow reserve
Fibrin	Strands formed from fibrinogen, which "catch" platelets as part of the clotting process

Fibrinogen	Inert form, or precursor, of fibrin
Fibrinolysis	Dissolving a blood clot
Fibromuscular dysplasia	Disease of unknown cause, affecting the medial (muscular) layer of an artery; well-known condition causing renal artery occlusive disease
First in Man (FIM)	Early clinical trial, with a small number of subjects, to test the basic safety and efficacy of the product
Fixed wire	Early design of angioplasty balloon in which the guide wire is permanently attached to the tip of the balloon
Flap	Section of the intima that has partly torn away from the vessel wall
Fluoroscopy	Examination that uses an X-ray source that projects through the patient onto an image intensifier and displays the images in real time on a monitor
FMD	Fibromuscular dysplasia
Foreshortening (of stents)	Difference in length of a stent when implanted compared when mounted on a balloon catheter or a delivery device
Fractional flow reserve	Maximal myocardial blood flow in the presence of a stenosis in the supplying coronary artery, divided by the normal blood flow
French	French gauge; unit used to measure diameter; 3F = 1 mm
Frequency response	Ability of the system to respond to changes in pressure at the measurement site
FRP	Functional refractory period
Functional refractory period	Minimum interval between two consecutively conducted impulses through that tissue
G	
Gadolinium	Contrast medium used in cardiac magnetic resonance angiography
Gangrene	Form of ischemic necrosis (death of tissue) due to insufficient blood flow
GCP	Good clinical practice
GFR	Glomerular filtration rate
Guide wire	Wire with a flexible, curved tip that can be threaded through a catheter and steered into position through a lesion. Balloon catheters, or other devices, are then threaded over this.
Guiding catheter	Catheter used to guide devices and contrast media to a vessel
H	
HBE	His bundle electrogram
HCM	Hypertrophic cardiomyopathy
HDE	Humanitarian device exemption

Heart attack	Myocardial infarction
Heart failure	Inability of the heart to pump enough blood
Heart rate	Number of ventricular contractions per minute, measured in beats per minute (bpm)
Hematoma	Accumulation of blood outside blood vessels
Hemodialysis	Procedure in which wastes are removed from the blood with a dialyzer (artificial kidney), used in treatment of kidney failure
Hemodynamics	Study of blood flow or circulation
Hemorrhage	Excessive bleeding
Hemostasis	Halting bleeding
Heparin	Antithrombin agent
HOCM	Hypertrophic obstructive cardiomyopathy
Holter ECG (monitoring)	Continuous recording of an ECG with a portable cassette recorder for at least 24 hours
HR	Heart rate
HRA	High right atrial
Hydrophilic	Water loving, high affinity for water; surface coating that absorbs moisture to become slippery
Hydrophobic	Water fearing, repelling; tending not to combine with, or unable to dissolve in, water
Hyperemia	Increase of blood flow to a part of the body
Hyperlipidemia	Elevated concentrations of any or all of the lipids in plasma
Hyperplasia	Excessive growth
Hypertension	High blood pressure; usually defined as a resting systolic pressure > 140 mmHg and/or a diastolic pressure > 95 mmHg
Hypertrophic cardiomyopathy	Thickening of the ventricle, often involving the septum that obstructs the left ventricular outflow tract
Hypotension	Low blood pressure
Hypoxemia	Insufficient concentration of dissolved oxygen in arterial blood
Hypoxia	The body, or region of the body, is deprived of an adequate oxygen supply

I

IABP	Intraaortic ballooning pump
Iatrogenic	Disease or injury resulting from medical treatment
ICD	Implantable cardioverter defibrillator
ICE	Intracardiac echocardiography

ICH	International Conference on Harmonization
IDE	Investigational device exemption
Idiopathic	Without a known cause
ICEG	Intracardiac electrogram
In segment	Within 5 mm proximal of, to 5 mm distal to, the stented lesion
In stent	Only within the stent
Inch ('')	Imperial measurement of length
IND	Investigational new drug
Inferior	Lower than, or below, the point of reference
Intercostal space	Space between two ribs
Intracardiac echocardiography	Catheter-based ultrasound with forward-oriented sensors for use within the heart
Infrapopliteal	Below the knee
INR	International normalized ratio
In-stent restenosis	Vessel lumen renarrowing within an implanted stent
Intensifier	Screen that shows an X-ray image as a real-time picture; also called image intensifier
International normalized ratio	Measures of the extrinsic pathway of coagulation; used to determine the clotting tendency of blood
Intermittent claudication	Muscle pain, cramp, numbness, or a sense of fatigue in the legs, classically in the calf muscle, which occurs during exercise and is relieved by a short period of rest
Internal	Within; away from the surface
Internal mammary artery	Artery that supplies the anterior chest wall and the breasts; there is one on each side of the body
Interventional cardiology	Medical discipline that diagnoses and treats cardiac or coronary disease using minimally invasive techniques and procedures
Intima	Innermost membrane of an organ or body part, such as an artery
Intra	Within a structure
Intraaortic ballooning pump	A cylindrical balloon in the aorta inflates in diastole, increasing blood flow to the coronary arteries, and deflates in systole, increasing forward blood flow by reducing afterload
Intracardiac electrogram	Recording of intrinsic electrical activity from an electrode within the heart
Intravascular ultrasound	Catheter-based device that bounces sound waves off the walls of a vessel from within. The resulting image shows the internal contours of the

	vessel and supplies information on the structure of tissue within the vessel walls.
Introducer sheath	Plastic tube, often with a haemostatic valve, that protects the vessel puncture site during a percutaneous procedure from multiple device insertions
Ipsilateral	At, or from, the same side
IRB	Institutional review board
Ischemia	A restriction in blood supply, with resultant damage or dysfunction of tissue
IVUS	Intravascular ultrasound

K

Kissing balloon technique	Angioplasty of bifurcation lesions with two balloons inflated simultaneously, one in each branch
Kissing stent technique	Simultaneous double-stent implantation technique to treat bifurcation lesions, with both stents touching (kissing) each other at the bifurcation

L

Lactate dehydrogenase	Cardiac enzyme that indicates the degree of anaerobic metabolism, resulting from ischemia
LAD	Left anterior descending coronary artery
LASER	Light amplification by the stimulated emission of radiation
Laser angioplasty	Debulking of atheroscleroric plaque with laser energy
Late loss	Difference in minimal luminal diameter between postprocedure, and follow-up, in mm
Late loss index	The fraction, or percent, of early gain that is lost at follow-up
Lateral	Toward the side, away from the midline
LBBB	Left bundle branch block
LDH	Lactate dehydrogenase
Left anterior descending artery	Coronary artery that supplies blood to most of the left ventricle
Left main coronary artery	Proximal section of left coronary artery between the aorta and where it branches into the LAD, CX, and intermedia branch (when present)
Left ventriculogram	X-ray study of the left ventricle using contrast medium; shows ventricle contraction and enables ejection fraction calculation
Left-sided heart failure	Failure of the left ventricle, with congestion of the pulmonary venous circuit

Lesion	Fatty, fibrous deposit in an artery that narrows the vessel and can reduce blood flow
Lesion Class (ACC/AHA)	Classification scheme of coronary lesion complexity
Type A	Minimally complex, discrete (length < 10 mm), concentric, readily accessible, nonangulated segment ($< 45°$), smooth contour, little or no calcification, less than totally occlusive, not ostial in location, no major side branch involvement, and an absence of thrombus
Type B	Type B lesions contain one, and Type B2 lesions contain two or more of the following: Moderately complex, tubular (length 10 to 20 mm), eccentric, moderate tortuosity of proximal segment, moderately angulated segment ($> 45°$, $< 90°$), irregular contour, moderate or heavy calcification, total occlusion < 3 months old, ostial in location, bifurcation lesions requiring double guide wires, and some thrombus present
Type C	Type C lesions contain one, and Type C2 contain two or more of the following: Severely complex, diffuse (length > 2 cm), excessive tortuosity of proximal segment, extremely angulated segment $> 90°$, total occlusions > 3 months old and/or bridging collaterals, inability to protect major side branches, and degenerated vein grafts with friable lesions
Lesion entry profile	Diameter of the most distal part of a balloon catheter/stent delivery system
Lipid	General term for body fats and fat-soluble substances
Local anaesthesia	Blocking of pain receptors in a small area
LRL	Lower rate limit
LSRA	Low septal right atrium
Luer lock	Form of syringe-connection, which can be locked in place by turning the connector
Lumen	Cavity or channel within a tubular structure
LVAD	Left ventricular assist device
LVOT	Left ventricular outflow tract
M	
MACCE	Major adverse cardiac and cerebral events; composite of myocardial infarction, stroke, death, TLR, TVR
MACE	Major adverse cardiac events; composite of myocardial infarction, death, TLR, TVR
Magnetic resonance imaging	Body tissue imaging based on the absorption or emission of electromagnetic radiation by electrons or atomic nuclei

Mainstem	Proximal section of left coronary artery between the aorta and where it branches into the LAD, CX, and intermedia branch (when present)
Malignant	Clinical course that progresses rapidly to death
Manifold	Tube with several inlets and outlets used to control the flow of fluids
Mean	The average; all results are added together, and this number is divided by the number of subjects
Mechanical recoil	Tendency of a stent to partially reduce its diameter after being expanded, due to the elasticity of the stent material and stent design
Media	Middle layer of blood vessels
Medial	Relating to, or extending toward, the middle or center
Memory	Ability of a device to hold its shape during use at body temperature; ability to return to a preformed shape after being stressed, straightened, or bent
MI	Myocardial infarction
Minimal luminal	Width of a lesion measured at its narrowest point diameter (MLD)
Mitral valve	Cardiac valve between the left atrium and the left ventricle
MLD	Minimal luminal diameter
Monorail design	Balloon catheter design whereby the guide wire enters at the tip and exits shortly after the balloon
Morbidity	Diseased state, disability, or poor health due to any cause
Morphology	Study of the structure, shape, or pathology of a structure
Mortality	Death
MR	Mitral regurgitation
MRA	Magnetic resonance angiography
MRI	Magnetic resonance imaging
MSCT	Multislice computed tomography
Myocardial infarction	Disease state that occurs when the blood supply to a part of the heart is interrupted
Myocardium	Middle (muscle) layer of the heart
N	
Naloxone	Opioid receptor antagonist; reverses the effects of opioids
NDA	New drug application
Neointimal hyperplasia	Excessive growth of new intimal cells
Neointimal hyperplasia volume	A measure of the volume of new tissue growth within a stent; measured by IVUS and expressed in mm3
Net gain	The difference in vessel (lesion) diameter between predilation and immediately after the procedure

NIPS	Noninvasive programmed stimulation
Nitinol	Alloy of nickel and titanium that has the ability to return to a predetermined shape
Nitroglycerin	A nitrate used to treat angina; improves myocardial oxygen delivery and decreases myocardial oxygen demand
Nominal diameter	Diameter to which a balloon is designed to expand to at its nominal pressure
Nominal pressure	Pressure at which a balloon reaches its nominal diameter
Noncompliant	Balloon which shows less than 10% growth in diameter in relation to an increase in pressure above the nominal pressure
Noninvasive programmed stimulation	Implanted device delivers pacing protocols to the heart in order to diagnose, initiate, or terminate arrhythmias
Non-Q wave MI	Elevation of postprocedure CK levels to > three times the upper limit of normal with CK-MB elevation, in the absence of pathological Q waves
NPO	*Nil per os* (Latin). Nil by mouth; fasting patient
NSAID	Nonsteroidal antiinflammatory drug

O

Occlusion	State of something that is normally open, is now totally closed
OCT	Optical coherence tomography
Oliguria	Decreased production of urine
Opioids	Analgesics derived from opium
Osmolarity	A measure of the number of particles in a solution
Ostium	Orifice; where a vessel emerges from another vessel, usually where a coronary artery emerges from the aorta
Over-the-wire (OTW)	Balloon catheter design whereby the guide wire goes through the entire length of the catheter

P

PA	Pulmonary artery
PA interval	P wave to atrium; obtained by measuring from the P wave on the surface ECG to the rapid deflection of the LSRA on the His bundle electrogram
PAD	Peripheral artery disease
Palliative	Therapy that provides relief of symptoms without curing the underlying disease
Partial thromboplastin time	Measuring the efficacy of both the "intrinsic" and the common coagulation pathways; used to monitor the treatment effects of heparin

Patency	Quality or state of being open or unobstructed
Patent ductus arteriosus	Congenital heart defect where the ductus arteriosus fails to close after birth
Patent foramen ovale	Congenital heart defect that enables blood to flow between the left and right atria via the interatrial septum
Pathology	Study of the traits, causes, and effects of disease
Pathophysiology	Process of disease
PCB	Percutaneous coronary bypass
PCI	Percutaneous coronary intervention
PCWP	Pulmonary capillary wedge pressure
PDA	Patent ductus arteriosus
Percutaneous	Procedure that involves puncturing the skin
Percutaneous coronary intervention	Minimally invasive technique by which coronary artery stenoses are treated
Percutaneous transluminal angioplasty	Minimally invasive technique by which stenoses of peripheral vessels are treated with a balloon catheter
Percutaneous transluminal coronary angioplasty	Minimally invasive technique by which stenoses of coronary vessels are dilated with a balloon catheter
Perforation	Puncturing of a material with a harder object to create a hole or aperture
Perfusion	Flow of blood or liquid through tissue
Pericardium	Double-walled sac that surrounds the heart and the roots of the great vessels
Peripheral artery disease	General term for disease of any blood vessel that is not part of the heart or brain; often a narrowing of vessels that carry blood to the legs, arms, stomach, or kidneys
Peripheral vascular disease	General term for disease of any blood vessel that is not part of the heart or brain; often a narrowing of vessels that carry blood to the legs, arms, stomach, or kidneys
PET	Positron emission tomography
PFO	Patent foramen ovale
Piezoelectric crystal	Crystal that emits electrical energy if bent
Plain old balloon angioplasty	Minimally invasive technique by which coronary artery stenoses are treated with balloon inflation only; no stenting
Plaque	Buildup of fatty deposits within the wall of a blood vessel
Platelet	Thrombocyte; small cytoplasmic body derived from cells
PMA	Premarket approval
PMT	Pacemaker-mediated tachycardia

POBA	Plain old balloon angioplasty
Positron emission tomography	Radioisotope detection technique, measuring the metabolic activity (perfusion) of tissue
Postdilation	Final balloon catheter dilation of an implanted stent to fully implant it in the vessel wall
Posterior	Toward the back of a structure
Power	Chance of failing to detect a difference between two results where one really does exist
PQ segment	Section of an ECG; represents AV-node and His-bundle depolarization
Preload	Volume of blood still in the ventricle at the end of diastole
Pressure gradient	A difference in pressure caused by an obstacle
Primary patency rate	Percent of vessels that remain patent after an intervention
Primary stenting	PCI where a stent is implanted without predilatation of the lesion with a balloon catheter
Profile	Diameter of balloon or catheter tip, used as a measure if its ability to cross lesions
Prospective study	A study that goes forward in time. Patients are enrolled, and their treatment is determined by the study protocol.
Prosthesis	Artificial extension or device that replaces a missing body part
Provisional stenting	Stenting only after suboptimal balloon angioplasty results
Proximal	Nearer to a central point of the body or a point of origin
PSA	Pacing system analyzer
Pseudoaneurysm	Outward pouching of a blood vessel, involving a defect in the two innermost layers (tunica intima and media), with continuity of the outermost layer (adventia)
PTCA	Percutaneous transluminal coronary angioplasty
PTT	Partial thromboplastin time
Pulmonary capillary wedge pressure	An approximation of the left atrial pressure, measured through the pulmonary tree from the pulmonary artery
Pulmonary atresia	Congenital malformation of the pulmonary valve in which the valve is closed completely
Pulmonary valve	Cardiac valve with three cusps between the right ventricle and the pulmonary artery
Pulse	Throbbing flow of blood in arteries due to contractions of the heart
Pulse width	Amount of time a pacemaker's electrical impulse is applied to the cardiac tissue

Pushability	Ability of an interventional device to transmit the proximally applied force to its distal tip with a minimal loss of axial energy
P-value	Likelihood that the difference between two results could have arisen by chance alone
PVARP	Postventricular atrial refractory period
PVD	Peripheral vascular disease
PVI	Peripheral vascular intervention
P-wave	Section of the ECG representing atrial contraction

Q

QCA	Quantitative coronary angiography
QRS complex	Section of the ECG representing ventricular depolarization
Quantitative coronary angiography	Diagnostic procedure in which a stenosis, or vessel segment, is analyzed and measured by a computer
Q-wave myocardial infarction	Development of new pathological Q waves in two or more contiguous ECG leads, with or without elevated CK or CK-MB levels.

R

Radial strength	Amount of pressure that it takes to collapse an expanded stent
Radiologist	Physician who specializes in the diagnosis of disease by using X-rays, MRI, ultrasound, and other imaging techniques
Radiology	Medical discipline that specializes in X-rays, MRI, ultrasound, and other imaging techniques
Radiolucent	Ability of a substance to absorb less radiation than its surroundings
Radiopacity	X-ray visibility of objects
Radiopaque	Ability of an object to absorb more radiation than its surroundings, visible in X-ray photographs and under fluoroscopy
Randomisation	Process by which subjects enrolled in a study are assigned to the treatment groups by chance
Rapid-exchange (Rx) design	Balloon catheter design whereby the guide wire enters at the tip and exits shortly after the balloon
RAS	Renal artery stenosis
Rashkind's procedure	Balloon atrial septostomy as palliative treatment for transposition of the great arteries
Rated burst pressure	Maximum pressure to which an angiography balloon can be inflated and be guaranteed not to burst
RAVC	Retrograde atrioventricular conduction
RBBB	Right bundle branch block

RBP	Rated burst pressure
RCA	Right coronary artery
Recanalization	Crossing/opening of a total occlusion or blockage of a vessel
Recoil	Tendency of a vessel or a stent to lose some of its inflated diameter when the balloon is deflated
Reendothelialisation	Regrowth of endothelium over an injured site, or over a foreign object, on the arterial wall
Reference vessel diameter (RVD)	Diameter of healthy vessel proximal and distal to the diseased segment
Registry	A single arm (one type of treatment for all subjects) study that includes a varied population, without inclusion/exclusion criteria
Relative refractory period	Longest coupling interval of a premature impulse that results in prolonged conduction of the premature impulse relative to that of the basic drive
Repolarization	Return of tissue to its initial resting state after depolarization
Restenosis	Medium-term (6 to 9 months) renarrowing of a vessel after dilatation or stenting
Retrograde	Opposite direction to the blood flow (upstream) in an artery or a vein
Retrospective study	A study that looks at events that have already occurred; data is extracted from patients' notes and other documentation
Revascularization	Opening of a narrowed or blocked artery
RF	Radio frequency
RFCA	Radiofrequency catheter ablation
Rheobase	Minimal electrical current that results in an action potential, or the contraction of a muscle
Right-sided heart failure	Inadequate pump action of the right ventricle, with congestion of the systemic venous circuit
Roadmapping	Special X-ray technique where a frame from an angiography is displayed on a extra monitor, and used to guide intravascular interventional devices to a lesion
Rotablator	Tool with a high-speed burr, which is introduced into the artery and used to remove vessel plaque
Rotational atherectomy	Use of the Rotablator to remove plaque and improve blood flow in vessels that are narrowed or blocked
RRP	Relative refractory period
RVA	Right ventricular apex
RVD	Reference vessel diameter
RVOT	Right ventricular outflow tract

S

SA	Sinoatrial
SACT	Sinoatrial conduction time
Safety	A measure of how much danger the treatment places the subject in; composed of death, MI, and stent thrombosis
Saphenous vein graft	Coronary artery bypass graft that uses a section of the saphenous vein to bridge the lesion
SAT	Subacute (stent) thrombosis
SCD	Sudden cardiac death
SDC	Strength-duration curve
Secondary patency rate	All vessels that remain patent, both with and without additional procedures
Secondary stenting	Interventional procedure that was initially planned as a balloon angioplasty, but a stent is implanted due to unsatisfactory results
Self-expanding stent	Stent is mounted on a delivery system that keeps it constrained by an outer sheath; outer sheath withdrawal allows the stent to expand to its predetermined size
Semilunar valve	Aortic valve and the pulmonary valve; flaps resemble a half moon
SEP	Systolic ejection period
SFA	Superficial femoral artery
Sheath	Plastic tube, often with a hemostatic valve, which protects the vessel puncture site during a percutaneous procedure from multiple device insertions
Shunt	Hole or passage that allows movement of fluid from one part of the body to another
Silent ischemia	Inadequate oxygen supply to myocardium, but without chest pain (angina)
Single blind study	A study in which the subjects do not know what treatment they are being given
Single photon emission computed tomography	Cardiac radioisotope detection technique providing tomographic cross-sectional images and 3-D-thallium images of the heart
Sinoatrial node	Impulse generating (pacemaker) tissue located in the right atrium
Sinus bradycardia	Slow heartbeat (< 60 bpm) with its origin in the SA node
Sinus tachycardia	Fast heartbeat (> 100 bpm) with its origin in the SA node
Slew rate	Rate of change of an electical signal
SMC	Smooth-muscle cells
Smooth-muscle cells	Type of nonstriated muscle cells; most common cells in neointimal hyperplasia

SNRT	Sinus node recovery time
Sonography	Using the reflections of high-frequency sound waves to construct an image of a body organ
SPECT	Single photon emission computed tomography
Stent	Fine mesh cylinder that acts as scaffolding, giving vessels added structural support
ST depression	Drop in the ST segment of the ECG below the baseline; can signify ischemia in that region
ST elevation	Elevation of the ST segment of the ECG above the baseline; can signify ischemia in the electrically opposite myocardial region
ST segment	Section of the ECG representing period between ventricular depolarization and depolarization
Standard deviation	Common measure of statistical dispersion, measuring how widely spread the values in a data set are. If the data points are close to the mean, then the standard deviation is small.
Stenosis	Abnormal narrowing in a blood vessel
Stent	A metallic scaffolding device implanted into a vessel to maintain its diameter
Stent jail	Blocking a side branch access with a stent overlapping the ostium of the side branch, making the coronary artery side branch inaccessible to further interventions.
Stent thrombosis	Formation of a thrombus within, or adjacent to, a previously successfully stented vessel
Stentgraft	Vascular endoprosthesis reinforced with a metallic stent
Sterile	Free of all living organisms, including bacterial spores and viruses
Sterile field	A specified area that is considered to be free of microorganisms
Stiffening wire	Metal wire within a shaft to give it stiffness and pushability; also referred to as a stylet
Strength-duration curve	Threshold amplitude plotted against threshold pulse duration
Stress test	A patient's ECG is measured while he or she is doing controlled exercise
Stroke	Rapidly developing loss of brain functions due to a disruption of the blood supply to the brain
Stylet	Metal wire within a shaft to give it stiffness and pushability
Subacute thrombosis	Formation of a thrombus within, or adjacent to, a stented vessel between 24 hours and 30 days after the index procedure
Sudden cardiac death	Death resulting from an abrupt loss of heart function (cardiac arrest)
Superior	Situated above or directed upward

Superior vena cava	Major vein that receives blood from the head, arms, and thorax, and empties into the right atrium
Supine	Lying flat on the back
SVC	Superior vena cava
SVG	Saphenous vein graft
SVT	Supraventricular tachycardia
Systole	Contraction phase of the cardiac cycle

T

Tachycardia	Rapid heartbeat; defined as a resting heart rate of > 100 bpm
Tamponade	Stoppage of blood flow through a blood vessel due to constriction by an outside force
Target lesion	Vessel section (narrowing) that is to receive intervention
Target lesion revascularization	Repeat revascularization—PTCA or bypass surgery—due to a stenosis within the lesion or within 5 mm of the stent
Target vessel	Index coronary artery that was in physical contact with any component (guiding catheter, guide wire, balloon catheter, etc.) of the angioplasty hardware during the initial procedure
Target vessel failure	Composite of: target vessel revascularization, Q wave or non-Q wave MI, and cardiac death that could not be clearly attributed to a vessel other than the target vessel
Target vessel revascularization	Revascularization—PTCA or bypass surgery—of any segment of the index coronary artery that was in physical contact with any component (guiding catheter, guide wire, balloon catheter, etc.) of the angioplasty hardware during the initial procedure
Technical success rate	Number (%) of procedures that could be successfully completed
TEE	Transesophageal echocardiogram
TGA	Transposition of the great arteries
Therapeutic	Action that remedies a health problem
Thrombectomy	Removal of a thrombus
Thrombocyte	Platelet
Thrombolytic	Pharmaceutical action that dissolves thrombus
Thrombosis	Formation of a blood clot in a blood vessel
Thrombotic	Related to, caused by, or of the nature of, a blood clot that obstructs a blood vessel or a cavity of the heart
Thrombus	Blood clot in an intact blood vessel; plural: thrombi
TIA	Transient ischemic attack
TIMI	Thrombolysis in Myocardial Infarction study

TIMI classification	A simple prognostication scheme that categorizes a patient's risk of death and ischemic events and provides a basis for therapeutic decision making
TIMI 0	No perfusion
TIMI 1	Penetration with minimal perfusion; contrast fails to opacify the entire bed distal to the stenosis for the duration of a cine run
TIMI 2	Partial perfusion; contrast opacifies the entire coronary bed distal to the stenosis. However, the rate of entry and/or clearance is slower in the coronary bed distal to the obstruction than in comparable areas not perfused by the dilated vessel.
TIMI 3	Complete perfusion. Filling and clearance of contrast equally rapid in the coronary bed distal to stenosis as in other coronary beds.
Tip	The distal end of a device
TIPS procedure	Transjugular intrahepatic portosystemic shunt is an artificial channel that is created in the liver; connects the portal circulation with the systemic circulation
TLR	Target lesion revascularization
Torque	Power of turning, twisting
Torque device, Torquer	Small device that is clamped or screwed onto a steerable guide wire, allowing the wire to be turned with the fingertips
Tortuous/tortuosity	Twisted, having many turns
Total occlusion	Complete blockage of a blood vessel
Total peripheral resistance	Sum of all forces that oppose blood flow through the systemic circulation; includes arterial diameter, vessel elasticity, obstruction or narrowing, blood viscosity, and vessel length
TPR	Total peripheral resistance
Trackability	Ability of a catheter or an interventional device to advance along a guide wire, negotiating vessel tortuosity and angulation
Transbrachial	Vessel access via the brachial artery
Transducer	Device that converts energy from one form into another
Transfemoral	Vessel access via the femoral artery or vein
Transient ischemic attack	Brief neurologic dysfunction caused by limited blood supply to the brain that persists for less than 24 hours
Transradial	Vessel access via the radial artery
Tricuspid valve	Cardiac valve between the right ventricle and the right atrium; consists of three segments (cusps)
Tunica adventitia	Outermost layer of a vessel or organ; continuous with the surrounding tissue

Tunica intima	Innermost layer of blood or lymphatic vessels
Tunica media	Medial layer of blood vessels; comprised of smooth-muscle cells
TVF	Target vessel failure
TVR	Target vessel revascularization
T wave	Section of the ECG representing ventricular depolarization

U

Ulcer	Loss of part or all of the top surface of the skin or membrane
Ultrasonography	Imaging structures by recording their reflection of high-frequency sound waves
Ultrasound	Inaudible, high-frequency sound waves
URL	Upper rate limit
Urticaria	Skin rash notable for red, raised, itchy bumps; hives

V

VA	Ventricle to atrium
Vein	Vessel that carries blood to the heart
Vein graft	A vein that is surgically removed and reattached elsewhere in the body to bypass a stenosis or blockage
Vena cava	Two large veins that return oxygen-depleted blood from the upper body and from the lower body to the right atrium
Ventricle	Pumping chamber of the heart
Ventricular fibrillation	Erratic and uncoordinated electrical discharge of the ventricle that results in no pumping action
Ventricular tachycardia	Fast heart beat (> 100 bpm) originating in the ventricles
VF	Ventricular fibrillation
Viscosity	Resistance of a liquid to flow, its "thickness"
Virtual histology IVUS	Spectral analysis of ultrasound amplitude to give additional information about plaque and tissue composition
VT	Ventricular tachycardia
Venules	Small veins

W

Winging	When a balloon catheter retains a wing-like shape following its initial inflation and subsequent deflation

X

X-ray	Method of viewing the interior of the body using electromagnetic radiation

INDEX

Italicized page locators indicate a photo/figure; tables are noted with a t.